D0765203

Recombinant Antibodies for Cancer Therapy

METHODS IN MOLECULAR BIOLOGY™

John M. Walker, SERIES EDITOR

METHODS IN MOLECULAR BIOLOGY™

Recombinant Antibodies for Cancer Therapy

Methods and Protocols

Edited by

Martin Welschof

Axaron Bioscience AG, Heidelberg, Germany

and

Jürgen Krauss

National Institutes of Health,
National Cancer Institute, Frederick, MD

Humana Press ✳ Totowa, New Jersey

Cover illustration: Figure 4B from Chapter 25, "Recombinant Adenoviruses for In Vivo Expression of Antibody Fragments," by Roland E. Kontermann et al.

Production Editor: Jessica Jannicelli.

Cover design by Patricia F. Cleary.

For additional copies, pricing for bulk purchases, and/or information about other Humana titles, contact Humana at the above address or at any of the following numbers: Tel.: 973-256-1699; Fax: 973-256-8341; E-mail: humana@humanapr.com; or visit our Website: www.humanapress.com

Printed in the United States of America. 10 9 8 7 6 5 4 3 2 1

Library of Congress Cataloging in Publication Data

Recombinant antibodies for cancer therapy : methods and protocols / edited by Martin Welschof and Jürgen Krauss.
       p. ; cm. -- (Methods in molecular biology ; v. 207)
    Includes bibliographical references and index.
    ISBN 0-89603-918-8 (alk. paper)
     1.Cancer--Immunotherapy. 2. Recombinant antibodies--Laboratory manuals. I.
   Welschof, Martin. II. Krauss, Jürgen. III. Methods in molecular biology (Clifton, N.J.) ;
   v. 207.
    [DNLM: 1. Antibodies--therapeutic use. 2. Neoplasms--therapy. 3.
    Antibodies--immunology. 4. Antigens, Neoplasm--immunology. 5. Antineoplastic
    Protocols. 6. Immunoglobulin Fragments--therapeutic use. 7. Immunotherapy--methods.
    8. Neoplasms--immunology. 9. Recombinant Proteins--therapeutic use. QZ 266 R311 2003]
    RC271.I45 R43 2003
     616.99'4061--dc21
                                                                    2002067889

Preface

Since the advent of hybridoma technology more than two decades ago, numerous antibodies have entered the clinical setting as potent therapeutic agents. Their repeated application in humans, however, is limited by the development of human antimouse antibodies (HAMA) in the recipient, leading to allergic reactions against the foreign murine protein and rapid neutralization. To circumvent these limitations many new antibodies have recently been tailored through recombinant antibody technology. The initial clinical data show encouraging results, thus demonstrating the potential of these new therapeutic agents.

The purpose of *Recombinant Antibodies for Cancer Therapy* is to present a collection of detailed protocols in recombinant antibody technology. It is primarily addressed to scientists working on recombinant antibodies as well as clinicians involved with antibody-based therapies. As with other volumes of this series, we placed the main focus on providing detailed protocols describing procedures step-by-step. Moreover, each protocol supplies a troubleshooting guide containing detailed information on possible problems and hints for potential solutions.

Antibody technology is a subject of constant and rapid change. This volume, therefore, does not attempt to cover all possible current experimental approaches in the field. Rather, we present carefully selected protocols, written by competent authors who have successfully verified the particular method described. Given our own professional backgrounds and interest in oncology, we chose to concentrate chiefly on therapeutic agents for cancer patients.

Recombinant Antibodies for Cancer Therapy: Methods and Protocols consists of five sections. First, concise reviews give an overview of the current status of recombinant antibodies in cancer therapy, and the generation of antibody molecules through antibody engineering. This is followed by protocols grouped according to subject into four sections: Hybridoma-Derived Recombinant Antibodies, Recombinant Antibody Fragments from Phagemid-Displayed Antibody Repertoires, Antibody Fragments with Additional Properties, and Large Scale Production of Recombinant Antibodies for Clinical Applications.

We would like to commend all contributing authors for the high quality and clarity of their respective manuscripts. We thank them for sharing their extensive experience in dealing with intricate experimental problems. Moreover, we are indebted to Prof. John Walker for his enthusiasm and encouragement, and Humana Press for publishing this volume. On a more personal level we are grateful to Mona, Lisa, Joshua, and Michaela for their patience and support.

Martin Welschof
Jürgen Krauss

Contents

Contributors

HINRICH ABKEN • *Tumorgenetik und Zellbiologie, Klinik I für Innere Medizin, University of Cologne, Germany*

LING-LING AN • *MedImmune, Inc., Gaithersburg, MD*

MICHAELA ARNDT • *National Cancer Institute at Frederick, Frederick, MD*

DANIELE ARNOLD-SCHILD • *Department of Immunology, Institute for Cell Biology, University of Tübingen, Germany*

ITAI BENHAR • *Department of Molecular Microbiology and Biotechnology, Tel-Aviv University, Ramat Aviv, Israel*

YEVGENY BERDICHEVSKY • *Department of Molecular Microbiology and Biotechnology, Tel-Aviv University, Ramat Aviv, Israel*

LIAT BINYAMIN • *Faculty of Biology, Technion-Israel Institute of Technology, Haifa, Israel*

MICHAEL BRAUNAGEL • *Affitech AS, Oslo, Norway*

OLE H. BREKKE • *Affitech AS, Oslo, Norway*

SILVANA CANEVARI • *Unit of Molecular Therapies, Department of Experimental Oncology, Istituto Nazionale per lo Studio e la Cura dei Tumori, Milano, Italy*

PARTHA S. CHOWDHURY • *Human Genome Sciences Inc., Rockville, MD*

CHRISTIANE CHRIST • *Department of Transplantation Immunology, Institute for Immunology, University of Heidelberg, Germany*

RIKKE CLAUSEN • *Department of Pharmacology, The Royal Danish School of Pharmacy, Copenhagen, Denmark*

CYRIL J. COHEN • *Faculty of Biology, Technion-Israel Institute of Technology, Haifa, Israel*

FRANCESCO COLOTTA • *Dompe Research Center, L'Aquila, Italy*

GALIT DENKBERG • *Faculty of Biology, Technion-Israel Institute of Technology, Haifa, Israel*

JAN ENGBERG • *Department of Pharmacology, The Royal Danish School of Pharmacy, Copenhagen, Denmark*

MARIANGELA FIGINI • *Istituto Nazionale per lo Studio e la Cura dei Tumori, Department of Experimental Oncology, Unit of Molecular Therapies, Milano, Italy*

xi

MARTINA FINGER • *Department of Transplantation Immunology, Institute for Immunology, University of Heidelberg, Germany*

RAINER FISCHER • *Fraunhofer Institute for Molecular Biology and Applied Ecology and Institut für Biologie VII, RWTH Aachen, Germany*

HANS HEINRICH FÖRSTER • *Labor Diagnostik GmbH, Leipzig, Germany*

JUNICHIRO FUTAMI • *Department of Bioscience and Biotechnology, Faculty of Engineering, University of Okayama, Japan*

ANDREW GREEN • *Unit of Molecular Therapies, Department of Experimental Oncology, Istituto Nazionale per lo Studio e la Cura dei Tumori, Milano, Italy*

HALLDIS HELLEBUST • *Affitech AS, Oslo, Norway*

INGRID HERMES • *Recombinant Antibody Unit (D0500), German Cancer Research Center, Heidelberg, Germany*

CLAUDIA HEUSER • *Tumorgenetik und Zellbiologie, Klinik I für Innere Medizin, University of Cologne, Germany*

ANDREAS HOMBACH • *Tumorgenetik und Zellbiologie, Klinik I für Innere Medizin, University of Cologne, Germany*

PETER J. HUDSON • *CRC for Diagnostic Technologies, CSIRO Health Sciences and Nutrition, Parkville, Australia*

LISELOTTE B. JENSEN • *Department of Pharmacology, The Royal Danish School of Pharmacy, Copenhagen, Denmark*

VALÉRIE JÉRÔME • *Vectron Therapeutics AG, Marburg, Germany*

TARRAN JONES • *AERES Biomedical Ltd., London, UK*

ARMIN KELLER • *Department of Technology, Axaron Bioscience AG, Heidelberg, Germany*

SERGEY M. KIPRIYANOV • *Affimed Therapeutics AG, Heidelberg, Germany*

CHRISTIAN KLEIST • *Department of Transplantation Immunology, Institute for Immunology, University of Heidelberg, Germany*

ROLAND E. KONTERMANN • *Vectron Therapeutics AG, Marburg, Germany*

PERNILLE KOPS • *Department of Pharmacology, The Royal Danish School of Pharmacy, Copenhagen, Denmark*

TINA KORN • *Institut für Molekularbiologie und Tumorforschung, University of Marburg, Marburg, Germany*

ALEXANDER A. KORTT • *CSIRO Health Sciences and Nutrition, Parkville, Australia*

JÜRGEN KRAUSS • *National Cancer Institute at Frederick, Frederick, MD*

DIANNE L. NEWTON • *SAIC-Frederick, National Cancer Institute, Frederick, Frederick, MD*

REVITAL NIV • *Faculty of Biology, Technion-Israel Institute of Technology, Haifa, Israel*

SIOBHAN O'BRIEN • *AERES Biomedical Ltd., London, UK*

GERHARD OPELZ • *Department of Transplantation Immunology, Institute for Immunology, University of Heidelberg, Germany*

MICHAEL PFREUNDSCHUH • *Universitätskliniken des Saarlandes, Innere Medizin I, Homburg, Germany*

DANIEL PLAKSIN • *Molecular Biology Group, Peptor Ltd., Kiryat Weizmann, Israel*

BARBARA E. POWER • *CSIRO Health Sciences and Nutrition, Parkville, Australia*

HANS-GEORG RAMMENSEE • *Department of Immunology, Institute for Cell Biology, University of Tübingen, Germany*

YORAM REITER • *Faculty of Biology, Technion-Israel Institute of Technology, Haifa, Israel*

ERIK RIISE • *Department of Pharmacology, The Royal Danish School of Pharmacy, Copenhagen, Denmark*

DALE RUBY • *SAIC-Frederick, National Cancer Institute, Frederick, MD*

SUSANNA M. RYBAK • *National Cancer Institute at Frederick, Frederick, MD*

HANSJÖRG SCHILD • *Department of Immunology, Institute for Cell Biology, University of Tübingen, Germany*

DINA SEGAL • *Faculty of Biology, Technion-Israel Institute of Technology, Haifa, Israel*

PETER SØRENSEN • *Department of Pharmacology, The Royal Danish School of Pharmacy, Copenhagen, Denmark*

PETER TERNESS • *Department of Transplantation Immunology, Institute for Immunology, University of Heidelberg, Germany*

JOHN E. THOMMESEN • *Division of Cell Biology, Department of Biology, University of Oslo, Norway*

BARBARA UCHANSKA-ZIEGLER • *Institut für Immungenetik, Universitätsklinikum Charité, Humboldt-Universität zu Berlin, Germany*

CARMEN VAQUERO-MARTIN • *Institut für Biologie VII, RWTH Aachen, Germany*

GEORGE VASMATZIS • *Cancer Center and Division of Experimental Pathology, Mayo Clinic, Rochester, MN*

MARTIN WELSCHOF • *Department of Technology, Axaron Bioscience AG, Heidelberg, Germany*

ANNA M. WU • *Department of Molecular Biology, Beckman Research Institute of the City of Hope, Duarte, CA*

HERREN WU • *MedImmune Inc., Gaithersburg, MD*

PAUL J. YAZAKI • *Department of Molecular Biology, Beckman Research Institute of the City of Hope, Duarte, CA*

ALI F. YENIDUNYA • *Department of Pharmacology, The Royal Danish School of Pharmacy, Copenhagen, Denmark*

ANDREAS ZIEGLER • *Institut für Immungenetik, Universitätsklinikum Charité, Humboldt-Universität zu Berlin, Germany*

I

INTRODUCTION

1

Generation of Antibody Molecules
Through Antibody Engineering

Sergey M. Kipriyanov

1. Introduction

Twenty-five years ago, Georges Köhler and César Milstein invented a means of cloning individual antibodies, thus opening up the way for tremendous advances in the fields of cell biology and clinical diagnostics *(1)*. However, in spite of their early promise, monoclonal antibodies (MAbs) were largely unsuccessful as therapeutic reagents resulting from insufficient activation of human effector functions and immune reactions against proteins of murine origin. These problems have recently been overcome to a large extent using genetic-engineering techniques to produce chimeric mouse/human and completely human antibodies. Such an approach is particularly suitable because of the domain structure of the antibody molecule *(2)*, where functional domains carrying antigen-binding activities (Fabs or Fvs) or effector functions (Fc) can be exchanged between antibodies (*see* **Fig. 1**).

On the basis of sequence variation, the residues in the variable domains (V-region) are assigned either to the hypervariable complementarity-determining regions (CDR) or to framework regions (FR). It is possible to replace much of the rodent-derived sequence of an antibody with sequences derived from human immunoglobulins without loss of function. This new generation of "chimeric" and "humanized" antibodies represents an alternative to human hybridoma-derived antibodies and should be less immunogenic than their rodent counterparts. Furthermore, genetically truncated versions of the antibody may be produced ranging in size from the smallest antigen-binding unit or Fv through Fab' to $F(ab')_2$ fragments. More recently it has become possible to produce totally human recombinant antibodies derived either from antibody libraries *(3)* or single immune B cells *(4)*, or from transgenic mice bearing human immunoglobulin loci *(5,6)*.

From: *Methods in Molecular Biology, vol. 207: Recombinant Antibodies for Cancer Therapy: Methods and Protocols*
Edited by: M. Welschof and J. Krauss © Humana Press Inc., Totowa, NJ

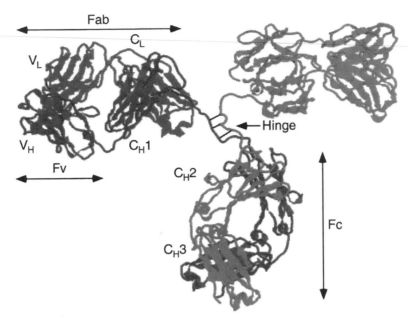

Fig. 1. Domain organization of an IgG molecule. Antigen-binding surface is formed by variable domains of the heavy (V_H) and light (V_L) chains. Effector functions are determined by constant C_H2 and C_H3 domains. The picture is based on the crystal structure of an intact IgG2 anti-canine lymphoma MAb231 *(2)* (pdb entry 1IGT). The drawing was generated using a molecular visualization program RasMac Molecular Graphics, version 2.7.1 (R. Sayle, Biomolecular Structure, Glaxo Research and Development, Greenford, Middlesex, UK).

2. Cloning the Antibody Variable Regions

Significant progress has been made in the in vitro immunization of human B cells *(7)* and in the development of transgenic mice containing human immunoglobulin loci (for review, *see* **refs. 5,8**). Recombinant DNA technology can also be employed for generating human MAbs from human lymphocyte mRNA. The genetic information for antibody variable regions is generally retrieved from total cDNA preparations using the polymerase chain reaction (PCR) with antibody-specific primers *(9,10)*. As a source of immunoglobulin-specific mRNA, one can use hybridoma cells *(11)*, human peripheral blood lymphocytes (PBL) *(3)*, and even a single human B cell *(4,12)*. Using the latter approach, it is possible to avoid the cumbersome hybridoma technology and obtain human antibody fragments with the original V_H/V_L pairing. Single bacterial colonies expressing antigen-specific antibody fragments can be identified by colony screening using antigen-coated membranes *(13)*. Novel high-throughput selection technologies allow screening thousands of different antibody clones at a time *(14)*. The appropriate V_H/V_L combination may also be selectively enriched from a phage-displayed antibody library through a series of immunoaffinity steps referred to as "library panning" *(15,16)*.

3. Genetically Engineered Monoclonal Antibodies

3.1. Chimeric Antibodies with Human Constant Regions

The first generation of recombinant monoclonal antibodies consisted of the rodent-derived V-regions fused to human constant regions (**Fig. 2**). It is thought that the most immunogenic regions of antibodies are the conserved constant domains *(17)*. Because the antigen-binding site of the antibody is localized within the variable regions, the chimeric molecules retain their binding affinity for the antigen and acquire the function of the substituted constant regions. The human constant regions allow more efficient interaction with human complement-dependent cytotoxicity (CDC) and antibody-dependent cell-mediated cytotoxicity (ADCC) effector mechanisms. Rituximab (Rituxan; IDEC Pharmaceuticals, San Diego, and Genentech, Inc., San Francisco, CA) is a chimeric anti-CD20 MAb containing the variable regions of the CD20-binding murine IgG1 MAb, IDEC-2B8, as well as human IgG1 and kappa constant regions *(18,19)*. Rituximab was the first monoclonal antibody to be approved for therapeutic use for any malignancy. Its approval was based on a single-agent pivotal trial in patients with indolent B-cell lymphoma, in which 166 patients were enrolled from 31 centers in the United States and Canada. Administration of this antibody induced remissions in 60% of patients with relapsed follicular lymphomas, including 5%–10% complete remissions *(20)*.

As a further step to reduce the murine content in an antibody, procedures have been developed for humanizing the Fv regions.

3.2. Antibody Humanization (Reshaping)

3.2.1. Humanization by CDR Grafting

CDRs build loops close to the antibody's N-terminus, where they form a continuous surface mounted on a rigid scaffold provided by the framework regions. Crystallographic analyses of several antibody/antigen complexes have demonstrated that antigen-binding mainly involves this surface (although some framework residues have also been found to take part in the interaction with antigen). Thus, the antigen-binding specificity of an antibody is mainly defined by the topography and by the chemical characteristics of its CDR surface. These features in turn are determined by the conformation of the individual CDRs, by the relative disposition of the CDRs, and by the nature and disposition of the side chains of the amino acids comprising the CDRs *(21)*.

A large decrease in the immunogenicity of an antibody can be achieved by grafting only the CDRs of xenogenic antibodies onto human framework and constant regions *(22,23)* (**Fig. 2**). However, CDR grafting *per se* may not result in the complete retention of antigen-binding properties. Indeed, it is frequently found that some framework residues from the original antibody need to be preserved in the humanized molecule if significant antigen-binding affinity is to be recovered *(24,25)*. In this case, human V regions showing the greatest sequence homology to murine V regions are chosen from a database in order to provide the human framework. The selection of human FRs can be made either from human consensus sequences or from individual human antibodies. In some rare examples, simply transferring CDRs onto the most identical human

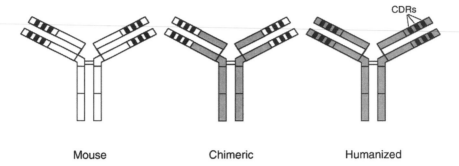

Mouse   Chimeric   Humanized

Fig. 2. Humanization of an IgG molecule. The mouse sequences are shown in white and the human sequences are shown in gray. In a chimeric antibody, the mouse heavy- and light-chain variable region sequences are joined onto human heavy-chain and light-chain constant regions. In a humanized antibody, the mouse CDRs are grafted onto human V-region FRs and expressed with human C-regions.

V-region frameworks is sufficient for retaining the binding affinity of the original murine MAb *(26)*. However, in most cases, the successful design of high-affinity CDR-grafted antibodies requires that key murine residues be substituted into the human acceptor framework to preserve the CDR conformations. Computer modeling of the antibody is used to identify such structurally important residues that are then included in order to achieve a higher binding affinity. The process of identifying the rodent framework residues to be retained is generally unique for each reshaped antibody and can therefore be difficult to foresee.

Such approach was successfully used for humanizing a MAb 4D5 against the product of protooncogene HER2 *(27)*. HER2 is a ligand-less member of the human epidermal growth factor receptor (EGFR) or ErbB family of tyrosine kinases. HER2 overexpression is observed in a number of human adenocarcinomas and results in constitutive HER2 activation. Specific targeting of these tumors can be accomplished with antibodies directed against the extracellular domain of the HER2 protein. The MAb 4D5, has been fully humanized and is termed trastuzumab (Herceptin; Genentech, San Francisco, CA). Treatment of HER2-overexpressing breast cancer cell lines with trastuzumab results in a number of phenotypic changes, such as downmodulation of the HER2 receptor, inhibition of tumor cell growth, reversed cytokine resistance, restored E-cadherin expression levels, and reduced vascular endothelial growth factor production. Interaction of trastuzumab with the human immune system via its human IgG1 Fc domain may potentiate its anti-tumor activities. In vitro studies demonstrate that trastuzumab is very effective in mediating antibody-dependent cell-mediated cytotoxicity against HER2-overexpressing tumor targets *(28)*. Trastuzumab treatment of mouse xenograft models results in marked suppression of tumor growth. When given in combination with standard cytotoxic chemotherapeutic agents, trastuzumab treatment generally results in statistically superior anti-tumor efficacy compared with either agent given alone *(28)*.

3.2.2. Humanization by Resurfacing (Veneering)

A statistical analysis of unique human and murine immunoglobulin heavy- and light-chain variable regions revealed that the precise patterns of exposed residues are different in human and murine antibodies, and most individual surface positions have a strong preference for a small number of different residues *(29,30)*. Therefore, it may be possible to reduce the immunogenicity of a nonhuman Fv, while preserving its antigen-binding properties, by simply replacing exposed residues in its framework regions that differ from those usually found in human antibodies. This would humanize the surface of the xenogenic antibody while retaining the interior and contacting residues that influence its antigen-binding characteristics and interdomain contacts. Because protein antigenicity can be correlated with surface accessibility, replacement of the surface residues may be sufficient to render the mouse variable region "invisible" to the human immune system. This procedure of humanization is referred to as "veneering" because only the outer surface of the antibody is altered, the supporting residues remain undisturbed *(31)*.

Variable domain resurfacing maintains the core murine residues of the Fv sequences and probably minimizes CDR-framework incompatibilities. This procedure was successfully used for the humanization of murine MAb N901 against the CD56 surface molecule of natural killer (NK) cells and MAb anti-B4 against CD19 *(26,32)*. A direct comparison of engineered versions of N901 humanized either by CDR grafting or by resurfacing showed no difference in binding affinity for the native antigen *(26,30)*. For the anti-B4 antibody, the best CDR-grafted version required three murine residues at surface positions to maintain binding, while the best resurfaced version needed only one surface murine residue *(26)*. Thus, even though the resurfaced version of anti-B4 has 36 murine residues in the Fv core, it may be less immunogenic than the CDR-grafted version with nine murine residues in the Fv core because it has a pattern of surface residues that is more identical to a human surface pattern.

3.3. Choice of Constant Region

The construction of chimeric and humanized antibodies offers the opportunity of tailoring the constant region to the requirements of the antibody. IgG is preferred class for therapeutic antibodies for several practical reasons. IgG antibodies are very stable, and easily purified and stored. In vivo they have a long biological half-life that is not just a function of their size but is also a result of their interaction with the so-called Brambell receptor (or FcRn) *(33)*. This receptor seems to protect IgG from catabolism within cells and recycles it back to the blood plasma. In addition, IgG has subclasses that are able to interact with and trigger a whole range of humoral and cellular effector mechanisms. Each immunoglobulin subclass differs in its ability to interact with Fc receptors and complement and thus to trigger cytolysis and other immune reactions. Human IgG1, for example, would be the constant region of choice for mediating ADCC and probably also CDC *(34,35)*. On the other hand, if the antibody were required simply to activate or block a receptor then human IgG2 or IgG4 would probably be more appropriate. For example, the humanized versions of the immunosuppressive anti-human CD3 MAb OKT3 were prepared as IgG4 antibodies *(36,37)*.

However, all four human IgG subclasses mediate at least some biological functions. To avoid the unwanted side effects of a particular isotype, it is possible to remove or modify effector functions by genetic engineering. For example, amino acid substitutions in the C_H2 portion of an anti-CD3 antibody led to the retention of its immunosuppressive properties, but markedly reduced the unwanted biological side effects associated with Fc receptor binding *(38–40)*. An alternative strategy has recently been described whereby potent blocking antibodies could be generated by assembly the C_H2 domain from sequences derived from IgG1, IgG2, and IgG4 subclasses *(41)*.

3.4. Alternative Strategies for Producing "Human" Antibodies

Other strategies for the production of "fully human" antibodies include phage libraries *(42,43)* or transgenic mice *(5,8)*, both utilizing human V-region repertoires.

3.4.1. Mice Making "Human" Antibodies

Several strains of mice are now available that have had their mouse immunoglobulin loci replaced with human immunoglobulin gene segments *(6,44,45)*. Transgenic mice are able to produce functionally important human-like antibodies with very high affinities after immunization. Cloning and production can be carried out employing the usual hybridoma technology. For example, high-affinity human MAbs obtained against the T-cell marker CD4 are potential therapeutic agents for suppressing adverse immune activity *(44)*. Another human MAbs with an affinity of 5×10^{-11} *M* for human EGFR was able to prevent formation and eradicate human epidermoid carcinoma xenografts in athymic mice *(46)*. However, during affinity maturation, the antibodies from transgenic mice accumulate somatic mutations both in FRs and CDRs *(45)*. It means that they are no longer 100% identical to inherited human germline genes and can, therefore, be potentially immunogenic in humans *(47)*. Besides, "human antibodies" from mice can be distinguished from human antibodies produced in human cells by their state of glycosylation, particularly with respect to their $Gal_\alpha1$–3Gal residue, against which human serum contains IgG antibody titers of up to 100 μg/ml. It has been argued that an antibody containing such residues would not survive very long in the human circulation *(48)*.

3.4.2. Human Antibodies from Phage Libraries

A rapid growth in the field of antibody engineering occurred after it was shown that functional antibody fragments could be secreted into the periplasmic space and even into the medium of *Escherichia coli* by fusing a bacterial signal peptide to the antibody's N-terminus *(49,50)*. These findings opened the way for transferring the principles of the immune system for producing specific antibodies to a given antigen into a bacterial system. It was now possible to establish antibody libraries in *E. coli* that could be directly screened for binding to antigen.

In order to screen large antibody libraries containing at least 10^8 individual members, it was necessary to develop a selection system as efficient as that of the immune system, in which the antibody receptor is bound to the surface of a B lymphocyte.

After binding its antigen, the B lymphocyte is stimulated to proliferate and mature into an IgG-producing plasma cell. A similar selection system could be imitated in microorganisms by expressing antibodies on their surface. Millions of microorganisms could then be simultaneously screened for binding to an immobilized antigen followed by the propagation and amplification of the selected microorganism. Although protein display methods have been developed for eukaryotic systems, e.g., retroviral *(51)*, baculoviral *(52)*, yeast *(53,54)* and even cell-free ribosome display *(55,56)*, the most successful surface expression system has been created using filamentous bacteriophages of the M13 family *(57)*. The phage display was originally reported for scFv fragments *(15)*, and later for Fab fragments *(58)* and other antibody derivatives such as diabodies *(59)*. Now it became possible to generate antibody libraries by PCR cloning the large collections of variable-region genes, expressing each of the binding sites on the surface of a different phage particle and selecting the antigen-specific binding sites by in vitro screening the phage mixture on a chosen antigen. The phage display technology could be used to select antigen-specific antibodies from libraries made from human B cells taken from individuals either immunized with antigen *(60)*, or exposed to infectious agents *(61)*, or with autoimmune diseases *(3)*, or with cancer *(62)*. Moreover, it was demonstrated that antibodies against many different antigens could be selected from "naive" binding-site library, prepared from the V_L and V_H IgM-V-gene pools of B cells of a non-immunized healthy individuals *(16,63)*. It was also shown that libraries of synthetic antibody genes based on human germline segments with randomized CDRs behave in a similar way to "naive" antibody libraries *(64,65)*. It became, therefore, possible to use primary ("naive" or "synthetic") antibody libraries with huge collections of binding sites of different specificity for in vitro selection of "human" antibody fragments against most antigens, including nonimmunogenic molecules, toxic substances and targets conserved between species (for review, *see* **refs.** *42,66*).

However, for some therapeutic applications whole IgGs are the preferred format as a result of their extended serum half-life and ability to trigger the humoral and cellular effector mechanisms. This necessitates recloning of the phage-display derived scFvs or Fabs into mammalian expression vectors containing the appropriate constant domains and establishing stable expressing cell lines. The specificity and affinity of the antibody fragments are generally well retained by the whole IgG, and, in some cases, the affinity may significantly improve due to the bivalent nature of the IgG *(67,68)*. In the past few years, four phage-derived antibodies have begun clinical trials *(69)*.

4. Recombinant Antibody Fragments

The Fv fragment consisting only of the V_H and V_L domains is the smallest immunoglobulin fragment available that carries the whole antigen-binding site (**Fig. 1**). However, Fvs appear to have lower interaction energy of their two chains than Fab fragments that are also held together by the constant domains C_H1 and C_L *(70)*. To stabilize the association of the V_H and V_L domains, they have been linked with peptides *(71,72)*, disulfide bridges *(70)* and "knob-into-hole" mutations *(73)* (**Fig. 3**).

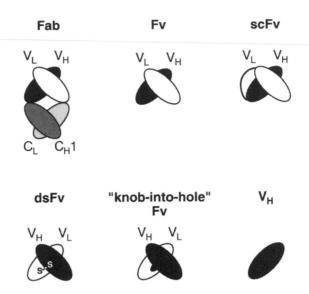

Fig. 3. Monovalent immunoglobulin fragments. Fab, Fv, disulfide-stabilized Fv (dsFv), and Fv fragments with remodeled V_H/V_L interface ("knob-into-hole" Fv) consist of two separate chains, while the single V_H domain and single chain Fv (scFv) fragments are made from a single gene.

4.1. Monovalent Antibody Fragments

4.1.1. Single Chain Fv Fragments (scFv)

Peptide linkers of about 3.5 nm are required to span the distance between the carboxy terminus of one domain and the amino terminus of the other (72). Both orientations, V_H-linker-V_L or V_L-linker-V_H, can be used. The small scFvs are particularly interesting for clinical applications (for review, *see* **ref. 74**). They are only half the size of Fabs and thus have lower retention times in nontarget tissues, more rapid blood clearance, and better tumor penetration. They are also potentially less immunogenic and are amenable to fusions with proteins and peptides.

Unlike glycosylated whole antibodies, scFv can be easily produced in bacterial cells as functional antigen-binding molecules. There are two basic strategies to obtain recombinant antibody fragments from *E. coli*. The first is to produce antibody proteins as cytoplasmic inclusion bodies followed by refolding in vitro. In this case the protein is expressed without a signal sequence under a strong promoter. The inclusion bodies contain the recombinant protein in a non-native and non-active conformation. To obtain functional antibody, the recombinant polypeptide chains have to be dissolved and folded into the right shape by using a laborious and time-consuming refolding procedure (for review, *see* **ref. 43**). The second approach for obtaining functional antibody fragments is to imitate the situation in the eukaryotic cell for secreting a correctly folded antibody. In *E. coli*, the secretion machinery directs proteins carrying a specific signal sequence to the periplasm (75). The scFv fragments are usually correctly processed in the periplasm, contain intramolecular disulfide bonds, and are soluble. However, the high-level expression of a recombinant protein with a bacterial signal peptide in *E. coli* often results in the accumulation of insoluble antibody fragments after transport to the periplasm *(76,77)*.

It is now recognized that aggregation in vivo is not a function of the solubility and stability of the native state of the protein, but of those of its folding intermediates in their particular environment *(78,79)*. The degree of successful folding of antibody fragments in the bacterial periplasm appears to depend to a large extent on the primary sequence of the variable domains *(80,81)*. The overexpression of some enzymes of the *E. coli* folding machinery such as cytoplasmic chaperonins GroES/L, periplasmic disulfide-isomerase DSbA as well as periplasmic peptidylprolyl *cis,trans*-isomerases (PPIase) PpiA and SurA did not increase the yield of soluble antibody fragments *(82–84)*. In contrast, the coexpression of either bacterial periplasmic protein Skp/OmpH or PPIase FkpA increased the functional yield of both phage-displayed and secreted scFv fragments *(84,85)*. Modifications in bacterial growth and induction conditions can also increase the proportion of correctly folded soluble scFv. For example, lowering the bacterial growth temperature has been shown to decrease periplasmic aggregation and increase the yield of soluble antibody protein *(78,86)*. Additionally, the aggregation of recombinant antibody fragments in the *E. coli* periplasm can be reduced by growing the induced cells under osmotic stress in the presence of certain nonmetabolized additives such as sucrose *(87,88)* or sorbitol and glycine betaine *(89)*. Moreover, inducing the synthesis of recombinant antibody fragments in bacteria under osmotic stress promotes the formation of domain-swapped scFv dimers *(89)*.

Single-chain Fv antibody fragments produced in bacteria provide new possibilities for protein purification by immunoaffinity chromatography. Their advantages include lower production costs, higher capacity for antigen on a weight basis, and better penetration in a small-pore separation matrix. Such recombinant immunosorbent proved to be useful for the one-step purification of a desired antigen from complex protein mixtures *(90)*. Another interesting possible application is the purification or separation of toxic compounds, which cannot be used for immunization of animals, using antibodies selected from phage-displayed antibody libraries.

4.1.2. Disulfide-Stabilized Fv Fragments (dsFv)

Another strategy for linking V_H and V_L domains has been to design an intermolecular disulfide bond (**Fig. 3**). The disulfide-stabilized (ds) Fv fragment appeared to be much more resistant to irreversible denaturation caused by storage at 37°C than the unlinked Fv. It was more stable than the scFv fragment and a chemically crosslinked Fv *(70)*. The two most promising sites for introducing disulfide bridges appeared to be $V_H 44$-$V_L 100$ connecting FR2 of the heavy chain with FR4 of the light chain and $V_H 105$-$V_L 43$ that links FR4 of the heavy chain with FR2 of the light chain *(91)*.

4.1.3. Single Antibody-Like Domains

To obtain even smaller antibody fragments than those described earlier, antigen-binding V_H domains were isolated from the lymphocytes of immunized mice *(92)*. However, one problem of the V_H domains is their "sticky patch" for interactions with

V_L domains. Since naturally occurring camel antibodies lack light chains *(93)*, the solubility of human V_H domains has been improved by mimicking camelid heavy chain sequences *(94)*. In addition, other non-antibody proteins with a single fold have been engineered for new specificity, including an alpha-helical protein domain of staphylococcal protein A (affibody *[95]*), an alpha-amylase inhibitor tendamistat *(96)*, domains of fibronectin *(97)*, lipocalins *(98)*, and the extracellular domain of CTLA-4 *(99)*. Potential advantages of such single-domain binding molecules might be their easy production, enhanced stability, targeting certain antigen types (e.g., ligand-binding pockets of receptors), and their fast engineering into multimeric or multivalent reagents. However, it appears that not all kinds of protein scaffold that may appear attractive for the engineering of loop regions will indeed permit the construction of independent ligand-binding sites with high affinity and specificity. Nevertheless, such single immunoglobulin fold and other artificial binding sites might eventually become major competitors for antibodies in many of the present applications *(100)*.

4.2. Bivalent and Multivalent Fv Antibody Constructs

One disadvantage of scFv antibody fragments is the monovalency of the product, which precludes an increased avidity due to polyvalent binding. Several therapeutically important antigens have repetitive epitopes resulting in a higher avidity for antibodies and antibody fragments with two or more antigen-binding sites. Another drawback of scFv fragments is their small size resulting in fast clearance from the blood stream through the kidneys. Recently, attention has focused upon the generation of scFv-based molecules with molecular weights in the range of the renal threshold for the first-pass clearance. In one approach, bivalent $(scFv')_2$ fragments have been produced from scFv containing an additional C-terminal cysteine by chemical coupling *(101,102)* or by the spontaneous site-specific dimerization of scFv containing an unpaired C-terminal cysteine directly in the periplasm of *E. coli (77,103)* (**Fig. 4**). Affinity measurements demonstrated that covalently linked $(scFv')_2$ have binding constants quite close to those of the parental MAbs and fourfold higher than scFv monomers *(77)*. In vivo, bivalent $(scFv')_2$ fragments demonstrated longer blood retention and higher tumor accumulation in comparison to scFv monomers *(101)*.

Alternatively, the scFv fragments can be forced to form multimers by shortening the peptide linker. Single-chain Fv antibody fragments are predominantly monomeric (~30 kDa) when the V_H and V_L domains are joined by polypeptide linkers of more than 12 residues. Reduction of the linker length to 3–12 residues prevents the monomeric configuration of the scFv molecule and favors intermolecular V_H-V_L pairings with formation of a 60 kDa noncovalent scFv dimer "diabody" *(104)*. Prolonged tumor retention in vivo and higher tumor to blood ratios reported for diabodies over scFv monomers result both from the reduced kidney clearance and higher avidity *(105)*. Reducing the linker length still further below three residues can result in the formation of trimers ("triabody", ~90 kDa *[106]*) or tetramers ("tetrabody," ~120 kDa *[107]*) (**Fig. 4**). A comparison of the in vitro cell-binding characteristics of the diabody, triabody and tetrabody specific to CD19 B-cell antigen demonstrated 1.5- and 2.5-fold higher affinities of the diabody and tetrabody in comparison with scFv monomer *(107)*.

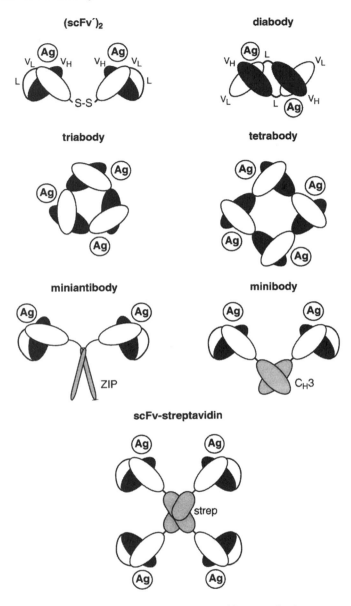

Fig. 4. Schematic representation of multivalent recombinant antibody constructs. (scFv')$_2$ is formed by covalent linking of two unpaired cysteine residues. Appearance of the noncovalent scFv dimer (diabody), trimer (triabody), and tetramer (tetrabody) depends on length of the linker between V_H and V_L domains and on the stability of V_H-V_L associations. The miniantibody, minibody, and scFv-streptavidin oligomers are formed due to the adhesive self-associating peptide or protein domains (leucine zipper-derived amphipathic helix, C_H3, streptavidin). The antibody variable domains (V_H, V_L), peptide linkers (L), intermolecular disulfide bond (S-S), and antigen-binding sites (Ag) of Fv modules are indicated.

This increase in avidity of the tetrabody combined with its larger size could prove to be particularly advantageous for tumor imaging and the radioimmunotherapy.

Construction of bivalent scFv molecules can also be achieved by genetic fusion with protein dimerizing motifs such as amphipathic helices ("miniantibody" *[108]*) or immunoglobulin C_H3 domains ("minibody" *[109]*) (**Fig. 4**). In a similar fashion, tetravalent scFv were produced by fusing them with streptavidin *(110,111)* (**Fig. 4**). The purified scFv-streptavidin tetramers demonstrated both antigen- and biotin-binding activity, were stable over a wide range of pH and did not dissociate at high temperatures (up to 70°C). Surface plasmon resonance measurements showed that the pure scFv-streptavidin tetramers bound immobilized antigen very tightly and no dissociation was observed. The association rate constant for scFv-streptavidin tetramers was also higher than those were for scFv monomers and dimers. This was also reflected in the apparent constants, which was found to be two orders of magnitude higher for pure scFv-streptavidin tetramers than monomeric single-chain antibodies *(111)*. It was also shown that most of the biotin binding sites of the scFv-streptavidin tetramers were accessible and not blocked by biotinylated bacterial proteins or free biotin from the medium. These sites should therefore facilitate the construction of bispecific multivalent antibodies by the addition of biotinylated ligands.

4.3. Bispecific Recombinant Antibodies

Bispecific antibodies (BsAb) comprise two specificities, and can redirect effector cells towards therapeutic targets. These molecules can limit complement activation, which is responsible for side effects in many therapeutic settings, and profoundly enhance target selectivity. BsAb were used initially to direct lymphocyte effector cells to specific targets. More recently, attention focused on other effector populations, such as dendritic cells and erythrocytes (for review, *see* **ref. *112***).

4.3.1. Bivalent Bispecific Antibodies

So far, bispecific antibodies have mainly been constructed by fusion of two hybridoma lines, generating so called quadromas. A major limitation of this procedure is the production of inactive antibodies due to the random L-H and H-H associations. Only about 15% of the antibody produced by the quadroma are of the desired specificity *(113)*. The correct BsAb must then be purified in a costly procedure from a large quantity of other very similar molecules. A further limitation of the quadroma BsAb from rodent cell lines is their immunogenicity. Recent advances in recombinant antibody technology have provided several alternative methods for constructing and producing BsAb molecules *(114,115)* (**Fig. 5**). For example, nearly quantitative formation and efficient recovery of bispecific human IgG (BsIgG) can be achieved by remodeling C_H3 domains of the heavy chains using "knob-into-hole" mutations in conjunction with engineered disulfide bonds *(116)*. Using an identical light chain for each arm of the BsIgG circumvented light chain mispairing. Smaller bispecific F(ab')₂ have been created either by chemical coupling from Fab' fragments expressed in *E. coli (117)* or by heterodimerization through leucine zippers *(118)*. Analogously, scFv fragments have been genetically fused either with Fos and Jun leucine zippers *(119)* or CH1 and

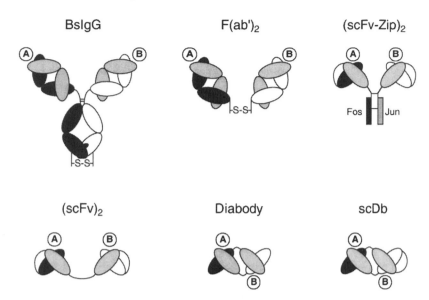

Fig. 5. Recombinant bivalent BsAb formats. The heavy chains of BsIgG were remodeled so that they heterodimerize but do not homodimerize using "knob-into-hole" mutations and an engineered disulfide bond between C_H3 domains. In this molecule, both specificities share the same light chain. The F(ab')$_2$ heterodimers are constructed by chemical coupling of Fab' fragments at the hinge region. Double scFvs can be formed either by interaction of Fos and Jun leucine zippers ([scFv-Zip]$_2$) or by connecting them in a tandem via linker ([scFv]$_2$). Noncovalent association of two hybrid scFv fragments comprising V_H and V_L domains of different specificity forms a bispecific diabody. In a single-chain diabody (scDb), these hybrid scFvs are connected with a long flexible linker. The antigen-binding sites of different specificity (**A** and **B**) are indicated.

CL antibody constant domains *(120,121)* to facilitate the formation of heterodimers. The genetic engineering of scFv-scFv tandems [(scFv)2)] linked with a third polypeptide linker has also been carried out in several laboratories *(122,123)*. An alternative bispecific antibody fragment is the scFv heterodimer diabody *(104)*. The bispecific diabody was obtained by the noncovalent association of two single chain fusion products consisting of the V_H domain from one antibody connected by a short linker to the V_L domain of another antibody *(124,125)* (**Fig. 5**). The two antigen-binding domains have been shown by crystallographic analysis to be on opposite sides of the diabody molecule such that they are able to cross-link two cells *(126)*. Diabodies are potentially less immunogenic than quadroma-derived BsAb and can be easily produced in bacteria in relatively high yields *(127,128)*.

Bispecific diabodies appeared to be more effective than quadroma-derived BsAb in mediating T cell *(125,128)* and NK cell *(129)* cytotoxicity in vitro against tumor cells. However, the ultimate goal of any anti-tumor immunotherapy is the in vivo eradication of tumor cells. The CD30 × CD16 diabody was able to induce a marked regression of xenotransplanted human Hodgkin's lymphoma in severe combined immunodeficiency (SCID) mice due to the recruitment of human NK cells *(129)*. Analogously, the potency of a CD3 × CD19 diabody to mediate T cell-dependent tumor lysis was tested in a fairly stringent in vivo model of immunodeficient mice bearing a s.c. growing human B cell lymphoma *(128)*. Mice receiving the diabody had a longer mean survival time twice as long as the control animals. The administration of the diabody together with the anti-CD28 MAb further prolonged the survival. Although bispecific diabody was relatively rapidly cleared from the blood stream through the kidneys, its anti-tumor activity was fairly similar to that of the quadroma-derived BsAb *(128,129)*. The fast clearance was probably compensated by a better tumor penetration and more efficient induction of cell lysis.

However, co-secretion of two hybrid scFv fragments forming bispecific diabody can give rise to two types of dimer: active heterodimers and inactive homodimers. Another problem is that two chains of diabodies are held together by noncovalent associations of the V_H and V_L domains and can diffuse away from one another. The stability of bispecific diabody can be enhanced by introduction of a disulfide bridge or "knob-into-hole" mutations into the V_H/V_L interface *(73,130)*. An alternative way to stabilize bivalent bispecific diabody is the formation of single chain diabody (scDb) where two hybrid scFv fragments are connected with a peptide linker *(89,131)* (**Fig. 5**).

4.3.2. Tetravalent Bispecific Molecules

In contrast to native antibodies, all aforementioned BsAb formats have only one binding domain for each specificity. However, bivalent binding is an important means of increasing the functional affinity and possibly the selectivity for particular cell types carrying densely clustered antigens. Therefore, a number of tetravalent bispecific antibody-like molecules of different molecular weight have been developed (**Fig. 6**). For example, scFv fragment was genetically fused either to the C_H3 domain of an IgG molecule or to Fab fragment through a hinge region. The IgG-(scFv)$_2$ antibody was bispecific, retained Fc associated effector functions, and had as long half-life in vivo as human IgG3 *(132)*. Alternatively, tetravalent bispecific IgG-like molecules have been created by fusion of bispecific scDb either to human Fc region or to C_H3 domain *(133)*. In another approach, two scFvs of different specificity were fused to the first constant domain of human heavy chain (C_H1) and to the constant domain of human κ chain (C_L), to form two polypeptides, (scFv)$_A$-C_H1-C_H2-C_H3 and (scFv)$_B$-C_L, respectively *(121)*. Coexpression of these polypeptides in mammalian cells resulted in the formation of a covalently linked bispecific heterotetramer, (scFv)$_4$-IgG (**Fig. 6**).

Smaller tetravalent bispecific molecules can be formed by dimerization of either scFv-scFv tandems with a linker containing a helix-loop-helix motif (DiBi miniantibody *[134]*) or a single chain molecule comprising four antibody variable domains (V_H and V_L) in an orientation preventing intramolecular pairing (tandem diabody *[89]*). Compared to bispecific diabody, the tandem diabody (Tandab; **Fig. 6**) exhibited a higher apparent affinity to both antigens and enhanced biological activity both in vitro and in vivo *(89,135)*. Unlike many other BsAb formats, the Tandab comprises only antibody variable domains without the need of extra self-associating structures.

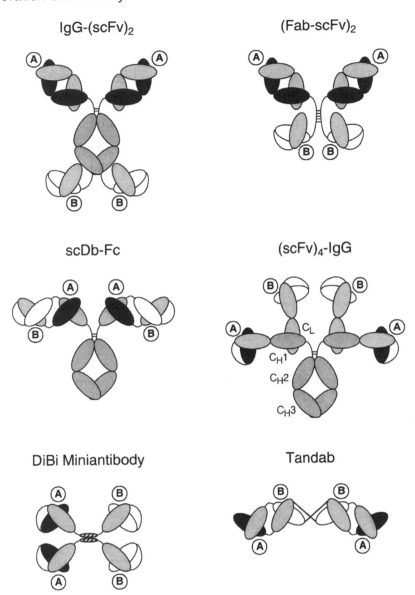

Fig. 6. Recombinant tetravalent bispecific antibodies. In IgG-(scFv)$_4$ and (Fab-scFv)$_4$, the scFv fragments are fused either to the C-terminus of C_H3 domain or to the hinge region, respectively. ScDb-Fc molecules are obtained by joining scDb and Fc part of an IgG. In (scFv)$_4$-IgG, the V_H and V_L domains of a human IgG1 molecule are replaced by two scFv fragments of different specificity. DiBi miniantibody is formed by dimerization of scFv-scFv tandem through the linker between two scFv moieties. Tandem diabody (Tandab) is also a homodimer stabilized by V_H/V_L associations. The antigen-binding sites of different specificity (**A** and **B**) are indicated.

5. Conclusion and Perspectives

Recombinant antibody technology is paving a new way for the development of therapeutic and diagnostic agents. For example, human antigen-binding fragments derived from antibody libraries or transgenic mice are being engineered to target and cure a variety of illnesses. In spite of the rapid advances of the last few years, several problems such as the routine production of experimental amounts of stable recombinant antibodies from selected clones need to be resolved. Recombinant antibodies also need to be tested in a clinical setting. Initial optimistic estimates that this technology would make previous antibody-based pharmaceuticals redundant almost overnight have now been modified. It will take somewhat longer. Nevertheless, the number of recombinant antibody-based products now entering clinical trials indicates an exponential growth of activities in this field. Furthermore, the development of complementary novel biotechniques such as ribosome display (56), molecular breeding (136,137) and antibody arrays for high-throughput screening of antibody-antigen interactions (14,138) are opening up many more potential applications for recombinant antibodies.

References

1. Köhler, G. and Milstein, C. (1975) Continuous cultures of fused cells secreting antibody of predefined specificity. *Nature* **256**, 495–497.
2. Harris, L. J., Larson, S. B., Hasel, K. W., and McPherson, A. (1997) Refined structure of an intact IgG2a monoclonal antibody. Biochemistry **36**, 1581–1597.
3. Welschof, M., Terness, P., Kipriyanov, S. M., Stanescu, D., Breitling, F., Dörsam, H., et al. (1997) The antigen-binding domain of a human IgG-anti-F(ab')2 autoantibody. *Proc. Natl. Acad. Sci. USA* **94**, 1902–1907.
4. Terness, P., Welschof, M., Moldenhauer, G., Jung, M., Moroder, L., Kirchhoff, F., et al. (1997) Idiotypic vaccine for treatment of human B-cell lymphoma. Construction of IgG variable regions from single malignant B cells. *Hum. Immunol.* **56**, 17–27.
5. Green, L. L. (1999) Antibody engineering via genetic engineering of the mouse: XenoMouse strains are a vehicle for the facile generation of therapeutic human monoclonal antibodies. *J. Immunol. Methods* **231**, 11–23.
6. Tomizuka, K., Shinohara, T., Yoshida, H., Uejima, H., Ohguma, A., Tanaka, S., et al. (2000) Double trans-chromosomic mice: mai0ntenance of two individual human chromosome fragments containing Ig heavy and kappa loci and expression of fully human antibodies. *Proc. Natl. Acad. Sci. USA* **97**, 722–727.
7. Borrebaeck, C. A., Danielsson, L., and Moller, S. A. (1988) Human monoclonal antibodies produced by primary in vitro immunization of peripheral blood lymphocytes. *Proc. Natl. Acad. Sci. USA* **85**, 3995–3999.
8. Little, M., Kipriyanov, S. M., Le Gall, F., and Moldenhauer, G. (2000) Of mice and men: hybridoma and recombinant antibodies. *Immunol. Today* **21**, 364–370.
9. Marks, J. D., Tristem, M., Karpas, A., and Winter, G. (1991) Oligonucleotide primers for polymerase chain reaction amplification of human immunoglobulin variable genes and design of family-specific oligonucleotide probes. *Eur. J. Immunol.* **21**, 985–991.
10. Welschof, M., Terness, P., Kolbinger, F., Zewe, M., Dübel, S., Dörsam, H., et al. (1995) Amino acid sequence based PCR primers for amplification of rearranged human heavy and light chain immunoglobulin variable region genes. *J. Immunol. Methods* **179**, 203–214.

11. Kipriyanov, S. M., Kupriyanova, O. A., Little, M., and Moldenhauer, G. (1996) Rapid detection of recombinant antibody fragments directed against cell-surface antigens by flow cytometry. *J. Immunol. Methods* **196,** 51–62.
12. Lagerkvist, A. C., Furebring, C., and Borrebaeck, C. A. (1995) Single, antigen-specific B cells used to generate Fab fragments using CD40-mediated amplification or direct PCR cloning. *Biotechniques* **18,** 862–869.
13. Dreher, M. L., Gherardi, E., Skerra, A., and Milstein, C. (1991) Colony assays for antibody fragments expressed in bacteria. *J. Immunol. Methods* **139,** 197–205.
14. de Wildt, R. M., Mundy, C. R., Gorick, B. D., and Tomlinson, I. M. (2000) Antibody arrays for high-throughput screening of antibody-antigen interactions. *Nature Biotechnol.* **18,** 989–994.
15. McCafferty, J., Griffiths, A. D., Winter, G., and Chiswell, D. J. (1990) Phage antibodies: filamentous phage displaying antibody variable domains. *Nature* **348,** 552–554.
16. Marks, J. D., Hoogenboom, H. R., Bonnert, T. P., McCafferty, J., Griffiths, A. D., and Winter, G. (1991) By-passing immunization. Human antibodies from V-gene libraries displayed on phage. *J. Mol. Biol.* **222,** 581–597.
17. Khazaeli, M. B., Conry, R. M., and LoBuglio, A. F. (1994) Human immune response to monoclonal antibodies. *J. Immunother.* **15,** 42–52.
18. McLaughlin, P., Hagemeister, F. B., and Grillo-Lopez, A. J. (1999) Rituximab in indolent lymphoma: the single-agent pivotal trial. *Semin. Oncol.* **26,** 79–87.
19. Maloney, D. G. (1999) Preclinical and phase I and II trials of rituximab. *Semin. Oncol.* **26,** 74–78.
20. Press, O. W. (1999) Radiolabeled antibody therapy of B-cell lymphomas. *Semin. Oncol.* **26,** 58–65.
21. Padlan, E. A. (1994) Anatomy of the antibody molecule. *Mol. Immunol.* **31,** 169–217.
22. Jones, P. T., Dear, P. H., Foote, J., Neuberger, M. S., and Winter, G. (1986) Replacing the complementarity-determining regions in a human antibody with those from a mouse. *Nature* **321,** 522–525.
23. Verhoeyen, M., Milstein, C., and Winter, G. (1988) Reshaping human antibodies: grafting an anti-lysozyme activity. *Science* **239,** 1534–1536.
24. Queen, C., Schneider, W. P., Selick, H. E., Payne, P. W., Landolfi, N. F., Duncan, J. F., et al. (1989) A humanized antibody that binds to the interleukin 2 receptor. *Proc. Natl. Acad. Sci. USA* **86,** 10,029–10,033.
25. Co, M. S. and Queen, C. (1991) Humanized antibodies for therapy. *Nature* **351,** 501-502.
26. Roguska, M. A., Pedersen, J. T., Henry, A. H., Searle, S. M., Roja, C. M., Avery, B., et al. (1996) A comparison of two murine monoclonal antibodies humanized by CDR-grafting and variable domain resurfacing. *Protein Eng.* **9,** 895–904.
27. Carter, P., Presta, L., Gorman, C. M., Ridgway, J. B., Henner, D., Wong, W. L., et al. (1992) Humanization of an anti-p185HER2 antibody for human cancer therapy. *Proc. Natl. Acad. Sci. USA* **89,** 4285–4289.
28. Sliwkowski, M. X., Lofgren, J. A., Lewis, G. D., Hotaling, T. E., Fendly, B. M., and Fox, J. A. (1999) Nonclinical studies addressing the mechanism of action of trastuzumab (Herceptin). *Semin. Oncol.* **26,** 60–70.
29. Padlan, E. A. (1991) A possible procedure for reducing the immunogenicity of antibody variable domains while preserving their ligand-binding properties. *Mol. Immunol.* **28,** 489–498.
30. Pedersen, J. T., Henry, A. H., Searle, S. J., Guild, B. C., Roguska, M., and Rees, A. R. (1994) Comparison of surface accessible residues in human and murine immunoglobulin Fv domains. Implication for humanization of murine antibodies. *J. Mol. Biol.* **235,** 959–973.

31. Mark, G. E. and Padlan, E. A. (1994) Humanization of monoclonal antibodies, in *Handbook of Experimental Pharmacology, vol. 113: The Pharmacology of Monoclonal Antibodies* (Rosenberg, M. and Moore, G. P., eds.); Springer-Verlag, Berlin, Heidelberg, pp. 105–134.

32. Roguska, M. A., Pedersen, J. T., Keddy, C. A., Henry, A. H., Searle, S. J., Lambert, J. M., et al. (1994) Humanization of murine monoclonal antibodies through variable domain resurfacing. *Proc. Natl. Acad. Sci. USA* **91,** 969–973.

33. Ghetie, V. and Ward, E. S. (1997) FcRn: the MHC class I-related receptor that is more than an IgG transporter. *Immunol. Today* **18,** 592–598.

34. Liu, A. Y., Robinson, R. R., Hellström, K. E., Murray, E. D., Chang, C. P., and Hellström, I. (1987) Chimeric mouse-human IgG1 antibody that can mediate lysis of cancer cells. *Proc. Natl. Acad. Sci. USA* **84,** 3439–3443.

35. Riechmann, L., Clark, M., Waldmann, H., and Winter, G. (1988) Reshaping human antibodies for therapy. *Nature* **332,** 323–327.

36. Adair, J. R., Athwal, D. S., Bodmer, M., Bright, S. M., Collins, A., Pulito, V. L., et al. (1994) Humanization of the murine anti-human CD3 monoclonal antibody OKT3. *Hum. Antibodies Hybridomas* **5,** 41–47.

37. Woodle, E. S., Thistlethwaite, J. R., Jolliffe, L. K., Zivin, R. A., Collins, A., Adair, J. R., et al. (1992) Humanized OKT3 antibodies: successful transfer of immune modulating properties and idiotype expression. *J. Immunol.* **148,** 2756–2763.

38. Alegre, M.-L., Collins, A., Pulito, V. L., Brosius, R. A., Olson, W. C., Zivin, R. A., et al. (1992) Effect of a single amino acid mutation on the activating and immunosuppressive properties of a "humanized" OKT3 monoclonal antibody. *J. Immunol.* **148,** 3461–3468.

39. Alegre, M.-L., Peterson, L. J., Xu, D., Sattar, H. A., Jeyarajah, D. R., Kowalkowski, K., et al. (1994) A non-activating "humanized" anti-CD3 monoclonal antibody retains immunosuppressive properties *in vivo. Transplantation* **57,** 1537–1543.

40. Cole, M. S., Anasetti, C., and Tso, J. Y. (1997) Human IgG2 variants of chimeric anti-CD3 are nonmitogenic to T cells. *J. Immunol.* **159,** 3613–3621.

41. Armour, K. L., Clark, M. R., Hadley, A. G., and Williamson, L. M. (1999) Recombinant human IgG molecules lacking Fcgamma receptor I binding and monocyte triggering activities. *Eur. J. Immunol.* **29,** 2613–2624.

42. Winter, G., Griffiths, A. D., Hawkins, R. E., and Hoogenboom, H. R. (1994) Making antibodies by phage display technology. *Annu. Rev. Immunol.* **12,** 433–455.

43. Kipriyanov, S. M. and Little, M. (1999) Generation of recombinant antibodies. *Mol. Biotechnol.* **12,** 173–201.

44. Fishwild, D. M., O'Donnell, S. L., Bengoechea, T., Hudson, D. V., Harding, F., Bernhard, S. L., et al. (1996) High-avidity human IgG kappa monoclonal antibodies from a novel strain of minilocus transgenic mice. *Nature Biotechnol.* **14,** 845–851.

45. Mendez, M. J., Green, L. L., Corvalan, J. R., Jia, X. C., Maynard-Currie, C. E., Yang, X. D., et al. (1997) Functional transplant of megabase human immunoglobulin loci recapitulates human antibody response in mice. *Nature Genet.* **15,** 146–156.

46. Yang, X. D., Jia, X. C., Corvalan, J. R., Wang, P., Davis, C. G., and Jakobovits, A. (1999) Eradication of established tumors by a fully human monoclonal antibody to the epidermal growth factor receptor without concomitant chemotherapy. *Cancer Res.* **59,** 1236–1243.

47. Clark, M. (2000) Antibody humanization: a case of the 'Emperor's new clothes'? *Immunol. Today* **21,** 397–402.

48. Borrebaeck, C. A. (1999) Human monoclonal antibodies: the emperor's new clothes? *Nature Biotechnol.* **17,** 621.

49. Better, M., Chang, C. P., Robinson, R. R., and Horwitz, A. H. (1988) *Escherichia coli* secretion of an active chimeric antibody fragment. *Science* **240,** 1041–1043.
50. Skerra, A. and Plückthun, A. (1988) Assembly of a functional immunoglobulin Fv fragment in *Escherichia coli. Science* **240,** 1038–1041.
51. Russel, S. J., Hawkins, R. E., and Winter, G. (1993) Retroviral vectors displaying functional antibody fragments. *Nucleic Acids Res.* **21,** 1081–1085.
52. Boublik, Y., Di Bonito, P., and Jones, I. M. (1995) Eukaryotic virus display: engineering the major surface glycoprotein of the Autographa californica nuclear polyhedrosis virus (AcNPV) for the presentation of foreign proteins on the virus surface. *Biotechnology* **13,** 1079–1084.
53. Kieke, M. C., Cho, B. K., Boder, E. T., Kranz, D. M., and Wittrup, K. D. (1997) Isolation of anti-T cell receptor scFv mutants by yeast surface display. *Protein Eng.* **10,** 1303–1310.
54. Boder, E. T. and Wittrup, K. D. (1997) Yeast surface display for screening combinatorial polypeptide libraries. *Nature Biotechnol.* **15,** 553–557.
55. Hanes, J., and Plückthun, A. (1997) In vitro selection and evolution of functional proteins by using ribosome display. *Proc. Natl. Acad. Sci. USA* **94,** 4937–4942.
56. Schaffitzel, C., Hanes, J., Jermutus, L., and Plückthun, A. (1999) Ribosome display: an *in vitro* method for selection and evolution of antibodies from libraries. *J. Immunol. Methods* **231,** 119–135.
57. Smith, G. P. (1985) Filamentous fusion phage: novel expression vectors that display cloned antigens on the virion surface. *Science* **228,** 1315–1317.
58. Hoogenboom, H. R., Griffiths, A. D., Johnson, K. S., Chiswell, D. J., Hudson, P., and Winter, G. (1991) Multi-subunit proteins on the surface of filamentous phage: methodologies for displaying antibody (Fab) heavy and light chains. *Nucleic Acids Res.* **19,** 4133–4137.
59. McGuinness, B. T., Walter, G., FitzGerald, K., Schuler, P., Mahoney, W., Duncan, A. R., and Hoogenboom, H. R. (1996) Phage diabody repertoires for selection of large numbers of bispecific antibody fragments. *Nature Biotechnol.* **14,** 1149–1154.
60. Persson, M. A. A., Caothien, R. H., and Burton, D. R. (1991) Generation of diverse high-affinity human monoclonal antibodies by repertoire cloning. *Proc. Natl. Acad. Sci. USA* **88,** 2432–2436.
61. Burton, D. R., Barbas, C. F., Persson, M. A., Koenig, S., Chanock, R. M., and Lerner, R. A. (1991) A large array of human monoclonal antibodies to type 1 human immunodeficiency virus from combinatorial libraries of asymptomatic seropositive individuals. *Proc. Natl. Acad. Sci. USA* **88,** 10,134–10,137.
62. Cai, X. and Garen, A. (1995) Anti-melanoma antibodies from melanoma patients immunized with genetically modified autologous tumor cells: selection of specific antibodies from single-chain Fv fusion phage libraries. *Proc. Natl. Acad. Sci. USA* **92,** 6537–6541.
63. Dörsam, H., Rohrbach, P., Kurschner, T., Kipriyanov, S., Renner, S., Braunagel, M., et al. (1997) Antibodies to steroids from a small human naive IgM library. *FEBS Lett.* **414,** 7–13.
64. Barbas, C. F., Bain, J. D., Hoekstra, D. M., and Lerner, R. A. (1992) Semisynthetic combinatorial antibody libraries: a chemical solution to the diversity problem. *Proc. Natl. Acad. Sci. USA* **89,** 4457–4461.
65. Nissim, A., Hoogenboom, H. R., Tomlinson, I. M., Flynn, G., Midgley, C., Lane, D., and Winter, G. (1994) Antibody fragments from a 'single pot' phage display library as immunochemical reagents. *EMBO J.* **13,** 692–698.
66. Hoogenboom, H. R. and Chames, P. (2000) Natural and designer binding sites made by phage display technology. *Immunol. Today* **21,** 371–378.

67. Xie, M. H., Yuan, J., Adams, C., and Gurney, A. (1997) Direct demonstration of MuSK involvement in acetylcholine receptor clustering through identification of agonist scFv. *Nature Biotechnol.* **15**, 768–771.
68. Huls, G. A., Heijnen, I. A., Cuomo, M. E., Koningsberger, J. C., Wiegman, L., Boel, E., et al. (1999) A recombinant, fully human monoclonal antibody with antitumor activity constructed from phage-displayed antibody fragments. *Nature Biotechnol.* **17**, 276–281.
69. McCafferty, J. and Glover, D. R. (2000) Engineering therapeutic proteins. *Curr. Opin. Struct. Biol.* **10**, 417–420.
70. Glockshuber, R., Malia, M., Pfitzinger, I., and Plückthun, A. (1990) A comparison of strategies to stabilize immunoglobulin Fv-fragments. *Biochemistry* **29**, 1362–1367.
71. Bird, R. E., Hardman, K. D., Jacobson, J. W., Johnson, S., Kaufman, B. M., Lee, S. M., et al. (1988) Single-chain antigen-binding proteins. *Science* **242**, 423–426.
72. Huston, J. S., Levinson, D., Mudgett Hunter, M., Tai, M. S., Novotny, J., Margolies, M. N., et al. (1988) Protein engineering of antibody binding sites: recovery of specific activity in an anti-digoxin single-chain Fv analogue produced in *Escherichia coli. Proc. Natl. Acad. Sci. USA* **85**, 5879–5883.
73. Zhu, Z., Presta, L. G., Zapata, G., and Carter, P. (1997) Remodeling domain interfaces to enhance heterodimer formation. *Protein Sci.* **6**, 781–788.
74. Huston, J. S., McCartney, J., Tai, M. S., Mottola Hartshorn, C., Jin, D., Warren, F., et al. (1993) Medical applications of single-chain antibodies. *Int. Rev. Immunol.* **10**, 195–217.
75. Pugsley, A. P. (1993) The complete general secretory pathway in gram-negative bacteria. *Microbiol. Rev.* **57**, 50–108.
76. Whitlow, M., and Filpula, D. (1991) Single-chain Fv proteins and their fusion proteins. *Methods Companion Methods Enzymol.* **2**, 97–105.
77. Kipriyanov, S. M., Dübel, S., Breitling, F., Kontermann, R. E., and Little, M. (1994) Recombinant single-chain Fv fragments carrying C-terminal cysteine residues: production of bivalent and biotinylated miniantibodies. *Mol. Immunol.* **31**, 1047–1058.
78. Plückthun, A. (1994) Antibodies from *Escherichia coli*, in *Handbook of Experimental Pharmacology, vol. 113: The Pharmacology of Monoclonal Antibodies* (Rosenberg, M. and Moore, G. P., eds.); Springer-Verlag, Berlin, Heidelberg, pp. 269–315.
79. Hockney, R. C. (1994) Recent developments in heterologous protein production in *Escherichia coli. Trends Biotechnol.* **12**, 456–463.
80. Knappik, A. and Plückthun, A. (1995) Engineered turns of a recombinant antibody improve its in vivo folding. *Protein Eng.* **8**, 81–89.
81. Kipriyanov, S. M., Moldenhauer, G., Martin, A. C. R., Kupriyanova, O. A., and Little, M. (1997) Two amino acid mutations in an anti-human CD3 single chain Fv antibody fragment that affect the yield on bacterial secretion but not the affinity. *Protein Eng.* **10**, 445–453.
82. Duenas, M., Vazquez, J., Ayala, M., Soderlind, E., Ohlin, M., Perez, L., et al. (1994) Intra- and extracellular expression of an scFv antibody fragment in *E. coli*: effect of bacterial strains and pathway engineering using GroES/L chaperonins. *Biotechniques* **16**, 476–477.
83. Knappik, A., Krebber, C., and Plückthun, A. (1993) The effect of folding catalysts on the *in vivo* folding process of different antibody fragments expressed in *Escherichia coli. Biotechnology* **11**, 77–83.
84. Bothmann, H., and Plückthun, A. (2000) The periplasmic *Escherichia coli* peptidylprolyl *cistrans*-isomerase FkpA. I. Increased functional expression of antibody fragments with and without cis-prolines. *J. Biol. Chem.* **275**, 17,100–17,105.
85. Bothmann, H. and Plückthun, A. (1998) Selection for a periplasmic factor improving phage display and functional periplasmic expression. *Nature Biotechnol.* **16**, 376–380.

86. Skerra, A. and Plückthun, A. (1991) Secretion and in vivo folding of the Fab fragment of the antibody McPC603 in *Escherichia coli*: influence of disulphides and *cis*-prolines. *Protein Eng.* **4,** 971–979.

87. Sawyer, J. R., Schlom, J., and Kashmiri, S. V. S. (1994) The effect of induction conditions on production of a soluble anti-tumor sFv in *Escherichia coli*. *Protein Eng.* **7,** 1401–1406.

88. Kipriyanov, S. M., Moldenhauer, G., and Little, M. (1997) High level production of soluble single chain antibodies in small-scale *Escherichia coli* cultures. *J. Immunol. Methods* **200,** 69–77.

89. Kipriyanov, S. M., Moldenhauer, G., Schuhmacher, J., Cochlovius, B., Von der Lieth, C. W., et al. (1999) Bispecific tandem diabody for tumor therapy with improved antigen binding and pharmacokinetics. *J. Mol. Biol.* **293,** 41–56.

90. Kipriyanov, S. M. and Little, M. (1997) Affinity purification of tagged recombinant proteins using immobilized single chain Fv fragments. *Anal. Biochem.* **244,** 189–191.

91. Reiter, Y., Brinkmann, U., Jung, S. H., Pastan, I., and Lee, B. (1995) Disulfide stabilization of antibody Fv: computer predictions and experimental evaluation. *Protein Eng.* **8,** 1323–1331.

92. Ward, E. S., Gussow, D., Griffiths, A. D., Jones, P. T., and Winter, G. (1989) Binding activities of a repertoire of single immunoglobulin variable domains secreted from *Escherichia coli*. *Nature* **341,** 544–546.

93. Hamers-Casterman, C., Atarhouch, T., Muyldermans, S., Robinson, G., Hamers, C., Songa, E. B., et al. (1993) Naturally occurring antibodies devoid of light chains. *Nature* **363,** 446–448.

94. Davies, J. and Riechmann, L. (1996) Single antibody domains as small recognition units: design and *in vitro* antigen selection of camelized, human VH domains with improved protein stability. *Protein Eng.* **9,** 531–537.

95. Hansson, M., Ringdahl, J., Robert, A., Power, U., Goetsch, L., Nguyen, T. N., et al. (1999) An in vitro selected binding protein (affibody) shows conformation-dependent recognition of the respiratory syncytial virus (RSV) G protein. *Immunotechnology* **4,** 237–252.

96. McConnell, S. J. and Hoess, R. H. (1995) Tendamistat as a scaffold for conformationally constrained phage peptide libraries. *J. Mol. Biol.* **250,** 460–470.

97. Koide, A., Bailey, C. W., Huang, X., and Koide, S. (1998) The fibronectin type III domain as a scaffold for novel binding proteins. *J. Mol. Biol.* **284,** 1141–1151.

98. Beste, G., Schmidt, F. S., Stibora, T., and Skerra, A. (1999) Small antibody-like proteins with prescribed ligand specificities derived from the lipocalin fold. *Proc. Natl. Acad. Sci. USA* **96,** 1898–1903.

99. Hufton, S. E., van Neer, N., van den Beuken, T., Desmet, J., Sablon, E., and Hoogenboom, H. R. (2000) Development and application of cytotoxic T lymphocyte-associated antigen 4 as a protein scaffold for the generation of novel binding ligands. *FEBS Lett.* **475,** 225–231.

100. Skerra, A. (2000) Engineered protein scaffolds for molecular recognition. *J. Mol. Recog.* **13,** 167–187.

101. Adams, G. P., McCartney, J. E., Tai, M. S., Oppermann, H., Huston, J. S., Stafford, W. F., et al. (1993) Highly specific *in vivo* tumor targeting by monovalent and divalent forms of 741F8 anti-c-erbB-2 single-chain Fv. *Cancer Res.* **53,** 4026–4034.

102. McCartney, J. E., Tai, M. S., Hudziak, R. M., Adams, G. P., Weiner, L. M., Jin, D., et al. (1995) Engineering disulfide-linked single-chain Fv dimers [(sFv')$_2$] with improved solution and targeting properties: anti-digoxin 26-10 (sFv')$_2$ and anti-c-erbB-2 741F8 (sFv')$_2$ made by protein folding and bonded through C-terminal cysteinyl peptides. *Protein Eng.* **8,** 301–314.

103. Kipriyanov, S. M., Dübel, S., Breitling, F., Kontermann, R. E., Heymann, S., and Little, M. (1995) Bacterial expression and refolding of single-chain Fv fragments with C-terminal cysteines. *Cell Biophys.* **26,** 187–204.

104. Holliger, P., Prospero, T., and Winter, G. (1993) "Diabodies": small bivalent and bispecific antibody fragments. *Proc. Natl. Acad. Sci. USA* **90,** 6444–6448.

105. Adams, G. P., Schier, R., McCall, A. M., Crawford, R. S., Wolf, E. J., Weiner, L. M., and Marks, J. D. (1998) Prolonged in vivo tumour retention of a human diabody targeting the extracellular domain of human HER2/neu. *Br. J. Cancer* **77,** 1405–1412.

106. Kortt, A. A., Lah, M., Oddie, G. W., Gruen, C. L., Burns, J. E., Pearce, L. A., et al. (1997) Single-chain Fv fragments of anti-neuraminidase antibody NC10 containing five- and ten-residue linkers form dimers and with zero-residue linker a trimer. *Protein Eng.* **10,** 423–433.

107. Le Gall, F., Kipriyanov, S. M., Moldenhauer, G., and Little, M. (1999) Di-, tri- and tetrameric single chain Fv antibody fragments against human CD19: effect of valency on cell binding. *FEBS Lett.* **453,** 164–168.

108. Pack, P. and Pluckthun, A. (1992) Miniantibodies: use of amphipathic helices to produce functional, flexibly linked dimeric Fv fragments with high avidity in *Escherichia coli. Biochemistry* **31,** 1579–1584.

109. Hu, S., Shively, L., Raubitschek, A., Sherman, M., Williams, L. E., Wong, J. Y., et al. (1996) Minibody: a novel engineered anti-carcinoembryonic antigen antibody fragment (single-chain Fv-CH3) which exhibits rapid, high-level targeting of xenografts. *Cancer Res.* **56,** 3055–3061.

110. Kipriyanov, S. M., Breitling, F., Little, M., and Dübel, S. (1995) Single-chain antibody streptavidin fusions: tetrameric bifunctional scFv-complexes with biotin binding activity and enhanced affinity to antigen. *Hum. Antibodies Hybridomas* **6,** 93–101.

111. Kipriyanov, S. M., Little, M., Kropshofer, H., Breitling, F., Gotter, S., and Dübel, S. (1996) Affinity enhancement of a recombinant antibody: formation of complexes with multiple valency by a single-chain Fv fragment-core streptavidin fusion. *Protein Eng.* **9,** 203–211.

112. van Spriel, A. B., van Ojik, H. H., and van De Winkel, J. G. (2000) Immunotherapeutic perspective for bispecific antibodies. *Immunol. Today* **21,** 391–397.

113. Milstein, C. and Cuello, A. C. (1983) Hybrid hybridomas and their use in immunohistochemistry. *Nature* **305,** 537–540.

114. Carter, P., Ridgway, J., and Zhu, Z. (1995) Toward the production of bispecific antibody fragments for clinical applications. *J. Hematother.* **4,** 463–470.

115. Dall'Acqua, W. and Carter, P. (1998) Antibody engineering. *Curr. Opin. Struct. Biol.* **8,** 443–450.

116. Merchant, A. M., Zhu, Z., Yuan, J. Q., Goddard, A., Adams, C. W., Presta, L. G., and Carter, P. (1998) An efficient route to human bispecific IgG. *Nat. Biotechnol.* **16,** 677–681.

117. Shalaby, M. R., Shepard, H. M., Presta, L., Rodrigues, M. L., Beverley, P. C., Feldmann, M., and Carter, P. (1992) Development of humanized bispecific antibodies reactive with cytotoxic lymphocytes and tumor cells overexpressing the HER2 protooncogene. *J. Exp. Med.* **175,** 217–225.

118. Kostelny, S. A., Cole, M. S., and Tso, J. Y. (1992) Formation of a bispecific antibody by the use of leucine zippers. *J. Immunol.* **148,** 1547–1553.

119. de Kruif, J. and Logtenberg, T. (1996) Leucine zipper dimerized bivalent and bispecific scFv antibodies from a semi-synthetic antibody phage display library. *J. Biol. Chem.* **271,** 7630–7634.

120. Müller, K. M., Arndt, K. M., Strittmatter, W., and Plückthun, A. (1998) The first constant domain (C$_H$1 and C$_L$) of an antibody used as heterodimerization domain for bispecific miniantibodies. *FEBS Lett.* **422,** 259–264.

121. Zuo, Z., Jimenez, X., Witte, L., and Zhu, Z. (2000) An efficient route to the production of an IgG-like bispecific antibody. *Protein Eng.* **13,** 361–367.

122. Gruber, M., Schodin, B. A., Wilson, E. R., and Kranz, D. M. (1994) Efficient tumor cell lysis mediated by a bispecific single chain antibody expressed in *Escherichia coli.* *J. Immunol.* **152,** 5368–5374.

123. Kurucz, I., Titus, J. A., Jost, C. R., Jacobus, C. M., and Segal, D. M. (1995) Retargeting of CTL by an efficiently refolded bispecific single-chain Fv dimer produced in bacteria. *J. Immunol.* **154,** 4576–4582.

124. Holliger, P., Brissinck, J., Williams, R. L., Thielemans, K., and Winter, G. (1996) Specific killing of lymphoma cells by cytotoxic T-cells mediated by a bispecific diabody. *Protein Eng.* **9,** 299–305.

125. Kipriyanov, S. M., Moldenhauer, G., Strauss, G., and Little, M. (1998) Bispecific CD3 × CD19 diabody for T cell-mediated lysis of malignant human B cells. *Int. J. Cancer* **77,** 763–772.

126. Perisic, O., Webb, P. A., Holliger, P., Winter, G., and Williams, R. L. (1994) Crystal structure of a diabody, a bivalent antibody fragment. *Structure* **2,** 1217–1226.

127. Zhu, Z., Zapata, G., Shalaby, R., Snedecor, B., Chen, H., and Carter, P. (1996) High level secretion of a humanized bispecific diabody from *Escherichia coli. Biotechnology* **14,** 192–196.

128. Cochlovius, B., Kipriyanov, S. M., Stassar, M. J. J. G., Christ, O., Schuhmacher, J., Strauss, G., et al. (2000) Treatment of human B cell lymphoma xenografts with a CD3 × CD19 diabody and T cells. *J. Immunol.* **165,** 888–895.

129. Arndt, M. A., Krauss, J., Kipriyanov, S. M., Pfreundschuh, M., and Little, M. (1999) A bispecific diabody that mediates natural killer cell cytotoxicity against xenotransplanted human Hodgkin's tumors. *Blood* **94,** 2562–2568.

130. FitzGerald, K., Holliger, P., and Winter, G. (1997) Improved tumour targeting by disulphide stabilized diabodies expressed in *Pichia pastoris. Protein Eng.* **10,** 1221–1225.

131. Kontermann, R. E. and Müller, R. (1999) Intracellular and cell surface displayed single-chain diabodies. *J. Immunol. Methods* **226,** 179–188.

132. Coloma, M. J. and Morrison, S. L. (1997) Design and production of novel tetravalent bispecific antibodies. *Nature Biotechnol.* **15,** 159–163.

133. Alt, M., Müller, R., and Kontermann, R. E. (1999) Novel tetravalent and bispecific IgG-like antibody molecules combining single-chain diabodies with the immunoglobulin gamma1 Fc or CH3 region. *FEBS Lett* **454,** 90–94.

134. Müller, K. M., Arndt, K. M., and Plückthun, A. (1998) A dimeric bispecific miniantibody combines two specificities with avidity. *FEBS Lett.* **432,** 45–49.

135. Cochlovius, B., Kipriyanov, S. M., Stassar, M. J., Schuhmacher, J., Benner, A., Moldenhauer, G., and Little, M. (2000) Cure of Burkitt's lymphoma in severe combined immunodeficiency mice by T cells, tetravalent CD3 × CD19 tandem diabody, and CD28 costimulation. *Cancer Res.* **60,** 4336–4341.

136. Patten, P. A., Howard, R. J., and Stemmer, W. P. (1997) Applications of DNA shuffling to pharmaceuticals and vaccines. *Curr. Opin. Biotechnol.* **8,** 724–733.

137. Minshull, J. and Stemmer, W. P. (1999) Protein evolution by molecular breeding. *Curr. Opin. Chem. Biol.* **3,** 284–290.

138. Holt, L. J., Enever, C., de Wildt, R. M., and Tomlinson, I. M. (2000) The use of recombinant antibodies in proteomics. *Curr. Opin. Biotechnol.* **11,** 445–449.

2

Application of Recombinant Antibodies in Cancer Patients

Jürgen Krauss, Michaela Arndt, and Michael Pfreundschuh

1. Introduction

As a consequence of the invention of the hybridoma technology by Köhler and Milstein *(1)*, many monoclonal antibodies (MAbs) have been evaluated in clinical trials since the early 1980s. Clinical outcomes were generally poor *(2–5)*, with the notable exception of marked tumor responses, including long-term remissions of patients with malignant B-cell lymphoma who were treated with patient-specific antiidiotypic antibodies *(6–8)*. The main factors responsible for these initial shortcomings were related to the immunogenicity of the murine protein, to modulation of targeted antigens, and to the poor ability of these antibodies to sufficiently mediate antibody-dependent effector functions in humans.

The advent of recombinant antibody technology led to an enormous revival in the use of antibodies as therapeutic agents in cancer therapy. This review provides a brief historical sketch of the development of recombinant antibodies for immunotherapy of cancer, which is followed by the most significant clinical data, as exemplified by the two clinically most established recombinant antibodies to date. Finally, we will focus on future prospects for antibody-based therapeutic concepts in oncology.

2. The Development of Recombinant Antibodies for Cancer Therapy

2.1. Chimeric Antibodies

The first reports of the successful cloning of immunoglobulin gene segments were published in 1977 *(9,10)*, nearly one decade after the discovery of the existence of restriction endonucleases, which enable microorganisms to cleave foreign DNA in a highly specific manner *(11)*. It took another several years until the first recombinant antibodies were constructed as "chimeric" molecules by fusing the rearranged murine variable V(D)J gene segments of a mouse MAb to human constant domains *(12,13)* or were generated as a recombinant Fab fusion protein by replacing the Fc fragment with

From: *Methods in Molecular Biology, vol. 207: Recombinant Antibodies for Cancer Therapy: Methods and Protocols*
Edited by: M. Welschof and J. Krauss © Humana Press Inc., Totowa, NJ

an enzyme moiety *(14)*. Chimerized antibodies retained the specificity of the mono-clonal ancestor and proved to be immunogenic in only a very small subset of patients when administered in clinical trials *(15–19)*. Half lives of chimeric antibodies in human serum were shown to be significantly longer compared to the respective paren-tal murine MAbs *(15,16,18,20,21)* and even increased after repetitive administrations *(18,20,21)*. Moreover, chimeric antibodies were capable of mediating antibody-dependent cellular cytotoxicity (ADCC) with human effector cells and/or to activate the complement cascade very efficiently, both in vitro *(22–25)* and in vivo *(26,27)*.

2.2. Humanized Antibodies

In order to further decrease the immunogenicity of murine antibodies, the first monoclonal antibody was "humanized" in 1986 by grafting the gene segments coding for the antigen binding loops onto human framework regions. Although the expressed antibody retained its full specificity, a substantial decrease of affinity was observed *(28)*. Subsequent cristallographic X-ray diffractions of many antibody variable region binding domains and computer modeling studies based on these crystal structures, allowed, with exception of loop H3, the identification of a small number of "key resi-dues" located either in the loops itself or in the framework regions. These residues determine the main chain conformation ("canonical structure") of the antigen binding loops *(29,30)*. Based on these fundamental insights into antibody structure, antibodies were successfully modified by retaining murine residues within the acceptor frame-work regions *(31–33)* or by secondary directed mutagenesis to restore observed decreases in affinity after humanization *(34,35)*. More recently, antibodies were humanized by "resurfacing" the variable domains. In this case, only accessible resi-dues are of human origin whereas buried, structure-maintaining backbone residues remain murine *(36)*.

Many chimeric and humanized antibodies have been employed in clinical trials (reviewed in **ref.** *37*) and, as a result of these studies, two cancer-specific reagents have been approved by the American Food and Drug Administration (FDA) for the treatment of non-Hodgkin's lymphoma and metastatic breast cancer, respectively.

In order to extend effector functions, chimeric or humanized antibodies were con-jugated to radionuclides and drugs and successfully employed in Phase I/II clinical trials *(38–43)*. As a consequence, the first humanized antibody-drug conjugate (Gemtuzumab Ozogamicin = Myelotarg™) was recently FDA-approved as an orphan drug for the treatment of acute myeloid leukemia of patients 60 yr or older and who are not considered candidates for cytotoxic chemotherapy *(44)*.

To retarget effector cells of the immune system, bispecific chimeric or humanized antibody molecules have been developed to activate cytotoxic T cells *(45–48)* or myeloid effector cells *(49)*. The latter construct has been administered in clinical Phase I trials to patients with a variety of solid tumors *(50–52)*.

2.3. Recombinant Antibody Fragments

The successful expression of functional antigen-binding domains in *E. coli (53,54)* provided the basis for the rapid development of a new generation of antibody based molecules with potentially great therapeutic impact. Noncovalently linked V_H and V_L domains tend to dissociate from each other, particularly at low protein concentrations *(55)*. In order to stabilize the assoziation of the two domains, a synthetic linker peptide has been introduced connecting both variable domains *(56)*. These "single-chain" molecules were shown to retain their full binding specificity and affinity *(57)*. To further enhance the stability of these fragments, intermolecular disulfide bonds were generated by introducing cystein residues in the V_H and V_L framework regions, respectively, and were shown to increase the stability markedly while retaining the full antigen binding properties *(55,58,59)*. ScFv fragments were engineered as fusion molecules to employ artificial effector functions, since they are unable to mediate natural effector functions owing to the lack of the Fc portion of whole antibodies. This was accomplished by linking them to toxins *(60–64)* cytotoxic ribonucleases *(65–67)*, enzymes for activation of prodrugs *(68–72)*, radionuclides (reviewed in **ref.** *73*), cytokines *(74,75)*, or chemokines *(76)*. Recombinant antibody fragments have been generated as bispecific molecules by various techniques *(77–81)* to retarget human cytotoxic T cells *(77,80,82–85)* or natural killer cells *(86)*. Several methods were employed to increase the avidity of bispecific antibody fragments by constructing them as tetravalent bispecific molecules *(87–89)*.

One approach for combining antibody targeting and activation of cellular effector cells is the construction of chimeric receptor molecules ("T-Body"), consisting of a tumor specific single chain antibody and a signal domain for activation of a cytotoxic effector cell. Engrafting of the constructs into cytotoxic T cells results in the MHC independent destruction of scFv-targeted tumor cells *(90–94)*.

From these third generation antibodies, recombinant immunotoxins are now beginning to enter clinical trials and initial data confirm them as very potent *(95,96)*.

2.4. Phage Display-Derived Antibodies

Parallel to the rapid development of engineering the described variants of functional hybridoma derived MAbs, new methods were developed to eventually bypass hybridoma technology. In 1985 was shown that peptides could be expressed on the surface of filamentous bacteriophage. The gene fragments encoding the foreign DNA were inserted into the filamentous phage gene III in order to encode a fusion protein displayed on the surface of the phage without disrupting its capability of infection upon binding of pIII to the F pilus of the bacteria. These phages could be enriched more than 1000-fold after a single round of selection through binding of the displayed peptide to a MAb *(97)*. In 1990 McCafferty and colleagues successfully expressed the variable domains of an antibody on the surface of filamentous phage. The phage-derived antibody retained its full binding and specificity to its antigen *(98)*. Antibody variable gene segments of different subgroups could be amplified by the polymerase chain reaction (PCR) *(99)*, using either degenerated primers *(100,101)*, a set of family-specific oligonucleotides *(102)*, or primers based on the amino acid sequences of immunoglobulin variable domains *(103)*. This allowed the construction of antibody libraries by cloning the PCR-amplified V_H and V_L repertoire of B lymphocytes into suitable phagemid vectors *(104–106)* for expression and screening of randomly associated variable domain fragments on the phage surface. Binding phage antibodies were isolated from a large number of nonbinders by enrichment of the particles through multiple rounds of in vitro-panning against the antigen of choice and extensive washing steps to remove nonbinders. Phage antibody technology has since become the most powerful tool for isolating highly specific antibodies with high affinities to predefined antigens. Antibody libraries have been constructed from patients *(107–109)*, immunized mice *(110–112)*, as naive libraries from (multiple) healthy donors *(113–116)*, and as (semi)synthetic libraries by randomizing sequences in one or more hypervariable regions *(117–123)*. Antibody repertoires were recently also displayed on ribosomes *(124,125)*, allowing for the generation of very large libraries to be screened within a short period of time.

The natural antibody repertoire of camels and other camelid species contains a large number of functional antibodies devoid of a light chain *(126)*. A phage display library from the V_H repertoire of an immunized camel has been constructed *(127)* and single V_H domain antibodies with subnanomolar affinities were isolated *(128)*.

Functional single V_H domains with high affinities have recently also been isolated from a human V_H repertoire phage display library *(129)*.

Phage display-derived antibody fragments have begun to be introduced in clinical trials as radioimaging reagents in cancer patients *(130,131)*.

2.5. Recombinant Antibodies from Transgenic Mice

Many attempts to generate human antibodies by employing the hybridoma technology have been unsuccessful, mainly from the lack of a suitable human myeloma cell line to immortilize B cells (reviewed in **ref.** *132*). Alternately, human antibodies were produced in transgenic mice by replacing the murine immunoglobulin loci of the host genome with the respective human counterpart *(133–137)*. Hyperimmunization of the transgenic animals with (tumor) antigens of choice results in the clonal activation of B lymphocytes producing human antibodies. Upon rechallenge of the mice with the antigen of interest, affinity maturated antibodies can be generated in vivo. Immortalization of B cells expressing these antibodies can be achieved by standard hybridoma technology, resulting in the production of entirely human antibodies from established cell lines.

3. Clinical Data

It took more than 10 years from the initial development of the first generation of recombinant antibodies to become an integrated part of treatment concepts in oncology today.

3.1. Rituximab (Rituxan™, Mabthera™)

The chimeric antibody Rituximab (Rituxan™, Mabthera™) binds to the transmembrane antigen CD20, which is strongly overexpressed in most B cell lymphomas *(138)*. In two independent Phase II clinical multicenter studies, Rituximab has been administered to more than 200 patients with refractory or relapsed low grade B-cell non-Hodgkin's lymphoma (B-NHL) in four weekly doses of 375 mg/m². Overall response rates in 185 evaluable patients were around 50% with complete remissions of 9% and 6%, respectively, by a medium time to progression of 10.2 and 13 mo, respectively *(18,139)*. A favorable tumor response was associated with a histology of follicular NHL, sustained high serum levels of antibody after the first infusion, and a longer remission after prior chemotherapy *(18)*. Treatment-related side effects, mostly observed in the first course of treatment, were low and reversible, and in most cases consisted of fever, chills and headache. These side effects were usually reversible by merely lowering the infusion rate. Only two patients developed an antibody response against the chimeric antibody. Most patients exhibited increasing serum concentrations of the chimeric antibody throughout the treatment courses, associated with progressively longer half lives from 76.3 h to 205.8 h after the fourth infusion *(21)*. The impressive results of these clinical trials led to the FDA approval of Rituximab in 1997 as the first recombinant antibody for tumor therapy.

Rituximab proved its potency also on patients with intermediate and high grade B-NHL. In a Phase II study of 54 patients with relapsing intermediate- and high-grade lymphomas single-agent therapy with Rituximab achieved 5 complete and 12 partial responses. Patients with diffuse large B-cell lymphoma achieved a favorable response rate of 37%, and the median time to progression exceeded 246 d for the responding patients *(140)*. These results formed the basis of a randomized trial in elderly patients (60–80 yr of age) with diffuse large B-cell lymphoma, which compared 8 cycles of a three-weekly CHOP regimen with the same chemotherapy plus Rituximab 375 mg/m^2 given on day one of each CHOP cycle. The combination of CHOP and Rituximab reduced the rate of primary progressions by 17%. After a median time of observation of only 12 mo in 328 evaluable patients, event-free and overall-survival achieved with CHOP + Rituximab was significantly better than that after chemotherapy only *(141)*. Patients of the low and low-intermediate risk group according to the international prognostic index (IPI) profited more from Rituximab than patients in the high and high-intermediate risk group *(142)*. Ongoing trials will have to show whether these results can be confirmed in younger patients of the different risk groups. In a recently conducted Phase II clinical trial, similar encouraging results for the combination of Rituximab with standard CHOP chemotherapy in 33 previously untreated patients with high grade B-NHL were achieved. In this study 6 cycles CHOP at 3-wk intervals plus Rituximab 2 d prior to each chemotherapy course were administered. The overall response rate was 94% including 61% complete remissions and the median duration of response and time to progression had not been reached after a median observation time of 26 mo. 29 of 31 responding patients remained in remission during this follow-up period. No additional toxicity has been observed compared to patients when treated with CHOP alone *(143)*.

Good response rates with long lasting remissions were recently also reported for patients with indolent low-grade B-NHL being treated with Rituximab/CHOP in combination *(144)*. In contrast to chemotherapy alone, combined immunochemotherapy induced molecular remissions in some patients with follicular lymphoma. In those patients, the initial detection of bcl-2 translocation transcripts by PCR in bone marrow cells changed to bcl-2 negativity after treatment *(144)*. Favorable response rates observed in patients with less advanced stages of the disease suggested a most promising role of Rituximab in eradicating minimal residue disease in patients with low tumor burden. To prove this hypothesis, 49 patients with follicular B-NHL and low tumor burden were treated with 4 weekly infusions of Rituximab (375 mg/m^2) as a single-agent first-line therapy. The response rate was 73% including 20% complete remissions in 49 evaluable patients 1 mo after treatment. Molecular remissions in the bone marrow were observed in 31% of the patients on d 50 and were positively correlated to progression-free survival *(145)*.

Current studies suggest other important roles for Rituximab in radioimmunotherapy *(38)* and for the in vivo purging of tumor cells from hematopoetic stem cells prior to high dose chemotherapy and subsequent autologous stem cell transplantation *(146)*.

3.2. Trastuzumab (Herceptin™)

Growth factor receptors play an important role in the regulation of epithelial cell growth. In epithelial cancers dysregulation of these receptors is a common feature in the pathogenesis. The protooncogene Her-2 encodes the 185 kDa transmembrane glycoprotein receptor p185^{Her-2} with intrinsic tyrosine kinase activity and is highly homologous to the epidermal growth factor receptor family (ECFR) *(147)*. This protein is expressed in a variety of solid tumors including breast, lung, prostate and gastric cancer. In breast cancer p185^{Her-2} is expressed in more than 25% of the cases and is associated with a poor prognosis *(148,149)*. 4D5 is a MAb binding to p185^{Her-2} and interferes with growth factor receptor-mediated growth stimulation. In preclinical trials the antibody has been capable of inhibiting tumor growth in vitro *(150)* and in a breast cancer xenograft mouse model *(151)*. 4D5 has been humanized in order to reduce its immunogenicity and to enhance the capability to mediate additional toxicity via natural effector functions *(152)*. This antibody, termed Trastuzumab (Herceptin™), was employed in a Phase II clinical trial as a single agent in 46 patients with p185^{Her-2} overexpressing metastatic breast cancer. Most of the patients had been heavily pretreated and the reagent was administered with a loading dose of 250 mg, followed by 10 weekly doses of 100 mg. Patients without disease progression received a weekly maintenance dose of the antibody of 100 mg. The overall response rate was 11,6% in 43 evaluable patients including one complete remission and four partial responses. Toxicity consisted mainly of fever and chills, but no severe side effects were observed. No antibodies directed against the humanized antibody could be detected *(153)*. In a multinational Phase II clinical trial, 222 extensively pretreated patients with advanced p185^{Her-2} expressing metastatic breast cancer were enrolled. Patients received a loading dose of 4 mg/kg, followed by weekly infusions of 2 mg/kg antibody. In this study a 15% overall response rate with 8 complete and 26 partial remissions was observed in 213 evaluable patients. The median duration of response was 9.1 mo and the median duration of survival was 13 mo. Although higher response rates up to 49% have been reported for second line therapy with docetaxel in anthracycline resistant patients *(154)*, the median duration of survival (10 mo) was actually shorter compared to patients treated with Trastuzumab (13 mo). Patients with high expression of p185^{Her-2} and patients who relapsed more than 6 mo after prior chemotherapy showed higher response rates and a longer time to disease progression. The mean half life of the antibody was 6,2 d. Significant side effects were reported by 41% of the patients, consisting of pain, asthenia, fever, chills, nausea, and vomiting as the most frequent events. These side effects were reversible and occurred almost exclusively in the first cycle of treatment. In addition, the study reported serious cardiac dysfunction in a total of almost 5% of the patients, manifesting as congestive heart failure, cardiomyopathy and/or decrease in cardiac ejection fraction by more than 10%. Nine out of ten of these patients had previously received chemotherapies containing anthracyclines, and had one or more risk factors for anthracycline induced cardiomyopathy, such as cumulative doxorubicin dose of more than 400 mg/m^2, previous radiotherapy to the left chest, age over 70 yr or history of hypertension. This study also included a quality-of-life assessment, surveying the variables physical function, role function, social function, global quality-of-life and fatigue. Patients who responded to therapy reported improvements in all of the evaluated parameters *(155)*. Based on these results Trastuzumab was approved by the American FDA for treating patients with p185^{Her-2} overexpressing metastatic breast cancer in relapse.

Preclinical data suggested synergistic effects of Herceptin in combination with various chemotherapeutic agents in tumor xenografted athymic mice *(156,157)*. In a Phase III multinational clinical trial Trastuzumab has been administered to 464 previously untreated patients with metastatic p185^{Her-2} positive breast cancer either as a single agent or in combination with either doxorubicin plus cyclophosphamide or paclitaxel. The combination therapy significantly increased the overall reponse rates from 32% to 50% and prolonged the median time to progression from 6.1 (doxorubicin plus cyclophosphamide alone) to 7.8 mo (doxorubicin plus cyclophosphamide plus trastuzumab) and from 3.0 (paclitaxel alone) to 6.9 mo (paclitaxel plus trastuzumab), respectively. The relative risk of death could be reduced by 20% at a median follow-up of 30 mo. No patient developed antibodies against Trastuzumab. Adverse side effects were generally mild to moderate in severity and occurred more frequently in the combination therapy groups. The most severe side effect consisted of WHO grade 3–4 cardiac toxicity, most pronounced in the Trastuzumab/doxorubicin/cyclophosphamide therapy group (27%) and less common and severe in patients treated with doxorubicin/cyclophospamide without Trastuzumab (8%) or in the combination therapy group with Trastuzumab/paclitaxel (13%) or paclitaxel alone (1%) *(158)*. These data clearly provide evidence for synergistic toxicity of Trastuzumab in combination with cytostatic drugs by yet unknown mechanisms.

The role of Herceptin in an adjuvant setting is currently under investigation in a Phase III clinical trial *(159)*.

4. Future Prospects

4.1. HAMA Response

One of the major limitations in using monoclonal antibodies as therapeutic agents for treating cancer has been the immnunogenicity of murine antibodies. The development of human anti-mouse antibodies (HAMA) in patients treated with these reagents generally precluded repeated administrations due to allergic reactions and rapid elimination of the murine protein. Chimeric, humanized, and fully human recombinant antibodies or antibody fragment derivatives thereof were shown to reduce immunogenicity dramatically. However, the issue of immunogenicity is not understood in detail. It still remains unclear why the development of a HAMA response is not occurring in all patients treated with monoclonal murine antibodies. Moreover, the HAMA response is strongly variable for different MAbs and not always associated with an unfavorable clinical outcome *(6,8,160,161,162,163)*. According to Jerne's network hypothesis *(164)* the HAMA response has been proposed as being potentially beneficial for patients due to the generation of anti-idiotypic antibodies, eliciting a humoral and/or cellular immune response to the tumor in the recipients *(160)*. In a number of clinical trials involving small groups of patients, clinically favorable outcomes were attributed to vaccination effects generated by the HAMA response *(165–169)*. However, in a recent large randomized, multicenter clinical Phase III study involving colorectal carcinoma patients treated with the monoclonal 17-1A in an adjuvant setting, neither a positive or negative correlation between the development of a HAMA response and the clinical outcome could be observed *(163)*. Moreover, in large clinical trials with chimeric and humanized antibodies in cancer patients the development of antiidiotypic antibodies in treated patients was only rarely observed *(18,140,143,144,155,158)*, although the generation of anti-idiotypic antibodies should be focused to the murine residues of the antigen-binding domains.

4.2. Selection of Target Antigens

The ultimate goal in cancer therapy is the complete destruction of the tumor while sparing healthy tissue. These issues, efficiency and selectivity, have been extensively addressed in antibody-based therapeutic approaches ever since the first patient was treated with a MAb in 1979 *(170)*. Various factors have since been identified as influential to the success of immunotherapy with monoclonal and recombinant antibodies.

The selection of an appropriate target antigen is one of the most essential prerequisites in the employment of antibodies as therapeutic agents. The target antigen should be expressed on the malignant cells selectively, consistently, and with high density. A variety of cell surface antigens have been used as targets for therapeutic antibodies. Early clinical studies reported antigen modulations after antibody administration, thereby vacating therapy *(2,171,172)*. With the exception of patient-specific anti-idiotypic antibodies directed against clonally expressed immunoglobulin on lymphoma cells, target antigens are generally not tumor-specific but also expressed on subsets of normal cells. The overexpression of cell-surface antigens, physiologically involved in cell-growth regulation, represents a complex role of these molecules in the tumor pathogenesis and the underlying molecular mechanisms are often only poorly understood. Thus the effects antibodies trigger upon binding to these receptors is hardly predictable. Only recently has it become possible to identify truly tumor specific antigens through either the SEREX technology *(173)* or by methods of antibody phage display technology *(174–176)*. These antigens represent a novel class of most promising targets for antibody-based therapeutics.

4.3. "Classical" Effector Functions Mediated by Recombinant Antibodies

Murine MAbs of IgG2a isotype are capable to activate human complement and/or mediate antibody-dependent cytotoxicity (ADCC) *(177–182)*. This capability, however, is often quite limited and additionally hampered by the HAMA response leading to rapid neutralization and degradation of the murine protein. In contrast, recombinant antibodies mediate these "classical" effector functions much more effectively than the murine counterpart *(22,183,184)*. Based on the impressive clinical results observed in patients who were treated with Rituximab and Trastuzumab, the underlying mechanisms of "classical" and antibody-specific effector functions have been examined more in detail.

For Rituximab it has been shown that high coexpression of the cell surface complement inhibitors CD55 and CD59 on the malignant cell could abolish complement dependent cytotoxicity in vitro almost completely. Blocking of these molecules with MAbs resulted in restoration of complement-mediated cytotoxicity *(25)*.

The efficiacy of ADCC in vivo is largely dependent on the interaction of activating FcγRIII and inhibiting FcγRIIb receptors expressed on myeloid cells (reviewed in **refs. *185,186***). Mice deficient in the common γ chain (FcRγ$^{-/-}$), thus lacking the activating FcγRI/FcγRIII, and mice without the inhibiting FcγRIIb, were each mated with athymic nude mice for use in CD20$^+$ or p185^{Her-2} expressing human xenograft tumor models. In FcRγ$^{+/+}$ mice, the tumor mass of established p185^{Her-2} expressing carcinomas could be reduced by 96% and 90%, respectively, when treated with Trastuzumab or its murine ancestor 4D5. Similarly, tumor size of xenotransplanted CD20+ lymphomas in FcRγ$^{+/+}$ mice could be reduced by >99% by treatment with Rituximab. These effects could be enhanced in both tumor models in FcRγIIB$^{-/-}$ deficient xenotransplanted mice. In contrast, FcRγ$^{-/-}$ mice developed palpable tumors in both tumor models in almost all cases. To further investigate the role of Fc receptors, 4D5 was systematically mutated to disrupt Fc binding of the antibodies to its receptors. The resulting mutant retained the wild type characteristics of its half live in vivo, antigen binding properties, and p185^{Her-2} receptor blockade. However, all mice treated with the mutant antibody developed palpable tumors *(27)*. These results clearly demonstrate the crucial role of Fcγ receptor interactions with Fc fragments for the in vivo efficacy of recombinant antibodies.

4.4. Antibody-Specific Effector Functions

Besides the importance of successful recruitment of "classical"effector functions, some antibodies were shown to be capable of mediating tumor cell killing by interfering with cell-signaling pathways. Binding of natural ligands to cell-surface receptors can mediate signal transduction events by activation of protein kinases and phosphatases leading to the release of a second messenger and the subsequent transcription of genes involved in cell growth regulation and apoptosis. Ligation of cell-surface receptors with MAbs could mimic the natural ligand of these cell-surface receptors, thereby triggering signal-transduction events (reviewed in **ref. *187***). It has recently been reported that CD20 ligation with Rituximab activates the protein tyrosine kinases

(PTK) Lyn and Lck leading to downstream activation of PTK substrates, such as phospholipase C. Activation of these substrates increases intracellular calcium levels, which in turn might activate the caspase cascade directly or provide further downstream signals leading to subsequent apoptosis *(188,189)*. Enhancement of apoptosis could be achieved by crosslinking Rituximab with either secondary antibodies or Fc receptor-bearing cells *(188)*. Furthermore, hypercrosslinking of antigens with MAb homodimers could mediate tumor cell G_0/G_1 arrest or apoptosis very efficiently by not yet well-defined mechanisms *(190)*.

CD40, a member of the tumor necrosis factor receptor family, is essential for activating antigen presenting cells (APC) *(191,192)*. Ligation of CD40 with MAbs was recently shown to be capable of "priming" cytotoxic CD8[+] T cells independent of T-helper cells, leading to complete eradication of CD40[+] lymphomas in a syngeneic mouse model. Moreover, treated mice were protected upon rechallenge with tumor cells, suggesting a role of anti-CD40 antibodies as a vaccine. The authors suggest a mechanism by which crosslinking of CD40 with the antibody may stimulate neoplastic B cells to become effective APC and present processed tumor antigens to autologous cytotoxic T cells *(193)*.

Recent studies in some cases elucidated the molecular basis of clinically observed synergistic effects of MAbs conjugated to drugs or radionuclides. Treatment of p185[Her-2] expressing tumor cells with cisplatin followed by Trastuzumab blocked the removal of cisplatin-induced adducts by upregulation of p21/WAF1, an important mediator of DNA repair. This effect was most pronounced when cells were incubated with Herceptin in close temporal proximity to the treatment with cisplatin *(157)*. More recently, Trastuzumab was shown also to enhance radiosensitivity of p185[Her-2] expressing cells in a time-dependent manner, possibly due to p21WAF1 dysregulation *(194)*. These results suggest an interaction between signaling events triggered by the antibody and DNA repair pathways, thus underlining the importance of elucidating molecular mechanisms of drug interactions as crucial for optimizing administration schedules in chemo- and radioimmunotherapy regimens.

4.5. Biodistribution and Pharmacokinetics

The efficiacy of tumor targeting by antibody-based molecules in vivo is not only dependent on the targeted tumor antigen but also on the tumor characteristics, e.g., tumor type (hematological malignancies or solid tumors); tumor mass; accessibility and density of the target antigen; and on characteristics of the antibody molecule itself, e.g., size, charge, affinity, and avidity *(195–197)*.

Pharmacokinetics describes the temporal sequence of the distribution and metabolism of a molecule in the body. Molecules with low molecular weights undergo ultrafiltration from the plasma in the glomerulum of the kidney. The passage of molecules across the glomerular filtration barrier decreases progressively with increasing molecular size. In addition to the permeability of the glomerular filter the molecular charge of a molecule affects its clearance. Negatively charged molecules are retarded by repulsion from the negatively charged endothelium and glomerular basement membranes of the kidney *(198,199)*.

Intact chimeric and humanized IgG molecules (150 kDa) persist in the circulation for several days *(21,155)* and half lives are even prolonged after repetetive administrations *(18,20,21)*. The rapid clearance of murine antibodies can largely be attributed to the HAMA response which leads to rapid degradation of the immune complexes. Sequences in the CH2 and CH3 regions of IgG have been shown to regulate the rate of clearance through their interaction with the neonatal Fc receptor (FcRn) *(200)*, thus playing a most important role in "recycling" antibodies from the bloodstream *(201–203)*. However, catabolism of antibodies is not exclusively regulated by FcRn as shown for chimeric antibodies by constant domain shuffling *(204)*.

Antibody fragments lacking a constant domain such as scFv (27 kDa), (scFv')2 (55 kDa), Fab' (55 kDa) and diabodies (50 kDa) are cleared from the circulation more rapidly *(89,205–207)*. However, compared to whole IgGs, small antibody fragments have a more favorable tumor penetration capacity. The comparison of tumor penetration properties of a radiolabeled single-chain Fv with larger immunglobulin forms (IgG, F(ab')$_2$ and Fab'), derived from a MAb directed against the human pancarcinoma antigen TAG-72, showed a rapid and uniform tumor penetration for the scFv in human colon carcinoma xenografts in mice *(208)*. In contrast, a relatively restricted penetration pattern was observed for the F(ab')$_2$ (100 kDa) and the Fab' (55 kDa) fragments, respectively. Intact IgG molecules barely exceeded the perivascular regions of the tumor even at 24 h after administration *(208–210)* and intratumoral diffusion distances of IgGs in solid tumor tissue of only about 1 mm in 2 d were reported *(211)*. In contrast, small antibody molecules were retained at relatively low levels but with much higher specificity at the tumor site *(205,207,212,213)*. To address the short half lives of antibody fragments, they were chemically modified by conjugation to monomethoxy-polyethylene glycol (PEG) *(214–216)*. In the latter approach two PEG molecules were site-specifically attached to two hinge cysteine residues of an engineered Fab fragment. This resulted in a dramatic increase in the overall half life in rats and monkeys. Given the fact that PEG is of low immunogenicity *(217)*, this substance provides a valuable reagent in order to overcome the disadvantage of short half lives of antibody fragments when administered to humans.

Affinity describes the interaction of an antibody with its antigen, and plays an important role in the humoral immune response and affinity maturation. High-affinity antibodies can be generated by phage-display technology, and natural affinity maturation can be mimicked by various techniques of recombinant antibody technology such as chain shuffling *(218)* or site-directed mutagenesis *(219,220)*. The affinity of a phage display-derived scFv C6.5 with moderate affinity (1.6×10^{-8} *M*) against the p185[Her-2] antigen *(221)* could be enhanced sixfold (2.5×10^{-9} *M*) by light-chain shuffling, an affinity comparable to that of the hybridoma derived antibody against the same antigen *(222)*. By sequential site-directed mutagenisis of the CDR3 region of the heavy (VH) and light chain (VL) of the same scFv, different affinity mutants were generated with up to 1230-fold higher affinities (1.3×10^{-11} *M*) compared to the wild-type scFv C6.5 *(220)*. The in vivo performance of the anti-p185[Her-2]-scFv mutants in tumor bearing mice supported the concept that higher affinity scFvs could enrich in solid tumors much better than mutants with lower affinity *(197,223)*. Contrary to the theory that high affinity antibodies are preferable for successful tumor targeting in vivo there is evidence of an existing physical penetration barrier for antibody-based molecules with extremely high affinities. The term "binding site barrier" effect was first postulated by Weinstein and colleagues *(224)* describing the theory that a strong binding of high-affinity antibodies confined mainly to the periphery of the tumor, might thereby prevent a deeper tumor penetration. In the meantime this theory could be experimentally validated for antibody fragments with extremely high affinities (10^{-11} *M*) *(225)*, thus questioning their values as favorable therapeutics when rapid and uniform tumor penetration is required.

Naturally occurring antibodies differ from recombinant antibody fragments in their valency of antigen binding. The multi-valency of natural antibodies contributes to an increased functional affinity from simultaneous binding to the targeted antigen epitopes, the avidity effect *(226)*. As a consequence, multivalency has a significant influence on the dissociation kinetics, which is of particular importance under nonequilibrium conditions of antibody–antigen interactions. Multivalent recombinant antibody fragments with increased avidity were shown to enhance tumor targeting much more efficient compared to monovalent counterparts *(73,207,213,227–229)*, thus providing a promising role for these constructs as novel therapeutic agents with improved biodistribution characteristics and pharmacokinetics.

5. Concluding Remarks

In conclusion, recombinant antibody technology has provided the basis for the success of immunotherapeutic reagents in oncology today. These constructs have overcome some of the major limitations previously associated with murine MAbs when administered to cancer patients. In particular, first and second generation of these reagents now employed in larger clinical trials were shown to be immunogenic in only very rare cases. In addition, "classical" effector functions were shown to be mediated much more efficiently than by murine equivalents. A number of antibodies are able to kill tumor cells not only by "classical" effector functions but also by specific interference with cell signaling. This effect can often be enhanced by multimerization of the antigen-binding domains. It remains a task of critical importance to elucidate the molecular mechanisms of how tumor associated antigens are involved in cell-growth regulation, and the effects antibodies mediate after binding to these antigens in order to utilize this knowledge for the deductive design of therapeutic antibodies.

Clinical studies employing recombinant antibodies in cancer patients generally reported very low toxicities. However, these reagents could ocassionally mediate unexpected toxicities for yet unknown reasons. These side effects need to be monitored very carefully and possible molecular mechanisms need to be investigated.

Great progress has been made in identifying novel, truly tumor specific antigens. Isolating human antibody fragments from antibody phage display libraries by panning on novel tumor specific antigens will play a key role in the development of a new generation of highly promising reagents for cancer therapy.

It is only now that the third generation of antibodies and antibody fragments enters clinical trials. Based on preclinical data, antibody fragments can be expected to have an improved capability of penetrating solid tumors. On the other hand they do have very short half lives, which appears to be associated with a rapid first-pass clearance due to their smaller sizes. Engineering of these molecules to determine the optimized ratio between tumor retention and metabolism promises to provide the basis for improved antibody based reagents within the next few years.

In our opinion, the most promising role for antibody based therapeutics in oncology in the future will be the employment of combinations of (multivalent) molecules that target different epitopes, thus mediating different immunological effector functions and/or interfering with different growth mechanisms of the malignant cells.

References

1. Köhler, G. and Milstein, C. (1975) Continuous culture of fused cells secreting antibody of predefined specifity. *Nature* **256,** 495–497.
2. Ritz, J., Pesando, J. M., Sallan, S. E., Clavell, L. A., Notis-McConarty, J., Rosenthal, P., and Schlossman, S. F. (1981) Serotherapy of acute lymphoblastic leukemia with monoclonal antibody. *Blood* **58,** 141–152.
3. Miller, R. A., Oseroff, A. R., Stratte, P. T., and Levy, R. (1983) Monoclonal antibody therapeutic trials in seven patients with T-cell lymphoma. *Blood* **62,** 988–995.
4. Dillman, R. O., Shawler, D. L., Dillman, J. B., and Royston, I. (1984) Therapy of chronic lymphocytic leukemia and cutaneous T-cell lymphoma with T101 monoclonal antibody. *J. Clin. Oncol.* **2,** 881–891.
5. Foon, K. A., Schroff, R. W., Bunn, P. A., Mayer, D., Abrams, P. G., Fer, M., et al. (1984) Effects of monoclonal antibody therapy in patients with chronic lymphocytic leukemia. *Blood* **64,** 1085–1093.
6. Meeker, T. C., Lowder, J., Maloney, D. G., Miller, R. A., Thielemans, K., Warnke, R., and Levy, R. (1985) A clinical trial of anti-idiotype therapy for B cell malignancy. *Blood* **65,** 1349–1363.
7. Brown, S. L., Miller, R. A., Horning, S. J., Czerwinski, D., Hart, S. M., McElderry, R., et al. (1989) Treatment of B-cell lymphomas with anti-idiotype antibodies alone and in combination with alpha interferon. *Blood* **73,** 651–661.
8. Davis, T. A., Maloney, D. G., Czerwinski, D. K., Liles, T. M., and Levy, R. (1998) Anti-idiotype antibodies can induce long-term complete remissions in non-Hodgkin's lymphoma without eradicating the malignant clone. *Blood* **92,** 1184–1190.
9. Brack, C. and Tonegawa, S. (1977) Variable and constant parts of the immunoglobulin light chain gene of a mouse myeloma cell are 1250 nontranslated bases apart. *Proc. Natl. Acad. Sci. USA* **74,** 5652–5656.
10. Tonegawa, S., Brack, C., Hozumi, N., and Schuller, R. (1977) Cloning of an immunoglobulin variable region gene from mouse embryo. *Proc. Natl. Acad. Sci. USA* **74,** 3518–3522.
11. Meselson, M. and Yuan, R. (1968) DNA restriction enzyme from E. coli. *Nature* **217,** 1110–1114.
12. Boulianne, G. L., Hozumi, N., and Shulman, M. J. (1984) Production of functional chimaeric mouse/human antibody. *Nature* **312,** 643–646.
13. Morrison, S. L., Johnson, M. J., Herzenberg, L. A., and Oi, V. T. (1984) Chimeric human antibody molecules: mouse antigen-binding domains with human constant region domains. *Proc. Natl. Acad. Sci. USA* **81,** 6851–6855.
14. Neuberger, M. S., Williams, G. T., and Fox, R. O. (1984) Recombinant antibodies possessing novel effector functions. *Nature* **312,** 604–608.

15. LoBuglio, A. F., Wheeler, R. H., Trang, J., Haynes, A., Rogers, K., Harvey, E. B., et al. (1989) Mouse/human chimeric antibody in man: kinetics and immune response. *Proc. Natl. Acad. Sci. USA* **86**, 4220–4224.

16. Khazaeli, M. B., Saleh, M. N., Liu, T. P., Meredith, R. F., Wheeler, R. H., Baker, T. S., et al. (1991) Pharmacokinetics and immune response of 131I-chimeric mouse/human B72.3 (human gamma 4) monoclonal antibody in humans. *Cancer Res.* **51**, 5461–5466.

17. Maloney, D. G., Liles, T. M., Czerwinski, D. K., Waldichuk, C., Rosenberg, J., Grillo-Lopez, A., and Levy, R. (1994) Phase I clinical trial using escalating single-dose infusion of chimeric anti-CD20 monoclonal antibody (IDEC-C2B8) in patients with recurrent B-cell lymphoma. *Blood* **84**, 2457–2466.

18. Maloney, D. G., Grillo-Lopez, A. J., White, C. A., Bodkin, D., Schilder, R. J., Neidhart, J. A., et al. (1997) IDEC-C2B8 (Rituximab) anti-CD20 monoclonal antibody therapy in patients with relapsed low-grade non-Hodgkin's lymphoma. *Blood* **90**, 2188–2195.

19. Davis, T. A., White, C. A., Grillo-Lopez, A. J., Velasquez, W. S., Link, B., Maloney, D. G., et al. (1999) Single-agent monoclonal antibody efficacy in bulky non-Hodgkin's lymphoma: results of a phase II trial of rituximab. *J. Clin. Oncol.* **17**, 1851–1857.

20. Maloney, D. G., Grillo-Lopez, A. J., Bodkin, D. J., White, C. A., Liles, T. M., Royston, I., et al. (1997) IDEC-C2B8: results of a phase I multiple-dose trial in patients with relapsed non-Hodgkin's lymphoma. *J. Clin. Oncol.* **15**, 3266–3274.

21. Berinstein, N. L., Grillo-Lopez, A. J., White, C. A., Bence-Bruckler, I., Maloney, D., et al. (1998) Association of serum Rituximab (IDEC-C2B8) concentration and anti-tumor response in the treatment of recurrent low-grade or follicular non- Hodgkin's lymphoma. *Ann. Oncol.* **9**, 995–1001.

22. Bruggemann, M., Williams, G. T., Bindon, C. I., Clark, M. R., Walker, M. R., Jefferis, R., et al. (1987) Comparison of the effector functions of human immunoglobulins using a matched set of chimeric antibodies. *J. Exp. Med.* **166**, 1351–1361.

23. Shaw, D. R., Khazaeli, M. B., and LoBuglio, A. F. (1988) Mouse/human chimeric antibodies to a tumor-associated antigen: biologic activity of the four human IgG subclasses. *J. Natl. Cancer Inst.* **80**, 1553–1559.

24. Abdullah, N., Greenman, J., Pimenidou, A., Topping, K. P., and Monson, J. R. (1999) The role of monocytes and natural killer cells in mediating antibody- dependent lysis of colorectal tumour cells. *Cancer Immunol. Immunother.* **48**, 517–524.

25. Golay, J., Zaffaroni, L., Vaccari, T., Lazzari, M., Borleri, G. M., Bernasconi, S., et al. (2000) Biologic response of B lymphoma cells to anti-CD20 monoclonal antibody rituximab in vitro: CD55 and CD59 regulate complement-mediated cell lysis. *Blood* **95**, 3900–3908.

26. Steplewski, Z., Sun, L. K., Shearman, C. W., Ghrayeb, J., Daddona, P., and Koprowski, H. (1988) Biological activity of human-mouse IgG1, IgG2, IgG3, and IgG4 chimeric monoclonal antibodies with antitumor specificity. *Proc. Natl. Acad. Sci. USA* **85**, 4852–4856.

27. Clynes, R. A., Towers, T. L., Presta, L. G., and Ravetch, J. V. (2000) Inhibitory Fc receptors modulate in vivo cytoxicity against tumor targets. *Nat. Med.* **6**, 443–446.

28. Jones, P. T., Dear, P. H., Foote, J., Neuberger, M. S., and Winter, G. (1986) Replacing the complementarity-determining regions in a human antibody with those from a mouse. *Nature* **321**, 522–525.

29. Chothia, C. and Lesk, A. M. (1987) Canonical structures for the hypervariable regions of immunoglobulins. *J. Mol. Biol.* **196**, 901–917.

30. Chothia, C., Lesk, A. M., Tramontano, A., Levitt, M., Smith-Gill, S. J., Air, G., et al. (1989) Conformations of immunoglobulin hypervariable regions. *Nature* **342**, 877–883.

31. Queen, C., Schneider, W. P., Selick, H. E., Payne, P. W., Landolfi, N. F., Duncan, J. F., et al. (1989) A humanized antibody that binds to the interleukin 2 receptor. *Proc. Natl. Acad. Sci. USA* **86**, 10,029–10,033.
32. Kettleborough, C. A., Saldanha, J., Heath, V. J., Morrison, C. J., and Bendig, M. M. (1991) Humanization of a mouse monoclonal antibody by CDR-grafting: the importance of framework residues on loop conformation. *Protein Eng.* **4**, 773–783.
33. Co, M. S., Avdalovic, N. M., Caron, P. C., Avdalovic, M. V., Scheinberg, D. A., and Queen, C. (1992) Chimeric and humanized antibodies with specificity for the CD33 antigen. *J. Immunol.* **148**, 1149–1154.
34. Roberts, S., Cheetham, J. C., and Rees, A. R. (1987) Generation of an antibody with enhanced affinity and specificity for its antigen by protein engineering. *Nature* **328**, 731–734.
35. Riechmann, L., Clark, M., Waldmann, H., and Winter, G. (1988) Reshaping human antibodies for therapy. *Nature* **332**, 323–327.
36. Roguska, M. A., Pedersen, J. T., Keddy, C. A., Henry, A. H., Searle, S. J., Lambert, J. M., et al. (1994) Humanization of murine monoclonal antibodies through variable domain resurfacing. *Proc. Natl. Acad. Sci. USA* **91**, 969–973.
37. Glennie, M. J. and Johnson, P. W. (2000) Clinical trials of antibody therapy. *Immunol. Today* **21**, 403–410.
38. Behr, T. M., Wormann, B., Gramatzki, M., Riggert, J., Gratz, S., Behe, M., et al. (1999) Low- versus high-dose radioimmunotherapy with humanized anti-CD22 or chimeric anti-CD20 antibodies in a broad spectrum of B cell-associated malignancies. *Clin. Cancer Res.* **5**, 3304s–3314s.
39. Juweid, M. E., Stadtmauer, E., Hajjar, G., Sharkey, R. M., Suleiman, S., Luger, S., et al. (1999) Pharmacokinetics, dosimetry, and initial therapeutic results with 131I- and (111)In-/90Y-labeled humanized LL2 anti-CD22 monoclonal antibody in patients with relapsed, refractory non-Hodgkin's lymphoma. *Clin. Cancer Res.* **5**, 3292s–3303s.
40. Sievers, E. L., Appelbaum, F. R., Spielberger, R. T., Forman, S. J., Flowers, D., Smith, F. O., et al. (1999) Selective ablation of acute myeloid leukemia using antibody-targeted chemotherapy: a phase I study of an anti-CD33 calicheamicin immunoconjugate. *Blood* **93**, 3678–3684.
41. Steffens, M. G., Boerman, O. C., de Mulder, P. H., Oyen, W. J., Buijs, W. C., Witjes, J. A., vet al. (1999) Phase I radioimmunotherapy of metastatic renal cell carcinoma with 131I- labeled chimeric monoclonal antibody G250. *Clin. Cancer Res.* **5**, 3268s–3274s.
42. Tolcher, A. W., Sugarman, S., Gelmon, K. A., Cohen, R., Saleh, M., Isaacs, C., et al. (1999) Randomized phase II study of BR96-doxorubicin conjugate in patients with metastatic breast cancer. *J. Clin. Oncol.* **17**, 478–484.
43. Saleh, M. N., Sugarman, S., Murray, J., Ostroff, J. B., Healey, D., Jones, D., et al. (2000) Phase I trial of the anti-Lewis Y drug immunoconjugate BR96-doxorubicin in patients with lewis Y-expressing epithelial tumors. *J. Clin. Oncol.* **18**, 2282–2292.
44. Miller, J. L. (2000) FDA approves antibody-directed cytotoxic agent for acute myeloid leukemia. *Am. J. Health Syst. Pharm.* **57**, 1202, 1204.
45. Shalaby, M. R., Shepard, H. M., Presta, L., Rodrigues, M. L., Beverley, P. C., Feldmann, M., and Carter, P. (1992) Development of humanized bispecific antibodies reactive with cytotoxic lymphocytes and tumor cells overexpressing the HER2 protooncogene. *J. Exp. Med.* **175**, 217–225.
46. Zhu, Z., Lewis, G. D., and Carter, P. (1995) Engineering high affinity humanized anti-p185HER2/anti-CD3 bispecific F(ab')2 for efficient lysis of p185HER2 overexpressing tumor cells. *Int. J. Cancer* **62**, 319–324.

47. Luiten, R. M., Coney, L. R., Fleuren, G. J., Warnaar, S. O., and Litvinov, S. V. (1996) Generation of chimeric bispecific G250/anti-CD3 monoclonal antibody, a tool to combat renal cell carcinoma. *Br. J. Cancer* **74,** 735–744.

48. Ridgway, J. B., Presta, L. G., and Carter, P. (1996) 'Knobs-into-holes' engineering of antibody CH3 domains for heavy chain heterodimerization. *Protein Eng.* **9,** 617–621.

49. Keler, T., Graziano, R. F., Mandal, A., Wallace, P. K., Fisher, J., Guyre, P. M., et al. (1997) Bispecific antibody-dependent cellular cytotoxicity of HER2/neu-overexpressing tumor cells by Fc gamma receptor type I-expressing effector cells. *Cancer Res.* **57,** 4008–4014.

50. van Ojik, H. H., Repp, R., Groenewegen, G., Valerius, T., and van de Winkel, J. G. (1997) Clinical evaluation of the bispecific antibody MDX-H210 (anti-Fc gamma RI × anti-HER-2/neu) in combination with granulocyte-colony-stimulating factor (filgrastim) for treatment of advanced breast cancer. *Cancer Immunol. Immunother.* **45,** 207–209.

51. Posey, J. A., Raspet, R., Verma, U., Deo, Y. M., Keller, T., Marshall, J. L., et al. (1999) A pilot trial of GM-CSF and MDX-H210 in patients with erbB-2-positive advanced malignancies. *J. Immunother.* **22,** 371–379.

52. Lewis, L. D., Cole, B. F., Wallace, P. K., Fisher, J. L., Waugh, M., Guyre, P. M., et al. (2001) Pharmacokinetic-pharmacodynamic relationships of the bispecific antibody MDX-H210 when administered in combination with interferon gamma: a multiple-dose phase-I study in patients with advanced cancer which overexpresses HER-2/neu. *J. Immunol. Methods* **248,** 149–165.

53. Skerra, A. and Pluckthun, A. (1988) Assembly of a functional immunoglobulin Fv fragment in Escherichia coli. *Science* **240,** 1038–1041.

54. Better, M., Chang, C. P., Robinson, R. R., and Horwitz, A. H. (1988) *Escherichia coli* secretion of an active chimeric antibody fragment. *Science* **240,** 1041–1043.

55. Glockshuber, R., Malia, M., Pfitzinger, I., and Plückthun, A. (1990) A comparison of strategies to stabilize immunoglobulin Fv fragments. *Biochemistry* **29,** 1362–1367.

56. Huston, J. S., Levinson, D., Mudgett-Hunter, M., Tai, M. S., Novotny, J., Margolies, M. N., et al. (1988) Protein engineering of antibody binding sites: recovery of specific activity in an anti-digoxin single-chain Fv analogue produced in *Escherichia coli*. *Proc. Natl. Acad. Sci. USA* **85,** 5879–5883.

57. Bird, R. E., Hardman, K. D., Jacobson, J. W., Johnson, S., Kaufman, B. M., Lee, S. M., et al. (1988) Single-chain antigen-binding proteins [published erratum appears in Science 1989 Apr 28;244(4903):409]. *Science* **242,** 423–426.

58. Brinkmann, U., Reiter, Y., Jung, S. H., Lee, B., and Pastan, I. (1993) A recombinant immunotoxin containing a disulfide-stabilized Fv fragment. *Proc. Natl. Acad. Sci. USA* **90,** 7538–7542.

59. Reiter, Y., Brinkmann, U., Jung, S. H., Lee, B., Kasprzyk, P. G., King, C. R., and Pastan, I. (1994) Improved binding and antitumor activity of a recombinant anti-erbB2 immunotoxin by disulfide stabilization of the Fv fragment. *J. Biol. Chem.* **269,** 18,327–18,331.

60. Chaudhary, V. K., FitzGerald, D. J., Adhya, S., and Pastan, I. (1987) Activity of a recombinant fusion protein between transforming growth factor type alpha and Pseudomonas toxin. *Proc. Natl. Acad. Sci. USA* **84,** 4538–4542.

61. Chaudhary, V. K., Queen, C., Junghans, R. P., Waldmann, T. A., FitzGerald, D. J., and Pastan, I. (1989) A recombinant immunotoxin consisting of two antibody variable domains fused to Pseudomonas exotoxin. *Nature* **339,** 394–397.

62. Batra, J. K., Fitzgerald, D. J., Chaudhary, V. K., and Pastan, I. (1991) Single-chain immunotoxins directed at the human transferrin receptor containing Pseudomonas exotoxin A or diphtheria toxin: anti-TFR(Fv)- PE40 and DT388-anti-TFR(Fv). *Mol. Cell. Biol.* **11,** 2200–2205.

63. Brinkmann, U., Pai, L. H., FitzGerald, D. J., Willingham, M., and Pastan, I. (1991) B3(Fv)-PE38KDEL, a single-chain immunotoxin that causes complete regression of a human carcinoma in mice. *Proc. Natl. Acad. Sci. USA* **88,** 8616–8620.

64. Siegall, C. B. (1995) Targeted therapy of carcinomas using BR96 sFv-PE40, a single-chain immunotoxin that binds to the Le(y) antigen. *Semin. Cancer Biol.* **6,** 289–295.

65. Newton, D. L., Nicholls, P. J., Rybak, S. M., and Youle, R. J. (1994) Expression and characterization of recombinant human eosinophil-derived neurotoxin and eosinophil-derived neurotoxin-anti-transferrin receptor sFv. *J. Biol. Chem.* **269,** 26,739–26,745.

66. Newton, D. L., Xue, Y., Olson, K. A., Fett, J. W., and Rybak, S. M. (1996) Angiogenin single-chain immunofusions: influence of peptide linkers and spacers between fusion protein domains. *Biochemistry* **35,** 545–553.

67. Zewe, M., Rybak, S. M., Dubel, S., Coy, J. F., Welschof, M., Newton, D. L., and Little, M. (1997) Cloning and cytotoxicity of a human pancreatic RNase immunofusion. *Immunotechnology* **3,** 127–136.

68. Bosslet, K., Czech, J., Lorenz, P., Sedlacek, H. H., Schuermann, M., and Seemann, G. (1992) Molecular and functional characterisation of a fusion protein suited for tumour specific prodrug activation. *Br. J. Cancer* **65,** 234–238.

69. Goshorn, S. C., Svensson, H. P., Kerr, D. E., Somerville, J. E., Senter, P. D., and Fell, H. P. (1993) Genetic construction, expression, and characterization of a single chain anti-carcinoma antibody fused to beta-lactamase. *Cancer Res.* **53,** 2123–2127.

70. Rodrigues, M. L., Presta, L. G., Kotts, C. E., Wirth, C., Mordenti, J., Osaka, G., et al. (1995) Development of a humanized disulfide-stabilized anti-p185HER2 Fv-beta-lactamase fusion protein for activation of a cephalosporin doxorubicin prodrug. *Cancer Res.* **55,** 63–70.

71. Michael, N. P., Chester, K. A., Melton, R. G., Robson, L., Nicholas, W., Boden, J. A., Pet, al. (1996) In vitro and in vivo characterisation of a recombinant carboxypeptidase G2:anti-CEA scFv fusion protein. *Immunotechnology* **2,** 47–57.

72. Haisma, H. J., Sernee, M. F., Hooijberg, E., Brakenhoff, R. H., vd Meulen-Muileman, I. H., Pet al. (1998) Construction and characterization of a fusion protein of single-chain anti-CD20 antibody and human beta-glucuronidase for antibody-directed enzyme prodrug therapy. *Blood* **92,** 184–190.

73. Colcher, D., Pavlinkova, G., Beresford, G., Booth, B. J., and Batra, S. K. (1999) Single-chain antibodies in pancreatic cancer. *Ann. NY Acad. Sci.* **880,** 263–280.

74. Rosenblum, M. G., Horn, S. A., and Cheung, L. H. (2000) A novel recombinant fusion toxin targeting HER-2/NEU-over-expressing cells and containing human tumor necrosis factor. *Int. J. Cancer* **88,** 267–273.

75. Xu, X., Clarke, P., Szalai, G., Shively, J. E., Williams, L. E., Shyr, Y., Shi, E., et al. (2000) Targeting and therapy of carcinoembryonic antigen-expressing tumors in transgenic mice with an antibody-interleukin 2 fusion protein. *Cancer Res.* **60,** 4475–4484.

76. Biragyn, A., Tani, K., Grimm, M. C., Weeks, S., and Kwak, L. W. (1999) Genetic fusion of chemokines to a self tumor antigen induces protective, T-cell dependent antitumor immunity. *Nature Biotechnol.* **17,** 253–258.

77. Kostelny, S. A., Cole, M. S., and Tso, J. Y. (1992) Formation of a bispecific antibody by the use of leucine zippers. *J. Immunol.* **148,** 1547–1553.

78. Pack, P. and Pluckthun, A. (1992) Miniantibodies: use of amphipathic helices to produce functional, flexibly linked dimeric FV fragments with high avidity in *Escherichia coli. Biochemistry* **31,** 1579–1584.

79. Holliger, P., Prospero, T., and Winter, G. (1993) "Diabodies": Small bivalent and bispecific antibody fragments. *Proc. Natl. Acad. Sci. USA* **90,** 6444–6448.

80. Gruber, M., Schodin, B. A., Wilson, E. R., and Kranz, D. M. (1994) Efficient tumor cell lysis mediated by a bispecific single chain antibody expressed in *Escherichia coli. J. Immunol.* **152,** 5368–5374.

81. Zhu, Z., Presta, L. G., Zapata, G., and Carter, P. (1997) Remodeling domain interfaces to enhance heterodimer formation. *Protein Sci.* **6,** 781–788.

82. Holliger, P., Brissinck, J., Williams, R. L., Thielmans, K., and Winter, G. (1996) Specific killing of lymphoma cells by cytotoxic T-cells mediated by a bispecific diabody. *Prot. Eng.* **9,** 299–305.

83. Zhu, Z., Zapata, G., Shalaby, R., Snedecor, B., Chen, H., and Carter, P. (1996) High-Level secretion of a humanized bispecific diabody from *Escherichia coli. Biotechnology* **14,** 192–196.

84. Kipriyanov, S. M., Moldenhauer, G., Srauss, G., and Little, M. (1998) Bispecific CD3 × CD19 diabody for T cell-mediated lysis of malignant human B cells. *Int. J. Cancer* **77,** 763–772.

85. Manzke, O., Fitzgerald, K. J., Holliger, P., Klock, J., Span, M., Fleischmann, B., H., et al. (1999) CD3X anti-nitrophenyl bispecific diabodies: universal Immunother.apeutic tools for retargeting T cells to tumors. *Int. J. Cancer* **82,** 700–708.

86. Arndt, M. A., Krauss, J., Kipriyanov, S. M., Pfreundschuh, M. ,and Little, M. (1999) A bispecific diabody that mediates natural killer cell cytotoxicity against xenotransplantated human Hodgkin's tumors. *Blood* **94,** 2562–2568.

87. Coloma, M. J. and Morrison, S. L. (1997) Design and production of novel tetravalent bispecific antibodies. *Nature Biotechnol.* **15,** 159–163.

88. Alt, M., Muller, R., and Kontermann, R. E. (1999) Novel tetravalent and bispecific IgG-like antibody molecules combining single-chain diabodies with the immunoglobulin gamma1 Fc or CH3 region. *FEBS Lett.* **454,** 90–94.

89. Kipriyanov, S. M., Moldenhauer, G., Schuhmacher, J., Cochlovius, B., Von der Lieth, C. W., Matys, E. R., and Little, M. (1999) Bispecific tandem diabody for tumor therapy with improved antigen binding and pharmacokinetics. *J. Mol. Biol.* **293,** 41–56.

90. Gross, G. and Eshhar, Z. (1992) Endowing T cells with antibody specificity using chimeric T cell receptors. *FASEB J.* **6,** 3370–3378.

91. Eshhar, Z., Waks, T., Gross, G., and Schindler, D. G. (1993) Specific activation and targeting of cytotoxic lymphocytes through chimeric single chains consisting of antibody-binding domains and the gamma or zeta subunits of the immunoglobulin and T-cell receptors. *Proc. Natl. Acad. Sci. USA* **90,** 720–724.

92. Hwu, P., Shafer, G. E., Treisman, J., Schindler, D. G., Gross, G., Cowherd, R., et al. (1993) Lysis of ovarian cancer cells by human lymphocytes redirected with a chimeric gene composed of an antibody variable region and the Fc receptor gamma chain. *J. Exp. Med.* **178,** 361–366.

93. Hombach, A., Heuser, C., Sircar, R., Tillmann, T., Diehl, V., Kruis, W., et al. (1997) T cell targeting of TAG72+ tumor cells by a chimeric receptor with antibody-like specificity for a carbohydrate epitope. *Gastroenterology* **113,** 1163–1170.

94. Hombach, A., Schneider, C., Sent, D., Koch, D., Willemsen, R. A., Diehl, V., et al. (2000) An entirely humanized CD3 zeta-chain signaling receptor that directs peripheral blood T cells to specific lysis of carcinoembryonic antigen- positive tumor cells. *Int. J. Cancer* **88**, 115–120.

95. Kreitman, R. J., Wilson, W. H., Bergeron, K., Raggio, M., Stetler-Stevenson, M., FitzGerald, D. J., and Pastan, I. (2001) Efficacy of the anti-CD22 recombinant immunotoxin BL22 in chemotherapy-resistant hairy-cell leukemia. *N. Engl. J. Med.* **26**, 241–247.

96. Kreitman, R. J., Wilson, W. H., White, J. D., Stetler-Stevenson, M., Jaffe, E. S., Giardina, S., et al. (2000) Phase I trial of recombinant immunotoxin anti-Tac(Fv)-PE38 (LMB-2) in patients with hematologic malignancies. *J. Clin. Oncol.* **18**, 1622–1636.

97. Smith, G. P. (1985) Filamentous fusion phage: novel expression vectors that display cloned antigens on the virion surface. *Science* **228**, 1315–1317.

98. McCafferty, J., Griffiths, A. D., Winter, G., and Chiswell, D. J. (1990) Phage antibodies: filamentous phage displaying antibody variable domains. *Nature* **348**, 552–554.

99. Saiki, R. K., Scharf, S., Faloona, F., Mullis, K. B., Horn, G. T., Erlich, H. A., and Arnheim, N. (1985) Enzymatic amplification of beta-globin genomic sequences and restriction site analysis for diagnosis of sickle cell anemia. *Science* **230**, 1350–1354.

100. Orlandi, R., Gussow, D. H., Jones, P. T., and Winter, G. (1989) Cloning immunoglobulin variable domains for expression by the polymerase chain reaction. *Proc. Natl. Acad. Sci. USA* **86**, 3833–3837.

101. Sastry, L., Alting-Mees, M., Huse, W. D., Short, J. M., Sorge, J. A., Hay, B. N., et al. (1989) Cloning of the immunological repertoire in *Escherichia coli* for generation of monoclonal catalytic antibodies: construction of a heavy chain variable region-specific cDNA library. *Proc. Natl. Acad. Sci. USA* **86**, 5728–5732.

102. Marks, J. D., Tristem, M., Karpas, A., and Winter, G. (1991) Oligonucleotide primers for polymerase chain reaction amplification of human immunoglobulin variable genes and design of family-specific oligonucleotide probes. *Eur. J. Immunol.* **21**, 985–991.

103. Welschof, M., Terness, P., Kolbinger, F., Zewe, M., Dubel, S., Dorsam, H., et al. (1995) Amino acid sequence based PCR primers for amplification of rearranged human heavy and light chain immunoglobulin variable region genes. *J. Immunol. Methods* **179**, 203–214.

104. Barbas, C. F., 3rd, Kang, A. S., Lerner, R. A., and Benkovic, S. J. (1991) Assembly of combinatorial antibody libraries on phage surfaces: the gene III site. *Proc. Natl. Acad. Sci. USA* **88**, 7978–7982.

105. Breitling, F., Dubel, S., Seehaus, T., Klewinghaus, I., and Little, M. (1991) A surface expression vector for antibody screening. *Gene* **104**, 147–153.

106. Hoogenboom, H. R., Griffiths, A. D., Johnson, K. S., Chiswell, D. J., Hudson, P., and Winter, G. (1991) Multi-subunit proteins on the surface of filamentous phage: methodologies for displaying antibody (Fab) heavy and light chains. *Nucleic Acids Res.* **19**, 4133–4137.

107. Cai, X. and Garen, A. (1995) Anti-melanoma antibodies from melanoma patients immunized with genetically modified autologous tumor cells: selection of specific antibodies from single-chain Fv fusion phage libraries. *Proc. Natl. Acad. Sci. USA* **92**, 6537–6541.

108. Pereira, S., Van Belle, P., Elder, D., Maruyama, H., Jacob, L., Sivanandham, M., et al. (1997) Combinatorial antibodies against human malignant melanoma. *Hybridoma* **16**, 11–16.

109. Welschof, M., Terness, P., Kipriyanov, S. M., Stanescu, D., Breitling, F., Dorsam, H., et al. (1997) The antigen-binding domain of a human IgG-anti-F(ab')2 autoantibody. *Proc. Natl. Acad. Sci. USA* **94**, 1902–1907.

110. Clackson, T., Hoogenboom, H. R., Griffiths, A. D., and Winter, G. (1991) Making antibody fragments using phage display libraries. *Nature* **352**, 624–628.

111. Chester, K. A., Begent, R. H. J., Robson, L., Keep, P., Pedley, R. B., Boden, J. A., et al. (1994) Phage libraries for generation of clinically useful antibodies. *Lancet* **343**, 455–456.

112. Kettleborough, C. A., Ansell, K. H., Allen, R. W., Rosell-Vives, E., Gussow, D. H., and Bendig, M. M. (1994) Isolation of tumor cell-specific single-chain Fv from immunized mice using phage-antibody libraries and the re-construction of whole antibodies from these antibody fragments. *Eur. J. Immunol.* **24**, 952–958.

113. Marks, J. D., Hoogenboom, H. R., Bonnert, T. P., McCafferty, J., Griffiths, A. D., and Winter, G. (1991) By-passing immunization. Human antibodies from V-gene libraries displayed on phage. *J. Mol. Biol.* **222**, 581–597.

114. Sheets, M. D., Amersdorfer, P., Finnern, R., Sargent, P., Lindquist, E., Schier, R., et al. (1998) Efficient construction of a large nonimmune phage antibody library: the production of high-affinity human single-chain antibodies to protein antigens. *Proc. Natl. Acad. Sci. USA* **95**, 6157–6162.

115. de Haard, H. J., van Neer, N., Reurs, A., Hufton, S. E., Roovers, R. C., Henderikx, P., et al. (1999) A large non-immunized human Fab fragment phage library that permits rapid isolation and kinetic analysis of high affinity antibodies. *J. Biol. Chem.* **274**, 18,218–18,230.

116. Little, M., Welschof, M., Braunagel, M., Hermes, I., Christ, C., Keller, A., et al. (1999) Generation of a large complex antibody library from multiple donors. *J. Immunol. Methods* **231**, 3–9.

117. Barbas, C. F., 3rd, Bain, J. D., Hoekstra, D. M., and Lerner, R. A. (1992) Semisynthetic combinatorial antibody libraries: a chemical solution to the diversity problem. *Proc. Natl. Acad. Sci. USA* **89**, 4457–4461.

118. Hoogenboom, H. R. and Winter, G. (1992) By-passing immunisation. Human antibodies from synthetic repertoires of germline VH gene segments rearranged in vitro. *J. Mol. Biol.* **227**, 381–388.

119. Garrard, L. J. and Henner, D. J. (1993) Selection of an anti-IGF-1 Fab from a Fab phage library created by mutagenesis of multiple CDR loops. *Gene* **128**, 103–109.

120. Griffiths, A. D., Williams, S. C., Hartley, O., Tomlinson, I. M., Waterhouse, P., Crosby, W. L., et al. (1994) Isolation of high affinity human antibodies directly from large synthetic repertoires. *EMBO J.* **13**, 3245–3260.

121. Nissim, A., Hoogenboom, H. R., Tomlinson, I. M., Flynn, G., Midgley, C., Lane, D., and Winter, G. (1994) Antibody fragments from a 'single pot' phage display library as immunochemical reagents. *EMBO J.* **13**, 692–698.

122. Braunagel, M. and Little, M. (1997) Construction of a semisynthetic antibody library using trinucleotide oligos. *Nucleic Acids Res.* **25**, 4690–4691.

123. Knappik, A., Ge, L., Honegger, A., Pack, P., Fischer, M., Wellnhofer, G., et al. (2000) Fully synthetic human combinatorial antibody libraries (HuCAL) based on modular consensus frameworks and CDRs randomized with trinucleotides. *J. Mol. Biol.* **296**, 57–86.

124. Hanes, J. and Pluckthun, A. (1997) In vitro selection and evolution of functional proteins by using ribosome display. *Proc. Natl. Acad. Sci. USA* **94**, 4937–4942.

125. He, M. and Taussig, M. J. (1997) Antibody-ribosome-mRNA (ARM) complexes as efficient selection particles for in vitro display and evolution of antibody combining sites. *Nucleic Acids Res.* **25**, 5132–5134.

126. Hamers-Casterman, C., Atarhouch, T., Muyldermans, S., Robinson, G., Hamers, C., Songa, E. B., et al. (1993) Naturally occurring antibodies devoid of light chains. *Nature* **363**, 446–448.

127. Arbabi Ghahroudi, M., Desmyter, A., Wyns, L., Hamers, R., and Muyldermans, S. (1997) Selection and identification of single domain antibody fragments from camel heavy-chain antibodies. *FEBS Lett.* **414,** 521–526.
128. Muyldermans, S. and Lauwereys, M. (1999) Unique single-domain antigen binding fragments derived from naturally occurring camel heavy-chain antibodies. *J. Mol. Recognit.* **12,** 131–140.
129. Reiter, Y., Schuck, P., Boyd, L. F., and Plaksin, D. (1999) An antibody single-domain phage display library of a native heavy chain variable region: isolation of functional single-domain VH molecules with a unique interface. *J. Mol. Biol.* **290,** 685–698.
130. Begent, R. H., Verhaar, M. J., Chester, K. A., Casey, J. L., Green, A. J., Napier, M. P., (1996) Clinical evidence of efficient tumor targeting based on single-chain Fv antibody selected from a combinatorial library. *Nat. Med.* **2,** 979–984.
131. Mayer, A., Chester, K. A., Flynn, A. A., and Begent, R. H. (1999) Taking engineered anti-CEA antibodies to the clinic. *J. Immunol. Methods* **231,** 261–273.
132. Carson, D. A. and Freimark, B. D. (1986) Human lymphocyte hybridomas and monoclonal antibodies. *Adv. Immunol.* **38,** 275–311.
133. Bruggemann, M., Spicer, C., Buluwela, L., Rosewell, I., Barton, S., Surani, M. A., and Rabbitts, T. H. (1991) Human antibody production in transgenic mice: expression from 100 kb of the human IgH locus. *Eur. J. Immunol.* **21,** 1323–1326.
134. Taylor, L. D., Carmack, C. E., Schramm, S. R., Mashayekh, R., Higgins, K. M., Kuo, C. C., et al. (1992) A transgenic mouse that expresses a diversity of human sequence heavy and light chain immunoglobulins. *Nucleic Acids Res.* **20,** 6287–6295.
135. Lonberg, N., Taylor, L. D., Harding, F. A., Trounstine, M., Higgins, K. M., Schramm, S. R., et al. (1994) Antigen-specific human antibodies from mice comprising four distinct genetic modifications. *Nature* **368,** 856–859.
136. Nicholson, I. C., Zou, X., Popov, A. V., Cook, G. P., Corps, E. M., Humphries, S., et al. (1999) Antibody repertoires of four- and five-feature translocus mice carrying human immunoglobulin heavy chain and kappa and lambda light chain yeast artificial chromosomes. *J. Immunol.* **163,** 6898–6906.
137. Tomizuka, K., Shinohara, T., Yoshida, H., Uejima, H., Ohguma, A., Tanaka, S., et al. (2000) Double trans-chromosomic mice: maintenance of two individual human chromosome fragments containing Ig heavy and kappa loci and expression of fully human antibodies. *Proc. Natl. Acad. Sci. USA* **97,** 722–727.
138. Stashenko, P., Nadler, L. M., Hardy, R., and Schlossman, S. F. (1980) Characterization of a human B lymphocyte-specific antigen. *J. Immunol.* **125,** 1678–1685.
139. McLaughlin, P., Grillo-Lopez, A. J., Link, B. K., Levy, R., Czuczman, M. S., Williams, M. E., et al. (1998) Rituximab chimeric anti-CD20 monoclonal antibody therapy for relapsed indolent lymphoma: half of patients respond to a four-dose treatment program. *J. Clin. Oncol.* **16,** 2825–2833.
140. Coiffier, B., Haioun, C., Ketterer, N., Engert, A., Tilly, H., Ma, D., et al. (1998) Rituximab (anti-CD20 monoclonal antibody) for the treatment of patients with relapsing or refractory aggressive lymphoma: a multicenter phase II study. *Blood* **92,** 1927–1932.
141. Coiffier, B., Lepage, E., Herbrecht, R., Tilly, H., Solal-Celigny, P., Munck, J. N., et al. (2000) Mabthera (Rituximab) plus CHOP is superior to CHOP alone in elderly patients with diffuse large B-cell lymphoma (DLCL): Interim results of a randomized GELA trial. Abstract #950 *American Society of Hematology (ASH)*.
142. Coiffier, B., Lepage, E., Gaulard, P., Quesnel, A., Bosly, A., Christian, B., et al. (2001) Prognostic factors affecting the efficacy of Rituximab plus CHOP (R-CHOP) therapy in

elderly patients with diffuse large B-cell lymphoma (DLCL): results of a randomized GELA trial. Abstract #1131 *Annual Meeting of American Society of Clinical Oncologists (ASCO)*.

143. Vose, J. M., Link, B. K., Grossbard, M. L., Czuczman, M., Grillo-Lopez, A., Gilman, P., et al. (2001) Phase II study of rituximab in combination with chop chemotherapy in patients with previously untreated, aggressive non-Hodgkin's lymphoma. *J. Clin. Oncol.* **19,** 389–397.

144. Czuczman, M. S., Grillo-Lopez, A. J., White, C. A., Saleh, M., Gordon, L., LoBuglio, A. F., et al. (1999) Treatment of patients with low-grade B-cell lymphoma with the combination of chimeric anti-CD20 monoclonal antibody and CHOP chemotherapy. *J. Clin. Oncol.* **17,** 268–276.

145. Colombat, P., Salles, G., Brousse, N., Eftekhari, P., Soubeyran, P., Delwail, V., et al. (2001) Rituximab (anti-CD20 monoclonal antibody) as single first-line therapy for patients with follicular lymphoma with a low tumor burden: clinical and molecular evaluation. *Blood* **97,** 101–106.

146. Buckstein, R., Imrie, K., Spaner, D., Potichnyj, A., Robinson, J. B., Nanji, S., et al. (1999) Stem cell function and engraftment is not affected by "in vivo purging" with rituximab for autologous stem cell treatment for patients with low- grade non-Hodgkin's lymphoma. *Semin. Oncol.* **26,** 115–122.

147. Coussens, L., Yang-Feng, T. L., Liao, Y. C., Chen, E., Gray, A., McGrath, J., et al. (1985) Tyrosine kinase receptor with extensive homology to EGF receptor shares chromosomal location with neu oncogene. *Science* **230,** 1132–1139.

148. Slamon, D. J., Clark. G. M., Wong, S. G., Levin, W. J., Ullrich A., and McGuire, W. L. (1987) Human breast cancer: correlation of relapse and survival with amplification of the HER-2/neu oncogene. *Science* **235,** 177–182.

149. Borg, A., Tandon, A. K., Sigurdsson, H., Clark, G. M., Ferno, M., Fuqua, S. A., et al. (1990) HER-2/neu amplification predicts poor survival in node-positive breast cancer. *Cancer Res.* **50,** 4332–4337.

150. Hudziak, R. M., Lewis, G. D., Winget, M., Fendly, B. M., Shepard, H. M., and Ullrich, A. (1989) p185HER2 monoclonal antibody has antiproliferative effects in vitro and sensitizes human breast tumor cells to tumor necrosis factor. *Mol. Cell Biol.* **9,** 1165–1172.

151. Shepard, H. M., Lewis, G. D., Sarup, J. C., Fendly, B. M., Maneval, D., Mordenti, J., et al. (1991) Monoclonal antibody therapy of human cancer: taking the HER2 proto-oncogene to the clinic. *J. Clin. Immunol.* **11,** 117–127.

152. Carter, P., Presta, L., Gorman, C. M., Ridgway, J. B., Henner, D., Wong, W. L., et al. (1992) Humanization of an anti-p185HER2 antibody for human cancer therapy. *Proc. Natl. Acad. Sci. USA* **89,** 4285–4289.

153. Baselga, J., Tripathy, D., Mendelsohn, J., Baughman, S., Benz, C. C., Dantis, L., et al. (1996) Phase II study of weekly intravenous recombinant humanized anti- p185HER2 monoclonal antibody in patients with HER2/neu-overexpressing metastatic breast cancer. *J. Clin. Oncol.* **14,** 737–744.

154. Vici, P., Belli, F., Di Lauro, L., Amodio, A., Conti, F., Foggi, P., et al. (2001) Docetaxel in patients with anthracycline-resistant advanced breast cancer. *Oncology* **60,** 60–65.

155. Cobleigh, M. A., Vogel, C. L., Tripathy, D., Robert, N. J., Scholl, S., Fehrenbacher, L., et al. (1999) Multinational study of the efficacy and safety of humanized anti-HER2 monoclonal antibody in women who have HER2-overexpressing metastatic breast cancer that has progressed after chemotherapy for metastatic disease. *J. Clin. Oncol.* **17,** 2639–2648.

156. Baselga, J., Norton, L., Albanell, J., Kim, Y. M., and Mendelsohn, J. (1998) Recombinant humanized anti-HER2 antibody (Herceptin) enhances the antitumor activity of paclitaxel and doxorubicin against HER2/neu overexpressing human breast cancer xenografts. *Cancer Res.* **58,** 2825–2831.

157. Pietras, R. J., Pegram, M. D., Finn, R. S., Maneval, D. A., and Slamon, D. J. (1998) Remission of human breast cancer xenografts on therapy with humanized monoclonal antibody to HER-2 receptor and DNA-reactive drugs. *Oncogene* **17,** 2235–2249.

158. Slamon, D. J., Leyland-Jones, B., Shak, S., Fuchs, H., Paton, V., Bajamonde, A., et al. (2001) Use of chemotherapy plus a monoclonal antibody against HER2 for metastatic breast cancer that overexpresses HER2. *N. Engl. J. Med.* **344,** 783–792.

159. Tan, A. R. and Swain, S. M. (2001) Adjuvant chemotherapy for breast cancer: an update. *Semin. Oncol.* **28,** 359–376.

160. Koprowski, H., Herlyn, D., Lubeck, M., DeFreitas, E., and Sears, H. F. (1984) Human anti-idiotype antibodies in cancer patients: Is the modulation of the immune response beneficial for the patient? *Proc. Natl. Acad. Sci. USA* **81,** 216–219.

161. LoBuglio, A. F., Saleh, M. N., Lee, J., Khazaeli, M. B., Carrano, R., Holden, H., and Wheeler, R. H. (1988) Phase I trial of multiple large doses of murine monoclonal antibody CO17-1A. I. Clinical aspects. *J. Natl. Cancer Inst.* **80,** 932–936.

162. Riethmuller, G., Schneider-Gadicke, E., Schlimok, G., Schmiegel, W., Raab, R., Hoffken, K., et al. (1994) Randomised trial of monoclonal antibody for adjuvant therapy of resected Dukes' C colorectal carcinoma. German Cancer Aid 17-1A Study Group. *Lancet* **343,** 1177–1183.

163. Gruber, R., van Haarlem, L. J., Warnaar, S. O., Holz, E., and Riethmuller, G. (2000) The human antimouse immunoglobulin response and the anti-idiotypic network have no influence on clinical outcome in patients with minimal residual colorectal cancer treated with monoclonal antibody CO17-1A. *Cancer Res.* **60,** 1921–1926.

164. Jerne, N. K. (1974) Towards a network theory of the immune system. *Ann. Immunol. (Paris)* **125C,** 373–389.

165. Frodin, J. E., Faxas, M. E., Hagstrom, B., Lefvert, A. K., Masucci, G., Nilsson, B., et al. (1991) Induction of anti-idiotypic (ab2) and anti-anti-idiotypic (ab3) antibodies in patients treated with the mouse monoclonal antibody 17-1A (ab1). Relation to the clinical outcome—an important antitumoral effector function? *Hybridoma* **10,** 421–431.

166. Wagner, U. A., Oehr, P. F., Reinsberg, J., Schmidt, S. C., Schlebusch, H. W., Schultes, B., et al. (1992) Immunotherapy of advanced ovarian carcinomas by activation of the idiotypic network. *Biotechnol. Ther.* **3,** 81–89.

167. Cheung, N. K., Cheung, I. Y., Canete, A., Yeh, S. J., Kushner, B., Bonilla, M. A., et al. (1994) Antibody response to murine anti-GD2 monoclonal antibodies: correlation with patient survival. *Cancer Res.* **54,** 2228–2233.

168. Schmolling, J., Reinsberg, J., Wagner, U., and Krebs, D. (1997) Anti-TAG-72 antibody B72.3 — immunological and clinical effects in ovarian carcinoma. *Hybridoma* **16,** 53–58.

169. Cheung, N. K., Guo, H. F., Heller, G., and Cheung, I. Y. (2000) Induction of Ab3 and Ab3' antibody was associated with long-term survival after anti-G(D2) antibody therapy of stage 4 neuroblastoma. *Clin. Cancer Res.* **6,** 2653–2660.

170. Nadler, L. M., Stashenko, P., Hardy, R., Kaplan, W. D., Button, L. N., Kufe, D. W., et al. (1980) Serotherapy of a patient with a monoclonal antibody directed against a human lymphoma-associated antigen. *Cancer Res.* **40,** 3147–3154.

171. Miller, R. A. and Levy, R. (1981) Response of cutaneous T cell lymphoma to therapy with hybridoma monoclonal antibody. *Lancet* **2**, 226–230.
172. Cobbold, S. P. and Waldmann, H. (1984) Therapeutic potential of monovalent monoclonal antibodies. *Nature* **308**, 460–462.
173. Sahin, U., Tureci, O., Schmitt, H., Cochlovius, B., Johannes, T., Schmits, R., et al. (1995) Human neoplasms elicit multiple specific immune responses in the autologous host. *Proc. Natl. Acad. Sci. USA* **92**, 11,810–11,813.
174. Barth, S., Weidenmuller, U., Tur, M. K., Schmidt, M. F., and Engert, A. (2000) Combining phage display and screening of cDNA expression libraries: a new approach for identifying the target antigen of an scFv preselected by phage display. *J. Mol. Biol.* **301**, 751–757.
175. Chames, P., Hufton, S. E., Coulie, P. G., Uchanska-Ziegler, B., and Hoogenboom, H. R. (2000) Direct selection of a human antibody fragment directed against the tumor T-cell epitope HLA-A1-MAGE-A1 from a nonimmunized phage-Fab library. *Proc. Natl. Acad. Sci. USA* **97**, 7969–7974.
176. Li, J., Pereira, S., Van Belle, P., Tsui, P., Elder, D., Speicher, D., et al. (2001) Isolation of the melanoma-associated antigen p23 using antibody phage display. *J. Immunol.* **166**, 432–438.
177. Herlyn, D. M., Steplewski, Z., Herlyn, M. F., and Koprowski, H. (1980) Inhibition of growth of colorectal carcinoma in nude mice by monoclonal antibody. *Cancer Res.* **40**, 717–721.
178. Hellstrom, I., Brown, J. P., and Hellstrom, K. E. (1981) Monoclonal antibodies to two determinants of melanoma-antigen p97 act synergistically in complement-dependent cytotoxicity. *J. Immunol.* **127**, 157–160.
179. Herlyn, D. and Koprowski, H. (1982) IgG2a monoclonal antibodies inhibit human tumor growth through interaction with effector cells. *Proc. Natl. Acad. Sci. USA* **79**, 4761–4765.
180. Adams, D. O., Hall, T., Steplewski, Z., and Koprowski, H. (1984) Tumors undergoing rejection induced by monoclonal antibodies of the IgG2a isotype contain increased numbers of macrophages activated for a distinctive form of antibody-dependent cytolysis. *Proc. Natl. Acad. Sci. USA* **81**, 3506–3510.
181. Herlyn, D., Herlyn, M., Ross, A. H., Ernst, C., Atkinson, B., and Koprowski, H. (1984) Efficient selection of human tumor growth-inhibiting monoclonal antibodies. *J. Immunol. Methods* **73**, 157–167.
182. Hellstrom, I., Beaumier, P. L., and Hellstrom, K. E. (1986) Antitumor effects of L6, an IgG2a antibody that reacts with most human carcinomas. *Proc. Natl. Acad. Sci. USA* **83**, 7059–7063.
183. Liu, A. Y., Robinson, R. R., Murray, E. D., Jr., Ledbetter, J. A., Hellstrom, I., and Hellstrom, K. E. (1987) Production of a mouse-human chimeric monoclonal antibody to CD20 with potent Fc-dependent biologic activity. *J. Immunol.* **139**, 3521–3526.
184. Caron, P. C., Co, M. S., Bull, M. K., Avdalovic, N. M., Queen, C., and Scheinberg, D. A. (1992) Biological and Immunological features of humanized M195 (anti-CD33) monoclonal antibodies. *Cancer Res.* **52**, 6761–6767.
185. Ravetch, J. V. and Clynes, R. A. (1998) Divergent roles for Fc receptors and complement in vivo. *Annu. Rev. Immunol.* **16**, 421–432.
186. Bolland, S. and Ravetch, J. V. (1999) Inhibitory pathways triggered by ITIM-containing receptors. *Adv. Immunol.* **72**, 149–177.
187. Cragg, M. S., French, R. R., and Glennie, M. J. (1999) Signaling antibodies in cancer therapy. *Curr. Opin. Immunol.* **11**, 541–547.

188. Shan, D., Ledbetter, J. A., and Press, O. W. (1998) Apoptosis of malignant human B cells by ligation of CD20 with monoclonal antibodies. *Blood* **91,** 1644–1652.

189. Shan, D., Ledbetter, J. A., and Press, O. W. (2000) Signaling events involved in anti-CD20-induced apoptosis of malignant human B cells. *Cancer Immunol. Immunother.* **48,** 673–683.

190. Ghetie, M. A., Podar, E. M., Ilgen, A., Gordon, B. E., Uhr, J. W., and Vitetta, E. S. (1997) Homodimerization of tumor-reactive monoclonal antibodies markedly increases their ability to induce growth arrest or apoptosis of tumor cells. *Proc. Natl. Acad. Sci. USA* **94,** 7509–7514.

191. Stout, R. D., Suttles, J., Xu, J., Grewal, I. S., and Flavell, R. A. (1996) Impaired T cell-mediated macrophage activation in CD40 ligand-deficient mice. *J. Immunol.* **156,** 8–11.

192. van Kooten, C. and Banchereau, J. (1997) Functions of CD40 on B cells, dendritic cells and other cells. *Curr. Opin. Immunol.* **9,** 330–337.

193. French, R. R., Chan, H. T., Tutt, A. L., and Glennie, M. J. (1999) CD40 antibody evokes a cytotoxic T-cell response that eradicates lymphoma and bypasses T-cell help. *Nat. Med.* **5,** 548–553.

194. Pietras, R. J., Poen, J. C., Gallardo, D., Wongvipat, P. N., Lee, H. J., and Slamon, D. J. (1999) Monoclonal antibody to HER-2/neureceptor modulates repair of radiation-induced DNA damage and enhances radiosensitivity of human breast cancer cells overexpressing this oncogene. *Cancer Res.* **59,** 1347–1355.

195. Goldenberg, D. M., Sharkey, R. M., Goldenberg, H., Hall, T. C., Murthy, S., Izon, D. O., et al. (1990) Monoclonal antibody therapy of cancer. *NJ Med.* **87,** 913–918.

196. Chester, K. A. and Hawkins, R. E. (1995) Clinical issues in antibody design. *Trends Biotechnol.* **13,** 294–300.

197. Adams, G. P., Schier, R., Marshall, K., Wolf, E. J., McCall, A. M., Marks, J. D., and Weiner, L. M. (1998) Increased affinity leads to improved selective tumor delivery of single- chain Fv antibodies. *Cancer Res.* **58,** 485–490.

198. Purtell, J. N., Pesce, A. J., Clyne, D. H., Miller, W. C., and Pollak, V. E. (1979) Isoelectric point of albumin: effect on renal handling of albumin. *Kidney Int.* **16,** 366–376.

199. Deen, W. M., Bridges, C. R., and Brenner, B. M. (1983) Biophysical basis of glomerular permselectivity. *J. Membr. Biol.* **71,** 1–10.

200. Vaughn, D. E., Milburn, C. M., Penny, D. M., Martin, W. L., Johnson, J. L., and Bjorkman, P. J. (1997) Identification of critical IgG binding epitopes on the neonatal Fc receptor. *J. Mol. Biol.* **274,** 597–607.

201. Junghans, R. P. and Anderson, C. L. (1996) The protection receptor for IgG catabolism is the beta2-microglobulin- containing neonatal intestinal transport receptor. *Proc. Natl. Acad. Sci. USA* **93,** 5512–5516.

202. Ghetie, V., Popov, S., Borvak, J., Radu, C., Matesoi, D., Medesan, C., et al. (1997) Increasing the serum persistence of an IgG fragment by random mutagenesis. *Nat. Biotechnol.* **15,** 637–640.

203. Ghetie, V. and Ward, E. S. (1997) FcRn: the MHC class I-related receptor that is more than an IgG transporter. *Immunol. Today* **18,** 592–598.

204. Zuckier, L. S., Chang, C. J., Scharff, M. D., and Morrison, S. L. (1998) Chimeric human-mouse IgG antibodies with shuffled constant region exons demonstrate that multiple domains contribute to in vivo half-life. *Cancer Res.* **58,** 3905–3908.

205. Milenic, D. E., Yokota, T., Filpula, D. R., Finkelman, M. A., Dodd, S. W., Wood, J. F., et al. (1991) Construction, binding properties, metabolism, and tumor targeting of a

single-chain Fv derived from the pancarcinoma monoclonal antibody CC49. *Cancer Res.* **51**, 6363–6371.

206. Huston, J. S., George, A. J., Adams, G. P., Stafford, W. F., Jamar, F., Tai, M. S., et al. (1996) Single-chain Fv radioimmunotargeting. *Q. J. Nucl. Med.* **40**, 320–333.

207. Adams, G. P., Schier, R., McCall, A. M., Crawford, R. S., Wolf, E. J., Weiner, L. M., and Marks, J. D. (1998) Prolonged in vivo tumour retention of a human diabody targeting the extracellular domain of human HER2/neu. *Br. J. Cancer* **77**, 1405–1412.

208. Yokota, T., Milenic, D. E., Whitlow, M., and Schlom, J. (1992) Rapid tumor penetration of a single-chain Fv and comparison with other immunoglobulin forms. *Cancer Res.* **52**, 3402–3408.

209. Boerman, O. C., Mijnheere, E. P., Broers, J. L., Vooijs, G. P., and Ramaekers, F. C. (1991) Biodistribution of a monoclonal antibody (RNL-1) against the neural cell adhesion molecule (NCAM) in athymic mice bearing human small-cell lung-cancer xenografts. *Int. J. Cancer* **48**, 457–462.

210. Kennel, S. J., Falcioni, R., and Wesley, J. W. (1991) Microdistribution of specific rat monoclonal antibodies to mouse tissues and human tumor xenografts. *Cancer Res.* **51**, 1529–1536.

211. Clauss, M. A. and Jain, R. K. (1990) Interstitial transport of rabbit and sheep antibodies in normal and neoplastic tissues. *Cancer Res.* **50**, 3487–3492.

212. Colcher, D., Bird, R., Roselli, M., Hardman, K. D., Johnson, S., Pope, S., et al. (1990) In vivo tumor targeting of a recombinant single-chain antigen-binding protein. *J. Natl. Cancer Inst.* **82**, 1191–1197.

213. Adams, G. P., McCartney, J. E., Tai, M. S., Oppermann, H., Huston, J. S., Stafford, W. F. D., et al. (1993) Highly specific in vivo tumor targeting by monovalent and divalent forms of 741F8 anti-c-erbB-2 single-chain Fv. *Cancer Res.* **53**, 4026–4034.

214. Kitamura, K., Takahashi, T., Yamaguchi, T., Noguchi, A., Takashina, K., Tsurumi, H., et al. (1991) Chemical engineering of the monoclonal antibody A7 by polyethylene glycol for targeting cancer chemotherapy. *Cancer Res.* **51**, 4310–4315.

215. Pedley, R. B., Boden, J. A., Boden, R., Begent, R. H., Turner, A., Haines, A. M., and King, D. J. (1994) The potential for enhanced tumour localisation by poly(ethylene glycol) modification of anti-CEA antibody. *Br. J. Cancer* **70**, 1126–1130.

216. Chapman, A. P., Antoniw, P., Spitali, M., West, S., Stephens, S., and King, D. J. (1999) Therapeutic antibody fragments with prolonged in vivo half-lives. *Nature Biotechnol.* **17**, 780–783.

217. Abuchowski, A., McCoy, J. R., Palczuk, N. C., van Es, T., and Davis, F. F. (1977) Effect of covalent attachment of polyethylene glycol on immunogenicity and circulating life of bovine liver catalase. *J. Biol. Chem.* **252**, 3582–3586.

218. Marks, J. D., Griffiths, A. D., Malmqvist, M., Clackson, T. P., Bye, J. M., and Winter, G. (1992) By-passing immunization: building high affinity human antibodies by chain shuffling. *Biotechnology (NY)* **10**, 779–783.

219. Hawkins, R. E., Russell, S. J., Baier, M., and Winter, G. (1993) The contribution of contact and non-contact residues of antibody in the affinity of binding to antigen. The interaction of mutant D1.3 antibodies with lysozyme. *J. Mol. Biol.* **234**, 958–964.

220. Schier, R., McCall, A., Adams, G. P., Marshall, K. W., Merritt, H., Yim, M., et al. (1996) Isolation of picomolar affinity anti-c-erbB-2 single-chain Fv by molecular evolution of the complementarity determining regions in the center of the antibody binding site. *J. Mol. Biol.* **263**, 551–567.

221. Schier, R., Marks, J. D., Wolf, E. J., Apell, G., Wong, C., McCartney, J. E., et al. (1995) In vitro and in vivo characterization of a human anti-c-erbB-2 single- chain Fv isolated from a filamentous phage antibody library. *Immunotechnology* **1,** 73–81.
222. Schier, R., Bye, J., Apell, G., McCall, A., Adams, G. P., Malmqvist, M., et al. (1996) Isolation of high-affinity monomeric human anti-c-erbB-2 single chain Fv using affinity-driven selection. *J. Mol. Biol.* **255,** 28–43.
223. Adams, G. P., Schier, R., McCall, A., Wolf, E. J., Marks, J. D., and Weiner, L. M. (1996) Tumor targeting properties of anti-c-erb-2 single-chain Fv molecules over a wide range of affinities for the same epitope. *Tumor Targeting* **2,** 154.
224. Weinstein, J. N., Eger, R. R., Covell, D. G., Black, C. D., Mulshine, J., Carrasquillo, J. A., et al. (1987) The pharmacology of monoclonal antibodies. *Ann. NY Acad. Sci.* **507,** 199–210.
225. Adams, G. P., Schier, R., McCall, A. M., Simmons, H. H., Horak, E. M., Alpaugh, R. K., Marks, J. D., and Weiner, L. M. (2001) High affinity restricts the localization and tumor penetration of single-chain Fv antibody molecules. *Cancer Res.* **61,** 4750–4755.
226. Crothers, D. M. and Metzger, H. (1972) The influence of polyvalency on the binding properties of antibodies. *Immunochemistry* **9,** 341–357.
227. Wu, A. M., Chen, W., Raubitschek, A., Williams, L. E., Neumaier, M., Fischer, R., et al. (1996) Tumor localization of anti-CEA single-chain Fvs: improved targeting by non-covalent dimers. *Immunotechnology* **2,** 21–36.
228. Goel, A., Colcher, D., Baranowska-Kortylewicz, J., Augustine, S., Booth, B. J., Pavlinkova, G., and Batra, S. K. (2000) Genetically engineered tetravalent single-chain Fv of the pancarcinoma monoclonal antibody CC49: improved biodistribution and potential for therapeutic application. *Cancer Res.* **60,** 6964–6971.
229. Nielsen, U. B., Adams, G. P., Weiner, L. M., and Marks, J. D. (2000) Targeting of bivalent anti-ErbB2 diabody antibody fragments to tumor cells is independent of the intrinsic antibody affinity. *Cancer Res.* **60,** 6434–6440.

II

HYBRIDOMA-DERIVED ANTIBODIES

3

DNA Immunization as a Means
to Generate Antibodies to Proteins

Partha S. Chowdhury

1. Introduction

For over a century now, antibodies have proven to be extremely useful reagents in biomedical research. They are also being tried as therapeutic agents for a number of intractable diseases. Their uses include identification and cloning of new genes from expression libraries, purification and structure-function analysis of proteins, histochemical localization of proteins, as diagnostic markers and/or probes, as targeting agents to deliver drugs and as magic bullets to bind and kill cells specifically among a long list of other uses to which they have been put.

The dawn of the functional genomics era has been accompanied by the surprising speed at which new protein coding genes are identified and cloned. To understand the basic biology of these new proteins such as their tissue and subcellular localization and association with other proteins one needs specific antibodies as tools. Many of these newly discovered proteins are also good targets for antibody-based drugs and the list of such proteins is increasing at a fast pace. As a result, the importance for generating antibodies against these proteins is great. The technology for raising antibodies has undergone radical change over the last few years. Currently there are two common ways to generate antibodies. One is by panning naïve phage antibody-display library on the relevant antigens. This technique has revolutionized the science of antibody development but is limited by the complexities of making and handling of large phage-display libraries and in some cases by the requirement for purified protein to pan the library. The other technique of procuring antibody is by xenogenic immunization with a purified protein or a cell line that expresses the protein. Although whole-cell immunization has been used successfully in several cases to raise antibodies against a particular antigen, it is usually a complicated process because a large number of antibodies to the irrelevant antigens of the cell are also generated. The method of choice therefore is to raise antibodies against a purified protein. While this has been practiced for a long time now, difficulty in raising desired antibodies against protein

From: *Methods in Molecular Biology, vol. 207: Recombinant Antibodies for Cancer Therapy: Methods and Protocols*
Edited by: M. Welschof and J. Krauss © Humana Press Inc., Totowa, NJ

antigens is quite frequent and the reasons can be attributed to the following facts *(1)*. Some proteins are difficult and sometimes impossible to purify, especially membrane-associated proteins *(2)*; sometime purification yields of proteins from natural sources are insufficient to support immunization procedures *(3)*; recombinant proteins made in *Escherichia coli* lack posttranslation modifications and folds differently to the extent that antibodies developed with these preparations fail to recognize the antigen in its natural form and *(4)* the whole process of purifying proteins for immunization is time-consuming and expensive.

Therefore, raising antibodies against native proteins and especially against membrane proteins is still not an easy task. These hurdles led to the technological development of the art of DNA immunization for the purpose of antibody development. The DNA used is simply a *E. coli*-derived plasmid DNA that is noninfectious and encode the protein of interest under the control of an eukaryotic constitutive promoter. The essence of the technique is that an animal injected with this eukaryotic expression vector takes up the plasmid into its cells, synthesizes the protein in its cell and presents it to the immune system *(1–2)*. Because the protein is made in a mammalian host, it is modified and folded in its native form and, because the protein is made in a xenogenic animal, it mounts an immune response. This development has made a large impact in the field of cell-mediated vaccine development and is gaining momentum in the field of humoral immunity. It is a good way to develop antibodies against a protein antigen without the necessity to purify the protein at all. Several successful studies have been reported about the use of DNA immunization to raise antibodies against specific proteins *(3–9)*. Most of these studies have been done in mice and a few in rabbits and nonhuman primates. It is evident from these studies that DNA immunization works both in small and large animals. Therefore, one can use it in mice to generate monoclonal antibodies (MAbs) or use it in large animals to generate large quantities of polyclonal antibodies (PAbs). Existing reports show that these antibodies can be used for a variety of purposes such as enzyme-linked immunosorbent assay (ELISA), Western blotting, and for cyto- and histochemical purpose both on fixed and live cells.

2. Materials

1. Plasmid: As the name indicates the plasmid containing the gene of interest is the foremost material required for DNA immunization. Typically it should contain an *E. coli* origin of replication, a mammalian origin of replication, an antibiotic resistance marker for *E. coli* and another for mammalian cell selection (e.g., Ampicillin and G418, respectively), a constitutive eukaryotic promoter (such as CMV) followed by a polycloning site to insert the cDNA of interest (*see* **Notes 1–3**).
2. *E. coli* strain: Any *E. coli* strain suitable for plasmid purification is sufficient (for example, DH5α).
3. Cell lines: HEK 293T, NIH 3T3, COS. Other cell lines negative for the cDNA of interest are also fine.
4. Transformation competent *E. coli* (e.g., DH5α).
5. Water bath.
6. LB plates with antibiotics for selection of the transformants.
7. 37°C incubators and shakers.

8. LB medium: To 900 mL of deionized water add 10 g Bacto-tryptone, 5 g Bacto-yeast extract, 10 g NaCl. Dissolve the solutes and adjust pH to 7.0 with 5 N NaOH. Adjust the volume to 1 L with deionized water. Sterilize by autoclaving for 20 min at 15 lb/sq. in on liquid cycle.

9. S.O.C. medium: To 80 mL water add 2 g Bacto-tryptone, 0.5 g Bacto-yeast extract, 54.4 mg NaCl, 18.64 mg potassium chloride, 95.2 mg magnesium chloride, 120 mg magnesium sulphate. Dissolve solutes. Adjust pH to 7.0 with 5 N NaOH. Adjust volume to 98 mL with deionized water. Sterilize by autoclaving for 20 min at 15 lb/sq. in on liquid cycle. Add 2 mL of a 1 M solution of sterile glucose and deionized water to make to volume to 100 mL.

10. 100 µg/mL Ampicillin for bacterial cultures.

11. DMEM and RPMI, fetal bovine serum (FBS), Penicillin-Streptomycin, Glutamine, G418 9 (or any other appropriate selection marker) for mammalian cell cultures. DMEM comes in many different formulations. Their use varies based on cell line being used and the laboratory. FBS is typically used at a concentration of 5–10%. Penicillin and Streptomycin are used at a concentration of 100 U/mL. L-Glutamine is typically used at 2 mM. G418 is used at 500 µg/mL.

12. Plasmid purification reagents: A number of commercial kits are available (e.g., Qiagen maxiprep kit).

13. 0.15 M NaCl, sterilize.

14. Insulin syringe.

15. Alcohol swabs.

16. ELISA plates.

17. Anti-mouse/anti-rabbit antibodies coupled to HRP/alkaline phosphatase. If a different animal other than mouse or rabbit is used for immunization, then a corresponding antibody should be available.

18. 35 mm Culture dishes or multi-chambered slides.

19. Animal restrainers.

20. ELISA reader.

21. Flurescence microscope.

22. Animals: Depends upon the preference of the investigator. The author has good experience using Balb/c female mice and Switzerland female rabbits.

3. Methods

In a DNA immunization experiment, one should be prepared for the following steps:

1. Actual immunization of animals with DNA;
2. Collection and screening/analysis of sera from the immunized animals for the production of the antibody; and, if necessary;
3. Cloning the antibody producing cells and genes.

The present chapter will deal with the immunization and screening of the animal sera only. Cloning of the antibody producing cells by the hybridoma technology and the genes by phage display or other technology are outside the scope of the current chapter and therefore will not be covered here.

DNA immunization for antibody generation can be done under several different situations. In one situation purified protein may be available that is insufficient for immunization (and hence the need for DNA immunization) but sufficient for screening by ELISA and/or Western blotting. In such a situation one may only need to immunize the animals and screen the sera for a humoral response by ELISA using the purified protein. In another situation there may not be any protein available for screening. Under such a circumstance one would have to either find out cell lines, one or more of which are positive and the others negative, for the antigen being encoded by the cDNA or generate positive and negative transfectants that can be used to screen the animal sera. Because mammalian cell transfections are not within the scope of this volumes, they will not be described here.

3.1. DNA Immunization

Prior to starting immunization, serum from every animal should be collected for use later on as control samples. Blood is usually collected from orbital sinus of mice and ear veins of rabbits. Let the blood clot at ambient temperature (22°C) or 37°C for about 2 h. Then keep it in ice for about 1 h. Collect the serum by centrifuging the clot at 11,000*g* in a microcentrifuge. Heat-inactivate the serum at 50°C for 20 min (*see* **Note 4**).

The DNA to be immunized should be purified with negligible or low endotoxin content.

1. Dose of DNA to be injected: The dose of DNA to be injected varies upon the animal used. Typically one can inject between 15–25 µg of DNA per mouse per injection for a total of 6–8 injections. In rabbits one may need to immunize with 300–400 µg DNA per immunization for a total of 4–5 immunizations.
   a. For immunizing mice dilute the plasmid DNA in 0.15 *M* NaCl to a concentration of 150–250 µg/mL just before use. Take 100 µL of this solution into 0.5 or 1 mL insulin syringe.
   b. For rabbit immunization dilute the DNA to 500 µg/mL. For each rabbit take 800 of this solution into a 1 mL hypodermic syringe with a 26G needle.
2. Route and site of injection: Irrespective of the animal used the DNA should be injected intradermally (*see* **Note 5**). The site of injection varies from one to another animal species. In mice good intradermal injections can be given in the tail. Elsewhere on a mouse the skin is so soft that it may be difficult and tricky to give an intradermal injection.
   a. Restrain the animals in a mouse holder pulling the tail out.
   b. Clean the tail with an alcohol swab.
   c. Insert the needle for injection about 2.5 cm from the base of the tail (where the tail joins the body) in the white area between the tail veins.
   d. Slowly inject 100 µL of the DNA solution (*see* **Note 6**). There should be no blood visible.
   In rabbits it is easier to give intradermal injections.
   a. Defoliate four 2 × 2 cm area on the thigh and back skin of a rabbit.
   b. Clean the area with an alcohol swab.
   c. Pull out the skin and gently insert the needle into the skin and inject the DNA solution. Again as in mouse it should be hard to push the plunger (*see* **Note 5**).
   d. Spacing of the injections: Typically at least 4–5 injections should be given 2–3 wk apart.

3.2. Analysis of Sera

About 1 wk after the last injection the sera should be analyzed for the presence of specific antibodies. Depending on the resources available, the sera can be analyzed by ELISA, Western blotting, and/or immunofluorescence. Because all these are common techniques, they are not described in detail in this chapter. The important points for each of these experiments are mentioned below.

1. ELISA: If purified protein is available, then ELISA should be done using this and one or more negative control proteins. If protein for ELISA is not available, then transfected and mock transfected cells can be used. Usually cells need to be fixed in 3.75% formaldehyde or glutaraldehyde in PBS before ELISA. For the first analysis, serum should be serially diluted starting from a dilution of about 1:25.
2. Western blotting: Western blotting can be done either with antigen positive and negative natural cells or transfected cells. A good dilution of antisera to start with is 1:20.
3. Immunoflurescence: As with Western blotting, this can be done either with natural cells or transfected cells. Immunoflurescence can be done either with live or fixed cells. If live cells are used, then the experiment needs to be done at 4°C (or on ice). If the antigen is intracellular, then the cells would have to be permeabilized with 0.1% saponin in PBS containing 4 mg/mL normal goat globulin (*see* **Note 7**) for 15 min at ambient temperature (22°C).
4. Booster immunizations: Once a response is detected fresh sera should be collected every week or alternate weeks and analyzed for the titer. With time one should see a drop in the titer of the serum samples. When the titer begins to drop, the animals should be immunized again and the sera analyzed 10–14 d later. This leads to a better immune response and therefore to the likelihood of getting better antibodies. **Figure 1A, B** shows the two different patterns of response the author has seen in his experiments.

4. Notes

1. The plasmid should preferably be high copy number plasmid to enable purification of sufficient amount of the plasmid without any difficulty.
2. The antibiotic resistance marker should specifically be for ampicillin. Studies have shown that ampicillin resistance gene contain CpG motifs that elicit a better immune response than others like kanamycin in DNA immunization studies.
3. In the authors experience pcDNA3/pcDNA3.1 from Clontech performs nicely in DNA immunization studies.
4. Heat-inactivation of the serum sometime (but not always) gives a high background in immunofluorescence experiments. The reason for this is not clearly understood. The author has found that using serum without inactivation do not cause any problem in live cells if the experiment is done at 4°C.
5. It is very important for the DNA to be injected intradermally for a good humoral response. The author and others have repeatedly found that subcutaneous and intramuscular injections do not elicit a very good response.
6. When injecting DNA intradermally into the tail of a mouse the skin should turn opaque as the solution goes in and the plunger of the syringe should be hard to push. If it goes in easily, be sure that it was not intradermal.
7. Normal goat globulin can be substituted by the globulin fraction from other common animal species. However, it should not crossreact with the secondary antibodies to globulin fraction of the sera being used.

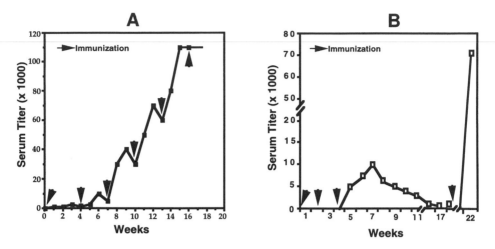

Fig. 1. Two different types of antisera response seen after DNA immunization into (**A**) mice and (**B**) rabbit. These responses were seen after immunization of pcDNA3 containing the cDNA for mesothelin. The pattern may vary from these for other antigens. The important point to note is that booster immunizations at a time when the serum titer drops leads to a remarkable antisera response.

References

1. Tang, D. C., DeVit, M., and Johnston, S. A. (1992) Genetic immunization is a simple method for eliciting an immune response. *Nature* **356**, 152–154.
2. Donnelly, J. J., Ulmer, J. B., Shiver, J. W., and Liu, M. (1997) DNA vaccines. *Annu. Rev. Immunol.* **15**, 617–648.
3. Sundaram, P., Xiao, W., and Brandsma, J. L. (1996) Particle-mediated delivery of recombinant expression vectors to rabbit skin induces high-titered polyclonal antisera (and circumvents purification of a protein immunogen). *Nucleic Acids Res.* **24**, 1375–1377.
4. Chowdhury, P. S., Viner, J. L., Beers, R., and Pastan, I. (1998) Isolation of a high-affinity stable single-chain Fv specific for mesothelin from DNA-immunized mice by phage display and construction of a recombinant immunotoxin with anti-tumor activity. *Proc. Natl. Acad. Sci. USA* **95**, 669–674.
5. Hinrichs, J., Berger, S., and Shaw, J. G. (1997) Induction of antibodies to plant viral proteins by DNA-based immunization. *J. Virol. Methods* **66**, 195–202.
6. Yeung, S. C., Anderson, J., Kobayashi, K., Oka, K., and Chan, L. (1997) Production of rabbit polyclonal antibody against apobec-1 by genetic immunization. *Lipid Res.* **38**, 2627–2632.
7. Gardsvoll, H., Solberg, H., Dano, K., and Hoyer-Hansen, G. (2000) Generation of high-affinity rabbit polyclonal antibodies to the murine urokinase receptor using DNA immunization. *J. Immunol. Methods* **234**, 107–116.
8. Chowdhury, P. S., Gallo, M., and Pastan, I. (2001) Generation of high titer antisera in rabbits by DNA immunization. *J. Immunol. Methods* **249**, 147–154.
9. Rozemuller, H., Chowdhury, P. S., Pastan, I., and Kreitman, R. J. (2001) Isolation of new anti-CD30 scFvs from DNA-immunized mice by phage display and biologic activity of recombinant immunotoxins produced by fusion with truncated pseudomonas exotoxin. *Int. J. Cancer* **92**, 861–870.

4

Chimerization of a Monoclonal Antibody for Treating Hodgkin's Lymphoma

Jürgen Krauss, Hans Heinrich Förster, Barbara Uchanska-Ziegler, and Andreas Ziegler

1. Introduction

Conventionally, monoclonal antibodies (MAbs) are generated by fusing B cells from an immunized animal with myeloma cells from the same species (*1*). Several murine MAb have already been employed for in vivo diagnosis and therapy, including Ber-H2 which recognizes the human CD30 molecule with high specificity and affinity (*2*). CD30, a member of the nerve growth factor (NGF) tumor necrosis factor receptor (TNFR) superfamily (*3*), is strongly expressed on the pathognomonic Hodgkin (H) and Reed-Sternberg (R-S) cells of Hodgkin's lymphoma (*4*) and various non-Hodgkin lymphomas of either T- or B-cell type origin (*5*). Its reaction pattern in normal lymphoid tissue is restricted to a population of blastoid cells located around B-cell follicles and at the rim of germinal centers (*2*). Consequently, Ber-H2 has been utilized as an immunotoxin by conjugating the antibody to the ribosome-inactivating toxin Saporin to treat four patients with refractory Hodgkin's lymphoma (*6*). However, despite remarkable tumor reductions of up to more than 75% were achieved after administration of one single dose of the reagent, patients developed an immune response against both the rodent immunoglobulin and the toxin moiety, precluding further application of the immunotoxin (*6*). In order to fully preserve the specificity of Ber-H2 and to overcome the aforementioned disadvantages, we have generated a chimeric mouse/human antibody.

Conventionally, chimeric antibodies are constructed by fusing the V_LJ- and V_HDJ-encoding cDNA to the C$\kappa_{/}\lambda$ and Cγ gene segments (*7–11*), respectively. In most cases, cDNA is amplified by PCR using degenerated primers (*12–14*). This approach modifies the 5' and 3' ends of the rearranged gene segments by introducing restriction sites for cloning, thus creating chimeric antibodies with non-authentic residues at both ends. Moreover, these constructs lack authentic leader peptide-V(D)J-C exon/intron junc-

From: *Methods in Molecular Biology, vol. 207: Recombinant Antibodies for Cancer Therapy: Methods and Protocols*
Edited by: M. Welschof and J. Krauss © Humana Press Inc., Totowa, NJ

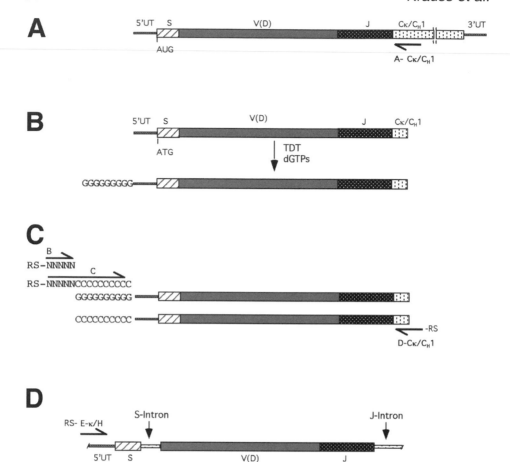

Fig. 1. Schematic representation of the isolation of rearranged genomic variable domains encoding gene segments from hybridoma cells by PCR. After isolation of RNA for the monoclonal antibody to be chimerized, cDNA synthesis of the rearranged variable gene segments of the L and H chains, respectively, is performed by using gene-specific primers A-Cκ/C$_H$1, matching the constant κ and C$_H$ domains, respectively (**A**). cDNA of V$_L$ and V$_H$, respectively, is extended by a poly-G-tail using Terminal Deoxynucleotidyl Transferase and dGTP's (**B**). Tailed cDNA is amplified by PCR using a combination of 5' primers B and C and gene specific primers D-Cκ/C$_H$1 matching the constant κ and C$_H$1 domains, respectively (**C**). For directional cloning and sequencing of the fragments, these primers introduce restriction cleavage sites. From sequence information of the 5'UT sequence and the rearranged J gene segment, primers Eκ/H binding in the 5'UT region of the L and H chains, respectively, and primers F-κ/H, matching part of the J-Intron sequence of the previously identified specific rearranged J gene segment of the L and H chains, respectively, can be designed. Thus, the PCR-amplified products contain the genomic rearranged V(D)J gene segments including the respective authentic leader peptide coding sequences of their murine counterparts (**D**).

tions with the respective splice sites, leading to low protein expression *(7,14)*, or even to nonexpression of the chimeric light chain due to the artificial signal peptide-VJ region fusion construct *(15)*. To circumvent these problems, we employed a method, first described by Weissenhorn and colleagues *(16)*, to isolate the genomic rearranged V(D)J gene segments including authentic leader peptide sequences of the light (L) and heavy (H) chains, respectively, by polymerase chain reaction (PCR).

We first deduced the authentic cDNA sequences of the mouse variable region gene segments including the 5'-untranslated (UT) region. This enabled us to design nondegenerated primers to amplify genomic V(D)J regions by PCR. The constructs contained the sequences coding for the original leader peptide and leader peptide intron, including authentic splice sites. Therefore, the expressed chimeric antibody contains the same authentic variable regions as the murine MAb. The schematic representation (*see* **Fig. 1**) summarizes the procedure for the chimerization of Ber-H2. To mediate natural effector functions (e.g., antibody-dependent cellular cytotoxicity, ADCC), we fused the variable regions to the human IgG1κ constant gene segments.

In conclusion, the chimerized reagent ChimBer-H2 has retained the antigen specificity of its murine ancestor, but can now be expected to be much less immunogenic with respect to its therapeutic application in humans. In addition, the chimerized reagent, unlike its murine ancestor, can be employed in ADCC (manuscript in preparation).

In principal, the procedure described below can be adapted to any other antibody of animal origin for eventual use in in vivo diagnostic or therapeutic procedures.

2. Materials
2.1. General Equipment

1. Miscellaneous: Appropriate biological hazard class II cabinets, freezers (–20°C, –80°C), refrigerators (4°C), liquid nitrogen tank for storage of cell lines.
2. Plastic material: Pipet tips, serological pipets, various types of disposable vessels and centrifuge tubes, multiple-well cell-culture plates, cell-culture flasks of various size.
3. Glassware: Clean and sterile Erlenmeyer flasks, beakers, bottles, etc., of various size.
4. Agarose gel electrophoresis supplies and respective power supplies.
5. Various centrifuges with fixed angle and swinging bucket rotors.
6. Ultracentrifuge (depending on method of mRNA isolation).
7. Cell culture incubator 37°C, 5% CO_2, humidified atmosphere.
8. Spectroalphotometer.
9. Various water baths.
10. Thermomixer (Eppendorf, Westbury, NY).
11. PCR Thermocycler (Perkin-Elmer, Branchburg, NJ).
12. Orbital shaker for bacterial cultures.
13. Electroporation apparatus (Gene Pulser II, Biorad, Life Science Research, Hercules, CA).
14. Enzyme-linked immunosorbent assay (ELISA) reader.
15. Flow cytometer (e.g., FACScan, Becton Dickinson) or fluorescence microscope.

2.2. Primers for cDNA Synthesis and PCR Amplification of V_H and V_L cDNA and Genomic DNA

1. A-$_C$κ: 5' AGATGGATACAGTTGGT
2. A-$_{CH1}$: 5' GGGGCCAGTGGATAGAC

3. B_{NotI}: 5' GCGCGGCCGCGGAGG
4. C_{NotI}: 5' GCGCGGCCGCGGAGGCCCCCCCCCCCCC
5. D-$C\kappa_{EcoRI}$: 5' GGAATTCGGATACAGTTGGTGCAGC
6. D-$CH1_{EcoRI}$: 5' GGAATTCGTGGATAGACAGATGGG
7. E-κ_{SalI}: 5' GATCGTCGACGGAAATGCATCAGACCAGCATGGGC
8. E-H_{SalI}: 5' CATAGTCGACAATACGATCAGCATCCTCTCCACAG
9. F-κ_{NotI}: 5' ATCAGCGGCCGCACTTAACAAGGTTAGACTTAGTG
10. F-H_{NotI}: 5' GATAGCGGCCGCATGCATTTAGAATGGGAGAAGTTAGG

2.3. Vectors

1. Cloning and sequencing vectors pGEM11zf+ and pGEM5zf+ (Promega, Madison, WI).
2. Expression vectors (*see* **Fig. 2**).

2.4. Preparation of Genomic DNA and Total RNA from Hybridoma Cells

1. Hybridoma cell line producing the MAb to be chimerized.
2. Eukaryotic cell growth medium: Dulbecco's modified Eagle's medium (DMEM) (Life Technologies, Rockville, MD) containing 10% heat-inactivated fetal calf serum (FCS) (*see* **Note 1**), 2 mM L-glutamine, 1 mM sodium pyruvate, 100 U/mL penicillin, 100 µg/mL streptomycin.
3. GT lysis buffer: 4 M guanidinium isothyocyanate, 25 mM sodium citrate, 0.5% (w/v) sodium dodecyl sulfate (SDS). Adjust pH to 7.0, filtrate through 0.22 µm filter, add 1% (v/v) 2-mercaptoethanol.
4. 20 mL Syringes and 0.8 × 40 mm canulas (Braun, Melsungen, Germany).
5. Cesium chloride density gradient: 2 mL 5.7 M CsCl, 1.5 mL 40% (w/v) CsCl, 1.5 mL 30% (w/v) CsCl, 1 mL 20% (w/v) CsCl.
6. PIC solution: 50 mL phenol, 2 mL isoamyl alcohol, 48 mL chloroform, vortex and store at room temperature [RT] in a light-protected bottle.
7. Double-distilled [dd]H$_2$O - Diethyl pyrocarbonate (DEPC) 0.1% (v/v).
8. Ethanol absolute and 70% (v/v).
9. 3 M Sodium acetate, pH 5.2.

2.5. cDNA Synthesis, "Tailing" and "Anchor"-PCR

1. Dimethyl sulfoxide (DMSO) (Sigma-Aldrich Corp., St. Louis, MO).
2. Ethanol absolute and 70% (v/v).
3. M-MLV Reverse Transcriptase and M-MLV Reverse Transcriptase 5X buffer (Life Technologies).
4. Dithiothreitol [DTT] (Sigma-Aldrich).
5. 6% Polyacrylamide gel containing 8 M urea.
6. [α-^{32}P]-dCTP (Amersham Pharmacia Biotech Inc., Piscataway, NJ).
7. dNTP (Roche Diagnostics Corp., Indianapolis, IN).
8. dGTP (Roche).
9. Ribonuclease Inhibitor (Stratagene, La Jolla, CA).
10. Ribonuclease A (Sigma).
11. PIC solution: *see* **Subheading 2.4.**, **item 6**.
12. ddH$_2$O.
13. 3MM Whatman paper (Whatman Inc., Clifton, NJ).
14. cDNA elution buffer: 0.5 M ammonium acetate, 1 mM EDTA, 0.1% (w/v) SDS.

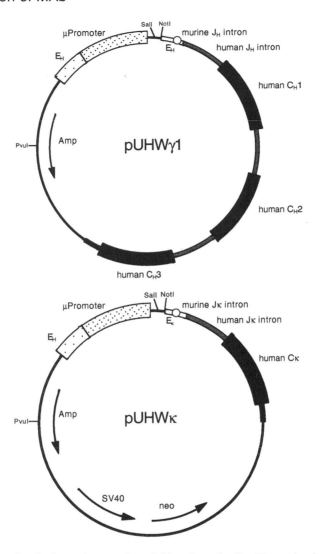

Fig. 2. Vectors for cloning and expression of chimeric antibodies. For equimolar expression of the chimeric L and H chains, both vectors contain a μ-heavy chain-promoter and a 5'μ-enhancer (EH). pUHWγ contains the human H chain constant regions and a mouse/human hybrid H chain intron including the mouse 3' H chain enhancer (EH). For selection in bacteria, the vector contains an ampicillin-resistance gene. For transfection, the plasmid can be linearized at its unique *Pvu*I restriction site. The PCR-amplified genomic V_LDJ gene segment can be cloned into pUHWγ as *Sal*I/*Not*I fragment. pUHWκ contains the human κ L chain constant region and a mouse/human hybrid L chain intron including the mouse 3' κ-enhancer (Eκ). The *neo* marker gene allows selection in eukaryotic cells under the control of an SV40 transcription unit. For selection in bacteria, the vector contains an ampicillin-resistance gene. For transfection, the plasmid can be linearized at its unique *Pvu*I restriction site. The PCR-amplified genomic V_LJ gene segment can be cloned into pUHWκ as *Sal*I/*Not*I fragment.

15. Terminal Deoxynucleotidyl Transferase and Terminal Deoxynucleotidyl Transferase 5X buffer (Life Technologies) (*see* **Note 2**).
16. Bovine serum albumin [BSA] (Life Technologies) (*see* **Note 1**).
17. *Vent* DNA polymerase and 10X PCR buffer (New England Biolabs Inc., Beverly, MA).
18. 1% (w/v) and 2% (w/v) agarose gels.
19. QIAquick gel extraction kit (Qiagen, Valencia, CA).
20. PCR purification kit (Qiagen).
21. Restriction endonucleases *Eco*RI, *Not*I, and respective buffers (New England Biolabs).
22. Calf intestine phosphatase [CIP] (Amersham Pharmacia Biotech) (*see* **Note 1**).
23. 0.5 M EDTA stock solution, pH 8.0.
24. Ethanol absolute and 70% (v/v).
25. T4 ligase and 10X ligase buffer (Roche).
26. Glycogen 35 mg/mL (Life Technologies).
27. Ampicillin: Prepare stock solution 100 mg/mL, sterilize by filtration through 0.22 µm filter, store at –20°C.
28. XLI Blue electroporation competent cells (Stratagene).
29. Electroporation cuvets 0.1 cm (Bio-Rad, Life Science Research, Hercules, CA).
30. SOC medium: 2% (w/v) tryptone, 0.5% (w/v) yeast extract, 10 mM NaCl, 2.5 mM KCl, 10 mM MgCl$_2$, 10 mM MgSO$_4$, 20 mM glucose.
31. LBA medium: Autoclave 10 g tryptone, 5 g yeast extract, and 5g NaCl in 1000 mL ddH$_2$O at 121°C for 15 min. Let cool down in a 45°C preheated water bath, add sterile ampicillin solution to a final concentration of 100 µg/mL.
32. LBA agar plates: Autoclave 10 g tryptone, 5 g yeast extract, 5g NaCl and 1.5% (w/v) bacto agar in 1000 mL ddH$_2$O at 121°C for 15 min. Let cool down in a 45°C preheated water bath, add sterile ampicillin solution to a final concentration of 100 µg/mL. Pour about 20 mL LBA agar solution into each of 85mm Ø Petri dish. Store agar plates at 4°C.
33. Plasmid preparation kits (Qiagen Mini and Midi kit, or similar kits).

2.6. PCR Amplification and Cloning of Genomic Rearranged Variable Gene Segments into Eukaryotic Expression Vectors

1. ddH$_2$O.
2. *Vent* DNA polymerase and 10X PCR buffer (New England Biolabs).
3. Restriction endonucleases *Sal*I, *Not*I and respective buffers (New England Biolabs).
4. Calf intestine phosphatase (CIP) (Amersham Pharmacia Biotech) (*see* **Note 1**).
5. 0.5 M EDTA stock solution, pH 8.0.
6. 0.8% (w/v) and 1,5% (w/v) agarose gels.
7. 0.5 M NaOH.
8. NA45-DEAE membrane (Schleicher & Schüll Inc., West Palm Beach, FL).
9. NA45-DEAE membrane washing buffer: 0.1 mM EDTA 20 mM Tris-HCl, 0.15 M NaCl, adjust pH to 8.0. Store at room temperature.
10. NA45-DEAE membrane elution buffer: 0.1 mM EDTA 20 mM Tris-HCl, 2.5 M NaCl, adjust pH to 8.0. Store at room temperature.
11. Ethanol absolute and 70% (v/v).
12. T4 ligase and 10X ligase buffer (Roche).
13. Glycogen 35 mg/mL (Life Technologies).
14. Ampicillin 100 mg/mL (*see* **Subheading 2.5.**, **item 27**)
15. XLI Blue electroporation competent cells (Stratagene).
16. Electroporation cuvets 0.1 cm (Bio-Rad, Life Science Research).

17. SOC medium: (*see* **Subheading 2.5.**, **item 30**).
18. LBA medium (*see* **Subheading 2.5.**, **item 31**).
19. LBA agar plates (*see* **Subheading 2.5.**, **item 32**).
20. Plasmid preparation kit (Qiagen Mini kit).
21. EndoFree® plasmid kit (Qiagen).

2.7. Stable Transfection of Eukaryotic Expression Vectors into Myeloma Cells

1. Restriction endonuclease *Pvu*I and respective buffer (New England Biolabs).
2. 0.8% (w/v) Agarose gel.
3. 0.5 *M* NaOH.
4. NA45-DEAE membrane (Schleicher & Schüll Inc.).
5. NA45-DEAE membrane washing buffer: 0.1 m*M* EDTA, 20 m*M* Tris-HCl, 0.15 *M* NaCl, adjust pH to 8.0. Store at room temperature.
6. NA45-DEAE membrane elution buffer: 0.1 m*M* EDTA, 20 m*M* Tris-HCl, 2.5 *M* NaCl, adjust pH to 8.0. Store at room temperature.
7. Ethanol absolute and 70% (v/v).
8. Mouse myeloma cell line Sp2/0-Ag14 (ATCC-CRL 1581).
9. 2X Transfection buffer: 40 m*M* HEPES, 274 m*M* NaCl, 10 m*M* KCl, 1.4 m*M* $Na_2HPO_4 \cdot 2H_2O$, 12 m*M* dextrose, adjust pH to 7.5.
10. Sterile ddH_2O.
11. Sterile electroporation cuvet 0.4 cm (Bio-Rad, Life Science Research).
12. 50-mL Cell-culture flasks.
13. Eukaryotic cell growth medium (*see* **Subheading 2.4.**, **item 2**).
14. Geneticin (G418): Prepare stock solution 1000 mg/mL, sterilize by filtration through 0.22 µm filter, store at 4°C.
15. 96-Well flat bottom tissue culture dish (Nalgene Nunc International, Rochester, NY).

2.8. Expression of Chimeric Antibodies

1. 96-Well ELISA microplates (Nalgene Nunc International).
2. ELISA coating buffer: 50 m*M* sodium hydrogen carbonate, adjust pH to 9,6.
3. ELISA washing buffer: 0.05% (v/v) Tween 20 in phosphate-buffered saline (PBS).
4. ELISA blocking buffer: 2% (w/v) nonfat dry milk in ELISA washing buffer.
5. ELISA substrate buffer: 0.1 *M* citric acid, 0.2 *M* Na2HPO4, adjust pH to 5.0. Add 9 mg orthophenyldiamine per 25 mL buffer and 6-10 µL H_2O_2. Prepare buffer shortly before use.
6. Goat-anti-human-Fcγ fragment-specific serum (Jackson Immuno Research Laboratories Inc., West Grove, PA).
7. Rabbit-anti-human-κ-human IgG, horseradish peroxidase conjugated (Dako Corp., Carpinteria, CA).
8. Goat-anti-human-Fcγ fragment-specific IgG, FITC conjugated (Jackson Immuno Research Laboratories Inc., West Grove, PA)
9. Serial dilution of human imunoglobulin (0.1–1000 ng) as a positive control.
10. 12.5% (v/v) H_2SO_4.

2.9. Upscaling of Chimeric Antibodies in Eukaryotic Cells

1. Eukaryotic cell growth medium (*see* **Subheading 2.4.**, **item 2**).
2. Balanced salt solution (BSS) (Life Technologies) (*see* **Note 3**).
3. Hank's balanced salt solution (HBSS) (Life Technologies) (*see* **Note 3**).

4. BSS or HBSS /0.1%NaN$_3$: BSS or HBSS containing 0.1% sodium azide. Store at 4°C.
5. BSS or HBSS /1%BSA/0.1% NaN$_3$: BSS or HBSS containing 1% BSA (*see* **Note 1**) and 0.1% sodium azide. Store at 4°C.
6. Cryopreservation medium: for freezing of $5 \times 10^6 - 1 \times 10^7$ cells use 1 mL medium composed of 90% FCS (*see* **Note 1**) and 10% DMSO prechilled to 4°C (*see* **Note 4**).
7. PFHM-II: Complete protein-free medium supporting hybridoma growth (Life Technologies).

3. Methods

3.1. Isolation of Genomic DNA and Total RNA

1. Grow $5 \times 10^7 - 1 \times 10^8$ cells of the MAb-producing hybridoma cell line at 37°C, 5% CO$_2$ in eukaryotic cell growth medium (*see* **Note 5**).
2. Centrifuge cells at 200g, 4°C, 10 min, discard supernatant, and resuspend pellet in 5 mL GT lysis buffer.
3. Push lysate 10–15 times through a 20 mL syringe equipped with a 0.8×40 mm hypodermic needle canula (*see* **Note 6**).
4. Transfer lysate onto cesium chloride density gradient (*see* **Note 7**).
5. Ultracentrifuge tube at 200,000g, 4°C, 16 h without braking.
6. Discard upper protein band.
7. Harvest genomic DNA, visualized as a distinct band, by slowly aspirating with a 5 mL serological pipet and transfer to a fresh 15 mL tube. Save the vial at 4°C! You will need it for the isolation of total RNA (*see* **Subheading 3.1.**, **step 13**).
8. Add one sample volume of ddH$_2$O to DNA suspension.
9. To remove remaining protein from the preparation, add an equal sample volume of PIC solution, vortex, and centrifuge at 20,000g, 20°C, 15 min. Collect the DNA-containing upper phase using a serological pipet and transfer to a fresh tube.
10. Precipitate DNA at room temperature for 60 min by adding one sample volume of isopropanole. Centrifuge sample at 20,000g, 20°C, 60 min.
11. Discard supernatant, wash pellet twice with 500 μL 70% ethanol, let air-dry for 10 min.
12. Resuspend genomic DNA in 100 μL ddH$_2$O. Determine OD$_{260}$ in a spectroalphotometer and calculate DNA concentration. Store sample at 4°C.
13. Discard remaining supernatant from the ultracentrifuge tube (*see* **Subheading 3.1.**, **step 7**) and harvest total RNA, visible as a glassy pellet at the bottom of the vial, by dissolving in 400 μL ddH$_2$O-DEPC (*see* **Note 8**).
14. Precipitate RNA at –20°C overnight by adding 2.5 sample volumes 100% ethanol and 1/10 sample volume of 3 M sodium acetate, pH 5.2.
15. Centrifuge at 20,000g, 4°C, 60 min. Discard supernatant, wash pellet twice with 500 μL 70% ethanol, let air-dry for 10 min.
16. Dissolve total RNA in 100 μL sterile ddH$_2$O-DEPC. Determine OD$_{260}$ in a spectroalphotometer and calculate total RNA concentration. Use 20–50 μg of total RNA for each subsequent cDNA synthesis reaction (*see* **Note 9**).
17. Store remainng RNA after precipitation (*see* **Subheading 3.1.**, **step 14**) at –80°C.

3.2. cDNA Synthesis

1. Denature RNA by adding 375 μL DMSO and incubate 20 min at 45°C in a water bath.
2. Add 2.5 sample volumes of 100% ethanol and 1/10 sample volume of 3 M sodium acetate pH 5.2 to the reaction tube, allow precipitation of RNA at –20°C overnight.
3. Centrifuge, wash, and let RNA air-dry as described in **Subheading 3.1.**, **step 15**.

4. Dissolve RNA in 10 μL 5X M-MLV Reverse transcriptase buffer.
5. For cDNA synthesis of V_L and V_H, carry out two different reactions by adding 50 pmol primer from **Subheading 2.2.**, **items 1** or **2**, matching the Cκ and C_H1 region, respectively, 0.1 mM DTT, 20 μCi [α-^{32}P]-dCTP, 200 U M-MLV-Reverse Transcriptase, 1 mM dNTPs and 2 U Ribonuclease Inhibitor (*see* **Note 10**).
6. Incubate at 37°C for 90 min in a water bath.
7. Digest RNA by adding 50 μg Ribonuclease A for 30 min at 37°C, remove enzyme by adding 1 sample volume PIC solution, vortex, and centrifuge sample at 20,000g, 20°C, 15 min. Transfer upper phase containing cDNA to a fresh tube.
8. Precipitate, centrifuge and wash synthesized cDNA as described for RNA in **Subheading 3.1.**, **steps 14** and **15**. Add 1 μL glycogen (35 mg/mL) prior to precipitation to help pellet identification. Dissolve in 8 μL ddH$_2$O.
9. Load sample on 6% polyacrylamide gel containing 8 M urea and run electrophoresis at 55 W and 54°C for 2 h. Use α^{32}P-labeled 100 bp ladder as a reference.
10. Transfer gel onto a precut 3MM Whatman paper, wrap into saran foil and expose to X-ray film for 12 h in a cassette (*see* **Note 11**). Develop film.
11. Excise gel fragments corresponding to the visualized bands representing the V_L and V_H fragments, respectively, and transfer into a clean 1.,5 mL tube.
12. Elute DNA by incubation with 2 M ammonium acetate for 3 h at 37°C and 250 rpm in an Eppendorf thermomixer.
13. Precipitate and wash cDNA (*see* **Subheading 3.1.**, **steps 14** and **15**). Add 1 μL glycogen (35 mg/mL) prior to precipitation to help pellet identification. Dissolve in 10 μL H$_2$O.

3.3. cDNA "Tailing"

1. For the "tailing" reaction, add 1 mM dGTPs, 4 μL Terminal Deoxynucleotidyl Transferase 5X buffer (*see* **Note 2**), 33 U Terminal Deoxynucleotidyl Transferase and 2 μg BSA to 5 μL of the dissolved cDNA from **Subheading 3.2.**, **step 13**. Add ddH$_2$O to a total volume of 20 μL.
2. Incubate reaction tube at 37°C for 1 h in a water bath. Add 1 sample volume PIC solution, vortex, and centrifuge sample at 20,000g, 20°C, 15 min. Aspirate aequeous upper phase and transfer to a fresh tube.
3. Precipitate, centrifuge and wash tailed cDNA as described in **Subheading 3.1.**, **steps 14** and **15**. Add 1 μL glycogen (35 mg/mL) prior to precipitation to help pellet identification. Dissolve in 20 μL ddH$_2$O.

3.4. "Anchor"-PCR

1. To amplify tailed V_L cDNA by PCR, add 10 pmol of primer from **Subheading 2.2.**, **item 4**, 25 pmol of primer **Subheading 2.2.**, **items 3** and **5** each, 2 μL 10X PCR buffer, 1 U *Vent* DNA polymerase to 5 μL of a serial dilution (*see* **Note 12**) of tailed cDNA from **Subheading 3.3.**, **step 3**. Add ddH$_2$O to a total volume of 10 μL.
2. To amplify tailed V_H cDNA by PCR, add 10 pmol of primer from **Subheading 2.2.**, **item 4**, 25 pmol of primer from **Subheading 2.2.**, **items 3** and **6**. each, 2 μL 10X PCR buffer, 1 U *Vent* DNA polymerase to 5 μL of a serial dilution (*see* **Note 12**) of tailed cDNA from **Subheading 3.3.**, **step 3**. Add ddH$_2$O to a total volume of 20 μL.
3. Run PCR with the following program: 94°C, 5 min; 30 cycles 94°C, 1 min, 50°C, 1 min, 72°C, 2 min; 72°C, 10 min; 4°C.
4. Analyze the PCR-amplified fragments by electrophoresis on a 2% agarose gel (*see* **Note 13**).

5. If fragment size is correct (V_L~450 bp, V_H~550 bp, depending on the length of the 5'UT region), run preparative 2% agarose gel prestained with ethidium bromide, excise fragments, and recover DNA by using a QIAquick gel extraction kit.

6. Digest 250 ng of the PCR products representing V_L and V_H with 20 U each of *Not*I and *Eco*RI, respectively, in the appropriate restriction endonuclease buffer in a total volume of 50 μL for 4 h at 37°C. To inactivate endonucleases incubate the digest for 20 min at 65°. Purify cleaved DNA by using a Qiagen PCR purification kit.

7. For directional cloning of the fragments into the sequencing vector pGem 11zf+ digest 5 μg plasmid DNA with 20 U each of *Not*I and *Eco*RI, respectively, in the appropriate restriction endonuclease buffer for 2 h at 37°C in a total volume of 50 μL. To dephosphorylate the vector, add 0.5 U CIP to the restriction digest. After 2 h incubation time, add another 0.5 U CIP to the reaction mix and continue incubation for 2 more h. To inactivate CIP and restriction endonucleases, add EDTA, pH 8.0, to a final concentration of 5 mM and incubate at 65°C for 20 min. Apply the restriction digest on a preparative 1% agarose gel prestained with ethidium bromide, excise the cleaved vector with a sharp scalpel, and recover the DNA by using a QIAquick gel extraction kit.

8. Determine DNA concentrations from preparations of **steps 6** and **7**.

9. Ligate inserts into 50 ng of sequencing vector pGEM 11zf+ in a molar ratio of vector:insert = 1:3 by adding 1 U T4 ligase, 1 μL 10X ligase buffer and ddH$_2$O to a total volume of 10 μL. Perform ligation overnight at 16°C.

10. Precipitate, spin, and wash DNA as described in **Subheading 3.1.**, **steps 14** and **15**. Add 1 μL glycogen (35 mg/mL) prior to precipitation to help pellet identification. Dissolve DNA in 10 μL ddH$_2$O.

11. For electroporation, mix 5 μL of ligation product and 5 μL electrocompetent *E. coli* cells on ice. Add ice-cold ddH$_2$O to a total volume of 50 μL and transfer to a 0.1 cm electroporation cuvet, precooled on ice.

12. Pulse cells using the following settings of the electroporation apparatus: 1700 V, 200 Ω, 25 μF. Add 1 mL SOC medium into the cuvet immediately after pulse delivery.

13. Transfer suspension into a clean 15 mL tube and shake cells at 37°C for 1 h. Plate 100 μL onto LBA agar plates and incubate plates at 37°C overnight.

14. Pick 10 clones each for V_H and V_L, respectively, prepare plasmid DNA using a Qiagen Miniprep kit and confirm successful insert ligation by restriction digest.

15. Sequence 5 clones each for V_H and V_L, respectively, by standard procedures.

16. Align deduced sequences of 5 clones of V_H and V_L, respectively, to each other to detect possible mutations introduced by PCR. As a reference, align sequences to the most homologous V_H/V_L subgroup sequence entries in the KABAT *(17,18)* or IMGT *(19)* database (*see* **Note 14**).

3.5. PCR Amplification and Cloning
of Rearranged Genomic V_H and V_L Gene Segments

1. Choose the sequence of a "non-mutated" V_H and V_L clone each without individual mutations for design of primers to amplify genomic rearranged V_HDJ and V_LJ gene segments. The 5' primers (from **Subheading 2.2.**, **item 7** for the light chain; from **Subheading 2.2.**, **item 8** for the heavy chain, respectively) match the deduced sequence in the 5'UT region. 3' primers (from **Subheading 2.2**, **item 9** for the light chain; from **Subheading 2.2.**, **item 10** for the heavy chain, respectively) anneal to the sequence of the respective invariant J segment intron of the identified rearranged J gene segments. All primers introduce overhanging restriction endonuclease cleavage sites for directional cloning into expression vectors.

2. To amplify chromosomal DNA by PCR, dilute sample from **Subheading 3.1.**, **step 12** 1:5, 1:10, 1:20, 1:50, 1:100, 1:200 1:500 and 1:1000 in ddH$_2$O (*see* **Note 12**).

3. Add 25 pmol of each primer (**Subheading 2.2.**, **items 7** and **9** for amplification of the light chain, from **Subheading 2.2.**, **items 8** and **10** for amplification of the heavy chain, respectively), 5 µL 10X PCR buffer, 1 U *Vent* DNA polymerase to 5 µL of diluted genomic DNA samples from **Subheading 3.5.**, **step 2**. Add ddH$_2$O to a total volume of 50 µL.

4. Run PCR with the following program: 94°C, 5 min; 25 cycles 94°C, 1 min, 50–55°C, 2 min, 72°C, 2 min; 72°C, 10 min; 4°C.

5. Analyze the PCR-amplified fragments by electrophoresis on a 1.5% agarose gel.

6. If fragments are of correct size (V$_L$~750 bp, V$_H$~600 bp, depending on the length of the leader peptide intron), run preparative 1.5% agarose gel prestained with ethidium bromide. Excise fragments representing the amplified genomic rearranged VL/VH gene segments from the gel, recover and subclone PCR products in vector pGEM 5zf+ as *Sal*I/*Not*I fragments (*see* **Note 15**) and determine sequence of the subclones as described in **Subheading 3.4.**, **steps 5–15**.

7. Align deduced sequences of 5 clones of V$_H$ and V$_L$, respectively, to each other to detect possible mutations introduced by PCR. As a reference, align sequences to the previously determined cDNA sequences.

8. Choose "nonmutated" V$_H$ and V$_L$ clones, respectively, for cloning into eukaryotic expression vectors (*see* **Fig. 2**) and perform plasmid preparations of these clones using a Qiagen Midi kit.

9. Digest 5 µg of sequenced plasmid DNA containing the selected VH and VL clones, respectively, by adding 20 U each of *Sal*I and *Not*I restriction endonucleases, 5 µL of the appropriate 10X restriction buffer and ddH$_2$O to a total volume of 50 µL. Incubate at 37°C for 4 h.

10. Run preparative 1.5% agarose gel, excise insert fragments, and recover DNA by using a QIAquick gel extraction kit.

11. Prepare plasmid DNA of expression vectors using a Qiagen Midi kit. Digest 5 µg plasmid DNA of vectors pUHWκ for expression of the light chain, and pUHWγ for expression of the heavy chain, respectively, by adding 15 U each of *Sal*I and *Not*I restriction endonucleases, 5 µL of the appropriate 10X restriction buffer, 0.25 U CIP and ddH$_2$O to a total volume of 50 µL. After incubation at 37°C for 2 h add 0.25 U CIP to the reaction and continue incubation for another 2 h. To inactivate CIP and restriction endonucleases, add EDTA, pH 8.0, to a final concentration of 5 m*M* and incubate at 65°C for 20 min.

12. To recover cleaved vector DNA by blotting, prepare NA45-DEAE membranes (*see* **Note 16**).

13. Size fraction vector DNA from **Subheading 3.5.**, **step 11**. on a 0.8% agarose gel prestained with ethidium bromide by electrophoresis at 90 V for 90 min. Visualize bands representing V$_H$ and V$_L$, respectively, by exposing the gel to UV light at 260 nm. Apply slit to the gel 3 mm above the V$_L$ and V$_H$ representing bands using a clean scalpel. Transfer the previously pretreated (*see* **Note 16**) and precut NA45-DEAE membrane into the slot.

14. To blot DNA onto the membrane, run electrophoresis with reverse polarity at 90 V for 10 min. Wash membrane with 300 µL NA45-DEAE membrane washing buffer and transfer to a fresh reaction tube. Elute DNA in NA45-DEAE membrane elution buffer at 65°C for 30 min.

15. Transfer eluted DNA into a fresh reaction tube and recover remaining membrane-bound DNA by repeating the elution step.

16. Precipitate DNA by adding 2.5 sample volumes of 100% ethanol at –20°C overnight. Add 1 µL glycogen (35 mg/mL) prior to precipitation to help pellet identification.

17. Centrifuge sample at 20,000g, 4°C, 60 min. Discard supernatant, wash pellet twice with 500 µL 70% ethanol, let air-dry for 10 min. Dissolve in 30 mL ddH$_2$O.
18. Determine DNA concentrations from preparations in **Subheading 3.5.**, **steps 10** and **17**.
19. Ligate inserts into 200–300 ng of expression vectors in a molar ratio of vector:insert = 1:10–1:50 (*see* **Note 17**) by adding 1 U T4 ligase, 1 µL 10X ligase buffer and ddH$_2$O to a total volume of 10 µL. Perform ligation overnight at 16°C.
20. Precipitate, spin and wash DNA as described in **Subheading 3.1.**, **steps 14** and **15**. Dissolve DNA in 10 µL ddH$_2$O.
21. Perform transformation in *E. coli* cells as described in steps **Subheading 3.4.**, **steps 11–13**.
22. Pick 10 clones each for the V$_H$ and V$_L$, respectively, prepare plasmid DNA using a Qiagen Miniprep kit and confirm successful insert ligation by restriction digest.
23. Prepare plasmid DNA of one clone each of V$_H$ and V$_L$ containing expression vectors using a Qiagen EndoFree® plasmid kit (*see* **Note 18**).

3.6. Stable Transfection of Eukaryotic Expression Vectors into Sp2/0-Ag14 Myeloma Cells

1. Linearize 8 µg of eukaryotic plasmids pUHWκ and pUHWγ, respectively, at their unique restriction sites (*see* **Fig. 2**) by adding 30 U *Pvu*I, 5 µL of the appropriate 10X restriction buffer and ddH$_2$O to a total volume of 50 µL. Incubate at 37°C for 2–4 h.
2. Recover DNA as described in **Subheading 3.5.**, **steps 12–17** and determine DNA concentration.
3. Use 4 µg of each linearized plasmid for subsequent cotransfection of the heavy chain and light chain into mouse myeloma cells.
4. Grow 1 × 10^6 Sp2/0-Ag14 cells per transfection at 37°C and 5%CO$_2$ in eukaryotic cell growth medium.
5. Centrifuge cells at 200g, 4°C, 10 min. Discard supernatant and perform all further steps on ice.
6. Resuspend cells in 400 µL ice cold 2X transfection buffer, add 4 µg of each linearized plasmid from **Subheading 3.6.**, **step 2** and ice cold ddH$_2$O to a total volume of 800 µL and transfer to a sterile 0.4 cm transfection cuvet, precooled on ice, and incubate for 10 min.
7. Insert cuvet into electroporation chamber and apply pulse at 0.27 kV, 0.675 kV/cm, and 960 µF (*see* **Note 19**).
8. Incubate transfected cells on ice for 10 min.
9. Transfer suspension to a 30 mL cell-culture flask, add 10 mL prewarmed eukaryotic cell growth medium containing 20% FCS (*see* **Note 1**) and incubate at 37°C/5% CO$_2$ in humidity for 48 h. Do not add selection antibiotic at this stage.
10. After 48 h, let cells grow under selection pressure by adding G418, starting with a concentration of 0.8 mg/mL of culture medium. Increase antibiotic concentration gradually up to 1.2 mg/mL within 14 d (*see* **Note 20**).

3.7. Expression of Chimeric Antibodies

1. Formation of resistant clones should be visible within 14–16 d after transfection. Clone cells as soon as possible to obtain the maximum amount of different clones being transfected.
2. For cloning of cells, prepare sterile 96-well plates, centrifuge tubes and pipets.
3. Warm up eukaryotic cell growth medium containing 10–20% FCS (*see* **Note 1**) without antibiotics at 37°C. Add G418 to a final concentration of 1.2 mg/mL just before use.

4. Take transfected cells from the 37°C/5%CO$_2$ humidified incubator, transfer them into a conical centrifuge tube and centrifuge at 170g at room temperature for 5 min.

5. Resuspend cells in a small volume of fresh medium and count them.

6. Prepare serial dilutions with fresh medium calculating 10 cells/well for the first 2 rows of a 96-well plate. The next 3 rows should contain 2 cells/well and the last 3 rows on average 0.4 cells/well in a total volume of 0.2 mL of the cell suspension per well. Feeder cells should be either distributed into the plates before cloning, or be contained in the medium used for the dilution steps (*see* **Note 21**).

7. Place plates into the humid incubator at 37°C/5%CO$_2$. Check every day for contaminations, keep cells outside of the incubator as short as possible.

8. In the meantime, grow cells expressing the target antigen (e.g., CD30) or prepare antigen for activity testing of culture supernatants (*see* **Note 22**).

9. The first colonies may already be visible 4 d after cloning, usually in the first 2 rows. For picking colonies, however, choose cells growing in the last 3 rows if possible, since they most likely originate from single clones. Usually, a change of medium is not required during the first 2 wk.

10. When single colonies cover one-third of the bottom of the well, collect supernatant for testing of the expression of the human heavy chain constant domains by ELISA (*see* **Note 23**).

11. Coat ELISA plates with 100 µL/well of a goat-anti-human IgG Fcγ fragment specific serum diluted in ELISA coating buffer in a final concentration of 10 µg/mL.

12. Incubate plates at 4°C for 12 h. Wash plates 3× with 200 µL/well ELISA washing buffer.

13. To prevent unspecific protein binding, block with 200 µL/well using ELISA blocking buffer. Incubate 1 h at room temperature. Wash plates 3× with 200 µL/well ELISA washing buffer.

14. Apply 100 µL/well of supernatants from reclones, serially diluted in ELISA blocking buffer (*see* **Note 24**), to the plates. Incubate 1 h at RT. Wash plates 3× with 200 µL/well of ELISA washing buffer.

15. Apply 100 µL/well of a horseradish peroxidase conjugated rabbit-anti-κ-human IgG, 1:5000 diluted in blocking buffer to the plates and incubate 1 h at room temperatureRT. Wash plates 3× with 200 µL/well of ELISA washing buffer.

16. Detect positive clones by adding 200 µL/well substrate buffer and stop reaction after 15 min by adding 50 µL/well 12.5% (v/v) H$_2$SO$_4$.

17. Determine absorbance in an ELISA microtiter plate reader using a serial dilution of human immunoglobin as a standard.

18. Choose the best MAb-producing clones to examine specific binding to cell surface antigens by, e.g., flow cytometry analysis. Remove all inactive clones to avoid cross-contamination.

19. Pick positive clones with a Pasteur pipet when they are about 50% confluent in the well, and transfer each clone into separate wells of a 24-well plate containing 0.5 mL of fresh eukaryotic cell growth/G418 medium. At this point, also new feeder cells may be added. Fill the original well again with medium and keep until positive growth is noticed in the 24-well plate.

20. Collect culture supernatants for testing of activity (ELISA, FACScan etc.) after the cells of each colony cover one-third of the bottom of the well.

21. Either split positive clones into new wells of a 24-well plate or take two-thirds of the volume of the well and transfer the cells into a small culture flask. Add fresh medium.

22. After 1 or 2 d of additional culture, enough cells will be available for preservation by freezing. Centrifuge cells at 4°C in a conical tube at 170g for 10 min, collect supernatant for activity testing. Discard supernatant, resuspend the cell pellet gently in 1 mL of freezing medium prechilled to 4°C, and transfer to freezing vials (*see* **Note 25**).

23. Positive clones have to be grown further for the production of antibody and for the freezing of at least 10 vials/clone containing 1×10^7 cells each.

24. For clinical applications, antibodies are required to grow under serum-free culture conditions. For this purpose, seed cells in 24-well plates. After cells start to double, remove half of the medium and substitute it with serum-free PFHM-II medium. Repeat several times until cells will grow in 100% serum-free medium. Give cells time to adjust to new culture conditions between each medium change. For each subculture, use different serum-free formulations. In case of the ChimBer-H2 antibody, we were able to establish clones growing in PFHM-II medium in 3 wk.

4. Notes

1. Recent epidemic study of bovine spongiform encephalopathy (BSE) illustrates that transmissions from species to species can occur, although this is probably a very rare event. Therefore, exercise caution when employing animal sera or serum-derived proteins.

2. The buffer contains the highly toxic substances potassium cacodylate and $CoCl_2$. Wear gloves and safety goggles when working with these substances.

3. Routinely, we use calcium- and magnesium-free BSS and Hank's BSS. Both solutions are commercially available.

4. Although expensive in terms of FCS used, this freezing medium has been shown to give good viability results with hybridoma cells, even after storing cells for more than 10 yr in liquid nitrogen.

5. To obtain the maximum amount of mRNA, cells should be harvested in the logarithmic growth phase.

6. Alternatively, cells can be sonicated (200 W, 20 s). Using this method, however, we found a substantial loss of mRNA.

7. By using a cesium chloride density gradient and ultracentrifugation, RNA and genomic DNA of high quality can be isolated at the same time. Alternatively, RNA and DNA can also simultaneously be extracted using the RNA/DNA system kit (Qiagen) or similar kits.

8. Work in a sterile environment during RNA preparation. Use only sterile equipment specially prepared to work with RNA.

9. The quality of RNA preparations can be assessed by applying a small aliquot of RNA onto a MOPS gel. Ribosomal subunits should be clearly visible.

10. For first strand cDNA synthesis followed by subsequent 5'RACE (rapid amplification of cDNA ends)–PCR, the Marathon™ cDNA amplification kit (Clontech) or similar kits can also be used.

11. Apply fluorescent markers onto the foil of the wrapped gel before exposure to X-ray film. This helps to identify correct positions of the visualized bands corresponding to the V_H and V_L bands, respectively, on the gel.

12. It is highly recommended to perform serial dilutions of either tailed cDNA or genomic DNA for PCR amplification. In our experience, the DNA concentration is the most important factor for the successful amplification of tailed cDNA or genomic DNA by PCR.

13. PCR amplification of tailed cDNA ocassionally proves to be difficult. In this case, primers should be designed such that they do not introduce restriction sites but rather match the template sequence completely. PCR fragments can subsequently be cloned as blunt-

ended fragments into a blunt-ended vector using the pMOS Blue blunt-ended cloning kit (Amersham Pharmacia Biotech Inc.) or similar kits for sequencing. Insert orientation can be checked by restriction digest of randomly picked individual clones.

14. Deduced sequences can be aligned online to entries of: the KABAT database (http://immuno.bme.nwu.edu/) (http://immuno.bme.nwu.edu/) *(18)* or the IMGT database (http://imgt.cnusc.fr:8104/v2/DNAP/index.htmL) *(19)*.

15. Direct cloning of PCR products into prokaryotic/eukaryotic shuttle vectors is not recommended due to a very low transformation efficiency and very poor sequencing results.

16. Compared to the use of a Qiaquick gel extraction kit for the recovery of cleaved expression vector DNA, we found NA45-DEAE membranes to have a higher capacity of binding DNA fragments >10 kb in very good quality. To increase binding capacities, membranes should be pretreated according to the recommendations of the manufacturer: Wash membranes for 10 min with 10 mM EDTA, pH 7.6, 5 min with 0.5 M NaOH, followed by several brief final washes with ddH$_2$O.

17. Among several tested ratios, a high molar excess of insert was required for successful cloning of the genomic fragments into the expression vectors pUHWκ and pUHWγ1.

18. Removal of bacterial endotoxin prior to transfection is recommended to maximally reduce the exposure of the vulnerable pulsed cells to cytotoxic agents.

19. Try different parameters around the values given. Parameters have to be optimized for every cell line being transfected. Numerous electroporation protocols are established for many cell lines and are available online (http://www.bio-rad.com).

20. Selection at high concentration of antibiotic after transfection is not as effective as the so called progressive selection. Thus, using cytotoxicity tests, determine the concentration of antibiotic that kills 100% and about 95% of cells being used for transfection. First, expose the transfected cells to the lower concentration of antibiotic. Expose the survivours further to a higher concentration, also stepwise if necessary, until stable mutants are obtained. After the transfected cells have been growing in antibiotic-containing medium long enough to establish a transfectant (usually about four cell generations), withdraw the antibiotic gradually and grow cells in normal culture medium. For the first two passages in this medium, it is advisable to check for antibody production.

21. Cloning under limiting dilution conditions is the method to be used whenever the number of cells secreting a specific antibody is very low, i.e., less than 1×10^3 viable cells. Freshly transfected cells and cells under selection pressure are very fragile and show a density-dependent growth behaviour that causes considerable problems. It can be overcome by addition of feeder cells into the culture. Mouse spleen cells or peritoneal macrophages can be used as feeders at a concentration of 1×10^5/mL or 4×10^4/mL, respectively. After obtaining positive clones, it is advisable to repeat the cloning procedure (recloning) at least once. Although this procedure is time-consuming, it is the only way to establish clonal cells secreting a specific antibody and not to lose the precious cell line. A possible alternative would be to pick individual cells, e.g., with a micro-manipulator, and to place them into feeder cells-containing wells. We have no experience with this technique, and cloning under limiting dilution conditions is simple, fast, and needs no special equipment.

22. If the antigen of interest is expressed on the cell surface, specific binding of the recombinant antibodies should rather be confirmed by flow cytometry on viable cell lines (including positive controls with the parental murine antibody and negative controls using cell lines not expressing the antigen to be targeted) than to use purified antigen and ELISA. Very often antibodies positive in ELISA do not recognize cell-surface antigens and anti-

bodies recognizing cell-surface antigens sometimes do not work in ELISA. Thus,s the most important step is to use a reliable screening method that would allow to identify active antibodies at a very early stage of the cloning procedure.

23. Since only the expression vector encoding the light chain contains an antibiotic selection marker gene, screening for expression of the heavy chain by ELISA is a convenient method to prove a successful cotransfection of both plasmids, allowing a preselection of clones. Even a positive ELISA however, does not say anything definitive about the specific binding of the recombinant antibody to its antigen.

24. The concentration of immunoglobulins within the supernatants should be determined by serial dilutions (up to 1:1000) using serially diluted human immunoglobulin of known concentration as a reference.

25. If you do not have automated cell-freezing equipment, put vials into a polystyrene box and place in a −80°C freezer. After 72 h, place the vial into liquid nitrogen. Do not keep cells at −80°C for longer, because you might have problems with reestablishing them in culture. Freeze at least 5×10^6 cells/mL of freezing medium.

Acknowledgments

We thank Dr. U. H. Weidle (Roche Diagnostics Inc., Penzberg, Germany) for kindly providing the expression vectors pUHWκ and pUHWγ1.

References

1. Köhler, G. and Milstein, C. (1975) Continuous culture of fused cells secreting antibody of predefined specifity. *Nature* **256,** 495–497.

2. Schwarting, R., Gerdes, J., Durkop, H., Falini, B., Pileri, S., and Stein, H. (1989) BER-H2: a new anti-Ki-1 (CD30) monoclonal antibody directed at a formol-resistant epitope. *Blood* **74,** 1678–1689.

3. Dürkop, H., Latza, U., Hummel, M., Eitelbach, F., Seed, B., and Stein, H. (1992) Molecular cloning and expression of a new member of the nerve growth factor receptor family that is charakteristic for Hodgkin's disease. *Cell* **68,** 421–427.

4. Schwab, U., Stein, H., Gerdes, J., Lemke, H., Kirchner, H., Schaadt, M., and Diehl, V. (1982) Production of a monoclonal antibody specific for Hodgkin and Sternberg-Reed cells of Hodgkin's disease and a subset of normal lymphoid cells. *Nature* **299,** 65–67.

5. Stein, H., Mason, D. Y., Gerdes, J., O'Connor, N., Wainscoat, J., Pallesen, G., et al. (1985) The expression of the Hodgkin's disease associated antigen Ki-1 in reactive and neoplastic lymphoid tissue: evidence that Reed-Sternberg cells and histiocytic malignancies are derived from activated lymphoid cells. *Blood* **66,** 848–858.

6. Falini, B., Bolognesi, A., Flenghi, L., Tazzari, P. L., Broe, M. K., Stein, H., et al. (1992) Response of refractory Hodgkin's disease to therapy with anti-CD30 monoklonal antibody linked to saporin (Ber-H2/SO6) immunotoxin. *Lancet* **339,** 1195–1196.

7. Liu, A. Y., Robinson, R. R., Hellstrom, K. E., Murray, E. D., Chang, C. P., and Hellstrom, I. (1987) Chimeric mouse-human IgG1 antibody that can mediate lysis of cancer cells. *Proc. Natl. Acad. Sci. USA* **84,** 3439–3443.

8. Hoogenboom, H. R., Raus, J. C., and Volckaert, G. (1990) Cloning and expression of a chimeric antibody directed against the human transferrin receptor. *J. Immunol.* **144,** 3211–3217.

9. Shitara, K., Kuwana, Y., Nakamura, K., Tokutake, Y., Ohta, S., Miyaji, H., et al. (1993) A mouse/human chimeric anti-(ganglioside GD3) antibody with enhanced antitumor activities. *Cancer Immunol. Immunother.* **36,** 373–380.

10. Krishnan, I. S., Hansen, H. J., Losman, M. J., Goldenberg, D. M., and Leung, S. O. (1997) Chimerization of Mu-9: a colon-specific antigen-p antibody reactive with gastrointestinal carcinomas. *Cancer* **80,** 2667–2674.

11. Hanai, N., Nakamura, K. and Shitara, K. (2000) Recombinant antibodies against ganglioside expressed on tumor cells. *Cancer Chemother. Pharmacol.* **46,** S13–S17.

12. Orlandi, R., Gussow, D. H., Jones, P. T., and Winter, G. (1989) Cloning immunoglobulin variable domains for expression by the polymerase chain reaction. *Proc. Natl. Acad. Sci. USA* **86,** 3833–3837.

13. Dübel, S., Breitling, F., Fuchs, P., Zewe, M., Gotter, S., Welschof, M., et al. (1994) Isolation of IgG antibody Fv-DNA from various mouse and rat hybridoma cell lines using the polymerase chain reaction with a simple set of primers. *J. Immunol. Methods* **175,** 89–95.

14. Liu, A. Y., Robinson, R. R., Murray, E. D., Ledbetter, J. A., Hellstrom, I., and Hellstrom, K. E. (1987) Production of a mouse-human chimeric monoclonal antibody to CD20 with potent Fc-dependent biologic activity. *J. Immunol.* **139,** 3521–3526.

15. Gillies, S. D., Lo, K. M., and Wesolowski, J. (1989) High-level expression of chimeric antibodies using adapted cDNA variable region cassettes. *J. Immunol. Methods* **125,** 191–202.

16. Weissenhorn, W., Weiss, E., Schwirzke, M., Kaluza, B., and Weidle, U. H. (1991) Chimerization of antibodies by isolation of rearranged genomic variable regions by the polymerase chain reaction. *Gene* **106,** 273–277.

17. Kabat, E. A. and Wu, T. T. (1971) Attempts to locate complementarity determing residues in the variable position of light and heavy chains. *Ann. NY Acad. Sci.* **190,** 382–393.

18. Kabat, E. A., Wu, T. T., Reid-Miller, M., Perry, H. M., and Gottesmann, K. (1987) Sequence of proteins of immunological interest. U.S. Department of Health and Human Services, U.S. Government Printing Office, Washington, DC.

19. Lefranc, M. P. (2001) IMGT, the international ImmunoGeneTics database. *Nucleic Acids Res.* **29,** 207–209.

5

Humanization of Monoclonal Antibodies by CDR Grafting

Siobhan O'Brien and Tarran Jones

1. Introduction

The discovery of the process for making rodent monoclonal antibodies (MAbs) 26 years ago by Kohler and Milstein has led to a revolution in the treatment of over 50 major diseases, and has borne an industry whose products today represent 6% of total biotechnology sales. The full potential of this industry has still to be reached.

This revolution has, however, been slow in fulfilling its expectations. The delay is partly owing to several major stumbling blocks to the use of rodent MAbs as therapeutic agents, including:

- Short half-life.
- Poor utilization of the constant region if the rodent antibody by human effector functions.
- Rapid onset of a human anti-globulin response to rat or mouse specific residues—also known as HAMA (Human Anti-Mouse Antibody) response.

Initially, in an effort to combat the immunogenicity problem associated with rodent antibody therapeutics, chimeric recombinant antibodies containing genetically-linked mouse variable domains and human constant domains were engineered. The chimerization process resulted in antibodies that could better utilize human effector functions, but had limited success in combating the problems associated with the HAMA response. To overcome these limitations, Dr. Greg Winter and his colleagues (1,2) developed the concept of creating functional human-like antibodies by grafting the antigen binding complementarity determining regions (CDRs) from the variable domains of rodent antibodies onto the framework regions (FRs) of human variable domains. Since then, several different research groups, including AERES Biomedical Ltd., have successfully developed and improved the methods for designing and constructing humanized antibodies via CDR grafting. Both the conservation of immunoglobulin structure and function across the species barrier as well as molecular modeling have contributed

From: *Methods in Molecular Biology, vol. 207: Recombinant Antibodies for Cancer Therapy: Methods and Protocols*
Edited by: M. Welschof and J. Krauss © Humana Press Inc., Totowa, NJ

greatly to the success of the humanization process. The wide base of knowledge acquired through each humanization project has made it possible to accurately predict key residues that are important for the humanized antibody even before making the antibody.

The following chapter outlines in detail the strategy used by AERES Biomedical for the optimal humanization of a murine antibody. An outline of the procedures involved is shown in **Fig. 1**.

1.1. Cloning of Murine V-Region Heavy- and Light-Chain Genes

The process begins with the isolation of mRNA from hybridoma cells that are expressing the antibody of interest. Following the preparation of first-strand cDNA, the murine V_K and V_H genes are polymerase chain reaction (PCR) amplified using a set of consensus leader sequences and constant region sequence specific primers (*see* **Tables 1** and **2**). Use of primers that are leader sequence and constant region sequence specific insures that the entire accurate immunoglobulin V-regions are amplified.

In most cases, a chimeric antibody is constructed and tested for its ability to bind to antigen prior to constructing a reshaped human antibody.

There are two reasons for this:

1. To confirm, in a functional assay, that the correct mouse variable regions have been cloned and sequenced.
2. To create a valuable positive control for evaluating the reshaped human antibody.

In a chimeric antibody, no alterations have been made to the protein domains that constitute the antigen-binding site. A bivalent chimeric antibody is expected, therefore, to bind to antigen as well as the parent bivalent mouse antibody. Because the chimeric antibody is usually constructed with the same human constant regions that will be used in the reshaped human antibody, it is possible to compare directly the chimeric and reshaped human antibodies in antigen-binding assays that employ anti-human constant region antibody-enzyme conjugates for detection.

As a first step in the construction of chimeric light and heavy chains, the cloned mouse leader-variable regions are modified at the 5'- and 3'-ends using PCR primers to create restriction enzyme sites for convenient insertion into the expression vectors, Kozak sequences for efficient eukaryotic translation *(3)*, and splice-donor sites for RNA splicing of the variable and constant regions (*see* **Table 3**). The adapted mouse light and heavy chain leader-variable regions are then inserted into vectors designed to express chimeric or reshaped human light- and heavy-chains in mammalian cells *(4)*. These vectors contain the human cytomegalovirus (HCMV) enhancer and promoter for transcription, a human light or heavy chain constant region, a gene such as neo for selection of transformed cells, and the SV40 origin of replication for DNA replication in cos cells *(5)*.

1.2. Analysis of Mouse V-Region Genes

Prior to actually beginning to design the reshaped human variable regions, it is important to analyze carefully the amino acid sequences of the mouse variable regions to identify the residues that are most critical in forming the antigen-binding site.

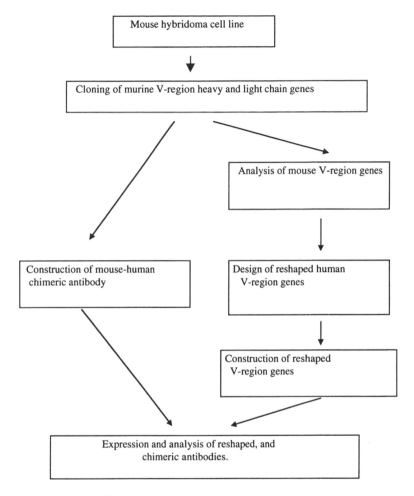

Fig. 1. AERES Biomedical Ltd. strategy for the "humanization" of a murine antibody via CDR grafting.

In addition to studying and comparing the primary amino acid sequences of the mouse variable regions, a structural model of the mouse variable regions is built based on homology to known protein structures, in particular, to the structures of other antibody variable regions. Molecular modeling is carried out using the AbM molecular modeling package supplied and utilized by Oxford Molecular Limited (OML). Antibody X-ray crystallographic structures, available from the brookhaven database along with some as yet unpublished immunoglobulin structures, were formatted to allow them to be used for modeling with AbM. As a first step in the modeling exercise, the FRs of the new variable regions are modeled on FRs from similar, structurally solved immunoglobulin variable regions. Testing of AbM with known structures has shown that FR backbone homology is an important factor in the quality of any model,

Table 1
PCR Primers for Cloning Mouse Kappa Light-Chain Variable Region Genes

Name	Sequence (5'→3')
MKV1 (30-mer)[a]	ATGAAGTTGCCTGTTAGGCTGTTGGTGCTG
MKV2 (30-mer)	ATGGAGWCAGACACACTCCTGYTATGGGTG
MKV3 (30-mer)	ATGAGTGTGCTCACTCAGGTCCTGGSGTTG
MKV4 (33-mer)	ATGAGGRCCCCTGCTCAGWTTYTTGGMWTCTTG
MKV5 (30-mer)	ATGGATTTWCAGGTGCAGATTWTCAGCTTC
MKV6 (27-mer)	ATGAGGTKCYYTGYTSAGYTYCTGRGG
MKV7 (31-mer)	ATGGGCWTCAAGATGGAGTCACAKWYYCWGG
MKV8 (25-mer)	ATGTGGGGAYCTKTTTYCMMTTTTTCAATTG
MKV9 (25-mer)	ATGGTRTCCWCASCTCAGTTCCTTG
MKV10 (27-mer)	ATGTATATATGTTTGTTGTCTATTTCT
MKV11 (28-mer)	ATGGAAGCCCCAGCTCAGCTTCTCTTCC
MKC (20-mer)[b]	ACTGGATGGTGGGAAGATGG

[a]MKV indicates primers that hybridize to leader sequences of mouse kappa chain variable region genes.

[b]MKC indicates the primer that hybridizes to the mouse kappa constant region gene.

Table 2
PCR Primers for Cloning Mouse Heavy-Chain Variable Region Genes

Name	Sequence (5'→3')
MHV1 (27-mer)[a]	ATGAAATGCAGCTGGGGCATSTTCTTC
MHV2 (26-mer)	ATGGGATGGAGCTRTATCATSYTCTT
MHV3 (27-mer)	ATGAAGWTGTGGTTAAACTGGGTTTTT
MHV4 (25-mer)	ATGRACTTTGGGYTCAGCTTGRTTT
MHV5 (30-mer)	ATGGACTCCAGGCTCAATTTAGTTTTCCTT
MHV6 (27-mer)	ATGGCTTGTCYTRGSGCTRCTCTTCTGC
MHV7 (26-mer)	ATGGRATGGAGCKGGRTCTTTMTCTT
MHV8 (23-mer)	ATGAGAGTGCTGATTCTTTTGTG
MHV9 (30-mer)	ATGGMTTGGGTGTGGAMCTTGCTATTCCTG
MHV10 (27-mer)	ATGGGCAGACTTACATTCTCATTCCTG
MHV11 (28-mer)	ATGGATTTTGGGCTGATTTTTTTTATTG
MHV12 (27-mer)	ATGATGGTGTTAAGTCTTCTGTACCTG
MHCG1 (21-mer)[b]	CAGTGGATAGACAGATGGGGG
MHCG2a (21-mer)	CAGTGGATAGACCGATGGGGC
MHCG2b (21-mer)	CAGTGGATAGACTGATGGGGG
MHCG3 (21-mer)	CAAGGGATAGACAGATGGGGC

[a]MHV indicates primers that hybridize to leader sequences of mouse heavy chain variable region genes.

[b]MHCG indicates primers that hybridize to mouse gamma constant region genes.

Table 3
Sequences Important for the Efficient Expression of Immunoglobulin Genes in Mammalian Cells

Name	Consensus DNA sequence[a]
	+1
Kozak translation initiation site	G C C G C C **R** C C **A U G G**
Kappa light chain splice donor site	A C : : **G T** R A G T
Heavy chain splice donor site	M A G : : **G T** R A G T
Immunoglobulin splice acceptor site	Y Y Y Y Y Y Y Y Y Y Y Y N **C A G** : : G

[a]Bases shown in bold are considered to be invariant within each consensus sequence.

because the use of FR structures that poorly match a sequence being modeled can significantly and adversely affect the position and orientation of the CDR loops. Most of the CDRs of the new variable regions are modeled based on the canonical structures for *(6–9)*. Testing of the performance of AbM predictions for known loop structures has shown that CDR loops that are created in this way are usually modeled very accurately, i.e., to within 1–1.5A RMS deviation. Those CDRs that do not appear to belong to any known group of canonical structures, for example CDR3 of the heavy-chain variable region, are modeled based on similar loop structures present in any structurally solved protein. After adjusting the whole model for obvious steric clashes, it was finally subjected to energy minimization, as implemented in MACROMODEL, both to relieve unfavorable atomic contacts and to optimize van der Waals and electrostatic interactions.

1.3. Design of Reshaped Human V-Region Genes

The first step in the design process is to select the human light- and heavy-chain variable regions that will serve as templates for the design of the reshaped human variable regions. In most cases, the selected human light and heavy chains come from two different human antibodies. By not restricting the selection of human variable regions to variable regions that are paired in the same antibody, it is possible to obtain much better homologies between the mouse variable regions to be humanized and the human variable regions selected to serve as templates. In practice, the use of human variable regions from different antibodies as the basis of the design of a reshaped human antibody has not been a problem. This is probably because the packing of light- and heavy-chain variable regions is highly conserved.

The next step in the design process is to join the mouse CDRs to the FRs from the selected human variable regions. The preliminary amino acid sequences are then carefully analyzed to judge whether or not they will recreate an antigen-binding site that mimics that present in the original mouse antibody. At this stage, the model of the mouse variable regions is particularly useful in evaluating the relative importance of each amino acid in the formation of the antigen-binding site. Within the FRs, each of amino acid differences between the mouse and the human sequences should be examined. In addition, any unusual amino acid sequences in the FRs of either the mouse or human sequences should be studied. Finally, any potential glycosylation sites in the FRs of either the mouse or human sequences should be identified and their possible influence on antigen binding considered. It is important to make the minimum number of changes in the human FRs. The goal is to achieve good binding to antigen while retaining human FRs that closely match the sequences from natural human antibodies.

1.4. Construction of Reshaped V-Region Genes

Once the amino acid sequences of the reshaped human variable regions have been designed, it is necessary to decide how DNA sequences coding for these amino acid sequences will be constructed.

There are two fundamental approaches:

1. Take an existing DNA sequence coding for a variable region that is very similar to the newly designed reshaped human variable region and modify the existing DNA sequence so that it will code for the newly designed reshaped human variable region. Modification to existing sequences are usually carried out using PCR and specially designed synthetic oligonucleotide *(10)*.
2. Synthetically make a DNA sequence that will code for the newly designed reshaped human variable region; this is the strategy routinely used by AERES Biomedical Ltd.

The method used is a variation on a gene assembly method first described by Stemmer et al. *(11)*. Oligonucleotides of 40 bp in size are synthesized, these oligos collectively encode both strands of the desired V gene, arranged such that upon assembly complementary oligos will overlap by 20 bp.

The process involves four steps:

1. Oligonucleotide synthesis
2. Gene assembly
3. Gene amplification
4. Cloning

An outline of the entire process can be seen in **Fig. 2.**

1.5. Expression and Analysis of Reshaped and Chimeric Antibodies

The reshaped human variable regions, together with their leader sequences, are cloned into mammalian cell vectors that already contain human constant regions. Each reshaped human variable region is linked via an intron to the desired human constant region. The expression vectors are identical or similar to the vectors that were described for the construction of chimeric light and heavy chains *(4,5)*.

The two mammalian cell expression vectors, one coding for the reshaped human light chain and one coding for the reshaped human heavy chain, are co-transfected into *cos* cells by electroporation using the method of Kettelborough et al. *(4)* (*see* **Subheading 3.4.1.**).

The vectors will replicate in the cos cells and transiently express and secrete reshaped human antibody. The medium is collected 3 d after transfection and analyzed by ELISA to determine the approximate amount of antibody present (*see* **Subheading 3.4.1.**).

In most cases, *cos* cells will also have been transfected with the vectors that express the chimeric antibody. The chimeric and reshaped human antibodies as produced in

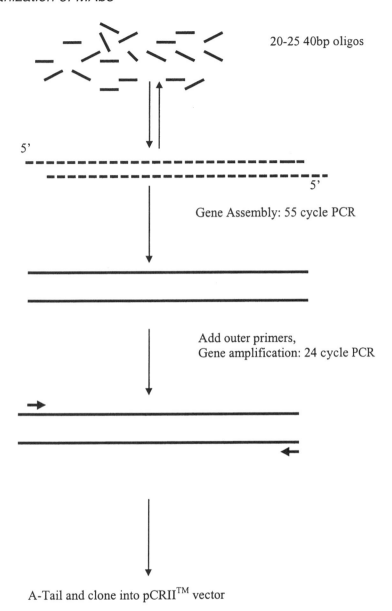

20-25 40bp oligos

5'

5'

Gene Assembly: 55 cycle PCR

Add outer primers,
Gene amplification: 24 cycle PCR

A-Tail and clone into pCRII^{TM} vector

Fig. 2. Schematic representation of the gene synthesis method used to make humanized V-genes.

the cos cells can be tested and compared for their relative abilities to bind to antigen. If purified antigen is available, the simplest approach is to use an ELISA format where the antigen is coated on the immunoplate and bound chimeric or reshaped human antibody is detected using a goat anti-human antibody-enzyme conjugate. However, more accurate binding and pharmacokinetic measurements can be obtained in real time, for example by using real-time BIA technology BIA (BIAcore), which uses the phenomonin of surface plasmon resonance to measure the K_{on} and K_{off} of the antibody.

2. Materials

2.1. Cloning and Sequencing of Murine V Region Genes

2.1.1. Preparation of cDNA from Hybridoma mRNA

1. RNA isolation kit (Stratagene, 2003345).
2. First strand cDNA synthesis kit (Pharmacea, 27-9261-01).
3. Glasstic® disposable cell-counting slide (Bio-stat Diagnostic, 887144).
4. Sterile water. Treat deionized, distilled water with 1 mL/L of DEPC (Sigma, D-5758) for 12 h at 37°C. Autoclave for 20 min at 115°C and 15 p.s.i.
5. 0.15 *M* Phosphate-buffered saline (PBS), pH 7.2.
6. 0.4% Trypan blue solution (Sigma, T8154).

2.1.2. PCR Amplification and Cloning of Murine V Region Genes

1. TA Cloning Kit (Invitrogen, K2000-01).
2. Biometra Thermoblock PCR machine.
3. GeneAmp™ PCR reaction tubes (Perkin-Elmer, N801-0180).
4. Sterile water. Treat deionized, distilled water with 1 mL/L of DEPC (Sigma, D-5758) for 12 h at 37°C. Autoclave for 20 min at 115°C and 15 p.s.i.
5. PCR-cloning primers (*see* **Tables 1** and **2**). Prepare separate 10 µ*M* stock solutions of MHV 1-12, MKV 1-11, MHC and MKC primers in sterile water.
6. AmpliTaq® DNA polymerase (5 U/µL; Perkin-Elmer, N801-0060).
7. 10X PCR buffer II: 500 m*M* KCl, 100 m*M* Tris-HCl, pH 8.3, 25 m*M* MgCl$_2$ (Perkin-Elmer, N808-0010).
8. GeneAmp® dNTPs; separate 10 m*M* stock solutions of dATP, dCTP, dGTP, and dTTP in distilled water, titrated to pH 7.0 with NaOH (Perkin-Elmer, N808-0007).
9. Mineral oil (Sigma, M-5904).
10. 10X TBE buffer: 1.337 *M* Tris-HCl base, 0.445 *M* boric acid, 26 m*M* EDTA, pH 8.8.
11. Agarose (UltraPure™) (Life Technologies, 15510-019).
12. 10 mg/mL Ethidium bromide (Sigma, E-1510).
13. TA Cloning® kit (Invitrogen, K2000-01).
14. LB agar plates.
15. Ampicillin (Sigma, A-2804). Prepare a 100 mg/mL stock solution in water and sterilize by filtration through a 0.22 mm filter. Store at –20°C.
16. X-Gal (Sigma, B-9146). Prepare a 40 mg/mL stock solution with dimethylformamide in a glass or polypropylene tube. Wrap the tube in aluminium foil and store at –20°C.

2.1.3. Identification of Positive Colonies by PCR Screening

1. Biometra Thermoblock PCR machine.
2. PCR screening primers that bracket the site of insertion.
3. Techne PHC-3 DNA thermal cycler with Techne Hi-temp 96 multiwell plate (Techne, FPHC3MD).
4. GeneAmp™ PCR reaction tubes (Perkin-Elmer, N801-0180).
5. Sterile water. Treat deionized, distilled water with 1 mL/L of DEPC (Sigma, D-5758) for 12 h at 37°C. Autoclave for 20 min at 115°C and 15 p.s.i.

6. AmpliTaq® DNA polymerase (5 U/μL; Perkin-Elmer, N801-0060).
7. 10X PCR buffer II: 500 m*M* KCl, 100 m*M* Tris-HCl, pH 8.3, 25 m*M* MgCl$_2$ (Perkin-Elmer, N808-0010).
8. GeneAmp® dNTPs; separate 10 m*M* stock solutions of dATP, dCTP, dGTP, and dTTP in distilled water, titrated to pH7.0 with NaOH (Perkin-Elmer, N808-0007).
9. Mineral oil (Sigma, M-5904).
10. 10X TBE buffer: 1.337 *M* Tris base, 0.445 *M* boric acid, 26 m*M* EDTA, pH 8.8.
11. Agarose (UltraPure™) (Life Technologies, 15510-019).
12. 10 mg/mL Ethidium bromide (Sigma, E-1510).

2.1.4. PCR Modification of Murine Variable Region Genes to Facilitate Expression as Chimeric Whole Antibody in Mammalian Cells

1. Biometra Thermoblock PCR machine.
2. PCR modification primers primers.
3. Techne PHC-3 DNA thermal cycler with Techne Hi-temp 96 multiwell plate (Techne, FPHC3MD).
4. GeneAmp PCR reaction tubes (Perkin-Elmer, N801-0180).
5. Sterile water. Treat deionized, distilled water with 1 mL/L of DEPC (Sigma, D-5758) for 12 h at 37°C. Autoclave for 20 min at 115°C and 15 p.s.i.
6. AmpliTaq DNA polymerase (5 U/μL; Perkin-Elmer, N801-0060).
7. 10X PCR buffer II: 500 m*M* KCl, 100 m*M* Tris-HCl, pH 8.3, 25 m*M* MgCl2 (Perkin-Elmer, N808-0010).
8. GeneAmp dNTPs; separate 10 m*M* stock solutions of dATP, dCTP, dGTP, and dTTP in distilled water, titrated to pH 7.0 with NaOH (Perkin-Elmer, N808-0007).
9. Mineral oil (Sigma, M-5904).
10. 10X TBE buffer: 1.337 *M* Tris-HCl base, 0.445 *M* boric acid, 26 m*M* EDTA, pH 8.8.
11. Agarose (UltraPure) (Life Technologies, 15510-019).
12. 10 mg/mL Ethidium bromide (Sigma, E-1510).

2.2. Design of the Reshaped Human Antibody

1. Genetics Computer Group (GCG) sequence analysis software package (University of Wisconsin Biotechnology Center, Madison, WI).
2. EMBL Data Library including the Kabat database (European Molecular Biology Laboratory, Heidelberg, Germany).
3. Leeds database of protein sequences (Department of Biochemistry and Molecular Biology, University of Leeds, Leeds, UK).
4. SPARC® station 1 (Sun Microsystems Inc., Mountain View, CA).
5. Molecular model of the mouse variable regions.

2.3. Construction of the Reshaped Human Antibody

1. Genetics Computer Group (GCG) sequence analysis software package (University of Wisconsin Biotechnology Center, Madison, WI).
2. EMBL Data Library including the Kabat database (European Molecular Biology Laboratory, Heidelberg, Germany).
3. Leeds database of protein sequences (Department of Biochemistry and Molecular Biology, University of Leeds, Leeds, UK).
4. TA Cloning Kit (Invitrogen, K2000-01).
5. Biometra Thermoblock PCR machine.

6. GeneAmp PCR reaction tubes (Perkin-Elmer, N801-0180).
7. Sterile water. Treat deionized, distilled water with 1 mL/L of DEPC (Sigma, D-5758) for 12 h at 37°C. Autoclave for 20 min at 115°C and 15 p.s.i.
8. Pfu DNA Polymerase (Stratagene #600154).
9. 10X Pfu reaction buffer: 100 mM KCl, 100 mM (NH$_4$)$_2$SO$_4$, 200 mM Tris-HCl, 20 mM MgSO$_4$, 1% Triton X-100, 1000 µg/mL BSA.
10. GeneAmp dNTPs; separate 10 mM stock solutions of dATP, dCTP, dGTP, and dTTP in distilled water, titrated to pH 7.0 with NaOH (Perkin-Elmer, N808-0007).
11. Mineral oil (Sigma, M-5904).
12. 10X TBE buffer: 1.337 M Tris-HCl base, 0.445 M boric acid, 26 mM EDTA, pH 8.8.
13. Agarose (UltraPure) (Life Technologies, 15510-019).
14. 10 mg/mL Ethidium bromide (Sigma, E-1510).
15. TA Cloning® kit (Invitrogen, K2000-01).
16. LB agar plates.
17. Ampicillin (Sigma, A-2804). Prepare a 100 mg/mL stock solution in water and sterilize by filtration through a 0.22 µm filter. Store at –20°C.
18. X-Gal (Sigma, B-9146). Prepare a 40 mg/mL stock solution with dimethylformamide in a glass or polypropylene tube. Wrap the tube in aluminium foil and store at –20°C.

2.4. Preliminary Expression and Analysis of Reshaped Human Antibodies

2.4.1. Transient Expression in cos Cells via Electroporation

1. 150 cm^2 Tissue culture flask (Bibby Sterilin, 25120-150).
2. Gene Pulser apparatus (Bio-Rad, 165-2078).
3. Gene Pulser cuvets (Bio-Rad, 165-2088).
4. io-Cult 100 × 20 mm multi-vented tissue culture dish (Bibby Tissue Culture, 25020B).
5. Cos-7 cells (American Type Culture Collection, CRL 1651).
6. Heavy variable region gene in heavy chain mammalian expression vector (10 µg) and kappa light chain variable region gene in kappa light-chain mammalian expression vector (10 µg). Or super-vector containing both heavy- and light-chain cassettes in a single expression vector (10 µg).
7. 0.15 M Phosphate-buffered saline (PBS) pH 7.2.
8. Dulbecco's modified eagle's medium (DMEM) (Life Technologies, 41966-029).
9. Fetal calf serum dialyzed (FCS) (Hyclone A 1101-L).
10. 58 mg/mL L-glutamine (Life Technologies, 25030-024).
11. 5000 U/mL Penicillin/5 mg/mL streptomycin (Life Technologies, 15070-022).
12. Trypsin-EDTA (Sigma T4049).

2.4.2. Determination of cos Cell Expression Levels by Capture ELISA

1. Nunc-Immuno Plate MaxiSorp (Life Technologies, 43945A).
2. Goat anti-human IgG antibody, Fcγ fragment-specific (Jackson ImmunoResearch Laboratories Inc. via Stratech Scientific, 109-005-098).
3. Human IgG1/kappa antibody (Sigma, I-3889).
4. Goat anti-human kappa light-chain peroxidase conjugate (Sigma, A-7164).
5. K-BLUE substrate (Sky Bio, KB176).
6. RED STOP solution (Sky Bio, RS20).
7. Sample enzyme conjugate beffer (SEC buffer): 0.02% (v/v) Tween-20, 0.2% (w/v) BSA, in 1X PBS.

3. Methods

3.1. Cloning of Murine V Region Heavy- and Light-Chain Genes

3.1.1. Preparation of cDNA from Hybridoma mRNA

1. Grow the mouse hybridoma cell line in an appropriate culture medium to provide a total viable cell count of at least 10^8 cells.
2. Pellet the cells in a bench top centrifuge ($250g$, 5 min). Gently resuspend the cells in 20 mL of PBS.
3. Add 100 μL of cells to 200 μL of PBS and 200 μL of trypan blue and mix gently. Pipet 10 μL of this mixture into a disposable cell-counting slide. Count the cells per square and determine the number of cells/mL according to the manufacturer's instructions.
4. Pellet approx 10^8 cells ($250g$, 5 min).
5. Use the RNA isolation kit as described by the manufacturer to purify total RNA from the cells. The kit uses a guanidinium thiocyanate phenol-chloroform single-step extraction procedure *(12)*.
6. Determine the quantity and quality of the total RNA by measuring the OD_{260} and OD_{280} and by testing 1–5 μg aliquots on a nondenaturing 1% (w/v) agarose gel in 1X TBE buffer containing 0.5 μg/mL ethidium bromide. The concentration of RNA = $OD_{260} \times 40$ μg/mL. The quality is satisfactory if $OD_{260} : OD_{280} >1.9$ and distinct bands are seen on the agarose gel representing 28S and 18S RNA, the 28S band being more intensely stained.
7. Following the manufacturer's instructions, use the first-strand cDNA synthesis kit to produce a single-stranded DNA copy of the hybridoma mRNA using the NotI-$(dT)_{18}$ primer. Use 5 μg of total RNA in a 33 μL final reaction volume.
8. Following the reaction, heat at 90°C for 5 min to denature the RNA-cDNA duplex and to inactivate the reverse transcriptase. Chill on ice.

3.1.2. PCR Amplification and Cloning of Murine V Region Genes

1. Label eleven Gene Amp PCR reaction tubes MKV1 to MKV11. In each tube prepare a 100 μL reaction mixture. PCR reaction mixture: 69.5 μL of sterile water, 10 μL of 10X PCR buffer, 6 μL of 25 m*M* MgCl$_2$, 2 μL each of the 10 m*M* stock solutions of dNTPs, 2.5 μL 10 m*M* MKC primer, 2.5 μL of one of the 10 m*M* MKV primers, 1 μL of RNA-cDNA template mix. Finally, add 0.5 μL of AmpliTaq DNA polymerase and overlay the reaction mix with 50 μL of mineral oil.
2. Prepare a similar series of reaction mixes to PCR clone the mouse heavy chain variable region gene using the twelve MHV primers and the appropriate MHC primer.
3. Place the reaction tubes into a DNA thermal cycler and cycle (after an initial melt at 94°C for 1.5 min) at 94°C for 1 min, 50°C for 1 min, and 72°C for 1 min over 25 cycles.
4. Follow the last cycle with a final extension step at 72°C for 10 min before cooling to 4°C. Use a ramp time of 2.5 min between the annealing (50°C) and extension (72°C) steps and a 30-s ramp time between all other steps of the cycle.
5. Run a 10 μL aliquot from each PCR reaction on a 1% (w/v) agarose/1X TBE buffer gel, containing 0.5 μg/mL ethidium bromide, to determine which of the leader primers produces a PCR product. Positive PCR products will be about 420–500 bp in size.
6. For those PCR reactions that appear to produce full-length PCR products, repeat the procedure (**steps 7–10**) to obtain at least two independent PCR reactions that give full-length PCR products.
7. Directly clone a 1 μL aliquot of any potential PCR product into the pCR™II vector provided by the TA Cloning kit as described in the manufacturer's instructions (This kit

allows the direct cloning of PCR products without prior purification and takes advantage of the preference of AmpliTaq DNA polymerase to insert a 3'-overhanging thymidine (T) at each end of the PCR product.). Pipet out 10.0% (v/v), 1.0% (v/v) and 0.1% (v/v) aliquots of the transformed *E. coli* cells onto individual 90 mm diameter LB agar plates containing 50 μg/mL ampicillin and overlaid with 25 mL of the X-Gal stock solution. Incubate overnight at 37°C.

8. Identify positive colonies by PCR screening as follows.

3.1.3. Identification of Positive Colonies by PCR Screening

1. Prepare a bulk solution of the PCR reaction mix (sufficient for 20 samples). PCR reaction mixture: 69.5 μL of sterile water, 10 μL 10X PCR buffer II, 2 μL each of 10 m*M* stock solutions of dNTPs, 2.5 μL 10 m*M* pCR™II forward primer, 2.5 μL 10 m*M* pCR™II back primers, 1 μL of mRNA-cDNA template mix. Finally add 0.5 μL of AmpliTaq DNA polymerase and overlay the reaction mix with 50 μL of mineral oil.

2. Dispense the above "mastermix" in 20 μL aliquots into the 96-well microplate.

3. Label twenty 30 μL universal containers and add to each 3 μL of LB media containing 50 μg/mL ampicillin.

4. Using an inoculating needle, gently "stab" an individual colony from a putative transformation mix grown overnight on selective agar plate. Then, stab the needle into one of the 20 μL aliquots of mastermix, making sure that the base of the microplate well is touched gently with the needle (*see* **Note 1**).

5. With the same needle, immediately inoculate a universal container (**step 3**) and incubate this culture overnight at 37°C and 300 rpm in the shaking incubator.

6. Prepare a negative control and a positive control where possible (as a positive control, add 1 μL of template DNA (5 ng/μL) to 20 μL of mastermix).

7. Overlay each of the inoculated PCR reactions with 2 drops of mineral oil per well.

8. Load the microplate into the Techne PHC-3 and cycle (after an initial melt at 94°C for 5 min) at 94°C for 1 min, 50°C for 1 min, and 72°C for 1 min over 25 cycles. Complete the PCR-reaction with a final extension step at 72°C for 10 min before cooling to 4°C. Use a ramp time of 30 s between each step.

9. Run a 10 μL aliquot from each PCR reaction on a 1% (w/v) agarose/1X TBE buffer gel containing 0.5 μg/mL ethidium bromide, and estimate the size of any PCR products (*see* **Note 2**).

10. Sequence the DNA from at least two independently isolated positive clones of each variable region to identify possible errors introduced by PCR.

3.1.4. PCR Modification of Murine Variable Region Genes to Facilitate Expression as Chimeric Whole Antibody in Mammalian Cells

1. In each PCR tube prepare a 100 μL reaction, each containing up to 41 μL of sterile water, 10 μL of 10X PCR buffer I, 8 μL of the 10 m*M* stock solution of dNTPs, 1 μL of 10 m*M* of 5' forward primer, 1 μL of the 10 m*M* 3' Reverse primer and 1 μL of a 1/10 dilution of template DNA. Finally, add 0.5 μL of AmpliTaq® DNA polymerase (2.5 U) before overlaying the completed reaction mix with 50 μL of mineral oil.

2. Load the reaction tubes into a DNA thermal cycler and cycle (after an initial melt at 94°C for 1 min) at 94°C for 30 s, 68°C for 30 s and 72°C for 50 s over 25 cycles. Follow the completion of the last cycle with a final extension step at 72°C for 7 min before cooling to 4°C.

3. Run a 10 μL aliquot from each PCR-reaction on a 1.2% (w/v) agarose/1X TBE buffer gel, containing 0.5 μg/mL ethidium bromide, to determine size and presence of a PCR-product. Positive PCR-clones will be about 420 bp in size.

4. Directly clone a 1 µL aliquot of any potential PCR-product into the pCR 2.1 TOPO vector, provided by the TOPO TA Cloning® kit, as described in the manufacturer's instructions. Pipet out 10.0% (v/v) and 90% (v/v) aliquots of the transformed *E.coli* cells onto individual 90 mm diameter LB agar plates containing 50 µg/mL ampicillin and overlaid with 25 µL of the X-Gal stock (TOP 10 cells do not require IPTG). Incubate overnight at 37°C. Colonies can be PCR screened for the presence of the correct size (*see* **Note 2**).
5. Selected 5 heavy-chain clones and 5 kappa light-chain clones for plasmid mini-preps and sequencing to identify any PCR-errors.
6. Once a positive clone has been identified, excise the reshaped gene out of the cloning vector and sub-clone it into an appropriate mammalian expression vector for whole antibody expression.

3.2. Design of the Reshaped Human Antibody

3.2.1. Analysis of the Amino Acid Sequences of the Mouse Variable Regions

1. Use the "SeqEd" program in the GCG package to create a series of files containing the consensus amino acid sequences of the subgroups of mouse and human light- and heavy-chain variable regions as defined by Kabat et al. (*13*).
2. With the same program, create two files containing the amino acid sequences of the light-chain and heavy-chain variable regions of the mouse antibody.
3. Compare the amino acid sequences of the mouse variable regions to the mouse consensus sequences using the "Gap" program in the GCG package and identify the mouse subgroups to which the mouse variable regions belong.
4. Analyze the amino acid sequences of the mouse variable regions and locate the following features within them:
   a. CDRs and FRs (*13*).
   b. Residues that are part of the canonical sequences for loop structure (*see* **Table 4**).
   c. Residues located at the V_L/V_H interface.
   d. Residues in the FRs that are unusual or unique for that position when compared to the consensus sequence for that mouse subgroup.
   e. Potential glycosylation sites (*see* **Note 3**).

3.2.2. Selection of the Human Variable Regions to Serve as Templates for Reshaping

Compare the amino acid sequences of the mouse variable regions to the human consensus sequences and identify the most similar human subgroup for each mouse variable region.

1. Compare the amino acid sequences of the mouse variable regions to all human variable region sequences in the databases and, for each mouse variable region, identify the 10 most similar human sequences. Use the "FastA" program in the GCG package.
2. Analyze the selected human variable regions for the following characteristics:
   a. Percent similarity with the mouse variable region.
   b. Percent identity with the mouse variable region noting the location of regions of non-identity.
   c. Length of the CDRs in comparison to the mouse CDRs.
   d. Identity to the mouse sequence in the residues in the FRs that are part of the canonical sequences for loop structure (*see* **Table 4**).
   e. Identity to the mouse sequence in the residues located at the V_L/V_H interface (*see* **Table 5**).

Table 4
Important Residues for the Maintenance of CDR Loop Conformation[a]

CDR loop	Canonical structure (loop size[b])	Residues important for loop conformation[c,d] (most common amino acids)
L1	1 (10)[e]	2(I), 25(A), 30(V), 33(M, L) and **71**(Y)
	2 (11)	2(I), 25(A), 29(V, I), 33(L) and **71**(F, Y)
	2 (12)[f]	2(I, N), 25(A), 28(V, I), 33(L) and **71**(F, Y)
	3 (17)	2(I), 25(S), 27b(V, L), 33(L) and **71**(F)
	4 (15)[f]	2(I), 25(A), 27b(V), 33(M) and **71**(F)
	4 (16)	2(V, I), 25(S), 27b(I, L), 33(L) and **71**(F)
L2	1 (7)	**48**(I), 51(A, T,), 52(S, T) and **64**(G)
L3	1 (9)	90(Q, N, H) and 95(P)
	2 (9)[e]	90(Q) and 94(P)
	3 (8)	90(Q) and 95(P)
H1	1 (5)	**24**(A,V, G), **26**(G), **27**(F, Y), **29**(F), 34(M, W, I) and **94**(R, K)
	2 (6)	**24**(V, F), **26**(G), **27**(F, Y, G), **29**(I, L), 35(W, C) and **94**(R, H)
	3 (7)	**24**(G, F), **26**(G), **27**(G, F, D), **29**(L, I, V), 35a(W, V) and **94**(R, H)
H2	1 (16)	55(G, D) and **71**(V, K, R)
	2 (17)	52a(P, T, A), 55(G, S) and **71**(A, T, L)
	3 (17)	54(G, S, N) and **71**(R)
	4 (19)	54(S), 55(Y) and **71**(R)
	5 (18)	52a(Y), 54(K), 55(W) and **71**(P)

[a]This table summarizes information presented in Chothia and Lesk *(6)*, Chothia et al. *(7)*, Tramontano et al. *(9)*, and Chothia et al. *(8)*.

[b]Loop size is the number of residues in the CDR loop as defined by Kabat et al. *(13)*.

[c]Numbering is according to Kabat et al. *(13)*. Note that in Chothia et al. *(8)* L1 and H1 are numbered differently.

[d]The residue numbers printed in bold are located within the FRs of the variable region. Residues 26–30 of the heavy-chain variable region are defined as FR residues by Kabat et al. *(13)*; however, structurally they are part of the H1 loop.

[e]These canonical structures have been observed only in mouse antibodies and not in human antibodies.

[f]Approximately 25% of human and 20% of mouse sequences have 13 residues in canonical structure 2 or 14 residues in canonical structure 4. These minor variations in loop size result in changes at the tip of the L1 loop but do not significantly alter loop conformation.

     f. Residues in the FRs that are unusual or unique for a particular position when compared to the consensus sequence for that human subgroup *(13)*.

     g. Potential glycosylation sites (*see* **Note 3**).

3. Make a subjective decision as to the most appropriate human sequences, one human light-chain variable region sequence and one human heavy-chain variable region sequence, to serve as templates for the design of a reshaped human antibody.

Table 5
Conserved Residues Found at the V$_L$/V$_H$ Interface[a]

Variable region	Residue position[b]	Number of sequences analyzed	Number of different amino acids observed	Principal amino acids at this position (number of occurrences[c])
VL	34	1365	16	A(326), H(306), N(280)
	36	1324	7	Y(1057), F(143)
	38	1312	11	Q(1158)
	44[d]	1244	14	P(1060)
	46	1252	17	L(827)
	87	1222	8	Y(874), F319)
	89	1238	16	Q(654)
	91	1234	17	W(275), Y(216), G(209), S(169)
	96[d]	1034	20	L(220), Y(203), W(196), R(121)
	98[d]	1066	6	F(1058)
VH	35	1459	19	H(378), N(356), S(287)
	37	1398	10	V(1212), I(151)
	39	1397	13	Q(1315)
	45[d]	1397	10	L(1362)
	47	1357	14	W(1252)
	91	1689	9	Y(1332), F(340)
	93	1683	16	A(1426)
	95	1451	20	D(285), G(212), S(187)
	100-100K[d,e]	1211	19	F(707), M(224)
	103d	1276	10	W(1251)

[a]The positions of interdomain residues were as defined by Chothia et al. *(7)*. The immunoglobulin sequences analyzed were from the database of Kabat et al. *(13)*.

[b]Numbering is according to Kabat et al. *(13)*. The residue numbers printed in bold are located within the FRs of the variable region.

[c]Only those residues that displayed a frequency of occurrence of >10% are shown.

[d]One of six residues that constitute the core of the V$_L$/V$_H$ interface as defined by Chothia et al. *(8)*.

[e]The residue that is immediately N-terminal to residue 101 in CDR3 is the amino acid that is part of the core of the V$_L$/V$_H$ interface. The numbering of this residue varies.

3.2.3. Design of the Additional Versions of Reshaped Human Variable Regions

Write out the sequences of the proposed reshaped human variable regions with the CDRs from the mouse variable regions joined to the FRs from the selected human variable regions.

1. Highlight the amino acids in the human FRs that are different from those that were present in the mouse FRs. Use the structural model of the mouse variable regions to help evaluate

the significance of the proposed amino acid changes. Consider conserving the following mouse residues:

  a. Residues that belong to canonical sequences for loop structure.
  b. Residues that the model suggests have a role in the supporting a CDR loop.
  c. Carefully examine buried residues and residues in the "Vernier" zone *(14)*.
  d. Carefully examine the H3 loop where there are no defined canonical structures to use for guidance.
  e. Residues that the model suggests are on the surface near the antigen-binding site.
  f. Residues located at the V_L/V_H interface.

2. Examine the revised sequences and consider the following points:

  a. Removing any potential N-glycosylation sites within the human FRs and conserving, or removing, any potential N-glycosylation sites that were present in the mouse FRs. Use the model to predict whether potential glycosylation sites are located at positions that are on the surface and accessible and, therefore, likely to be used.
  b. Role of mouse residues that are atypical when compared to the consensus sequence for that subgroup of mouse variable regions. It is possible that atypical amino acid residues have been selected for, at certain positions, to improve binding to antigen.
  c. Location of human residues that are atypical when compared to the consensus sequence for that subgroup of human variable regions. It is possible that the potential immunogenicity of the reshaped human antibody will be increased if the human FRs contain unusual human sequences.

3.2.4. Design of the Additional Versions of Reshaped Human Variable Regions

1. When preliminary assays indicate that the first reshaped human antibody has a binding affinity equal or better than the mouse or chimeric antibody, additional versions may be made to further reduce the number of substitutions of mouse residues into the human FRs.
2. When preliminary assays indicate that the first reshaped human antibody has a poor binding affinity, determine whether one or both reshaped human variable regions is the cause. As already described, express the reshaped human light and heavy chains in all combinations with the chimeric light and chains and determine the relative binding affinities of antibodies expressed.
3. Reanalyze the model and ask if any additional substitutions of mouse residues into the human FRs are required. Be particularly cautious about any amino acid differences between the mouse and human FRs that occur in buried residues.
4. Reconsider the removal or inclusion of any potential glycosylation sites (*see* **Note 3**).

3.3. Construction of the Reshaped Human Variable Regions

3.3.1. Design of the Oligonucleotides and Primers

1. Using the "SeqEd" program in the GCG package, create a file of the DNA sequence of the human leader-variable region that has been selected as the template for reshaping (*see* **Note 4**).
2. Substitute the DNA sequences coding for the mouse CDRs for the DNA sequences coding for the human CDRs. Make minor modifications in the DNA sequences coding for the human FRs as required to make any amino acid changes that were specified in the design of the reshaped human variable region. Base the codon usage on the mouse variable region or refer to the database of immunoglobulin genes *(13)* and try to avoid rare codon usage.

3. In order to function in the expression vectors previously described *(5)*, the reshaped human leader-variable region will require the following DNA sequences:

   a. Kozak translation initiation sequence.
   b. Splice donor sequence.
   c. Restriction sites for cloning.

4. Check the DNA sequence for the presence of unintentional splice donor sites that might interfere with RNA processing (*see* **Table 3**). Check that there are no internal restriction sites that will interfere with cloning into the expression vector. Remove undesirable DNA sequences by altering the codon usage.
5. The V gene is divided into oligonucleotides 40 bp in size, which overlap by 20 bp. Using the "Map" program in the GCG package, identify unique restriction sites already present in the DNA sequence and sites where unique restriction sites could be inserted without altering the amino acid sequence. Where possible, engineer a unique restriction sites into each overlapping region.
3. Using the "Stemloop" program in the GCG package, identify potential stemloops within the DNA sequence. Remove any potential stemloops with a melting temperature of over 40°C by modifying the codon usage.

3.3.2. PCR Assembly of the Oligonucleotides

1. Prepare an Oligo Mix containing 1 mL of each assembly primer at 250 m*M*.
2. Prepare PCR reactions containing: 15.2 µL of sterile water, 2.0 µL of 10X PCR buffer II, 0.6 µL of 100 m*M* MgCl$_2$, 1.6 µL of the 10 m*M* stock solutions of dNTPs, 0.25 µL of the Oligo Mix. Overlay each reaction with 50 µL of mineral oil and place in a DNA thermal cycler.
3. "Hot-start" the reactions by incubating for 5 min at 94°C, cooling to approx 80°C, and adding 0.5 µL of Pfu DNA polymerase to each reaction (*see* **Notes 5** and **6**).
4. Cycle at 94°C for 30 s and 52°C for 30 s and 72°C for 1 min, for 55 cycles.

3.3.3. PCR Gene Amplification of Assembled Gene

1. Prepare a 100 µL PCR reaction as follows: 65.5 µL of sterile water, 10 µL of 10X PCR buffer II, 3 µL of 25 m*M* MgCl$_2$, 8 µL each of the 10 m*M* stock solutions of dNTPs, 2.5 µL Gene assembly mix, 5 µL of each outer primer at 10 m*M*. Overlay each reaction with 50 µL of mineral oil and place in a DNA thermal cycler. "Hot start" adding 1 µL Pfu DNA polymerase to each reaction. Cycle at 94°C for 30 s, 50°C for 30 s and 72°C for 1 min for 24 cycles.
2. Immediately after the PCR reaction with Pfu polymerase add 1 mL of AmpliTaq polymerase, incubate at 72°C for 10 min (*see* **Note 7**).
3. Purify the resulting PCR products from using the the Qiaquick PCR purification kit according to the manufacturer's instructions.
4. Evaluate the quality and quantity of the PCR products by measuring the OD260 and by testing aliquots on a 1.5% (w/v) agarose gel in 1X TBE buffer containing 0.5 µg/mL ethidium bromide.
5. Clone the PCR product using the TA Cloning kit as already described.
6. PCR screen the transformants using as previously described.
7. Sequence the DNA from several clones that have inserts of the correct size. If errors are found in the DNA sequences, make use of the unique restriction sites within the reshaped human variable region to assemble one correct DNA sequence from a few sequences with errors in different sections of the sequence.

3.4. Preliminary Expression and Analysis
of Reshaped Human Antibodies

3.4.1. Transient Expression in cos Cells via Electroporation

1. All steps will be carried out in a tissue culture laboratory. Grow the *cos* cell line in DMEM supplemented with 10% (v/v) FCS, 580 µg/mL L-glutamine and 50 U/mL penicillin/ 50 µg/mL streptomycin in a 150 cm^2 flask until confluent.

2. Trypsinize the cells, spin them down in a bench top centrifuge (250 g for 5 min), then re-suspend the cells in 6 mL of media (**step 1**) before dividing them equally between three 150 cm^2 flasks, each containing 25 mL of fresh, prewarmed media (**step 1**). Incubate the cos cells overnight at 37°C in 5% CO_2 and then harvest them next day, while they are still growing exponentially. Each flask should contain approx 1×10^7 cells although this can be confirmed via a viable cell count.

3. Trypsinize the cells again, pellet (**step 2**) and wash the cells in 20 mL of PBS. Resuspend the cells in sufficient PBS to create a cell concentration of 1×10^7 cells/mL. Carefully pipet 700 mL of these washed *cos* cells into a Gene Pulser® cuvet.

4. Add X µL of both the heavy-chain and kappa light-chain expression vector DNA (each at 10 µg) to the cuvet and then deliver a 1900 V, 25 µFarad capacitance pulse to the mixture using the Bio-Rad Gene Pulser apparatus.

5. Repeat **step 4** for each experimental transfection and then also do a "no DNA" control where the *cos* cells are electroporated in the absence of any DNA.

6. Allow the *cos* cells to recover at room temperature for 10 min and then gently pipet the transfected cells into a 10 cm diameter tissue-culture dish containing 8 mL of prewarmed DMEM supplemented with 5% (v/v) γ-globulin free FBS, 580 µg/mL L-glutamine and 50 U/mL penicillin/50 µg/mL streptomycin.

7. Incubate in 5% CO_2 at 37°C for 72 h before harvesting the *cos* cell supernatant for analysis.

3.4.2. Determination of cos Cell Expression Levels
by Capture ELISA (see **Note 8**)

1. Coat each well of a 96-well immunoplate with 100 µL aliquots of 0.4 µg/mL goat anti-human IgG antibody, diluted in PBS, incubate overnight at 4°C (*see* **Note 9**).

2. Remove the excess coating solution and wash the plate three times with 200 µL/well of washing buffer (1X PBS, 0.1% Tween).

3. Dispense 100 µL of SEC buffer into all wells except the wells in column 2, rows B to G (*see* **Note 10**).

4. Prepare a 1 µg/mL solution of the human IgG1/kappa antibody in SEC buffer to serve as a standard. Pipet 200 µL/well into the wells in column 2, rows B and C (*see* **Note 11**).

5. Centrifuge the medium from transfected *cos* cells (250*g*, 5 min) and save the supernatant.

6. Pipet 200 µL of the supernatant from the "no DNA" control (where *cos* cells were transfected in the absence of DNA) into the well in column 2, row D.

7. Pipet 200 µL/well of experimental supernatants into the wells in column 2, rows E, F, and G.

8. Mix the 200 µL aliquots in the wells of column 2, rows B to G, and then transfer 100 µL to the neighboring wells in column 3. Continue to column 11 with a series of twofold dilutions of the standard, control, and experimental samples.

9. Incubate at 37°C for 1 h. Rinse all the wells six times with 200 µL aliquots of washing buffer.

10. Dilute the goat anti-human kappa light-chain peroxidase conjugate 5000-fold in SEC buffer and add 100 µL to each well (*see* **Note 11**). Repeat the incubation and washing steps (**step 9**).

11. Add 150 μL of K-BLUE substrate to each well, incubate in the dark at room temperature for 10 min.
12. Stop the reaction by adding 50 μL of RED STOP solution to each well. Read the optical density at 655 nm.

4. Notes

1. In **step 4**, do not swirl the needle in the solution or rub it along the inside of the microplate well as excess template DNA can have a negative effect on the efficiency of a PCR reaction.
2. Bands of 520–600 bp will be seen using the pCR™II forward and reverse primers (supplied with the TA™ Cloning kit) when the pCR™II vector contains a variable region gene. A negative result (i.e., no insert in the pCR™II vector) will produce an approx 100 bp band. Treat any bands smaller than 500 bp with caution as they may be psuedogenes.
3. The consensus sequence for N-glycosylation is Asn-Xaa-(Ser/Thr)-Yaa. When Yaa is a proline, the probability of glycosylation is reduced by approx 50%. When Xaa is a proline, the probability is reduced by approx 90%. When both Xaa and Yaa are proline, the probability of glycosylation is even further reduced *(5)*. There is no single consensus sequence for O-glycosylation. The Thr/Ser acceptor sites tend to reside in helical segments containing other serine or threonine residues and adjacent prolines. Four motifs that predict O-glycosylation *(15,16)* are:
   a. Xaa-Pro-Xaa-Xaa where at least one Xaa is Thr
   b. Thr-Xaa-Xaa-Xaa where at least one Xaa is Thr
   c. Xaa-Xaa-Thr-Xaa where at least one Xaa is Arg or Lys
   d. Ser-Xaa-Xaa-Xaa where at least one Xaa-Ser
4. If the DNA sequence of the selected human variable region is not available, use the DNA sequence from a closely related human variable region gene modifying the DNA sequence as necessary to obtain the required coding sequence.
5. Pfu polymerase has a proofreading facility that minimizes insertion of mutations due to PCR error.
6. The Pfu DNA polymerase is added last, i.e., after "hot start," because its 3'-5' exonuclease activity could potentially cause digestion of both primers and assembled gene products.
7. The AmpliTaq DNA polymerase adds a poly A tail to the 3'-ends of the PCR product, thus facilitating cloning using the TA Clining kit.
8. This assay is designed to detect human IgG1/kappa antibodies. It can be adapted to detect other isotypes of human, chimeric, or reshaped human antibodies. To assay for human IgG4/kappa antibodies, use human IgG4/kappa antibody (Sigma, I-4639) as the standard and dilute the antibody-enzyme conjugate 1000-fold. To assay for human IgG1/lambda antibodies, use human IgG1/lambda antibody (Sigma, I-4014) as the standard and goat anti-human lambda light-chain HRP conjugate(Sigma, A-2904), diluted 2500-fold in sample-enzyme conjugate buffer, as the antibody-enzyme conjugate. To assay for human IgG4/lambda antibodies, use human IgG4/lambda antibody (Sigma, I-4764) as the standard and the anti-human lambda antibody-enzyme conjugate described above diluted 1000-fold.
9. The immunoplates may be stored at this stage (**step 1**) for up to 1 mo at 4°C.
10. To avoid possible aberrant results caused by "edge effects," the wells on the outside edges of the immunoplate are not used.
11. The optimal dilution of any antibody or antibody-enzyme conjugate used should be determined for each lot.

Acknowledgments

The authors wish to acknowledge the contributions of all previous workers in the Antibody Engineering Group at the MRC Collaborative Centre in developing and testing the methods outlined in this chapter, especially MRC Collaborative Centre scientists Dr. C.A. Kettleborough, Dr. J. Saldanha, Dr. O.J. Léger, and Dr. Jon Chappel; and visiting scientists Dr. H. Maeda of Chemo-Sero-Therapeutics Research Institute, Dr. F. Kolbinger of Novartis, and Dr. M. Tsuchiya and Dr. K. Sato of Chugai Pharmaceuticals.

References

1. Jones, P. T., Dear, P. H., Foote, J., Neuberger, M. S., and Winter, G. (1986) Replacing the complementarity determining regions in a human antibody with those from a mouse. *Nature* **321,** 522–525.
2. Reichmann, L., Clark, M., Waldmann, H., Winter, G. (1988) Reshaping human antibodies for therapy. *Nature* **332,** 323–327.
3. Kozak, M. (1987) At least six nucleotides preceding the AUG initiator codon enhance translation in mammalian cells. *J. Mol. Biol.* **196,** 947–950.
4. Kettleborough, C. A., Saldanha, J., Heath, V. J., Morrison, C. J., and Bendig, M. M. (1991) Humanization of a mouse monoclonal antibody by CDR-grafting: the importance of framework residues on loop conformation.*Protein Eng.* **4,** 773–783.
5. Maeda, H., Matsushita, S., Eda, Y., Kimachi, K., Tokiyoshi, S., and Bendig, M. M. (1991) Humanization of a mouse monoclonal antibody by CDR-grafting: the importance of framework residues on loop conformation. *Hum. Antibod Hybridomas* **2,** 124–134.
6. Chothia, C. and Lesk, A. M. (1987) Canonical structures for the hypervariable regions of immunoglobulins. *J. Mol. Biol.* **196,** 901–917.
7. Chothia, C., Lesk, A. M., Gherardi, E., Tomlinson, I. M., Walter, G., Marks, J. D., et al. (1992) Structural repertoire of the human VH segments. *J. Mol. Biol.* **227,** 799–817.
8. Chothia, C., Lesk, A. M., Tramontano, A., Levitt, M., Smith-Gill, S. J., Air, G., et al. (1989) Conformations of immunoglobulin hypervariable regions. *Nature* **34,** 877–883.
9. Tramontano, A., Chothia, C., and Lesk, A. M. (1990) Framework residue 71 is a major determinant of the position and conformation of the second hypervariable region in the VH domains of immunoglobulins. *J. Mol. Biol.* **215,** 175–181.
10. Sato, K., Tsuchiya, M., Saldanha, J. Koishihara, Y., Ohsugi, Y., Kishimoto, T., and Bendig, M. M. (1993) Reshaping a human antibody to inhibit the interleukin 6-dependent tumor cell growth. *Cancer Res.* **53,** 851–856.
11. Stemmer, W. P. C. (1995) Single-step assembly of a gene and entire plasmid from large numbers of oligodeoxyribonucleotides. *Gene* **146,** 49–53.
12. Chomczynski, P. and Sacchi, N. (1987) Single step method of RNA isolation by acid guanidinium thiocyanate-phenol-chloroform extraction. *Anal. Biochem.* **162,** 156–159.
13. Kabat, E. A., Wu, T. T., Perry, H. M., Gottesman, K. S., and Foeller, C. (1991) Sequences of Proteins of Immunological Interest, 5th ed. U.S. Department of Health and Human Services, U.S. Government Printing Office, Washington, DC.
14. Foote, J. and Winter, G. (1992) Antibody framework residues affecting the conformation of the hypervariable loops. *J. Mol. Biol.* **224,** 487–499.
15. Mountain, A. and Adair, J. R. (1992) Engineering antibodies for therapy. *Biotechnol. Genet. Eng. Rev.* **10,** 1–142.
16. Pisano, A., Redmond, J. W., Williams, K. L., and Gooley, A. A. (1993) Glycosylatioin sited identified by solid-phase Edman degradation: O-linked glycosylation motifs on human glycophorin A. *Glycobiology* **3,** 429–435.

III

Recombinant Antibody Fragments
from Phagemid-Displayed Antibody Repertoires

6

Generation and Screening of a Modular Human scFv Expression Library from Multiple Donors

Martin Welschof, Christiane Christ, Ingrid Hermes, Armin Keller, Christian Kleist, and Michael Braunagel

1. Introduction

Human monoclonal antibodies (MAbs) are more suitable than MAbs of animal origin for clinical applications because of lower hypersensitivity reactions, less formation of circulating immune complexes, and lower anti-immunoglobulin responses. The classical production of human monoclonal antibodies via the hybridoma technique or Epstein-Barr virus (EBV) transformation is limited by the instability of cell lines, low antibody production, and the problems of immunizing humans with certain antigens *(1,2)*. A promising alternative is the production of human recombinant antibodies *(3)*. Recombinant DNA technology has made it possible to clone human antibody genes in vectors and to generate antibody expression libraries *(4–7)*. One approach has been to amplify and recombine the IgG repertoire of an "immunized" donor. This has been used to isolate several antibodies that were related to diseases *(8–10)*. In order to obtain more universal antibody libraries the naive IgM and the IgG repertoire of several "unimmunized" donors were pooled *(11–14)*. The complexity of the combinatorial libraries has been further increased by creating so called "semisynthetic" or "synthetic" antibody libraries *(15–20)*.

To prepare antibody DNA from peripheral lymphocytes, spleen lymphocytes or B cell lines, mRNA is first isolated by standard methods. After preparation of first strand cDNA the Fv-or Fab-encoding regions are amplified using the polymerase chain reaction (PCR) and a set of primers homologous to the variable region of the heavy (μ,γ) and light chains (κ,λ) *(14,21–25)*. The PCR products are randomly combined in an appropriate expression vector. For extra stability, the V_L and V_H domains of Fv fragments are often joined with a peptide linker *(26,27)*. The larger Fab fragment contains the V_L-C_L and V_H-C_{H1} segments linked by disulfide bonds. To facilitate the screening of these scFv-or Fab-antibody libraries, phagemid pIII display vectors are

From: *Methods in Molecular Biology, vol. 207: Recombinant Antibodies for Cancer Therapy: Methods and Protocols*
Edited by: M. Welschof and J. Krauss © Humana Press Inc., Totowa, NJ

commonly used *(28–30)*. These vectors contain a phage intergenic region to provide a packaging signal. The expression of the pIII-antibody fusion protein is regulated by a bacterial promoter under the control of a lac operator.

To display the antibody fragments on the phage surface, the phagemid must be packaged with proteins supplied by helper phages. First, *Escherichia coli* is transformed with the phagemid vector to which the PCR-products have been ligated. The phagemid-containing bacteria are infected with a helper phage such as M13KO7 to yield recombinant phage particles that display scFv or Fab fragments fused to the pIII protein. Phage displaying antibody fragments that bind to a specific antigen can be enriched from a large library of phages by panning over the antigen. Nonspecific phages are removed during the washing procedure, following which the remaining antigen-specific phages are eluted and used to reinfect exponentially growing *E. coli*. The specificity of the enriched phage particles can be confirmed in an enzyme-linked immunosorbent assay (ELISA). The screening procedure that is described in this chapter is outlined on a flowchart (**Fig. 1**).

This protocol describes the generation of individual libraries from both the IgM and IgG repertoires of multiple donors using a set of back primers which were based on V_H and V_L gene sequences from the V BASE *(31)* (**Tables 1–3B**). They correspond to the first nine amino acids of FR1. To allow for sequence variability, a representative choice of wobble nucleotides are included. These back primers are used in combination with a set of forward primers, which are homologous to the 5' end of DNA coding for the constant domains adjacent to the variable domains *(25)* (*see* **Table 4**). The primers are designed for a two-step PCR. After amplification of the Fv-regions the V_H and V_L genes are reamplified with homologous primers containing suitable restriction endonuclease sites for cloning into *pSEX81* *(10)*. These are *Nco*I (5') and *Hin*dIII (3') for V_H and *Mlu*I (5') and *Not*I (3') for V_L. In order to maximize the complexity and flexibility of the antibody library the antibody repertoire of each donor should be cloned and packaged separately. The individual phage-display libraries are only combined prior screening. Because the protocol described below recommends storing serum from each donor as reference for each individual antibody library, the combination of the individual antibody repertoires can be based on a ELISA-prescreening of the sera for the desired specificity.

2. Materials

2.1. RNA Extraction and cDNA Synthesis

1. Lymphoprep (Nyegaard & Co. AS, Oslo, Norway).
2. Optiprep.1 RNA isolation Kit (Biometra GmbH, Göttingen, Germany).
3. Optiprep.2 mRNA preparation Kit (Biometra GmbH).
4. First-strand cDNA synthesis Kit (Amersham, Amersham Place, Buckinghamshire, UK).

2.2. PCR-Amplification (of the Rearranged Variable Light- and Heavy-Chain Genes and Introduction of Restriction Sites)

1. Thermocycler PTC 150-16 (MJ Research, Watertown, MA).
2. Vent DNA polymerase (New England Biolabs, Inc., Beverly).
3. 10X Vent buffer (New England Biolabs).

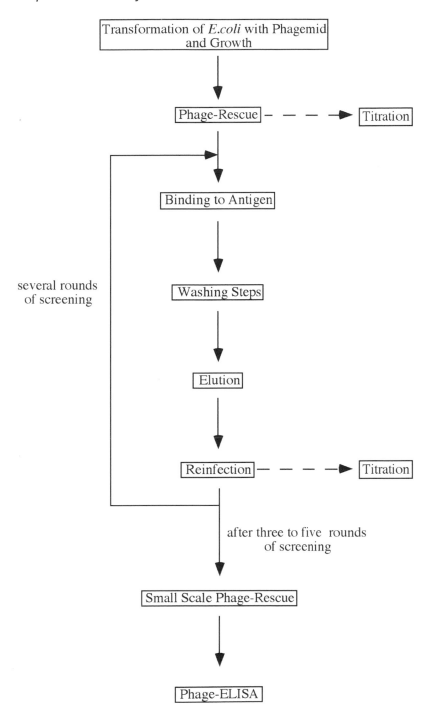

Fig. 1. Flow-chart of the screening procedure for isolating specific antibody clones.

Table 1
V$_H$-Primer for the First and Second Amplification

---

1. PCR

V$_H$-1 5' CAG GTG CAG CTG GTG CAG TCT GG 3'
           A C   A
          18 27   18%

V$_H$-2 5' CAG GTC ACC TTG AAG GAG TCT GG 3'
          A
        33%

V$_H$-3 5' GAG GTG CAG CTG GTG GAG TCT GG 3'
          C
        23%

V$_H$-4 5' CAG GTG CAG CTG CAG GAG TCG GG 3'
             C
          18%

V$_H$-5 5' GAG GTG CAG CTG GTG CAG TCT GG 3'
          A
        50%

V$_H$-6 5' CAG GTA CAG CTG CAG CAG TCA GG 3'

V$_H$-7 5' CAG GTG CAG CTG GTG CAA TCT GG 3'

2. PCR

V$_H$-1 5' GAA TAG GCC ATG GCG CAG GTG CAG CTG GTG CAG TCT GG 3'
                           A C   A
                          18 27   18%

V$_H$-2 5' GAA TAG GCC ATG GCG CAG GTC ACC TTG AAG GAG TCT GG 3'
                           A
                        33%

V$_H$-3 5' GAA TAG GCC ATG GCG GAG GTG CAG CTG GTG GAG TCT GG 3'
                           C
                      23%

V$_H$-4 5' GAA TAG GCC ATG GCG CAG GTG CAG CTG CAG GAG TCG GG 3'
                                C
                          18%

V$_H$-5 5' GAA TAG GCC ATG GCG GAG GTG CAG CTG GTG CAG TCT GG 3'
                           A
                      50%

V$_H$-6 5' GAA TAG GCC ATG GCG CAG GTA CAG CTG CAG CAG TCA GG 3'

V$_H$-7 5' GAA TAG GCC ATG GCG CAG GTG CAG CTG GTG CAA TCT GG 3'

Bases below the primer sequences represent substitutions at a given position and the number indicates the percentage of the substituted nucleotide. Restriction endonuclease recognition sequences are underlined.

4. H$_2$O *ad inj.* (Braun, Melsungen, Germany).
5. 100 mM dNTPs (New England Biolabs).
6. Bovine serum albumin (BSA), nonacetylated (10 mg/mL) (New England Biolabs).
7. 100 bp DNA molecular weight marker (Gibco-BRL, Gaithersburg, MD).

Table 2
Vκ-Primer for the First and Second Amplification

1. PCR

```
Vκ-1  5'  GAC  ATC  CAG  ATG  ACC  CAG  TCT  CC  3'
           C              G    T
           26             16   16%

Vκ-2  5'  GAT  ATT  GTG  ATG  ACC  CAG  ACT  CC  3'
           G                   T         T
           22                  44        44%

Vκ-3  5'  GAA  ATT  GTG  TTG  ACG  CAG  TCT  CC  3'
                A    A A       A
                29   14 43     43%

Vκ-4  5'  GAC  ATC  GTG  ATG  ACC  CAG  TCT  CC  3'
Vκ-5  5'  GAA  ACG  ACA  CTC  ACG  CAG  TCT  CC  3'
Vκ-6  5'  GAA  ATT  GTG  CTG  ACT  CAG  TCT  CC  3'
           T G            A    A
           33 33          33   33%
```

2. PCR

```
Vκ-1  5'  TA  CAG GAT CCA CGC GTA GAC ATC CAG ATG ACC CAG TCT CC  3'
                                        C           G    T
                                        26          16   16%

Vκ-2  5'  TA  CAG GAT CCA CGC GTA GAT ATT GTG ATG ACC CAG ACT CC  3'
                                        G                T        T
                                        22               44       44%

Vκ-3  5'  TA  CAG GAT CCA CGC GTA GAA ATT GTG TTG ACG CAG TCT CC  3'
                                            A   A A      A
                                            29  14 43    43%

Vκ-4  5'  TA  CAG GAT CCA CGC GTA GAC ATC GTG ATG ACC CAG TCT CC  3'
Vκ-5  5'  TA  CAG GAT CCA CGC GTA GAA ACG ACA CTC ACG CAG TCT CC  3'
Vκ-6  5'  TA  CAG GAT CCA CGC GTA GAA ATT GTG CTG ACT CAG TCT CC  3'
                                        T G           A    A
                                        33 33         33   33%
```

Bases below the primer sequences represent substitutions at a given position and the number indicates the percentage of the substituted nucleotide. Restriction endonuclease recognition sequences are underlined.

8. Agarose (AGS, Heidelberg, Germany).
9. 1X Tris-acetate electrophoresis buffer (1X TAE buffer): Prepare a stock solution of 50X TAE and dilute it 1:50 with water before use.
10. 50X TAE buffer: Dissolve 242 g Tris-base in distilled water. Add 57.1 mL glacial acetic acid, 100 mL 0.5 M EDTA and water to a total volume of 1 L.
11. 0.5 M EDTA, pH 8.0.
12. Ethidium bromide (10 mg/mL).

Table 3A
Vλ-Primer for the First Amplification (1. PCR)

```
Vλ-1   5' CAG TCT GTG CTG ACT CAG CCA CC   3'
                T       G       G
               20      40      40%
Vλ-2   5' CAG TCT GCC CTG ACT CAG CCT CC   3'
                                       GG
                                    40 20%
Vλ-3   5' TCC TAT GAG CTG ACT CAG CCA CC   3'
               C   T       TG      T
              13  13      13 13    13%
Vλ-4   5' CAG CCT GTG CTG ACT CAA TCC CC   3'
              T   T               C   T
             33  33              33  33%
Vλ-5   5' CAG CCT GTG CTG ACT CAG CCA CC   3'
              G                       G
             33%                      T
                                     33% each
Vλ-6   5' AAT TTT ATG CTG ACT CAG CCC CA   3'
Vλ-7   5' CAG ACT GTG GTG ACT CAG GAG CC   3'
              G
             50%
Vλ-8   5' CAG ACT GTG GTG ACC CAG GAG CC   3'
Vλ-9   5' CAG CCT GTG CTG ACT CAG CCA CC   3'
Vλ-10  5' CAG GCA GGG CTG ACT CAG CCA CC   3'
```

Bases below the primer sequences represent substitutions at a given position and the number indicates the percentage of the substituted nucleotide.

2.3. Cloning into pSEX81 (see Note 1)

1. Petri dishes, 85 mm and 145 mm diameter (Greiner, Frickenhausen, Germany).
2. Table-top microcentrifuge.
3. Clinical centrifuge with swinging-bucket rotor.
4. QIAquick Gel Extraction Kit (Quiagen, Hilden, Germany).
5. QIAquick-spin PCR Purification Kit (Quiagen).
6. XL1 blue electrocompetent *E. coli* (Stratagene Cloning Systems, La Jolla, CA).
7. *Hin*dIII restriction endonuclease (New England Biolabs).
8. *Nco*I restriction endonuclease (New England Biolabs).
9. *Mlu*I restriction endonuclease (Boehringer GmbH).
10. *Not*I restriction endonuclease (Boehringer GmbH).
11. 10X Restriction enzyme buffer 4 (New England Biolabs).
12. 10X Restriction enzyme buffer H (Boehringer GmbH).
13. RNaseA (Boehringer GmbH).
14. Calf intestine phosphatase, alkaline (CIP) (Boehringer GmbH).
15. T4 DNA-ligase (Boehringer GmbH).
16. 10X T4 DNA-ligase buffer (Boehringer GmbH).
17. 0.5 *M* EDTA, pH 8.0.

Table 3B
Vλ-Primer for the Second Amplification (2. PCR)

Vλ-1 5'-TACAGGATCC<u>ACGCGT</u>ACAGTCTGTGCTGACTCAGCCACC-3'
                             T   G   G
                            20   40   40%

Vλ-2 5'-TACAGGATCC<u>ACGCGT</u>ACAGTCTGCCCTGACTCAGCCTCC-3'
                                                 GG
                                           40 20%

Vλ-3 5'-TACAGGATCC<u>ACGCGT</u>ATCCTATGAGCTGACTCAGCCACC-3'
                             C   T   TG   T
                            13 13   13 13 13%

Vλ-4 5'-TACAGGATCC<u>ACGCGT</u>ACAGCCTGTGCTGACTCAATCCCC-3'
                             T   T   C   T
                            33   33   33   33%

Vλ-5 5'-TACAGGATCC<u>ACGCGT</u>ACAGCCTGTGCTGACTCAGCCACC-3'
                             G   G
                           33%   T
                                          33% each

Vλ-6 5'-TACAGGATCC<u>ACGCGT</u>AAAATTTT ATGCTGACTCAGCCCCA-3'

Vλ-7 5'-TACAGATCC<u>ACGCGT</u>ACAGACTGTGGTGACTCAGGAGCC-3'
                             G
                           50%

Vλ-8 5'-TACAGGATCC<u>ACGCGT</u>ACAGACTGTGGTGACCCAGGAGCC-3'

Vλ-9 5'-TACAGGATCC<u>ACGCGT</u>ACAGCCTGTGCTGACT CAGCCACC-3'

Vλ-10 5'-TACAGGATCC<u>ACGCGT</u>ACAGGCAGGGCTGACT CAGCCACC-3'

Bases below the primer sequences represent substitutions at a given position and the number indicates the percentage of the substituted nucleotide. Restriction endonuclease recognition sequences are underlined.

18. 100 bp DNA molecular weight marker (Gibco-BRL).
19. Lambda BstE II DNA molecular weight Marker (New England Biolabs).
20. Agarose (AGS).
21. 1X TAE buffer (*see* **Subheading 2.2.**).
22. 1 *M* Tris-HCl, pH 7.4.
23. Ethidium bromide (10 mg/mL).
24. 3 *M* Sodium acetate, pH 4.6.
25. Glycogen from mussels, molecular biology grade, (20 µg/µL) (Boehringer GmbH, Mannheim, Germany).
26. Ethanol p.A.
27. Ethanol p.A. (80%).
28. 2 *M* Glucose, sterile filtered.
29. Ampicillin (5 mg/mL), sterile filtered.
30. SOB-GA medium agar plates: To 15 g of Bacto-agar, 20 g of Bacto-tryptone, 5 g of Bacto-yeast extract, and 0.5 g of NaCl, add distilled water to 920 mL and autoclave. After the medium has cooled to 55°C, add 10 mL of sterile MgCl$_2$, 50 mL of sterile 2 *M* glucose, and 20 mL of sterile-filtered ampicillin (5 mg/mL). Pour plates quickly.

Table 4
Constant Domain-Primer for the First and Second Amplification

1. PCR

IgM	5' AAG GGT TGG GGC GGA TGC ACT 3'	
IgG	5' GAC CGA TGG GCC CTT GGT GGA 3'	
	G	
	50%	
cκ	5' GAA GAC AGA TGG TGC AGC CAC AGT 3'	
cλ	5' AGA GGA GGG CGG GAA CAG AGT GAC 3'	
	C T	
	25 30%	

2. PCR

IgM	5' CA GTC <u>AAG CTT</u> TGG GGC GGA TGC ACT 3'	
IgG	5' CA GTC <u>AAG CTT</u> TGG GCC CTT GGT GGA 3'	
cκ	5' TGA CAA GCT T<u>GC GGC CGC</u> GAA GAC AGA TGG TGC AGC CAC AGT	3'
cλ	5' TGA CAA GCT T<u>GC GGC CGC</u> AGA GGA GGG CGG GAA CAG AGT GAC	3'
	C T	
	25 30%	

Bases below the primer sequences represent substitutions at a given position and the number indicates the percentage of the substituted nucleotide. Restriction endonuclease recognition sequences are underlined.

31. SOB-GA medium: Dissolve 15 g of Bacto-agar, 20 g of Bacto-tryptone, 5 g of Bacto-yeast extract; and 0.5 g of NaCl in 800 mL distilled water, adjust the pH of the medium to 7.5 with 1 M NaOH, add distilled water to 920 mL and autoclave. Before use, add 10 mL of sterile $MgCl_2$, 50 mL of sterile 2 M glucose and 20 mL of sterile-filtered ampicillin (5 mg/mL).
32. Sterile glycerol.
33. Sterile glass spreader.

2.4. Phage Rescue, Panning, Reinfection, Small Scale Phage Rescue

1. Sterile glass Erlenmeyer flasks, 100 mL and 1000 mL.
2. Petri dishes, 85 mm and 145 mm diameter (Greiner, Frickenhausen, Germany).
3. Maxisorb® Immunotubes and caps (Nunc, Roskilde, Denmark).
4. Sterile polypropylene 96-deep-well microtiter plate (Beckmann, München, Germany) and sealing device (Beckman, Biomek™, Nr. 538619).
5. End-over-end shaker.
6. Table-top microcentrifuge.
7. Clinical centrifuge with swinging-bucket rotor.
8. IEC refrigerated centrifuge (or equivalent) with adaptors for microtiter plates.
9. ELISA plate shaker (e.g., IKA MTS-2).
10. Helper phage M13KO7-derived VCSM13 (Stratagene Cloning Systems, La Jolla, CA).
11. XL-1 blue bacteria (Stratagene Cloning Systems).
12. 2 M Glucose, sterile filtered.
13. Ampicillin (5 mg/mL), sterile filtered.
14. Kanamycin (10 mg/mL), sterile filtered.

15. M9-minimal medium agar plates: To 15 g of Bacto-agar add water to 750 mL and autoclave. After the solution has cooled to 55°C, add 200 mL of sterile 5X M9 salts, 50 mL of sterile 2 M glucose, and 10 mL of sterile-filtered 100X supplement. Pour plates quickly.

16. 5X M9 salts: To 37.4 g $Na_2HPO_4 \times 2 H_2O$, 11.75 g $NaH_2PO_4 \times H_2O$, 2.5 g NaCl and 5 g NH_4Cl, add distilled water to 1 L and autoclave.

17. 100X Supplement: To 1 mL of 1 M $MgSO_4 \times 7 H_2O$, 1 mL of 100 mM $CaCl_2 \times 2 H_2O$, 30 μL of 100 mM $Fe(III)Cl_3 \times 6 H_2O$ and 60 μL of 500 mM Thiamin, add distilled water to 10 mL and sterile filter.

18. SOB-GA medium agar plates: To 15 g of Bacto-agar, 20 g of Bacto-tryptone, 5 g of Bacto-yeast extract, and 0.5 g of NaCl, add distilled water to 920 mL and autoclave. After the medium has cooled to 55°C, add 10 mL of sterile $MgCl_2$, 50 mL of sterile 2 M glucose and 20 mL of sterile filtered ampicillin (5 mg/mL). Pour plates quickly.

19. 2XYT medium: Dissolve 15 g of Bacto-agar, 17 g of Bacto-tryptone, 10 g of Bacto-yeast extract, and 5 g of NaCl in 800 mL distilled water, adjust the pH of the medium to 7.5 with 1 M NaOH, add distilled water to 1 L total volume and autoclave.

20. 2XYT-GA medium: 2XYT medium containing 100 μg/mL ampicillin and 100 mM glucose.

21. 2XYT-AK medium: 2XYT medium containing 100 μg/mL ampicillin and 50 μg/mL kanamycin.

22. Sterile Glycerol.

23. PEG/NaCl: to 200 g Polyethylene glycol (PEG) 6000 and 146.1 g NaCl add distilled water to 1 L, heat to dissolve and autoclave.

24. Phage dilution buffer: 10 mM Tris-HCl, pH 7.5, 20 mM NaCl, 2 mM EDTA.

25. Coating buffer: 50 mM Na_2CO_3, pH 9.6.

26. PBS: 50 mM phosphate buffer, pH 7.2, 140 mM NaCl.

27. PBST: PBS, Tween 20 (0.1% v/v).

28. Blocking buffer: 2% (w/v) skimmed milk powder in PBS, use immediately.

29. 100 mM Triethylamine

30. 1 M Tris-HCl, pH 7.4.

2.5. Phage-ELISA

1. Anti-M13-antibody: rabbit-anti-M13-Sera, diluted 1:1000 in blocking buffer (Stratagene, No. 240210).

2. Second antibody: goat-anti-rabbit IgG, HRP-conjugated (Jackson Immuno Research Laboratories, Inc., West Grove, PA, No. 111-095-144).

3. Enzyme substrate: TMBKit from Kierkegaard-Perry-Labs, No. 507600.

4. ELISA-plates: Bibby-Dunn (Asbach, Germany), PVC, activated, flat bottom, No.: 77-173-05.

5. PBS: 50 mM phosphate buffer, pH 7.2, 140 mM NaCl.

6. PBST: PBS, Tween 20 (0.1% v/v).

7. Blocking buffer: 2% (w/v) skimmed milk powder in PBS, store at –20°C.

8. Coating buffer: 50 mM Na_2CO_3, pH 9.6.

9. *E. coli*-lysate-coated-nitocellulose:
   a. Pellet a 50 mL overnight culture of *E. coli* at 6000g for 10 min. Discard the supernatant.
   b. Resuspend the pellet in 10 mL PBS and lyse by sonification.
   c. Incubate a sheet of nitrocellulose (ca. 50 cm^2) with the cell lysate for 1 h at room temperature (RT) on a shaker.
   d. Wash the nitrocellulose 3×15 min in PBST.
   e. Cut the nitrocellulose sheet into 1 cm^2 pieces. Store them at –20°C.
   f. One piece of the *E. coli*-lysate-coated-nitrocellulose is enough to preabsorb up to 20 mL of diluted antibody.

3. Methods

3.1. RNA Extraction and cDNA Synthesis

1. Separate peripheral blood mononuclear cells (PBMC) by density gradient centrifugation on Lymphoprep starting with 50 mL blood from each donor. Two milliliters of serum from each donor is stored at –80°C as a reference for each antibody library.
2. Prepare total RNA by acid guanidium thiocyanate phenol chloroform (AGPC) extraction and isopropanol precipitation *(32,33)* using an Optiprep.1 RNA isolation kit (any other kit using the AGPC method is usable).
3. Poly (A)+ RNA was extracted from total RNA on oligo (dT) minicolumns using an Optiprep.2 mRNA preparation kit (any other kit for mRNA extraction is usable).
4. cDNA is prepared with a first-strand cDNA synthesis kit.

3.2. PCR-Amplification of the Rearranged Variable Light- and Heavy-Chain Genes (1. PCR)

1. Amplification by PCR is carried out in a total of 50 μL containing 5–50 ng (in 1–10 μL) cDNA, 10 or 25 pmol of each primer, 300 μM dNTPs, 5 μL of 10X PCR buffer, 5 μg BSA and 1 U *Vent* DNA polymerase.
2. Perform 24 separate reactions. Combine each variable heavy chain back primer with a IgM or -IgG forward primer and each κ and λ variable light chain back primer with the corresponding constant region forward primer. The genes Vh6,7 and Vλ6-10 are amplified in single reaction mixtures using 10 pmol of each primer.
3. Run 30 PCR cycles on a thermal cycler. The thermal cycle is 95°C for 0.5 min (denaturation), 55°C for 1 min (annealing), and 75°C for 1 min (extension). At the beginning of the first cycle incubate at 95°C for 3' and at the end of the last cycle incubate at 75°C for 5 min (*see* **Note 2**).
4. The amplified DNA fragments are analyzed by electrophoresis on a 1.5% agarose gel and stained with ethidium bromide (expected size for the HC and λLC is around 400 bp, for the κLC around 360 bp) (*see* **Note 2**).

3.3. Introduction of Restriction Sites (2.PCR)

1. Amplification by PCR is carried out in a total of 50 μL containing 1 μL 1.PCR (10–20 ng), 10 or 25 pmol of each primer, 300 μM dNTPs, 5 μL of 10X PCR Buffer, 5 μg BSA, and 1 U *Vent* DNA polymerase (*see* **Note 3**).
2. Perform 24 separate reactions. Combine each homologous second variable heavy chain back primer with the homologous second-IgM or -IgG forward primer and each homologous second κ and λ variable light chain back primer with the corresponding homologous second constant region forward primer.
3. Run 10–15 PCR cycles using an MJ Research thermal cycler. The thermal cycle is 95°C for 0.5 min (denaturation), 57°C for 1 min (annealing), and 75°C for 1 min (extension). At the beginning of the first cycle incubate at 95°C for 3 min and at the end of the last cycle incubate at 75°C for 5 min.
4. The amplified DNA fragments are analyzed by electrophoresis on a 1.5% agarose gel and stained with ethidium bromide (expected size for the HC and the κλLC is around 400 bp) (*see* **Note 4**).

3.4. Cloning into pSEX81

3.4.1. Light-Chain Sublibraries

1. Digest 10 µg pSEX81 (*see* **Note 5**) by adding 50 U of *Mlu*I, 50 U of *Not*I, 10 µg RNaseA (*see* **Note 5**), 0.5 U of alkaline phosphatase (CIP), restriction buffer H from Boehringer and H$_2$O. The final volume should be at least 10× the volume of the enzyme samples (*see* **Note 7**). Incubate for 2h at 37°C.
2. Add 0.5 U of alkaline phosphatase (CIP) and incubate for 2 h at 37°C.
3. Add EDTA, ph 8.0, to a final concentration of 5 m*M* (*see* **Note 8**) and incubate for 20 min at 65°C.
4. Add agarose gel electrophoresis sample buffer, load a 1% agarose gel with 2 µg/lane of the digest and run at 80 V. Cut out the gel band containing the *Mlu/Not*-pSEX81-fragment and extract the DNA (QIAquick gel extraction kit).
5. Remove PCR primers and nonspecific bands from the κ- and λ-light chain PCR products by agarose gel electrophoresis. Add 2 µg/lane of PCR products in sample buffer to 1.5% gels and run at 80 V. Cut out the gel bands containing the specific PCR products and extract the DNA (QIAquick gel extraction kit).
6. Digest 1 µg of the pooled κ- and λ-light chain PCR products, respectively, with 19 U of *Mlu*I and 14 U of *Not*I, restriction buffer H from Boehringer and H$_2$O. The final volume should be at least 10× the volume of the enzyme samples (*see* **Note 7**). Incubate for 4 h at 37°C followed by an incubation for 20 min at 65°C.
7. Remove stuffer fragments and purify the digested PCR products using the QIAquick-spin PCR purification kit.
8. Ligate the vector and insert using a molar ratio between 1:1 and 1:3. The reaction mixture consists of 50 ng DNA, 1 U of T4 ligase, ligation buffer from Boehringer and H$_2$O to a final volume of 10–15 µL. Incubate overnight at 16°C.
9. Precipitate the DNA by adding 1/10 vol 3 *M* sodium acetate, 20 µg glycogen, 2.5X vol absolute ethanol. Incubate for at least 1 h at –20°C. Sediment the precipitate by centrifugation for 30 min at 13,000 rpm (minifuge). Wash the pellet with 500 µL 80% ethanol and centrifuge for 10 min at 13,000 rpm (minifuge). Repeat this step 3×. Allow the pellet to dry at RT. Resuspend the dried pellet in 1–5 µL H$_2$O.
10. Use the products of one ligation reaction for the electroporation of 40 µL electrocompetent *E. coli* XL1blue according the suppliers protocol. Plate the bacteria on 3 or 4 SOB-GA agar plates of 145 mm diameter and incubate overnight at 30°C (*see* **Notes 9** and **10**).
11. Isolate the plasmid DNA by adding 10 mL 2X SOB-GA medium to each plate. Disperse the bacteria into the medium by scraping them off the agar with a sterile glass spreader. Pellet the bacteria at 4000 rpm for 15 min in a clinical centrifuge with a swinging-bucket rotor. Lyse the cells and isolate the plasmid DNA (*see* **Note 11**).

3.4.2. Cloning Heavy Chains into the Light Chain Sublibraries

1. To 10 µg of the light chain sublibrary in pSEX81 add 40 U of *Nco*I, 60 U of *Hind*III, 10 µg RNaseA (*see* **Note 6**), 0.5 U of akaline phosphatase, restriction buffer H from Boehringer and H$_2$O. The final volume should be at least 10× the volume of the enzyme samples (*see* **Note 7**). Incubate for 2h at 37°C.
2. Add 0.5 U of alkaline phosphatase (CIP) and incubate for 2 h at 37°C.

3. Add EDTA, pH 8.0, to a final concentration of 5 mM (*see* **Note 7**) and incubate for 20 min at 65°C.

4. Add agarose gel electrophoresis sample buffer, load a 1% agarose gel with 2 µg/lane of the digest and run at 80 V. Cut out the gel band containing the *Not*I/*Hin*dIII-pSEX81-fragment and extract the DNA (QIAquick gel extraction kit).

5. Remove PCR primers and nonspecific bands from the heavy chain PCR products by agarose gel electrophoresis. Add 2 µg/lane of PCR products in sample buffer to 1.5% gels and run at 80 V. Cut out the gel bands containing the specific PCR products and extract the DNA (QIAquick gel extraction kit).

6. Digest 1 µg of the pooled IgG- and IgM-heavy chain PCR products, respectively, with 32 U of *Nco*I and 19 U of *Hin*dIII, restriction buffer H from Boehringer and H$_2$O. The final volume should be at least 10× the volume of the enzyme samples (*see* **Note 7**). Incubate for 4 h at 37°C followed by an incubation for 20 min at 65°C.

7. Remove stuffer fragments and purify the digested PCR product using the QIAquick-spin PCR purification kit.

8. The ligation of the heavy chain PCR products into pSEX81 containing the light chain library was performed under the same conditions as used for cloning the light chains into pSEX81. The ligation product was also similarly purified as described in **Subheading 3.4.1.**, **step 9**. Use the products of one ligation reaction for the electroporation of 40 µL electrocompetent *E. coli* XL1blue (Stratagene) according the suppliers protocol.

3.5. Phage Rescue

1. Plate each transformation of the ligated DNA library onto three SOB-GA agar plates of 145 mm diameter and incubate overnight at 30°C (*see* **Note 9**).

2. Add 10 mL 2XYT-GA medium to each plate and scrape bacteria into the medium with a sterile glass spreader. Pool cells from all three plates and measure absorbance at 600 nm (A$_{600}$) in appropriate dilution.

3. Inoculate 400 mL of 2XYT-GA medium with bacteria from the plate to A600 of 0.025 (*see* **Note 12**).

4. To the remaining bacteria harvested from the plates add glycerol to a final concentration of 20% (v/v) and freeze in appropriate aliquots at –70°C. These are the library stock cultures and should be handled with care (*see* **Note 13**).

5. Grow the inoculated culture at 37°C with shaking at 280 rpm until an A$_{600}$ of 0.1 is reached.

6. Add M13KO7 helper phage at multiplicity of infection of 20 and mix gently (*see* **Notes 14** and **15**).

7. Incubate 15 min at 37°C without shaking, then 45 min at 37°C with shaking at 260 rpm.

8. Pellet infected bacteria for 10 min at 1500g.

9. Gently resuspend the bacteria in 400 mL of 2XYT-AK medium (no glucose) (*see* **Note 16**).

10. Grow at 37°C with shaking at 280 rpm for 5–8 h (*see* **Note 17**).

11. Take 1 mL of the culture and centrifuge in a microcentrifuge >13000g for 2 min, use supernatant for determination of number of infectious particles (titration) (*see* **Notes 17** and **18**).

12. Spin the rest of the culture at >6000g for 15 min at 4°C to pellet the cells. From now on keep everything on ice!

13. Add 1/5 vol ice cold PEG solution to the supernatant and place on ice for at least 30 min.

14. Spin at 10,000g for 20 min at 4°C (*see* **Note 20**).

15. Discard the supernatant and invert the tube over a clean paper towel to remove remaining buffer.

16. Resuspend the pellet in 4 mL of ice cold phage dilution buffer (*see* **Note 21**).
17. Transfer the resuspended phages to 1.5 mL tubes and spin in a microcentrifuge 5 min >13,000g at 4°C to pellet cellular debris.
18. Transfer supernatant to fresh tubes and place aliquots on ice. Take a 10 µL aliquot and determine the number of infectious particles (titration of phages) (*see* **Note 18**).
20. Proceed with panning to select for antigen-positive recombinant phage antibodies (*see* **Note 22**).

3.6. Panning to Select for Antigen-Binding Clones

1. Coat one Maxi Sorb® Immunotube with appropriate amounts of your protein diluted in 50 mM Na$_2$CO$_3$, pH 9.6 buffer or PBS. Coating can be performed for 2 h at RT or overnight at 4°C by rotating end-over-end (*see* **Note 23**). Always incubate one tube only with coating buffer but without antigen. This will be the negative control (*see* **Note 23**).
2. For each immunotube inoculate 20 mL of 2XYT-G medium with a colony from a minimal medium plate and incubate at 37°C with shaking at 280 rpm until the culture reaches an A$_{600}$ of 0.4. These bacteria are needed for reinfection with the enriched phage clones (*see* **Subheading 3.7.**).
3. Wash immunotubes 3× with 2 mL of PBS. For washing, add 2 mL of PBS to the tube, close it and vortex 2 s. Empty the tube completely after each wash (*see* **Note 25**).
4. Block with blocking buffer at RT by rotating end over end for 3 h (*see* **Note 26**).
5. Wash immunotubes 3× with PBS as in **step 3**.
6. Dilute 1×10^{11}–1×10^{12} of the recombinant phages in 5 mL of blocking buffer and incubate for 15 min at RT (*see* **Notes 27** and **28**).
7. Add the preincubated phage dilution to the antigen coated tube and incubate at RT by rotating end over end for 30 min, then leave it undisturbed for another 1.5 h.
8. Wash the tube 20× with PBS containing 0.1% Tween-20 and 20× with PBS as described in **step 3**.
9. To elute the bound phage antibodies add 1 mL of 100 mM triethylamine to the tube and agitate gently for 5 min. Make sure that all parts of the tube are rinsed. Neutralize phage solution with 1 mL of Tris-HCl, pH 7.5, and place it immediately on ice (*see* **Note 29**).

3.7. Reinfection of E. coli with Enriched Phage Clones

1. Each sample of phages eluted from an individual immunotube is added to 20 mL exponentially growing XL-1 blue or TG1 cells. These bacteria are prepared by transferring a colony from a minimal medium plate to 20 mL of 2XYT medium and incubating at 37°C with shaking at 280 rpm until the culture reaches an A$_{600}$ of 0.4.
2. Mix phages and bacteria by gently agitating the culture (*see* **Note 30**).
3. Leave the culture undisturbed for 15 min at 37°C, then shake at 260 rpm for 45 min at 37°C.
4. Remove 100 µL of the 20 mL cell suspension. Prepare 10-fold dilutions of the cell suspension in 2XYT-GA medium and plate onto separate SOB-GA agar plates (titer plates) (*see* **Note 31**). Incubate titer plates overnight at 30°C.
5. Centrifuge the reinfected cell suspension 5 min at 3400g.
6. Discard supernatant, resuspend the bacteria immediately in 1 mL of SOB-GA medium and plate them onto three SOB-GA medium agar plates of 145 mm diameter. When dry, invert the plates and incubate overnight at 30°C (*see* **Note 32**).
7. Next day resuspend the bacteria in 2XYT-GA medium as described in **Subheading 3.5.**, **step 2** and proceed with phage rescue. Plates can also be sealed and stored for up to 2 wk at 4°C before rescue (*see* **Note 33**).

8. For analyzing individual clones, take isolated colonies from your titer plates and proceed as described in the next subheading (*see* **Note 34**).

3.8. Small Scale Phage Rescue

1. Add 500 µL of 2XYT-GA medium to each well of a sterile polypropylene 96-deep-well microtiter plate (*see* **Note 35**).
2. Transfer individual isolated colonies (e.g., from your titer plates) to separate wells using sterile toothpicks or pipet tips.
3. Incubate overnight (18 h) at 37°C at 1100 rpm on an IKA MTS-2 ELISA shaker. This is the master plate (*see* **Notes 36** and **37**).
4. Transfer 5 µL of saturated culture from each well of the master plate to the corresponding well of a new plate containing 500 µL of 2XYT-GA medium.
5. Incubate at 1100 rpm on an IKA ELISA shaker for 3 h at 37°C if using XL-1 blue or 1.5 h if using TG1 cells.
6. Add 1×10^{10} M13KO7 helper phages to each well.
7. Place the microtiter plates onto the ELISA shaker, mix with 1100 rpm for 5 s and leave them undisturbed for 30 min at 37°C.
8. Incubate with shaking (1100 rpm) at 37°C for 1 h.
9. Centrifuge plates at 350*g* for 10 min at RT.
10. Carefully remove the supernatant and discard in an appropriate waste container.
11. Add 500 µL of prewarmed (RT or 37°C) 2XYT-AK medium (No Glucose) to each well.
12. Incubate at 37°C with shaking at 1100 rpm for 5–8 h (*see* **Note 17**).
13. Centrifuge 20 min at 1000*g* at 4°C to pellet the cells.
14. Transfer 400 µL of the supernatant to a polypropylene 96-deep-well microtiter plate precooled to 4°C.
15. Seal the plate and store on ice or 4°C until required for the phage ELISA (*see* **Note 22**).

3.9. Phage-ELISA

1. Add 1 µg antigen to 100 µL coating buffer per well. Incubate overnight at 4°C or 4 h at RT. Discard the coating solution and wash 1× with 200 µL PBS (*see* **Notes 38** and **39**).
2. Each well of the microwell titer plate is blocked with 200 µL of blocking buffer. Incubate 2 h at RT. Discard the blocking buffer and wash 3× with PBS (*see* **Note 26**).
3. Add 100 µL of rescued phagemids (containing 108–109 particles) to each well. Incubate 2 h at RT. Discard the phage solution and wash 5× with PBST (*see* **Note 40**).
4. Add an appropriate amount of anti-M13-antibody diluted in 100 µL blocking buffer. Incubate 2 h at RT. Discard the phage solution and wash 6× with PBST (*see* **Note 41**).
5. Add an appropriate amount of "second antibody" diluted in 100 µL blocking buffer. Incubate 2 h at RT. Discard the phage solution and wash 5× with PBST (*see* **Note 42**).
6. Add an appropriate amount of "enzyme substrate" in 100 µL solution and quantify the reaction with a ELISA reader (*see* **Notes 32** and **44**).

4. Notes

1. All reagents of Boehringer GmbH are now sold by Roche Molecular Biochemicals.
2. Fairly low stringent conditions are used in order to amplify a wide range of Ig genes. Because of length variations (especially in the CDR-3 of the HC variable region) one can not expect to see sharp bands in gel electrophoresis! Sharp bands instead of broad bands could be an indication that the complexity of the amplified Ab repertoire is not very high.
3. If there is more than one band (expected size for the HC and λLC ca. 400 bp, for the κLC ca, 360 bp) we recommend purifying the PCR products of the first PCR.

4. One clear band should be obtained. If this is not the case, we recommend testing different cycle numbers. Please remember that one should not expect sharp bands because of length variations in the CDR-3!

5. The above protocols were established using the phagemid vector pSEX81.

6. If your plasmid preparation is free of RNA the RNase-treatment is unnecessary.

7. The final volume should always be at least 10× more than that of the enzyme samples in order to dilute the glycerol concentration of the enzyme storage buffer below 5%. Higher concentrations of glycerol cause star activity.

8. Inactivation of the alkaline phosphatase is very important!

9. Both XL-1 blue and TG1 bacteria are suitable hosts for phagemid libraries, whereby TG1 grows faster than XL-1 blue. Plating transformed bacteria onto SOB-GA plates reduces the risk of losing slower growing clones.

10. One should obtain 107 transformants per ligation reaction obtaining a total complexity of 4×10^7 per donor after cloning of the heavy chains into the light chain sublibraries resulting in 4 repertoires per donor (IgG-κ, IgG-λ, IgM-κ, IgM-λ).

11. To prepare the plasmid DNA of 1 transformation reaction we used one tip 100 (Quiagen). Handle this DNA with care because it represents the light chain sublibrary.

12. For performing phage rescue on a smaller or larger scale adjust the volume of the media and the number of M13KO7 helper phages. It is important to use optimal growth conditions for the bacteria at all times. It is therefore important to use large flasks for better aeration.

13. Phage rescue can also be started from an overnight culture or with bacteria from a glycerol stock. In the latter case, the concentration of glycerol in the culture should not exceed 2% to avoid inhibition of bacterial growth.

14. Do not handle the cells too vigorously before and during superinfection with helper.

15. One mL of XL-1 blue at A_{600} of 0.1 corresponds to 5×10^8 bacteria. To obtain a multiplicity of infection of 20, add 1×10^{10} phages to each mL of the culture. One mL of TG1 at A_{600} of 0.1 corresponds to 1×10^8 bacteria, so 2×10^9 phages per mL are required.

16. It is very important to use glucose free medium at this step, since the presence of glucose will inhibit expression of the antibody genes.

17. Extended incubation increases the number of rescued phages (infectious particles), but decreases the ratio of functional recombinant antibody to phage particles. The binding capacity of the rescued phage antibodies is mainly lost due to protease activity in the culture.

18. Determination of the number of infectious particles defined as colony-forming units (cfu) can be performed according to standard methods (*see* **ref. 34**).

19. The number of infectious particles in the supernatant is usually about 1×10^{10} to 1×10^{11} cfu/mL. If it is less than 1×10^9 cfu/mL, the rescue should be repeated.

20. Take care, since the pellet may be hardly visible.

21. Rinse that side of the tube where the pellet is to be expected with 1 ml of buffer several times, pool in a polypropylene tube and repeat this procedure 4 times.

22. Panning should be performed as soon as possible following rescue, since some phage-displayed recombinant antibody preparations may be unstable. It is possible to freeze rescued phage antibodies at –20°C, although it is presently unknown whether some antibodies might possibly be denatured during freezing. In any case, repeated freezing and thawing should be avoided.

23. The optimal conditions for coating may differ for each antigen. Small-scale trials should therefore first be carried out. The present protocol is suitable for protein antigens. We use 200 μg of protein per tube if sufficient amounts are available, but the optimal amounts

may vary. Our suggestion is to make an empirical estimation of the amount of antigen necessary to coat a well of an ELISA plate. This amount can then be scaled up to the volume of the Immunotubes (5 mL).

The suitability of the plastic support for immobilization of the particular antigen should also be determined prior to panning. If possible, an immunoassay should be established prior to panning to ensure that under the conditions used for coating the antigen binds to the tube wall.

24. A negative control is always necessary to verify that an enrichment is due to binding of the recombinant phage antibodies to the antigen rather than to components of the blocking buffer. The tube used as negative control should be treated exactly like the antigen coated tubes.

25. The tube can be closed with Parafilm® or with the caps provided by the supplier of the tubes.

26. 2% Skimmed milk in PBS works very well as a blocking buffer. Some commercially available blocking buffers (e.g., Pierce Superblock™) give comparable results and should be used according to the manufacturers instructions. If the solid support is coated with a nonprotein antigen, other blocking buffers may be required. In this case, refer to the buffers used in a conventional ELISA. Take note that collagen, FCS or gelatine do not work well as blocking agents due to their interaction with phagemid particles.

27. The amount of rescued phagemid antibodies used for panning is dependent on the complexity of the library. Make sure that the number of phages is at least 10^3–1×10^4 times more than the complexity of the library.

28. To reduce nonspecific, hydrophobic protein-protein interactions between native M13 phage proteins and some antigens, Triton X-100 may be added to a final concentration of 0.1%.

29. Incubation with Triethylamine reduces the infectivity of the recombinant phage antibodies. Do not exceed an incubation time of more than 5–10 min.

30. Handle the cells gently before and during infection with eluted phages.

31. This titration is to determine the number of infectious phagemid particles eluted from the tube after panning. The number should be low after first round of panning and then increase after subsequent rounds as specific clones are enriched.

32. It is very important that the agar plates are well dried before plating the bacteria.

33. If there are only a few colonies on the plates, extend the incubation at 30°C until the colonies are fairly large. Resuspend the cells in a smaller volume.

34. After the third round of panning and reinfection, its possible to start analyzing single clones.

35. For the small-scale rescue of phagemids, we recommend the use of special polypropylene 96-deep-well microtiter plates (volume per well = 1 mL). However, these plates may require a special adaptor for centrifugation.

36. If another shaker is used, speed may have to be decreased in order to prevent spillage of the medium into adjacent wells.

37. The remaining master plate may be stored at 4°C for up to 2 wk. To store it longer, add sterile glycerol to the cultures to a final concentration of 20%, seal the plate and mix by inverting several times. Store at –70°C.

38. All incubation steps should be carried out in a wet chamber to prevent evaporation or contamination. For example, the microwell plate can be placed in a closed box containing moistened tissue paper.

39. These conditions work for most protein antigens or haptens bound to a protein carrier. The optimal amount of antigen may vary. Nonprotein antigens (e.g. lipopolysaccharides) may require a different buffer. In this case, refer to the buffers used in a conventional ELISA.

40. Both supernatant or PEG-precipitated phagemids may be used in phage-ELISA. PEG precipitation lowers the background and removes contaminants interferring with the binding.
41. The anti-M13-antibody is a polyclonal serum raised against M13 or fd phages. A commercial source is listed in Materials. The serum should be diluted according to the manufacturers instructions in the same solution used for blocking as described in **step 2**. The serum used here contains a high titer of antibodies against *E. coli* proteins and therefore cross-reacts with proteins in the phage supernatant. To avoid this, the serum must be preabsorbed. Incubate the diluted serum overnight with a piece of *E. coli*-lysate-coated nitrocellulose at 4°C. This can be done in parallel with the coating (**Subheading 3.9., step 1**).
42. The "second antibody" is a serum raised against the anti-M13-antibody linked to HRP. A commercial source is listed in **Subheading 2**. The serum should be diluted according to the supplier.
43. "Enzyme substrate" is a substrate for HRP. A commercial source is listed in Materials.
44. The detection limit of the phage-ELISA is about 10^5 bound phages/well.

References

1. Carson, D. A. and Freimark, B. D. (1986) Human lymphocyte hybridomas and monoclonal antibodies. *Adv. Immunol.* **38**, 275–311.
2. Glassy, M. C. and Dillman, R. O. (1988) Molecular biotherapy with human monoclonal antibodies. *Mol. Biother.* **1**, 7–13.
3. Winter, G. and Milstein, C. (1991) Man made antibodies. *Nature* **349**, 293–299.
4. McCafferty, J., Griffiths, A. D., Winter, G., and Chiswell, D. J. (1990) Phage antibodies: filamentous phage displaying antibody variable domains. *Nature* **348**, 552–554.
5. Mullinax, R. L., Gross, E. A., Amberg, J. R., Hay, B. N., Hogrefe, H. H., Kubitz, M. M., et al. (1990) Identification of human antibody fragment clones specific for tetanus toxoid in bacteriophage lambda immunoexpression library. *Proc. Natl. Acad. Sci. USA* **87**, 8095–8099.
6. Marks, J. D., Hoogenboom, H. R., Bonnert, T. P., McGafferty, J., Griffiths, A. D., and Winter, G. (1991) By-passing immunization. Human antibodies from V-gene libraries displayed on phage. *J. Mol. Biol.* **222**, 581–597.
7. Barbas, C. F., Rosenblum, J. S., and Lerner, R. A. (1993) Direct selection of antibodies that coordinate metals from semisynthetic combinatorial libraries. *Proc. Natl. Acad. Sci. USA* **90**, 6385–6389.
8. Barbas, C. F., 3rd, Collet, T. A., Amberg, W., Roben, P., Binley, J. M., Hoekstra, D., et al. (1993) Molecular profile of an antibody response to HIV-1 as probed by recombinatorial libraries. *J. Mol. Biol.* **230**, 812–823.
9. Rapoport, B., Portolano, S., and McLachlan, S. M. (1995) Combinatorial libraries: new insights into human organ-specific autoantibodies. *Immunol. Today* **16**, 43–49.
10. Welschof, M., Terness, P., Kipriyanov, S., Stanescu, D., Breitling, F., Dörsam, H., et al. (1997) The antigen-binding domain of a human IgG-anti-F(ab')2 autoantibody. *Proc. Natl. Acad. Sci. USA* **94**, 1902–1907.
11. Marks, J. D., Hoogenboom, H. R., Bonnert, T. P., McGafferty, J., Griffiths, A. D., and Winter, G. (1991) By-passing immunization. Human antibodies from V-gene libraries displayed on phage. *J. Mol. Biol.* **222**, 581–597.
12. Griffiths, A. D., Malmquist, M., Marks, J. D., Bye, J. M., Embleton, M. J., McCafferty, J., et al. (1993) Human anti-self antibodies with high specificity from phage display libraries. *EMBO Journal* **12**, 725–734.

13. Vaughan, T. J., Williams, A. J., Pritchard, K., Osbourn, J. K., Pope, A. R., Earnshaw, J. C., et al. (1996) Human antibodies with sub-nanomolar affinities isolated from a large non-immunized phage display library. *Nat. Biotechnol.* **14(3)**, 309–314.
14. Little, M., Welschof, M., Braunagel, M., Hermes, I., Christ, C., Keller, A., et al. (1999) Generation of a large complex antibody library from multiple donors. *J. Immunol. Methods* **231**, 3–9.
15. Hoogenboom, H. R. and Winter, G. (1992) By-passing immunisation. Human antibodies from synthetic repertoires of germline V_H gene segments rearranged in vitro. *J. Mol. Biol.* **227**, 381–388.
16. Barbas, C. F., Bain, J. D., Hoekstra, D. M., and Lerner, R. A. (1992) Semisynthetic combinatorial antibody libraries: A chemical solution to the diversity problem. *Proc. Natl. Acad. Sci. USA* **89**, 4457–4461.
17. Hayashi, N., Welschof, M., Zewe, M., Braunagel, M., Dübel, S., Breitling, F., and Little, M. (1994) Simultaneous mutagenesis of antibody CDR regions by overlap extension and PCR. *Bio/Techniques* **17**, 310–315.
18. Braunagel, M. and Little, M. (1997) Construction of a semisynthetic antibody library using trinucleotide oligos. *Nucleic Acids Res.* **25(22)**, 4690–4691.
19. Knappik, A., Ge, L., Honegger, A., Pack, P., Fischer, M., Wellnhofer, G., et al. (2000) Fully synthetic human combinatorial antibody libraries (HuCAL) based on modular consensus frameworks and CDRs randomized with trinucleotides. *J. Mol. Biol.* **296(1)**, 57–86.
20. Soderlind, E., Strandberg, L., Jirholt, P., Kobayashi, N., Alexeiva, V., Aberg, A. M., et al. (2000) Recombining germline-derived CDR sequences for creating diverse single-frame-work antibody libraries. *Nat. Biotechnol.* **18(8)**, 852–856.
21. Larrick, J. W., Danielsson, L., Brenner, C. A., Wallace, E. F., Abrahamson, M., Fry, K. E., and Borrebaeck, C. A. K. (1989) Polymerase chain reaction using mixed primers: cloning of human monoclonal antibody variable region genes from single hybridoma cells. *Biotechnology* **7**, 934–939.
22. Marks, J. D., Tristem, M., Karpas, A., and Winter, G. (1991) Oligonucleotide primers for polymerase chain reaction amplification of human immunoglobulin variable genes and design of family-specific oligonucleotide probes. *Eur. J. Immunol.* **21**, 985–991.
23. Campbell, M. J., Zelenetz, A. D., Levy, S., and Levy, R. (1992) Use of family specific leader region primers for PCR amplification of the human heavy chain variable region gene repertoire. *Mol. Immunol.* **29**, 193–203.
24. Barbas, C. F., Björling, E., Chiodi, F., Dunlop, N., Cababa, D., Jones, T. M., et al. (1992) Recombinant human Fab fragments neutralize human type I immunodeficiency virus *in vitro*. *Proc. Natl. Acad. Sci. USA* **89**, 9339–9343.
25. Welschof, M., Terness, P., Kolbinger, F., Zewe, M., Dübel, S., Dörsam, H., et al. (1995) Amino acid sequence based PCR primers for the amplification of human heavy and light chain immunoglobulin variable region genes. *J. Immunol. M.* **179**, 203–214.
26. Huston, J. S., Levinson, D., Mudgett-Hunter, M., Tai, M.-S., Novotny, J., Margolies, M. N., et al. (1988) Protein engineering of antibody binding sites: Recovery of specific activity in an anti-digoxin single-chain Fv analogue produced in *Escherichia coli*. *Proc. Natl. Acad. Sci. USA* **85**, 5879–5583.
27. Bird, R. E., Hardman, K. D., Jacobson, J. W., Johnson, S., Kaufman, B. M., Lee, S.-M., et al. (1988) Single-chain antigen-binding proteins. *Science* **242**, 423–426.
28. Breitling, F., Dübel, S., Seehaus, T., Klewinghaus, I., and Little, M. (1991) A surface expression vector for antibody screening. *Gene* **104**, 147–153.

29. Hoogenboom, H. R., Griffiths, A. D., Johnson, K. S., Chiswell, D. J., Hudson, P., and Winter, G. (1991) Multi-subunit proteins on the surface of filamentous phage: methodologies for displaying antibody (Fab) heavy and light chains. *Nucleic Acids Res.* **19,** 4133–4137.

30. Barbas, C. F., Kang, A. K., Lerner, R. A., and Benkovic, S. J. (1991) Assembly ofcombinatorial antibody libraries on phage surfaces: the gene III site. *Proc. Natl. Acad. Sci. USA* **88,** 7978–7982.

31. Tomlinson, I. M, Williams, S. C., Corbett, S. J., Cox, J. P. L., and Winter, G. (1995) MRC Centre for Protein Engineering, Cambridge, UK.

32. Chirgwin, J. M., Przybyla, A. E., MacDonald, R. J., and Rutter, W. J. (1979) Isolation of biologically active ribonucleic acid from sources enriched in ribonuclease. *Biochemistry* **18,** 5294–5299.

33. Chomczynski, P. and Sahi, N. (1987) Single-step method of RNA isolation by acid guanidium thiocyanate-phenol-chloroform extraction. *Anal. Biochem.* **162,** 156–159.

34. Sambrook, J., Fritsch, E. F., and Maniatis, T. (1989) *Molecular Cloning. A laboratory manual* (Nolan, C., ed.), Cold Spring Harbor Laboratory Press, Cold Spring Harbor, NY.

7

Construction of Semisynthetic Antibody Libraries

Michael Braunagel

1. Introduction

Antibody libraries expressed on the surface of filamentous phage are proven to be a valuable tool in isolating antibodies specific for a wide variety of antigens (for review, see **ref. 1**). As it is assumed that the probability of isolating high affinity binders is related to the initial library size *(2)*, the construction of large libraries representing a high diversity of molecules is a central goal of recombinant antibody technology. In addition to generate antibody libraries from naïve B-cell repertoires *(3–6)*, germline sequences *(7)* or immunized donors *(8)*, it is also possible to make use of the available information on antibody structure to generate diversity by including short stretches of random sequences in carefully chosen parts of the antibody.

It is long known that the contact points to the antigen are formed by the six hypervariable regions of the antibody, also known as complementarity determining regions (CDR) *(9)*. The sequence in these regions varies widely between different antibodies, determining their specificity *(10)*. The most variable portion is CDR3 of the heavy chain, which also contributes most to the antigen binding in the majority of examined cases.

By replacing amino acids in one or more CDR regions of one or more defined antibody(s) with random sequences using polymerase chain reaction (PCR) techniques, it is possible to construct highly diverse antibody libraries containing genes not found in vivo *(4,7,11–17)*. Such libraries are called semisynthetic libraries.

Semisynthetic libraries can be used to isolate binders to various antigens in the same manner as B-cell repertoire derived libraries *(4,7,11,15–17)*. It is important to note, though, that there are a few differences between these two types of libraries. A B-cell derived library has been preselected in several ways. As an example, antibodies recognizing self antigens have been removed from the repertoire. This is not the case with the semisynthetic library. Semisynthetic libraries, in contrast, have the disadvantage of containing always a certain amount of nonfunctional clones, stemming from PCR errors, stop codons in the random sequence, or inability to fold

From: *Methods in Molecular Biology, vol. 207: Recombinant Antibodies for Cancer Therapy: Methods and Protocols*
Edited by: M. Welschof and J. Krauss © Humana Press Inc., Totowa, NJ

properly. These effects get usually more pronounced if more than one CDR is randomized.

A second use for semisynthetic libraries is the improvement of a given antibody. In this case, the original antibody, which may have been isolated by selection out of a library or may be hybridoma derived, is considered as lead structure *(18–20)*. It is randomized in one or more CDRs, and the resulting secondary library is screened for binders with improved characteristics, like higher affinity or reduced crossreactivity. Especially, the successive randomization of several CDRs (CDR walking) may lead to dramatic improvements *(21–23)*.

The approach of using semisynthetic libraries has been taken further with the construction of fully synthetic libraries, in which a certain number of artificially designed antibody frameworks is used in combination with random sequences in all CDRs *(24)*.

In the following chapter, several issues crucial for the design of a random library will be discussed.

1.1. Choice of CDR to be Randomized

CDR3 of the heavy chain is an obvious candidate for randomization. It usually is the CDR with the largest contact surface to the antigen, so introduction of random sequences may show drastic effects. Furthermore, the CDR3 loop of the heavy chain is not known to have a specific conformation *(25)*, so randomization does not affect the structural integrity of this loop. CDR3 of the light chain is also a region suitable to randomization, as it often contributes much to the antigen binding also.

1.2. Number of Amino Acid Positions Randomized

Libraries described in literature vary strongly in the amount of amino acid positions randomized. In some cases, all CDR regions have been completely randomized *(14)*, in others only selected positions were chosen for introduction of diversity. It should be kept in mind, though, that all CDRs with exception of CDR3 of the heavy chain have certain structural constraints (canonical structures, *25–27*), which are connected to some key amino acids inside the CDRs. Randomization of these positions may lead to nonfunctional antibodies, limiting the effective complexity of the library. A full description of canonical structures is outside of the scope of this article, but the interested reader may check the relevant literature; the use of a special program for antibody modeling (AbM, *[28]*) might prove helpful.

As CDR3 of the heavy chain is less involved in structural interactions in the immunoglobulin, a complete randomization of this region is also less likely to result in a large number of nonfunctional clones. It may also be mentioned that randomizing only eight positions gives 2.56×10^{10} possible sequences. This is about the maximum library size that can be obtained using conventional cloning methods.

1.3. Length of the Randomized CDR

CDR regions vary considerably in length. Most libraries are keeping the length of the CDR given by the antibody they are based on, or use the length most often found in nature, leaving extremes out.

1.4. Use of Codons

If the triplet (NNN)n is used for introducing random sequences, three out of 64 codons will be stop codons, leading to a defective protein. If all CDRs are randomized, nearly no full sequences would be generated. If a total of 20 amino acids are randomized using $(NNN)_n$, only 38% will be without stop codon. Therefore, other mixtures have been devised. The two most used strategies are to use $(NNK)_n$, where K is G or T, or $(NNB)_n$, where B is G, C, or T. In both cases all amino acids are coded for, although at different rates, and the probability for stop codons is 1 out of 32 (NNK) or 1 out of 48 (NNB), respectively. For this reason $(NNB)_n$ is the most popular choice today. Stop codons can be completely avoided by using the sequence $(VNN)_n$, where V is A, G or C. However, with this strategy, tryptophan, cystein, tyrosin, and phenylalanin will not be included in the library. An interesting alternative is the use of trinucleotides. In this case, the synthesis of the oligonucleotide is not performed using mononucleotides, but presynthesized trinucleotidblocks *(29–31)*. There is one block for each amino acid, and by mixing the 20 blocks for each position in the randomized sequence, all amino acids can be introduced in the wished ratio, while completely avoiding stop codons.

A special case may arise if the semisynthetic library is made to improve an existing antibody. For this purpose it is possible to design the random sequence in a way that at each randomized position the original amino acid of the lead structure is prevalent *(22)*. This way, the number of mutations introduced in the lead sequence is limited, which may be of advantage for this special application.

1.5. Example for Construction of a Semisynthetic Library

As described earlier, semisynthetic libraries may differ considerably in their construction. For this reason it is impossible to give a general protocol applicable for all cases. Instead, an example will be given for randomizing CDR3 of the heavy chain. This method can be adapted with little effort (primer design) to all randomizations of CDR3 regions of single chain antibodies. In more general terms, this method requires a restriction site usable for cloning in less than 90-bp distance from the CDR to be randomized. If this is not the case, the reader is advised to check **ref. 8**. If a restriction site useful for cloning is nearby the CDR in question (<35 bp) the method described in **ref. 11** is recommended.

A semisynthetic library was constructed based on a scFv against 2-phenyloxazol-5-one (phOx) as outlined in **Fig. 1**. In a first step the "random oligo" containing the randomized CDR3 region was elongated with the primer "rnd back" in an overlap extension reaction. The product was gel-purified and used together with primer "rnd for" in a PCR. The template for this reaction was the heavy-chain variable domain of a human antibody against phOx *(32)*. The PCR product was gel-purified, digested with *NcoI/Hin*dIII (Boehringer Mannheim) and substituted for the heavy chain variable region of the phage display vector pSEX 81-phOx *(33)*.

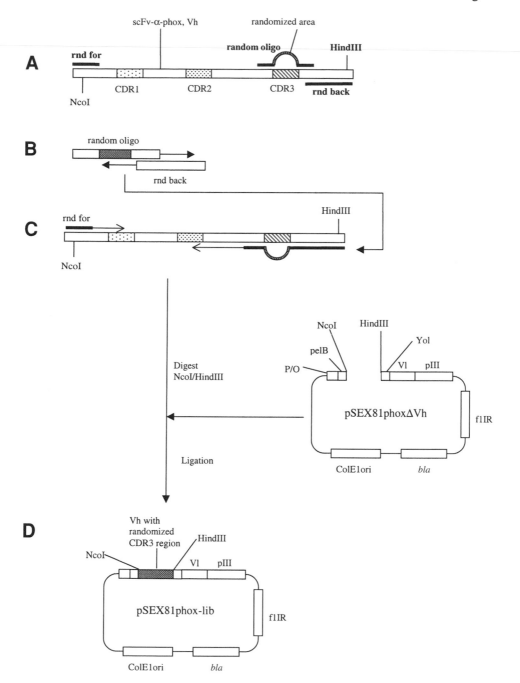

2. Materials

2.1. Elongation and PCR

1. Thermocycler PTC 150-16 (MJ Research, Watertown, MA).
2. *Vent* DNA Polymerase (New England Biolabs Inc., Beverly, MA).
3. 10X Vent buffer (New England Biolabs).
4. *Taq* polymerase (AmpliTaq, Perkin-Elmer, Branchburg, NJ).
5. TaqPCR buffer II (Perkin-Elmer).
6. 25 m*M* MgCl$_2$.
7. H$_2$O ad inj. (Braun, Melsungen, Germany).
8. 100 m*M* dNTPs (New England Biolabs).
9. Primers (*see* **Note 1**):
   a. "rnd for": 5'-CAGCCGG<u>CCATGG</u>CCCAGGTG-3', *Nco*I site underlined
   b. "rnd back": 5'-TTCTTC<u>AAGCTT</u>TGGGGCGGATGCACT
      CCCTGAGGAGACGGT<u>*GACCGTGGTCCCTTTGCCCCA*</u>-3, sequence
      overlapping with "random oligo" in italics, *Hin*dIII site underlined.
   c. "random oligo" 5'-
      GACACGGCCGTGTATTACTGTGTGAGA(Tri)$_8$*TGGGGCAAA*
      GGGACCACGGTC-3, sequence overlapping with "rnd back" in italics.
10. pSEX81-phox *(33)*.
11. 100 bp-DNA molecular weight marker (Gibco-BRL).
12. Agarose, NuSieve GTG, and Seakem (FMC, Rockland, MN).
13. 1X TAE buffer: Dilute 1:50 with water from 50X TAE stock solution.
14. 50X TAE buffer: Dissolve 242 g Tris base in distilled water. Add 57.1 mL glacial acetic
    acid, 100 mL 0.5 *M* EDTA, add water to a total volume of 1 L.
15. 0.5 *M* EDTA.
16. Ethidium bromide (10 mg/mL).
17. QIAquick Gel extraction kit (Qiagen, Hilden, Germany).

2.2. Cloning into pSEX81phox

1. Petri dishes, 85 and 145 mm diameter (Greiner, Frickenhausen, Germany).
2. Table-top microcentrifuge.
3. QIAquick Gel extraction kit (Qiagen).
4. QIAquick spin PCR purification kit.

Fig. 1. *(opposite page)* **(A)** Position of the used primers in respect to the template. **(B–D)** Steps in generating a semisynthetic library: **(B)** Elongation, **(C)** PCR, **(D)** Cloning. Rnd for, random oligo, rnd back: oligos described in the text. *Nco*I, *Hin*dIII: restriction sites used for cloning. CDR1, CDR2, CDR3: hypervariable regions. scFv-α-phox, Vh: variable domain of the heavy chain of a single chain Fv fragment directed against phox. pSex81phoxΔVh: Phagemidvector containing a scFv against phox, the heavy chain was removed by *Nco*I/*Hin*dIII digest. P/O: Promoter/operator lac wt. pelB: signal peptide of pectate lyase of *Erwinia carotovora*. Yol: Peptide linker of 18 amino acids connecting V$_H$ and V$_L$. V$_L$: light chain of a single chain Fv fragment directed against phox. pIII: sequence encoding the gene III product of bacteriophage M13. f1IR: intergenic region of phage f1. *bla*: β-lactamase gene. ColE1ori: origin of replication of plasmid ColE1. pSEX81phox-lib: semisynthetic library based on a scFv against phox in the vector pSEX81.

5. XL1 Blue electrocompetent cells (Stratagene, La Jolla, CA).
6. *Nco*I restriction endonuclease (New England Biolabs).
7. *Hin*dIII restriction endonuclease (New England Biolabs).
8. 10X Restriction enzyme buffer 2 (New England Biolabs).
9. Calf intestine phosphatase (CIP) (New England Biolabs).
10. T4 DNA-ligase (New England Biolabs).
11. 10X T4 DNA-ligase buffer (New England Biolabs).
12. 100 bp-DNA molecular weight marker (Gibco-BRL).
13. 1000 bp-DNA molecular weight marker (Gibco-BRL).
14. Agarose, Seakem (FMC, Rockland, MN).
15. 1X TAE buffer (*see* **Subheading 2.1.**).
16. 0.5 *M* EDTA.
17. Ethidium bromide (10 mg/mL).
18. 3 *M* Sodium acetate pH 5.2.
19. Glycogen from mussels, molecular biology grade, 20 mg/mL (Roche Diagnostics GmbH, Mannheim, Germany).
20. Ethanol p.A.
21. 70% Ethanol.
22. 2 *M* Glucose, sterile-filtered.
23. 1 *M* $MgCl_2$.
24. Ampicillin (5 mg/mL), sterile-filtered.
25. SOB-GA medium agar plates: To 15 g Bacto-agar, 20 g Bacto-tryptone, 5 g Bacto-yeast extract, and 0.5 g NaCl add distilled water to 920 mL and autoclave. After the medium has cooled to 55°C, add 50 mL 2 *M* glucose, 10 mL 1 *M* $MgCl_2$ and 20 mL ampicillin (5 mg/mL).
26. Sterile glass spreader.

3. Methods

3.1. Elongation and PCR

1. Elongation is carried out in five parallel reactions, each in a total volume of 100 µL, containing 75 pmol of each primer ("random oligo" and "rnd back"), 250 µ*M* of each nucleotide, 2.5 m*M* $MgCl_2$, 10 mL 10X PCR buffer II 2.5 U AmpliTaq, initial denaturation 94°C, 15 min, then 25 cycles: 94°C, 15 min; 55°C, 30 min; 72°C, 60 min, final extension 72°C, 120 min (*see* **Note 2**).
2. The amplified DNA is loaded on a 4% NuSieve GTG agarose gel and run at 4 V/cm distance between the electrodes for ca. 1 h.
3. Elute and purify the band corresponding to the elongated product (size 117 bp) from the gel using the QIAquick Gel extraction kit (*see* **Note 3**).
4. Amplification by PCR is carried out in five parallel reactions, each with a total volume of 50 µL containing 25 pmol of the PCR product eluted in **step 3**, 25 pmol primer "rnd for", 0.1 ng pSEX81phox as template, 300 µ*M* of each nucleotide, 10 µL 10X *Vent* buffer, 1 U AmpliTaq, initial denaturation 94°C, 15 min, then 25 cycles: 94°C, 15 min; 55°C, 30 min; 72°C, 60 min (*see* **Note 4**).
5. The amplified DNA is loaded on a 2% Seakem agarose gel and run at 4 V/cm distance between the electrodes for ca. 1 h.
6. Elute and purify the band corresponding to the amplified product (size 412 bp) from the gel using the QIAquick Gel extraction kit.

3.2. Cloning into pSEX81phox

1. Digest 5 mg of pSEX81phox by adding 20 U of *Nco*I, 30 U of *Hin*dIII and 0.5 U CIP, restriction buffer 2 (final concentration 1X) and H$_2$O. The final volume should be at least 10× the volume of the enzyme samples. Incubate for 2 h on 37°C (*see* **Note 5**).
2. Add 0.5 U of CIP and incubate for another 2 h at 37°C.
3. Add EDTA, pH 8.0, to a final concentration of 5 μ*M* and incubate for 20 min at 65°C to inactivate CIP.
4. The digest is loaded on a 1% Seakem agarose gel and run at 4 V/cm distance between the electrodes for ~1 h.
5. Elute and purify the band corresponding to the elongated product (size 4.4 kbp) from the gel using the QIAquick Gel extraction kit.
6. Digest 500 ng PCR product eluted in **Subheading 3.1.**, **step 6** by adding 16 U of *Nco*I, 19 U of *Hin*dIII, restriction buffer 2 (final concentration 1X) and H$_2$O. The final volume should be at least 10× the volume of the enzyme samples. Incubate for 4 h on 37°C (*see* **Note 5**).
7. Remove stuffer fragments and purify the digested DNA from **step 5** by using the QIAquick spin PCR purification kit.
8. Ligate vector (**step 4**) and insert (**step 6**) at a molecular ratio of 1:3. The reaction mixture contains 100 ng DNA, 1 U T4 ligase ligation buffer, and H$_2$O in a total volume of max 50 μL. Incubate overnight at 16°C.
9. Precipitate the DNA by adding 1/10 vol 3 *M* sodium acetate, pH 5.2, 20 μg glycogen, and 2.5 vol absolute ethanol. Incubate for >1 h at –20°C. Sediment the pellet centrifugation for 20 min in a microcentrifuge at >10,000*g*, 4°C. Wash the pellet with 500 μL ice-cold 70% ethanol and centrifuge again (same conditions). Repeat this washing step one more time. Allow the pellet to dry at room temperature. Resuspend the pellet in 6 μL H$_2$O.
10. The product of **step 9** is transformed into *E. coli*. Use 2 μL of the resuspended ligation product for 40 μL XL 1 blue electrocompetent cells according to the suppliers instruction. Plate the bacteria four SOB-GA agar plates of 145 mm diameter. Plate 1 and 10 μL on SOB-GA dishes 85 mm diameter (*see* **Note 6**).
11. The library is now finished and ready for phage rescue and screening, *see* **ref. 34**.

4. Notes

1. The primers listed here are specific for this special experiment. Other primers have to be designed by each researcher for his special setup. The primers need to have the following characteristics:
   a. The equivalent to primer "rnd for" should have perfect match to the template, contain the correct restriction site (*see* **Note 5**) and must be long enough to work in a PCR together with the elongated "random oligo."
   b. The equivalent to primer "rnd back" should have perfect match to the template, contain the correct restriction site (*see* **Note 5**) and must be long enough to work in a in an elongation with the "random oligo."
   c. The equivalent to primer "random oligo" should have perfect match to the template except in the randomized area, and must be long enough to work in an elongation with "rnd back" and in a PCR together in a with "rnd for."

   The quality of the primers used, especially the "random oligo" are absolute crucial for the experiment. A thorough quality check is recommended. For construction of the random area *see* **Subheading 1.**

2. The elongation step is the technically most demanding step in this protocol. Reaction conditions may have to be adjusted for each experiment and it may be worthwhile to find the optimal conditions in test experiments using 20 pmol of each primer in 50 µL volume. Use of proof reading polymerases is not recommended, as most of theses enzymes are also able to degrade oligos, which may be detrimental during elongation. The amount isolated from this elongation should be enough for several PCRs. As this reaction is an elongation (linear amplification) and not a PCR (exponential amplification) the chances of accumulating mistakes is rather low. If there is reason to believe that the elongation may not work, e.g., due to predicted secondary structures in one oligo, it can be circumvented by an alternative approach. For this method the "random oligo" is constructed as homolog to the counterstrand of the original antibody. The first step is then a PCR using "rnd for" and "random oligo" on the template vector using the conditions described in **Subheading 3.1., step 4**. The PCR product is purified and serves as template for a second PCR using the primers "rnd for" and "rnd back." The disadvantage of this method is a higher risk of getting a biased library as consequence of two sequential PCRs.

3. The QIAquick Gel extraction kit has a lower size limit for purification of DNA of about 80 bp. For fragments <100 alternative means of purification are optional, like elution low melting agarose.

4. The PCR is performed in five parallel reactions for two reasons: first to avoid a bias possible in a single PCR reaction; second, to obtain enough material for the following purification.

5. This protocol is devised for the use of pSEX81 as starting vector. Other vectors are most likely to have other restriction sites. The reaction volume should always be more 10× more than that of the combined enzyme samples in order to dilute the glycerol coming from the enzyme storage buffers to below 5%. Higher concentrations may cause star activity.

6. The small dishes are used to count the transformants. 10^6 to 5×10^6 transformants can be expected per transformation. Other vector systems than pSEX81 may require other medium and/or antibiotics for growth.

References

1. Hoogenboom, H. R., De Bruine, A. P., Hufton, S. E., Hort, R. M., Arends, J. W., and Roovers, R. C. (1998) Antibody phage display technology and its applications. *Immunotechniques* **4**, 1–20.

2. Perelson, A. S. (1989) Immune network theory. *Immunol. Rev.* **100**, 5–36.

3. Vaughan T. J, Williams, A. J., Pritchard, K., Osbourn, J. K., Pope, A. R., Earnshaw, J. C., et al. (1996) Human antibodies with sub-nanomolar affinities from a large non-immunized phage display library. *Nature Biotechnol.* **14**, 309–314.

4. Sheets, M. D., Amersdorfer, P., Finnern, R., Sargent, P., Lindqvist, E., Schier, R., et al. (1998) Efficient construction of a large non-immune phage antibody library – The production of high-affinity human single-chain antibodies to protein antigens. *Proc. Natl. Acad. Sci. USA* **95**, 6157–6162.

5. De Haard, H. J., Van Neer, N., Reurs, A, Hufton, S. E., Roovers, R. C., Henderikx, P., et al. (1999) A large non-immunized human Fab fragment phage library that permits rapid isolation and kinetic analysis of high affinity antibodies. *J. Biol. Chem.* **274**, 18,218–18,230.

6. Little, M., Welschof, M., Braunagel, M., Hermes, I., Christ, C., Keller, A., et al. (1999) Generation of a large complex antibody library from multiple donors. *J. Immunol. Methods* **231**, 3–9.

7. Griffiths, A. D., Williams, S. C., Hartley, O., Tomlinson, I. M., Waterhouse, P., Crosby, W. L., et al. (1994) Isolation of high affinity human antibodies directly from large synthetic repertoires. *EMBO J.* **13,** 3245–3260.

8. Barbas, C. F., Bain, J. D., Hoekstra, D. M., and Lerner, R. A. (1992) Semisynthetic combinatorial antibody libraries: a chemical solution to the diversity problem. *Proc. Natl Acad. Sci. USA* **89,** 4457–4461.

9. Poljak, R. J., Amzel, L. M., Avery, H, Chen, B. L., Phizackerley, R. P., and Saul, F. (1973) Three-dimensional structure of the Fab-fragment of a human immunoglobulin on 2,8Å resolution. *Proc. Natl. Acad. Sci. USA* **70,** 3305–3310.

10. Wu, T. and Kabat, E. (1971) Attempts to locate complementarity-determining regions residues in the variable positions of light and heavy chains. *Ann. NY Acad. Sci.* **190,** 382–393.

11. Hoogenboom, H. R. and Winter, G. (1992) By-passing immunisation: Human antibodies from synthetic repertoires of germline VH gene segments rearranged in vitro. *J. Mol. Biol.* **227,** 381–388.

12. Barbas, C. F., Bain J. D., Hoekstra, D. M., and Lerner, R. A. (1992) Semisynthetic combinatorial antibody libraries: a chemical solution to the diversity problem. *Proc. Natl Acad. Sci. USA* **89,** 4457–4461.

13. Barbas, C. F., Amberg, W., Simoncsits, A., Jones, T. M., and Lerner, R. A. (1993) Selection of human anti-hapten antibodies from semi-synthetic libraries. *Gene* **137,** 57–62.

14. Hayashi N., Welschof, M., Zewe, M., Braunagel, M., Dübel, S., Breitling, F., and Little, M. (1994) Simultaneous mutagenesis of antibody CDR regions by overlap extension and PCR. *Biotechniques* **17,** **310, 312,** 314–315.

15. Nissim, A., Hoogenboom, H. R., Tomlinson, I. M., Flynn, G., Midgley, C., Lane, D., and Winter, G. (1994) Antibody fragments from a 'single pot' phage display library as immunochemical reagents. *EMBO J.* **13,** 692–698.

16. De Kruif, J., Boel E., and Logtenberg, T. (1995) Selection and application of human single chain Fv antibody fragments from a semi-synthetic phage antibody display library with designed CDR3 regions. *J. Mol. Biol.* **248,** 97–105.

17. Braunagel, M. and Little, M. (1997) Construction of a semisynthetic antibody library using trinucleotide oligos. *Nucleic Acids Res.* **25,** 4690–4691.

18. Barbas, C. F., Hu, D., Dunlop, N., Sawyer, L., Cababa, D., Hendry, R. M., et al. (1994) *In vitro* evolution of a neutralizing human antibody to human immunodeficiency virus type 1 to enhance affinity and broaden strain cross-reactivity. *Proc. Natl. Acad. Sci. USA* **91,** 3809–3813.

19. Hemminki, A., Niemi, S., Hoffren, A. M., Hakalahti, L., Söderlund, H., and Takkinen, K. (1998) Specificity improvement of a recombinant anti-testosterone Fab fragment by CDRIII mutagenesis and phage display selection. *Protein Eng.* **11,** 311–319.

20. Lamminmaki, U., Pauperio, S., Westerlund-Karlsson, A., Karvinen, J., Virtanen P. L., Lovgren, T., and Saviranta, P. (1999) Expanding the conformational diversity by random insertions in CDRH2 results in improved anti-estradiol antibodies. *J. Mol. Biol.* **291,** 589–602.

21. Yang, W. P., Green, K., Pinz-Sweeney, S., Briones, A. T., Burton, D. R., and Barbas, C. F. (1995) CDR walking mutagenesis for the affinity maturation of a potent human anti-HIV-1 antibody into the picomolar range. *J. Mol. Biol.* **25,** 392–403.

22. Schier, R., McCall, A., Adams, G. P., Marhall, K. W., Merritt, H., Yim, M., et al. (1996b) Isolation of picomolar affinity anti-c-erbb-2 single-chain Fv by molecular evolution of the complementarity determining regions in the center of the antibody binding site. *J. Mol. Biol.* **263,** 551–567.

23. Wu, H., Beuerlein, G., Nie, Y., Smith, H., Lee, B. A., Hensler, M., et al. (1998) Stepwise in vitro affinity maturation of Vitaxin, an alpha(v)beta(3)-specific humanized Mab. *Proc. Natl Acad. Sci. USA* **95,** 6037–6042.

24. Knappik, A., Ge, L., Honegger, A., Pack, P., Fischer, M., Wellnhofer, G., et al. (2000) Fully synthetic human combinatorial libraries (HuCAL) based on modular consensus frameworks and CDRs randomized with trinucleotides. *J. Mol. Biol.* **296,** 57–86.

25. Chothia, C., and Lesk, A. M. (1987) Canonical structures for the hypervariable regions of immunoglobulins. *J. Mol. Biol.* **196,** 901–917.

26. Chothia, C., Lesk, A. M., Tramontano, A., Levitt, M., Smith-Gill, S. J., Air, G., et al. (1989) Conformations of immunoglobulin hypervariable regions. *Nature* **342,** 877–883.

27. Chothia, C., Lesk, A. M., Gherardi, E., Tomlinson, I. M., Walter, G., Marks, J. D., et al. (1992) Structural repertoire of the human VH segments. *J. Mol. Biol.* **227,** 799–817.

28. Rees, A. R., Martin, A. C. R., Pedersen, J. T., and Searle, S. M. J. (1992) *ABM™, A Computer Program for Modelling Variable Regions of Antibodies.* Oxford Molecular Ltd., Oxford, UK.

29. Virnekäs, B., Ge, L., Plückthun, A., Schneider, K. C., Wellnhofer, G., and Moroney S. E. (1994) Trinucleotide phosphoramidites: ideal reagents for the synthesis of mixed oligonucleotides for random mutagenesis. *Nucleic Acids Res.* **22,** 5600–5607.

30. Lyttle, M. H., Napolitano, E. W., Calio, B. L., and Kauvar, L. M. (1995) Mutagenesis using trinucleotide betacyanoethyl phosphoramidites. *Biotechniques* **19,** 274–281.

31. Kayushin, A. L., Korosteleva, M. D., Miroshnikov, A. I., Kosch, W., Zubov, D., and Piel, N. (1996) A convenient approach to the synthesis of trinucleotide phosphoramidites-synthons for the generation of oligonucleotide/peptide libraries. *Nucleic Acids Res.* **24,** 3748–3755.

32. Marks, J. D., Griffiths, A. D., Malmqvist, M., Clackson, T. P., Bye, J. M., and Winter, G. (1992) By-passing immunization: building high affinity human antibodies by chain shuffling. *Biotechnology (NY)* **10,** 779–783.

33. Welschof, M., Terness, P., Kipriyanov, S. M., Stanescu, D., Breitling, F., Dörsam, H., et al. (1997) The antigen-binding domain of a human IgG-anti-F(ab')2 autoantibody. *Proc. Natl. Acad. Sci. USA* **94,** 1902–1907.

34. Dörsam, H., Braunagel, M., Kleist, C., Moynet, D., and Welschof, M. (1996) Screening of phage-displayed antibody libraries in *Methods in Molecular Medicine, vol. 13: Molecular Diagnosis of Infectious Diseases,* (Reischl, U., ed.), Humana Press Inc., Totowa, NJ, pp. 605–614.

8

Single-Domain V$_H$ Antibody Fragments from a Phage Display Library

Liat Binyamin, Daniel Plaksin, and Yoram Reiter

1. Introduction

The interaction between antigens and antibodies can be viewed as a protein engineering system that was optimized by nature and is capable of recognizing any given molecular entity (antigen). Antigen recognition is conferred to the antibody by a limited number of hypervariable surface loops, differing in sequence and in length, which are connected to a conserved framework structure.

Understanding recognition of antigen targets at the molecular level is of fundamental and applied importance, because the ability to mimic these loops using small molecules is of important therapeutic value. In addition to the design of novel reagents that are based on antibody hypervariable loops, small and recombinant versions of antibodies are of fundamental importance in the field of targeted therapy and imaging (*1–3*).

Recent developments in antibody engineering and recombinant DNA technology have made it possible to generate recombinant antibodies with a high degree of specificity and affinity for theoretically any antigen by employing phage display technology and constructing very large repertoires of antibodies that are displayed on the surface of filamentous phage (*4–6*).

Panning and selection of individual phage clones can screen the phage population containing tens of millions of individual clones through binding to an immobilized antigen.

Several forms of recombinant antibody fragments can be designed and used for phage display to substitute for large intact immunoglobulin molecules. These options include Fab fragments or Fv fragments that are stabilized and/or covalently linked utilizing various strategies (*7–9*).

Fv fragments of antibodies, which consist of the heavy- and light-chain variable domains, are the smallest module of antibodies that contains the functional antigen-binding moiety without significant loss in antigen affinity and specificity (*7,9,10*).

From: *Methods in Molecular Biology, vol. 207: Recombinant Antibodies for Cancer Therapy: Methods and Protocols*
Edited by: M. Welschof and J. Krauss © Humana Press Inc., Totowa, NJ

Typically the hypervariable loops (CDRs) of both chains contribute to antigen binding. Smaller fragments of antibodies are advantageous for pharmaceutical applications, for example, cancer targeting and imaging when small antigen binding molecules are needed to penetrate into large solid tumors.

There are examples in which heavy chains alone retain a significant binding ability in the absence of light chain. It is also well-established, from structural studies, that the CDR3 of the heavy chain generally contributes the most to antigen binding because CDR3 residues are responsible for most of the surface contact area and molecular interaction with the antigen *(11–14)*. Less binding activity was observed for isolated light chains.

In view of these data, attempts were made to isolate single V_H domains. For example, V_H domains were isolated from expression libraries derived from immunized mice *(15)*. In another report, antigen-binding V_H domains were rescued from a human phage-displayed V_H library. In this case a human V_H/V_L interface of camelid immunoglobulin heavy chain was mimicked to prevent nonspecific binding of the V_H through its interface with the light chain variable domain. This was achieved through three mutations in the V_H/V_L interface that mimic camel heavy chains naturally devoid of light-chain partners *(16–25)*.

In this chapter we describe the generation and screening of a single-domain V_H phage-displayed library that is based on a natural framework scaffold of a mouse monoclonal antibody with a unique V_H/V_L interface and a randomized CDR3 *(24,25)*.

The V_H library is displayed on the phage without any mutations or modifications in the original interface framework residues. We have selected phage clones that bind specifically with affinity in the nanomolar range to protein antigens after several rounds of panning. After library selections on antigen, the V_H domains are produced in *Escherichia coli* at very high yields as soluble protein by in vitro refolding of insoluble inclusion bodies. The V_H domain can then be purified to homogeneity as a monomeric protein and be used for functional, structural, and biological studies.

2. Materials

2.1. PCR Amplification of V_H Randomized CDR3

1. Thermocycler Trioblock (Biometra).
2. High Fidelity Taq polymerase (Boehringer Mannheim, Germany).
3. 100 m*M* dNTPs (New England Biolabs, Inc).

2.2. Cloning into Phagemid Vector

1. Petri dishes, 85 and 145 mm diameter.
2. Table-top microcentrifuge.
3. QIAquick Gel Extraction kit (Qiagen).
4. QIAquick polymerase chain reaction (PCR) purification kit (Qiagen).
5. TG1 electrocompetent *E. coli* (Stratagene Cloning Systems, La Jolla, CA).
6. *Sfi*I restriction endonuclease (Boehringer Mannheim).
7. *Not*I restriction endonuclease (Boehringer Mannheim).
8. T4 DNA ligase (Boehringer Mannheim).
9. PCANTAB5E phagemid vector (Pharmacia).

10. Ampicillin (5 mg/mL) sterile.
11. 2XYT-GA medium agar plates.
12. 2XYT medium.
13. Sterile glycerol.

2.3. Panning of Library on Antigen

1. M13KO7 helper phage (Pharmacia).
2. Polystyrene sulfated latex beads (Interfacial Dynamics Corporation, Portland OR).
3. Magnetic-sterptavidin-coated polystyrene beads (Dynal, Oslo, Norway).
4. Tween-20 (Sigma).
5. Low-fat milk.
6. Glycine-HCl (Sigma).

2.4. Characterization of Phage Clones

1. 96-Well ELISA plates (Nalge Nunc).
2. Tween-20 (Sigma).
3. Low fat milk.
4. Blocking solution: PBS 0.05% Tween and 5% low-fat milk.
5. Anti-M13-HRP (Amersham).
6. Anti-E-tag-HRP (Amersham).
7. TMB (3',3',5',5'-tetramethylbezidine) (Sigma).
8. H_2O_2 (Sigma).

2.5. Production of Soluble V$_H$ Domain Protein

1. Thermocycler (Biometra).
2. High Fidelity Taq polymerase (Boehringer Mannheim).
3. 100 mM dNTPs (New England Biolabs, Inc).
4. QIAquick Gel Extraction kit (Qiagen).
5. QIAquick PCR purification kit (Qiagen).
6. Qiagen plasmid kit (Qiagen).
7. Expression vector pET21a (Novagen).
8. BL21(DE3) competent *E. coli* (Stratagene Cloning Systems).
9. IPTG (Sigma).
10. Superbroth (Terrific Broth).
11. Lysozyme (5 mg/mL) (Sigma).
12. Guanidine-HCl (Sigma).
13. Tris-HCl, pH 8.0 (Sigma).
14. EDTA (Sigma).
15. TE50/20 (50 mM Tris-HCl, pH 7.4, 20 mM EDTA).
16. Solubilization buffer: 6 M guanidine HCl, 100 mM Tris-HCl, pH 8.0, 2 mM EDTA.
17. 5 M NaCl (Sigma).
18. Triton X-100 (Sigma).
19. Gluthatione (oxidized) (GSSG) (Sigma).
20. DTE (Ditioeritherol) (Sigma).
21. Refolding buffer: 0.1 M Tris-HCl, pH 8.0, 1 mM EDTA, 0.5 M arginine, 0.09 mM Gluthatione, oxidized (GSSG).
22. Urea (Sigma).
23. MonoQ Column (Pharmacia).
24. TSK3000 Column (TosoHass).

3. Methods

3.1. PCR Amplification of V_H Randomized CDR3

1. The gene encoding the V_H domain scaffold (family I(A)) originated from a mouse hybridoma specific for H-2Dd+RGPGRAFVTI peptide *(28)*.
2. Amplify V_H by PCR using primers 1 and 2 described in **Table 1**. Amplification is carried out in a total volume of 50 µL containing 50–100 ng (1–5 µL) DNA, 100 pmol of each primer, 250 µM dNTPs, 5 µL 10X PCR buffer, and 1 U Taq DNA polymerase.
3. Run 30 PCR cycles. The thermal cycle is 1: 95°C, 1 min; 2: 55°C, 1 min; 3: 72°C, 1 min. At the beginning of the first cycle incubate at 95°C for 5 min and at the end of the last cycle at 72°C for 5 min.
4. Analyze the amplified DNA fragment by electrophoresis on a 1.5% agarose gel. Stain gel with ethidium bromide.
5. Purify PCR product with QIAquick PCR purification kit (Qiagen).

3.2. Construction of V_H Library

1. Reamplify 1 µg sample of PCR product (10 cycles) with the primers described in **Table 1** to avoid nonsymmetric pairing of strands due to primer exhaustion. Reamplification conditions are as described in **Subheading 3.1., step 2.**
2. Purify PCR product with QIAquick PCR purification kit (Qiagen).
3. Digest the final PCR product (1–2 µg) with 50 U *Sfi*I (5 h at 50°C) and 50 U *Not*I (4 h at 37°C) in a volume of 100–200 µL.
4. Ligate 0.5 µg into 1.0 µg phagemid vector pCANTAB 5 E (Amersham Pharmacia Biotech, Piscataway, NJ). Each ligation reaction mixture consists of 100 ng DNA, 1 U of T4 ligase, ligation buffer and water to a final volume of 10–15 µL. Incubate overnight at 16°C.
5. Precipitate the DNA by adding 1/10 vol 3 M sodium acetate, 20 µg glycogen, and 2.5 vol of absolute ethanol. Incubate for 4 h on dry ice and sediment the precipitate by centrifugation at 10,000g for 30 min at 4°C.
6. Wash pellet with 500 µL 70% ethanol, dry the pellet and resuspend in 20 µL water.
7. Electroporate ligated DNA is into 40 µL *E. coli* TG1. Electroporation conditions are: 2.5 kV, 200 Ω, 25 µF. After three ligations and 30 electroporations a library was obtained with a complexity of 4×10^8 independent clones.
8. Plate the bacteria on large 2XYT-GA medium agar plates and incubate overnight at 30°C.
9. Sequence randomly picked clones to verify the insert and the correct integration of CDR3.

3.3. Phage Selection on Antigen

3.3.1. Preparation of Phage for Selection

3.3.1.1. PHAGE RESCUE

1. Take 1 mL of library stock (frozen cells–Glycerol stock), dilute with 2X YT + Glucose 2% + Amp 100 µg/mL to 20 mL, determine OD_{600} nm.
2. Dilute to $OD_{600} = 0.3$ and grow at in a shaker at 37°C to $OD_{600} = 0.8$.
3. Infect with M13KO7 helper phage at multiplicity of infection (m.o.i) of 10–15 according to: $(5 \times 10^8$ cells/1 OD_{600} nm) × (m.o.i) × (OD_{600} nm of culture) × (culture vol) = number of M13KO7 pfu needed.
4. Add helper phage, incubate at 37°C, 45 min low-speed shake (150 rpm) and 45 min high speed (250 rpm).
5. Centrifuge cells 3000 rpm for 10 min at 20°C (to remove glucose).

Table 1
PCR Primers for V$_H$ Domain Scaffold Cloning and Randomization of CDR3

1. 5' primer for introduction of *Sfi*I cloning site:
   5'-AAGGAAAAAAGGCCCAGCCGGCCGATGTCCAGCTGCAGGAGTCAGGAC CGGC-3'
2. 3' primer for CDR3 randomization and introduction of *Nco*I cloning site:
   5'-TATCAAATGCGGCCGCGACGGTGACAGTGGTCCCTTGGCCCCAGTAGTC MNNMNNMNNMNNMNNMNNMNNMNNMNNTCTTGCACAGTAATATGTGGC TGT-3'
3. PCR primer for reamplification:
   *Sfi*I *short:* 5'-AAGGAAAAAAGGCCCAGCCGGCCGATGTCC-3'
   *Not*I *short:* 5'-TATCAAATGCGGCCGCGACGGTGACAGTGG-3'

6. Carefully remove all supernatant, gently resuspend in 10 mL 2XYT-AK (Amp 100 µg/mL and Kanamycin 50 µg/mL) in 50 mL sterile tubes (DO NOT ADD GLUCOSE).
7. Incubate overnight at 37°C, shake 250 rpm.
8. Spin cells at 3000 rpm, 20 min, transfer up to 50 mL tube, supernatant contains recombinant phage (save pellet at –70°C for safety).
9. Use supernatant for titration and phage precipitation.

3.3.1.2. PHAGE PRECIPITATION

1. Centrifuge supernatant at 3000 rpm for 10 min at 4°C.
2. Remove supernatant to a clean SS34 centrifuge tube.
3. Add 1/5 vol of PEG/NaCl (autoclaved 20% PEG8000 with 2.5 *M* NaCl), incubate on ice for 1 h.
4. Centrifuge at 10,000 rpm with SS34 rotor for 30 min at 4°C.
5. Remove as much supernatant as possible saving the phage pellet.
6. Resuspend phages carefully in 1 mL STE (TE, pH 7.4 + 100 m*M* NaCl).
7. Transfer phages to a new Eppendorf tube, centrifuge at top speed (10,000*g*) for 15 min at 4°C.
8. Transfer supernatant to a clean Eppendorf tube, add 1/5 vol of PEG/NaCl, incubate 15 min on ice.
9. Centrifuge at top speed (10,000*g*) for 15 min at 4°C.
10. Resuspend pellet in 1 mL STE, add 1/5 vol of PEG/NaCl, incubate 15 min on ice and perform subsequently a final centrifugation at top speed for 15 min, 4°C.
11. Resuspend pellet in 0.5–1 mL PBS.
12. Store phages at 4°C (or freeze at –70°C, add glycerol to frozen stocks).

3.3.2. Phage Selection on Antigen

1. Phage library (5 × 10^{11} cfu) was selected against antigens by panning four rounds on polystyrene sulfated latex beads (Interfacial Dynamics Corporation, Portland, OR) coated with antigen or with magnetic-streptavidin-coated polystyrene beads (DYNAL, Oslo, Norway) to which biotinylated antigen was immobilized.
2. To coat antigen on beads, coat beads overnight at room temperature with 1–5 µg of protein in 50–200 µL of PBS. Following antigen immobilization, block the beads with PBS containing 0.05% (v/v) Tween, and 5% (w/v) low-fat milk.

3. For attaching antigen onto magnetic beads biotinylation should be performed according to standard techniques and the activity of target protein should be determined.
4. Incubate phage pool for 1 h in blocking buffer and wash 10× with PBS/0.05% Tween.
5. Elute bound phage with 500 µL of 0.2 M glycine, pH 2.2, and neutralize with 75 µL of 1 M Tris-HCl, pH 9.5.
6. Infect eluted phages into TG1 cells and rescue phage for the next round of panning using the M13KO7 helper phage.
7. Titrate eluted phages by making 1:10 serial dilutions in 2XYT medium and infecting TG1 cells with diluted phage (30 min at 37°C).
8. Plate the infected TG1 cells on LB/Amp plates.

3.4. Characterization of Phage Clones

1. Screen single phage clones by ELISA assays using PEG-precipitated phages.
2. For phage precipitation add one-fifth the volume of phage-containing supernatant of 20% PEG8000 and incubate on ice for 30 min. Centrifuge at 12,000g (microfuge) for 30 min at 4°C and resuspend phage pellet in 1 mL of PBS.
3. Immobilize antigen onto 96-well Maxisorb microtiter plates using different concentrations of antige (0.1–1 µg/mL) 150–200 µL/well of carbonate buffer, pH 9.5 or PBS.
4. Block the plate with PBS 0.05% Tween and 5% low-fat milk (blocking solution).
5. Incubate with phage (109–1011) for 1 h at room temperature or at 37°C in a volume of 150–200 µL.
6. Wash plate 10× with PBS/0.05% Tween.
7. Detection is with a second antibody anti-M13-HRP (Amersham Pharmacia Biotech, Piscataway, NJ) according to the instructions for phage analysis or anti-E-tag-HRP (Amersham Pharmacia Biotech, Piscataway, NJ) for soluble protein analysis.
8. Incubate with anti-M13-HRP diluted according to the manufacturer instructions for 30 min at room temperature.
9. Wash plate well (10×) with PBS/0.05% Tween.
10. Develop ELISA assays with 3', 3', 5',5',-tetramethylbenzidine (TMB).

3.5. Cloning of Isolated V_H Domain Phage Clone into Expression Vector

1. For large-scale protein production, reamplify plasmid DNA from positive binding clones with the oligonucleotides described in **Table 2**. These insert cloning sites enabled subcloning into the T7 promotor-based pET-21a expression vector.
2. Amplification is carried out in a total volume of 50 µL containing 50–100 ng (1–5 mL) DNA, 100 pmol of each primer, 250 μM dNTPs , 5 µL 10X PCR buffer and 1 U Taq DNA polymerase. Run 30 PCR cycles. The thermal cycle is 1: 95°C, 1 min; 2: 55°C, 1 min; 3: 72°C, 1 min. At the beginning of the first cycle incubate at 95°C for 5 min and at the end of the last cycle at 72°C for 5 min.
3. Analyze the amplified DNA fragment by electrophoresis on a 1.5% agarose gel. Stain with ethidium bromide.
4. Purify PCR product with QIAquick PCR purification kit (Qiagen).
5. Digest purified PCR (1–2 µg) with 5 U NdeI and XhoI (1 h at 37°C) in a volume of 20–50 µL. Ligate 1–2 µg into 2 µg Expression vector pET21a (Novagen) in a final volume of 10–15 µL. Incubate overnight at 16°C.
6. Transform DH5α competent cells with DNA and isolate plasmid by Qiagen mini-plasmid prep kit.

Table 2
Primers for Cloning V$_H$ Domain DNA into Expression Cector

V$_H$ 5' *Nde*I primer: 5'-GGGAATTCCATATGGATGTCCAGCTGCAGGAGTC-3'
V$_H$ 3' *Xho*I primer: 5'GGGAATTCCTCGAGCTATGCGGCA CGCGGTTCCA-3'

7. Verify the correct insert size by DNA restriction using *Nde*I and *Xho*I and verify sequence by DNA sequencing.

3.6. Production of Soluble V$_H$ Domain Protein

1. The methods described here for plasmid expression in *E. coli* BL21/λDE3 cells is applicable for plasmids containing the T7 promoter and the ampicillin resistance gene. Upon induction of the T7 RNA polymerase in *E. coli* BL21/λDE3 cells by IPTG, large amounts of recombinant protein are produced. The overexpressed V$_H$ protein accumulate in insoluble intracellular inclusion bodies, which can subsequently be isolated, purified, solubilized, and prepared for in vitro refolding.
2. Transform DNA into BL21(DE3) competent *E. coli*. Use 3–5 μg of DNA (0.5–1.0 mg/mL) to transform 100 μL competent cells and plate transformation on 85 mm LB/Amp plates.
3. Inoculate 2–3 plates full of colonies into 0.5 L flask of superbroth containing 20 mL/L 20% glucose, 1.68 mL/L 1 *M* MgSO$_4$ and 100 μg/mL ampicillin. OD$_{600}$ nm after inoculation should be 0.15–0.2.
4. Incubate at 37°C shaking at ~250 rpm, check the OD$_{600}$ nm in 30–40 min intervals.
5. At OD$_{600}$ = 2.0–2.5 add 5 mL 0.1 *M* IPTG to each flask (final concentration of 1 m*M*). (dilute 1:10 in superbroth when OD readings are above 0.6). Save 1 mL culture as preinduction control sample.
6. Continue shaking incubation at 37°C for 90–120 min.
7. Save 1 mL aliquot of culture as postinduction sample.
8. Harvest bacteria by centrifugation at 1500*g* for 30 min, 4°C.
9. Discard supernatant. Cell pellet may be frozen at –70°C.
10. Analyze aliquots from **steps 5** and **7** by sodium dodecyl polyacrylamide gel electrophoresis (SDS-PAGE). Resuspend cell pellets in 1 mL TE buffer. Sonicate 20 s in bath sonicator and centrifuge at top speed in Eppendorf centrifuge. Resuspend pellet in 0.1 mL TE. Sonicate 10–20 s and resuspend in 0.1 mL TE. Determine protein concentration and run equal amounts of protein on reduced SDS-PAGE to verify induction.
11. Resuspend pellet cells from each liter of culture into 160 mL TE50/20. Transfer suspension to 250 mL Sorvall centrifuge bottle.
12. Add 6.5 mL lysozyme at 5 mg/mL, mix well and incubate for 30 min at room temperature. Shake by hand frequently.
13. Add 20 mL of 25% Triton X-100 and 20 mL of 5 *M* NaCl, mix well, and incubate for 30 min at room temperature. Shake by hand frequently.
14. Centrifuge 27,500*g* for 60 min at 4°C in Sorvall GSA rotor.
15. Discard supernatant and resuspend pellet by using a tissuemizer (tissue homogenizer) in 180 mL TE50/20.
16. Repeat **steps 14** and **15** 3–4 times. Keep a small amount of inclusion bodies pellet after last wash to be analyzed on SDS-PAGE as described in **step 10**.

17. Transfer inclusion bodies pellet into 50 mL Oak Ridge Centrifuge Tubes (Nunc) and resuspend in solubilization buffer. 1.5–1.8 g wet inclusion bodies solubilized into 10 solubilization buffer will give a protein concentration of ~10 mg/mL.

18. Dissolve inclusion bodies in solubilization buffer (if required use tissuemizer with a small probe) until completely dissolved. Centrifuge solubilized inclusion bodies at 10,000g, 20 min, 4°C in Sorvall SS34 rotor.

19. Take supernatant containing solubilized inclusion bodies, determine protein concentration with pierce Coomassie plus reagent.

20. Dilute the protein to 10 mg/mL with solubilization buffer and add DTE (Dithioerithritol) to 10 mg/ mL (65 mM final concentration), mix, and incubate for at least 2 h at room temperature.

21. Prepare 100-fold more buffer then the volume of the denatured protein solution and chill to 10°C.

22. Add 551 mg/L oxidized glutathion (GSSG).

23. Briskly stir the chilled refolding buffer by using a pipet, add the denatured protein from stage 20 quickly over 10–20 s. Mix well for 2–3 min, stop stirring and allow refolding at 10°C for 36–48 h.

24. Dialyze protein at 4°C in 25-fold of the initial refolding volume against 20 mM Tris-HCl, pH 7.4, 100 mM urea with 2–3 changes until conductivity measures 3–4 mM HO.

3.7. Purification of V_H Protein

3.7.1. Ion-Exchange Chromatography

1. Purification of V_H domain protein is performed on an ion-exchange column Q-Sepharose or S-Sepharose (depending on the V_H domain PI charge and pH) applying an elusion gradient of sodium chloride.

2. All chromatography steps are performed at 4°C. Load the dialyzed protein on a 5–8 mL Q-Sepharose or S-Sepharose column (Pharmacia) previously equilibrated and washed with 10 column volumes of buffer A, 10 column volumes of buffer B, and then 20 vol of buffer A. The protein is loaded at 2–4 mL/min.

3. After loading the protein (1–3 h), wash the column with buffer A until no protein is present in the flowthrough.

4. Elute protein with a linear gradient of 0–40% buffer B in buffer A at a flow rate of 2 mL/min over 10 column volumes. Collect 2 mL fractions. This will yield a gradient with a 1% increase in buffer B per 1 mL of elution.

5. Evaluate the peak fractions of protein individually for protein concentration and for purity by SDS-PAGE under reducing conditions.

6. Pooled fractions should be >90% pure and not be contaminated with proteins of similar molecular weight, otherwise these contaminants will still be present after the size-exclusion chromatography step.

3.7.2. Size Exclusion Chromatography

1. Concentrate the pooled protein, purified on the Q-Sepharose/S-Separose anion-exchange chromatography, by centricon 30 (Amicon) to a concentration of 2–3 mg/mL.

2. Load protein on a 7.5 × 60 cm TSK G3000SW column (equipped with a respective guard column), equilibrated with PBS. Elute the column with PBS. The protein usually elutes at 18–20 mL. The column can be previously calibrated with molecular-weight standard protein kit (Pharmacia) to verify the apparent elution size of the recombinant protein.

3. Analyze fractions from size exclusion chromatography, pooled, and stored at –70°C, by reducing conditions on SDS-PAGE. A typical yield of scFv or dsFv-immunotoxin is 5–10% and 10–15%, respectively, of total recombinant protein renatured.

4. Notes

1. For best expression results, fresh transformation of expression plasmids into competent *E. coli* BL21/λDE3 cells should be performed. The transformation should not precede the expression by more then 18 h. The expression system has some leakyness and can result in protein expression and in some cases bacterial lysis prior to induction by IPTG. This may result in reduced growth and viability of the bacteria during culture and poor expression after induction with IPTG.

2. In some cases premature protein expression occurs while bacteria are growing on the LB/Amp plates, leading to smaller than normal colonies. To decrease the leakyness of the expression system, an episome containing a repressor (*lac*Iq, *lac* repressor) can be added to the BL21/λDE3 cells.

3. In some cases protein expression may be poor because the eukaryotic DNA to be expressed in the bacteria contains codons that are rare for gram negative bacteria, such as AGA and AGG. This problem can be solved by using a plasmid encoding tRNA for these codons as well as a *lac* repressor. The BL21/λDE3 cells are simply transformed with the episome, which contains a kanamycin resistance gene, and competent cells prepared for transformation with plasmid-encoding recombinant V$_H$. The BL21-CodonPlus™ Competent Cells from Stratagene can be also used. They are designed for high-level expression of difficult heterologous proteins and eliminate additional procedures to express recombinant genes that encode rare codons. They contain extra copies of the genes that encode tRNAs for codons in *E. coli* that are rarely used. BL21-CodonPlus-RIL cells contain extra argU, ileY, and leuW tRNA genes and BL21-CodonPlus-RP cells contain extra argU and proL tRNA genes.

4. An alternative to transform DNA for producing a particular protein each time, is to prepare a master cell bank. To produce a master cell bank, a single colony obtained from a fresh transformation is cultured in a shake flask with 200 mL of superbroth containing 100 µg/mL ampicillin. When the culture reaches an OD$_{600}$ nm of ~3, the cells are placed on ice, mixed with a 50% volume of 86% glycerol in water, and frozen at –70°C in 1.5 mL aliquots. Future fermentations can be started from a single aliquot.

5. A problem with some recombinant proteins is that their inclusion bodies often dissolve in detergents, such as the Triton X-100 that is being used to wash the inclusion bodies (**Subheading 3.3., step 3**). In these cases the number of washes with detergent must be minimized.

6. The protein concentration in the denaturing solution must be measured accurately because protein concentration in the final refolding is critical for successful renaturation of the recombinant protein. The protein in the denaturing solution (solubilization buffer) should be diluted 20-fold in solubilization buffer rather than water just prior to adding to the cuvet, since precipitation of protein will occur after dilution in water, leading to an inaccurate measurement of protein concentration. Measuring protein concentration in the refolding solution is difficult because of the presence of large concentration of L-arginine, but it can be measured accurately after the dialysis step of the refolding solution.

7. Stirring during the entire 36–48 h incubation of refolding at 10°C should not be done because it leads to increased and severe aggregation of the protein.

8. Isolated and purified inclusion bodies can be stored for prolonged periods at $-70°C$ as a paste or in a solubilized form but without the reducing agent (DTE). After thawing, the inclusion bodies can be solubilized then add DTE. Storage of solubilized inclusion bodies in the presence of DTE will cause a significant decrease in refolding efficiencies.

9. Recombinant proteins after the Q-Sepahrose column need to be evaluated by reducing conditions on SDS-PAGE to rule out contamination with disulfide-bonded impurities that might comigrate with the V_H protein on a nonreducing gel but appear as lower molecular weight impurities on a reducing gel. The protein may be contaminated with dimeric or multimeric V_H, which will not be apparent on a reducing gel, but these multimers can be removed subsequently by the size exclusion chromatography step.

References

1. Reiter, Y. and Pastan, I. (1998) Fv fragments of antibodies as novel reagents for cancer therapy and diagnosis. *Trends Biotechnol.* **16**, 513–520.
2. Vitetta, E. S., Thorpe, P. E., and Uhr, J. (1993) Immunotoxins: magic bullets or misguided missiles. *Trends Pharmacol. Sci.* **14**, 148–154.
3. Haard, H., Henderikx, P., and Hoogenboom, H. R. (1998) Creating and engineering human antibodies for immunotherapy. *Advan. Drug Del. Rev.* **31**, 5–31.
4. Winter, G., Griffith, A. D., Hawkins, R. E., and Hoogenboom, H. R. (1994) Making antibodies by phage display technology. *Annu. Rev. Immunol.* **12**, 433–455.
5. Barbas, C. F. (1995) Synthetic human antibodies. *Nature Med.* **1**, 837–839.
6. Hoogenboom, H. R., Bruine, A. P., Hufton, S. E., Hoet, R. M., Arends, J., and Roovers, R. C. (1998) Antibody phage display technology and its applications. *Immunotechnology* **4**, 1–20.
7. Bird, R. E., Hardman, K. D., Jacobson, J. W., Johnson, S., Kaufman, B. M., and Lee, S. M. (1988) Single-chain antigen binding proteins. *Science* **242**, 423–426.
8. Huston, J. S., Levinson, D., Mudghett-Hunter, M., Tai, M. S., Novotny, J., and Margolies, M. N. (1988) Protein enginnering of antibody binding sites: recovery of specific activity in an anti dogoxigenin single-chain Fv analogue produced in *Escherichia coli. Proc. Natl Acad. Sci. USA* **85**, 5879–5883.
9. Glockshuber, R., Malia, M., Pfitzinger, I., and Pluckthun A. (1990) A comparision of strategies to stabilize immunoglobulin Fv fragments. *Biochemistry* **29**, 1362–1376.
10. Reiter, Y., Brinkmann, U., Lee, B. K., and Pastan, I. (1996) Engineering antibody Fv fragments for cancer detection and therapy: Disulfide-stabilized Fv fragments. *Nature Biotechnol.* **14**, 1239–1245.
11. Padlan, E. A. (1994) Anatomy of the antibody molecule. *Mol. Immunol.* **31**, 169–217.
12. Webster, D. M., Henry, A. H., and Rees, A. R. (1994) Antibody-antigen interactions. *Curr. Opin. Struct. Biol.* **4**, 123–129.
13. Chothia, C. and Lesk, A. (1987) Canonical structures of the hypervariable regions of immunoglobulins. *J. Mol. Biol.* **196**, 904–917.
14. Chothia, C., Novotny, J., Bruccoleri, R., and Karplus, M. (1985) Domain association in immunoglobulin molecules. The packing of variable domains. *J. Mol. Biol.* **186**, 651–663.
15. Ward, E. S., Gussow, D., Griffith, A. D., Jones, P. T., and Winter, G. (1989) Binding activities of a repertoire of single immunoglobulin variable domains secreted from *Escherichia coli. Nature* **341**, 544–546.
16. Muyldermans, S., Atarhouch, T., Saldanha, J., Barbosa, J. A., and Hamers, R. (1994) Sequence and structure of V_H domain from naturally occuring camel heavy chain immunoglobulins lacking light chains. *Protein Eng.* **7**, 1129–1135.

17. Davies, J. and Riechmann, L. (1995) Antibody V$_H$ domains as small recognition units. *Biotechnology* **13,** 475–479.
18. Davies, J. and Riechmann, L. (1996) Affinity improvement of single antibody V$_H$ domains. Residues in all three hypervariable regions affect antigen binding. *Immunotechnology* **2,** 169–179.
19. Kortt, A. A., Guthrie, R. E., Hinds, M. G., Power, B. E., Ivancic, N., Caldwell, B. J., et al. (1995) Solution properties of *Escherichia coli*-expressed V$_H$ domain of anti-neuraminidase antibody NC41. *J. Protein Chem.* **14,** 167–178.
20. Ghahroudi, M. A., Desmyter, A., Wyns, L., Hamers, R., and Muyldermans, S. (1997) Selection and identification of single domain antibody fragments from camel heavy-chain antibodies. *FEBS Lett.* **414,** 521–526.
21. Lauwereys, M., Ghahroudi, M. A., Desmyter, A., Kinne, J., Holzer, W., DeGenst, E., et al. (1998) Potent enzyme inhibitors derived from dromedary heavy-chain antibodies. *EMBO J.* **17,** 3512–3520.
22. Martin, F,. Volpari, C., Steinkuhler, C., Dimasi, N., Brunetti, M., Biasiol, G. et al. (1997) Affinity selection of a camelized V$_H$ domain antibody inhibitor of hepatitis C virus NS3 protease. *Protein Eng.* **10,** 607–614.
23. Sheriff, S. and Constantine, K. L. (1996) Redefining the minimal antigen-binding fragment. *Nature Struct. Biol.* **3,** 733–736.
24. Reiter, Y., Schuck, P., Boyd, L., and Plaksin, D. (1999) An Antibody Single-domain Phage Display Library of a Native Heavy Chain Variable Region: Isolation of Functional Single-domain V$_H$ Molecules with a Unique Interface. *J. Mol. Biol.* **292,** 685–698.
25. Polakova, K., Plaksin, D., Chung, D. H., Belyakov, I. M., Berzofsky, J. A., and Margulies, D. H. (2000) Antibodies directed against the MHC-I molecule H-2D(d) complexed with an antigenic peptide: similarities to a T cell receptor with the same specificity. *J. Immunol.* **165,** 5703–5712.

9

Isolation of Human Fab Fragments Against Ovarian Carcinoma Using Guided Selection

Mariangela Figini, Andrew Green, Francesco Colotta, and Silvana Canevari

1. Introduction

Ovarian cancer remains a major health problem in the United States and most Western European countries. Despite the availability of several effective chemotherapeutic agents for the treatment of ovarian cancer, survival is still poor. Major problems in ovarian cancer chemotherapies are a failure to consolidate response, acquired/intrinsic drug resistance, and dose-limiting toxicity. Thus new therapeutic treatment modalities have been developed, most of which are based on the targeting ability of monoclonal antibodies (MAbs) that detect tumor-associated antigens. After early disappointments, some relevant clinical success has recently been achieved, and several alternative and/or supplementary approaches are being explored. For detailed information on aspects such as mechanisms of action, preclinical screening, and clinical results, *see* specific references in **Table 1** and an excellent recent review *(1)*.

For any MAb-based cancer therapy, target selection is crucial and the probability of success ultimately depends on a thorough knowledge of the function of the selected target antigen/epitope in physiological and pathological conditions. **Table 1** lists the more promising therapeutic MAb applications in ovarian carcinoma patients.

Of particular interest is the generation of human antibodies against the surface antigens of ovary tumor cells, since these reagents are more likely to allow repeated injections without the toxicity associated with immunogenicity of rodent components (*see* reviews in this volume and **ref. 2**). Recent phage technology now readily allows the generation of fully human MAb. Standard procedures for screening phage-display antibody libraries are based on the use of soluble antigens coated directly or indirectly on different solid matrices, although any target suitable for affinity interaction with phage can be used. In particular, the use of whole live cells as a direct source of target antigen *(3–7)* promises that the physiological status and correct conformation of the

From: *Methods in Molecular Biology, vol. 207: Recombinant Antibodies for Cancer Therapy: Methods and Protocols*
Edited by: M. Welschof and J. Krauss © Humana Press Inc., Totowa, NJ

Table 1
Target Antigens Potentially Suited for Antibody-Based Immunotherapy of Ovarian Carcinoma[a]

Target antigen overexpressed by	Antibody entered into clinic[b]	Product type	Type of therapy	Trial status	References
Ovarian and few other carcinomas					
FR[c] (a isoform)	MOV 18	Murine	Radioimmunotherapy	I/II	(22)
		Murine-bispecific	CTL retargeting	I/II	(23)
		Chimeric	Radioimmunotherapy	I/II	(24)
Ca-125	B43. 13 (OVAREX)	Murine	Naked Ab	II/III	(25)
	OC-125	Murine	Radioimmunotherapy	I/II	(26)
Ovarian and many other carcinomas					
HER2/neu	Trastuzumab (HERCEPTIN)[d]	Humanized	Naked Ab	I/II	(27)
PEM/MUC1	HMFG-1 (THERAGYN)	Murine	Radioimmunotherapy	III	(28)
	hCTMO1	Chimeric	Radioimmunotherapy	I	(29)
CEA	MN-14	Murine	Radioimmunotherapy	I	(30,31)
TAG-72	B72. 3	Murine	Radioimmunotherapy	I/II	(32)
	CC49	Murine	Radioimmunotherapy	I/II	(33)
Not defined	88BV59 (HUMARAD)	Human	Radioimmunotherapy	I/II	

[a]For details on target antigen characteristics and biodistribution and rationale for therapeutic approach, *see* specific references cited in the clinical trial reports. For trial status, *see also* individual company websites.

[b]In parenthesis the commercial name of the reagent.

[c]FR, folate receptor; PEM/MUC1, polymorphic epithelial mucin, product of MUC1 gene; CEA, carcinoembryonic antigen.

[d]FDA-approved (1998) for metastatizing breast tumors; phase III for early breast cancer tumors.

relevant cell-surface molecule are retained. However the selection of phage antibodies against unpurified cell-surface markers by panning on whole cells has proved very difficult due to the huge number of different antigens with different expression levels. Thus, a general methodology, originally called epitope imprinting selection and now defined as "guided selection" *(8–10)* was developed involving the use of a mouse template antibody chain (either light or heavy chain) to drive selection of a human antibody with corresponding specificity from a preassembled human antibody repertoire. With this methodology, the antigen- as well as epitope-specificity of an MAb with desired properties is retained. The procedure has been tailored to specific needs, such as the derivation of an antibody against a predefined epitope on a cell surface antigen for which a rodent MAb is available but the purified antigen is not. The combined use of guided selection and panning on whole cells might be particularly relevant for the target antigens listed in **Table 1** or for other tumor-associated antigens for which mouse MAb have already demonstrated clinical utility. In addition to the theoretical advantages of the method, it also avoids the need for cumbersome purification of antigens.

Using this procedure on a naive human antibody phage repertoire, we have selected an Fab fragment specifically directed against the folate receptor, which is overexpressed in ovarian carcinomas *(5)*. Selection for other tumor-associated antigens can be achieved using the following sequential procedures described in this chapter and schematized in **Fig. 1**:

1. Amplification of immunoglobulin repertoires (V_HC_H1 and V_LC_L) from human PBL.
2. Preparation of human antibody libraries using phage and phagemid vectors.
3. Cloning murine MAb V_LC_L gene to be used in "guided selection."
4. Preparation of half-human library by infection of *E. coli* containing the murine guiding (V_LC_L) chain with the V_HC_H1 human library.
5. First selection by panning on monolayer cultures of the most appropriate carcinoma cells.
6. Screening by phage enzyme-linked immunosorbent assay (ELISA) and FACS.
7. Selection of the human light chain.
8. Characterization of human Fab binders.

2. Materials

In addition to the materials and equipment listed below, standard reagent and equipment for RT and PCR, tumor cell lines expressing or not expressing the ovarian carcinoma-associated antigen of interest and a murine hybridoma secreting the MAb against the antigen of interest, standard reagents (RPMI 1640, heat-inactivated FCS, glutamine, trypsin-EDTA, antibiotics) and equipment for cell culture maintenance and sterile handling are required.

2.1. Cell Culture and Testing

1. Cell-culture Petri dishes (Costar).
2. 96-Well flat-bottom plates for cell culture (Costar).
3. Poly-L-lysine.
4. Glutaraldehyde (Polysciences, Inc.).

A SELECTION OF HUMAN VH

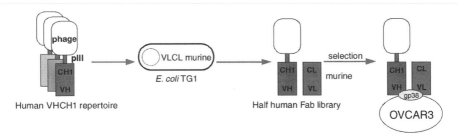

B CLONING OF THE SELECTED IN A PHAGEMIDE VECTOR CONTAINING HUMAN VLCL REPERTOIRE

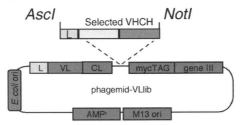

C SELECTION OF HUMAN VL

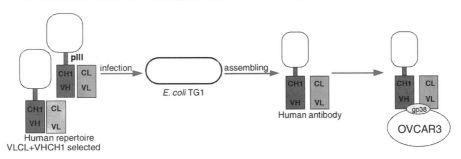

Fig. 1.

2.2. Phage Preparation

1. *Escherichia coli* TG1.
2. Square plates (243 × 243 mm).
3. TYE plates (2XTY, 1% glucose and 15 g agar/L).
4. Sterile glycerol.
5. PEG/NaCl: 20% polyethylene glycol 6000 and 2. 5 *M* NaCl.
6. P/C/I: phenol/Chloroform/isoamyl alcohol.
7. C/I: chloroform/isoamyl alcohol.
8. Gene Pulser Plus (Bio-Rad).

2.3. Phage Testing

1. MPBS: nonfat dry milk in PBS.
2. Anti-M13 HRP (horseradish peroxidase)-conjugated antibody (Pharmacia Biotech, cat. no. 27-9411-01).
3. TMB (tetramethyl-benzidine dihydrochloride).
4. Anti-M13 sheep antibody (Pharmacia Biotech, cat. no. 27-9410-01).
5. FITC (fluorescein-isothiocyanate)-conjugated anti-sheep antibody.
6. ELISA multichannel reader.
7. FACS scan.

3. Methods

3.1. Amplification of $V_H C_H 1$ and $V_L C_L$ Repertoires from Human PBL

A critical step in determining the success of the guided selection procedure is the use of large chain-shuffled repertoires with a high number of functional inserts. Because the aim of guided selection is to recapitulate the properties of binding specificity and affinity of the rodent antibody in its human equivalent, maximization of library sizes during chain-shuffling ensures that as many permutations of heavy-light chain pairings as possible are available for antigen selection. The ease with which a high-affinity antibody can be isolated by phage display correlates with the size of the starting repertoire *(11,12)*.

3.1.1. Extraction of RNA from Human PBL *(see **Note 1**)*

Total RNA is extracted from human PBL using a commercial kit (for example the Qiagen kit) according to the manufacturer's instructions. Usually the yield of RNA extracted from lymphocytes is low compared to the yield from other cell types as also reported in the kits' datasheet.

3.1.2. RT

RT-PCR is carried out using a commercial kit (e.g., the Perkin-Elmer GeneAmp RNA PCR Kit) according to the manufacturer's instructions.

The entire amount of RNA obtained is used to produce three separate cDNA syntheses using HuIgMFOR, HuCLFOR, and HuCKFOR, respectively as downstream primer (*see* **Table 2** for primer sequences).

1. Set up the following assembly RT reaction: RNA X μL, 10X reaction buffer 10 μL, dNTP 10 μL each, downstream primer (10 pmol/μL) 10 μL, $MgCl_2$ 20 μL, H_2O to 98 μL.
2. Keep at 65°C for 5 min.
3. Add 1 μL of RNasin inhibitor (20 U/μL) and 1 μL of MuLV reverse transcriptase (50 U/μL).
4. Keep at 42°C for 1 h.

3.1.3. Primary PCR of Human V Genes

One-third of the cDNA obtained in **Subheading 3.1.2.** is used to amplify each of the three antibody libraries (V_H, $V_\kappa C_\kappa$ and $V\lambda C\lambda$). The 3' primers are the same as those used in **Subheading 3.1.2.**; 5' primers are from the set of 42 primers suggested by the

Table 2
Sequence of Primers Used

Primer	Sequence
HuIgMFOR	TGGAAGAGGCACGTTGAAGCTCTT
HuCLFOR	TGAAGATTCTGTAGGGGCCACTGTCTT
HuCKFOR	AGACTCTCCCCTGTTGAAGCTCTT
HuJH1-2FOR	TGAGGAGACGGTGACCAGGGTGCC
HuJH3FOR	TGAAGAGACGGTGACCATTGTCCC
HuJH4-5FOR	TGAGGAGACGGTGACCAGGGTTCC
HuJH6FOR	TGAGGAGACGGTGACCGTGGTCCC
G3LASCGTGBACK	GTCCTCGCAACTGGCGCGCCACAATTTCACAGT
	AAGGAGGTTTAACTTGTGAAAAAATTATTATTCGCAATT
FdSEQ1	GAATTTTCTGTATGAGG

V-Base repertoire (available online at: http://www.mrc-cpe.cam.ac.uk/imt-doc/restricted/PRIMERS.html).

1. Set up the following PCR reactions (one for each pairs of primers): cDNA X μL, 5 mM dNTP 5 μL, 10 pmol/μL BACK primer 2 μL, 10 pmol/μL FOR primer 2 μL, 10X buffer 5 μL, Taq DNA polymerase (5 U/μL) 1 μL, H$_2$O to 50 μL.
2. PCR amplify for 30 cycles of 94°C for 1 min, 55°C for 1 min, 72°C for 2 min followed by incubation at 72°C for 10 min.

3.1.4. Secondary PCR of Human V Genes

A second PCR is necessary to introduce restriction sites suitable for cloning in the appropriate vectors. *Apa*lI-*Sal*I and *Sfi*I-*Not*I restriction sites are chosen for V$_H$ and V$_L$ chains, respectively, since they are rare in the germline immunoglobulin V genes (http://www.mrc-cpe.cam.ac.uk/imt-doc/restricted/RESTRICTION.html). For the heavy chain, only the V$_H$ is amplified since ApalI is present at the beginning of the C$_H$1; we have described a strategy in which only the V$_H$ are cloned and then inserted into a vector containing a human C$_H$1 in which the *Apa*lI site has been removed *(8)*.

1. Estimate the quantities of V$_H$ and V$_L$ DNA prepared in the primary PCR on an agarose gel.
2. Carry out secondary PCR using the same scheme as for the primary PCR. For light chains, use the 5' and 3' primers as in **Subheading 3.1.3.**, with the appropriate restriction site tails; for heavy chain, use the different JH primers in **Table 1** in 3' and the primers in **Subheading 3.1.3.** in 5' with the appropriate restriction tails.
3. PCR-amplify using 25 cycles of 94°C for 1 min, 55°C for 1 min, 72°C for 2 min followed by incubation at 72°C for 10 min.
4. Check each PCR amplification with a 5-μL sample on a 1.5% agarose gel.
5. Gel-purify fragments on a 1.5% LMP (low melting point) agarose/TBE gel. Carefully excise the VH (350 bp) and VL (600 bp) bands (using a different sterile scalpel or razor blade for each) and transfer each slice to a separate sterile microfuge tube.
6. Purify fragments from the agarose using the Geneclean Kit (Bio 101).

3.2. Preparation of Human Antibody Libraries

The procedure below allows the expression of a repertoire of human heavy-chain genes (V_HC_H1) in an fd filamentous phage and of a V_LC_L repertoire in a phagemid vector as a fusion protein with the pIII protein (8).

3.2.1. Ligation Protocol (see **Note 2**)

1. Set up the following ligation reactions: digested vector DNA (6 µg) X µL, digested fragment (5 µg) X µL, 10X ligase buffer 10 µL, H_2O to 95 µL (we suggest the use of vectors prepared by the cesium chloride method).
2. Mix and spin briefly in a microfuge.
3. Add 5 µL T4 DNA ligase (400 U/µL).
4. Incubate overnight at 16°C.
5. Precipitate with high salt and ethanol, pellet the ligated DNA in a microfuge (14,000 rpm for 10 min); aspirate ethanol, wash pellet once in 70%, ethanol and dry pellet briefly.
6. Resuspend pellet in 10 µL H_2O and either store at –20°C or use directly for electroporation.

3.2.2. Electroporation of Ligation Reactions

1. If frozen TG1 are used, thaw the appropriate number of aliquots on ice (allow 50 µL of cells per 2 µL of ligation reaction).
2. Transfer to a prechilled 0. 2-cm cuvet that is compatible with the Bio-Rad electroporator. Set up controls with 1 ng of vector DNA to evaluate the competence of TG1 cells.
3. Set up Bio-Rad electroporator for a 2. 5-kV pulse, with a 25-µF capacitor and the pulse controller set to 200 Ω.
4. Dry cuvet with tissue and place in the electroporation chamber.
5. Pulse once. The registered time constant should be 4.5–5.0.
6. Immediately add 1 mL fresh 2X TY 1% glucose, resuspend cells and transfer to a disposable culture tube.
7. Incubate with shaking at 37°C for 1 h to allow cells to recover and to express antibiotic resistance.
8. Plate appropriate dilutions (in 2X TY) on 90-mm TYE + antibiotic plates for the titration of the library. Plate the entire library on 243 × 243 mm (Nunc) TYE + antibiotic plates.
9. Grow overnight at 30°C.
10. Harvest repertoire by flooding plates with 2–10 mL 2X TY and detaching cells with a sterile scraper. Transfer cells to sterile polypropylene tube and disperse clumps using a vortex.

3.2.3. Phage Production

1. Titrate the rescue.
2. Inoculate a 2-L conical flask containing 500 mL of 2X TY and 12. 5 mg/mL tetracycline with an amount of bacteria representing at least 10× the number of the colonies you obtain to be sure to have the possibility to grow all the clones you rescued.
3. Grow at 30°C for 16–24 h.
4. Store remaining culture at –70°C.
5. Centrifuge overnight culture at 10,800g for 10 min or at 3300g for 30 min.
6. Add PEG/NaCl to supernatant at 1:5 (vol/vol); mix well and incubate at 4°C for 1 h or more.
7. Centrifuge at 10,800g for 10 min or 3300g for 30 min and carefully aspirate supernatant.

8. Resuspend in 10 mL of PBS and add 2.5 mL of PEG/NaCl. Mix and incubate at 4°C for 20 min or more.
9. Spin again briefly and aspirate any remaining trace of PEG/NaCl.
10. Resuspend in 2 mL of PBS and centrifuge at 11,600g for 10 min to remove most of the remaining bacterial debris.
11. Store phage at 4°C for short-term storage or in PBS and 15% glycerol for longer term storage at −70°C.
12. Titrate phage stock.

3.3. Cloning Murine Monoclonal Antibody V_LC_L Gene

This step allows cloning of the selected murine $V_L\ C_L$ gene into a plasmid vector, enabling secretion of the murine light chain into the bacterial periplasm (*see* **Note 3**).

3.3.1. PCR Amplification of Murine V_LC_L Gene

1. Set up the following PCR reaction: 50 ng cDNA X µL, 5 mM dNTP 5 µL, 10 pM BACK primer 2. 5 µL, 10 pM FOR primer 2. 5 µL, 10X *Taq* buffer 5 µL, *Taq* DNA polymerase (5 U/mL) 1 µL, H_2O to 50 µL.
2. Amplify by PCR using 30 cycles at 94°C for 1 min, 55°C for 1 min, 72°C for 2 min followed by incubation at 72°C for 10 min.

3.3.2. Ligation Protocol

1. Set up the following ligation reaction: Vector DNA (50 ng) X µL, digested fragment (150 ng) X µL, 10X ligase buffer 2 µL, H_2O to 19 µL.
2. Mix and spin briefly in a microfuge.
3. Add 1 µL of T4 DNA ligase (400 U/µL).
4. Incubate at overnight 16°C.

3.3.3. Transformation of E. coli with V_LC_L Gene

Transformation is performed by electroporation of ligation reactions using the Bio-Rad Gene Pulser Plus as described above.

3.4. Preparation of Half-Human Library

A half-human library is obtained by infection of *E. coli* containing the plasmid with murine guiding chain (V_LC_L) with phage containing the V_HC_H1 human repertoire.

Since the heavy chains, fused at their C-terminus to pIII, associate spontaneously in the periplasmic space to light chain, the resulting phage particles display hybrid Fab fragments (human V_HC_H-murine V_LC_L) on their surface (**Fig. 1A**) *(13)*.

1. Prepare 10 mL of log-phase E. coli TG1 bearing the VLCL plasmid and 1012 TU of phage from the VH library; incubate for 30 min at 37°C without shaking.
2. Use 0.5 mL to make serial dilutions in 2X TY broth; plate 100 mL of the dilutions (from 10-4 to 10-8) on TYE Amp-Tet 1% glu plates to determine the titer of the library.
3. Centrifuge the remaining 9.5 mL at 3300g for 10 min and resuspend the pellet in about 0. 6 mL of 2X TY.
4. Plate the resuspended pellet in a 243 × 243-mm plate containing TYE-Amp-Tet1% glu.
5. Grow overnight at 30°C.

6. Rescue bacteria with a sterile scraper; the next day, inoculate 500 mL of 2X TY Amp-Tet for phage production using a number of bacteria representing at least 10 times more than the number of colonies scraped; grow overnight at 30°C with shaking.

3.5. First Selection by Panning on Monolayer Cultures of Carcinoma Cells

The hybrid murine/human Fab-phage repertoire is selected by panning on a monolayer of cells overexpressing the target antigen. Phage that bind to the cells are used to directly infect bacteria cells containing the light chain, and bacteria are grown to produce more Fab-phage. After 3–6 rounds of positive selection, at least one human $V_H C_H 1$ should be identifiable and, in combination with the original murine light chain used as the guide probe, can bind to the target antigen (*see* **Note 4**).

3.5.1. Preparation of Cells (see **Note 5**)

1. Select the most appropriate carcinoma cells expressing the target antigen. Routinely confirm cell surface expression of the antigen by FACS analysis.
2. Maintain cultures in complete culture medium in a humidified 5% CO_2 atmosphere at 37°C and recover cells by detachment with trypsin-EDTA.
3. For panning purposes, seed cells in 100-mm cell culture Petri dishes at a concentration of 4×10^5/mL (depending on cell size and growth rate) and grow as monolayers (80% confluent).
4. For phage-ELISA selection, seed $1–3 \times 10^5$ cells in 200 µL in 96-well flat-bottom and grow as monolayers.
5. If necessary, fix cells with glutaraldehyde.

3.5.2. Panning on Cell Monolayers (see **Note 6**)

1. Incubate cells in 20 mL of 2% MPBS for 2 h at 37°C to block any remaining unsaturated binding sites on the plastic.
2. Aspirate MPBS.
3. Add ~10^{12} t. u. of phage library displaying hybrid Fab fragments in 10 mL of 2% MPBS; shake slowly at room temperature for 1 h.
4. Wash 5× with 10 mL of 0. 1% Tween-20/PBS and then 10× with 10 mL of PBS alone. In each washing step, gently add the buffer, briefly swirl in the plate, and immediately remove (*see* **Note 7**).

3.5.3. Infection with Bound Phage (see **Note 8**)

All rescues should be checked for the presence of insert (by PCR), and the number of positive clones should scored.

1. Prepare 10 mL of log-phase *E. coli* TG1 bearing the $V_L C_L$ plasmid and add it directly to the tumor cells used for panning.
2. Incubate for 30 min at 37°C without shaking.
3. Use 0. 5 mL to make serial dilutions in 2X TY broth; plate 100 µL of the dilutions (from 10^{-4} to 10^{-8}) on TYE-Amp-Tet 1% glu plates to determine the titer of rescue.
4. Centrifuge the remaining 9.5 mL at 3300g for 10 min and resuspend the pellet in 0. 6 mL of 2X TY.

5. Plate the resuspended pellet in a 243 × 243-mm plate containing TYE-Amp-Tet 1% glu.
6. Grow overnight at 30°C.
7. Rescue bacteria with a sterile scraper and monitor the extent of enrichment.

3.5.4. Phage Production

Perform as in **Subheading 3.2.3.** and after every round of infection:

1. Check phage titer and phage binding by polyclonal phage-ELISA (*see* **Subheading 3.6.1.**).
2. Repeat the panning until a positive signal is detected.
3. Grow single colonies in a 96-well plate to isolate single positive clones.

3.6. Screening by Phage ELISA and FACS Analysis

3.6.1. Single-Clone ELISA

1. Pick individual colonies with a sterile toothpick. Place the toothpick into 200 μL of 2X TY broth with the appropriate antibiotic in a 96-well plate and grow with shaking (300 rpm) at 30°C until culture saturation (10^{10} t. u phage/mL), generally reached in 16–20 h (*see* **Note 9**).
2. Centrifuge the 96-well plate with growing bacteria at 3300g for 10 min.
3. Test the single clone on ELISA plates containing monolayers of cells overexpressing the antigen of interest and on other plates containing antigen-negative cells.
4. Rinse ELISA plates 3× with PBS and block unsaturated sites on the plastic by adding 200 μL of 2% MPBS to each well; incubate at 37°C for 2 h.
5. Remove the 2% MPBS by aspiration and add 25 μL of 10% MPBS to each well.
6. Using a multichannel pipet, transfer 80 ml of bacterial culture supernatant from **step 2** above to the ELISA plate, mix, and leave at room temperature for 1 h.
7. Wash wells 3× with 0. 1% Tween-20/PBS and then 3× with PBS.
8. Add 100 μL of HRP-anti-M13 conjugated antibody (1:5000 dilution) to each well.
9. Wash wells 3× with 0. 1% Tween-20/PBS and then 3× with PBS.
10. Add 100 μL of TMB to each well and leave at room temperature for 10–20 min.
11. Block the reaction with 1 *M* H_2SO_4 and read absorbance at 450 nm in an ELISA multichannel reader.

3.6.2. FACS Analysis

1. For each sample, add 100 μL of PBS+1% of BSA containing ~5 × 10^9 antibody-bearing phage particles to a pellet of 3 × 10^5 cells overexpressing the antigen of interest and to other negative cells; incubate at room temperature for 1 h.
2. Wash 3× with PBS.
3. Add 100 μL of sheep anti-M13 antibody (1:5000 dilution) and incubate on ice for 30 min.
4. Wash 3× with PBS.
5. Add 100 μL of FITC-conjugated anti-sheep antibody (1:1000 dilution) and incubate on ice for 30 min.
6. Wash 3× with PBS.
7. Analyze cells with a FAC scan.

3.7. Selection of the Human Light Chain

To obtain a completely human Fab, the selected V_HC_H1 is amplified and inserted into the phagemid display vector containing precloned repertoires of human kappa and human lambda light-chain genes (**Fig. 1B**). The resulting human Fab phagemid repertoire is rescued by infection with helper phage and the phagemid particles are again selected on cell monolayers (*see* **Note 10**).

3.7.1. Cloning

1. Amplify the $V_H C_H 1$ using primers Fdseq and G3LASCGTGBACK (the latter encodes a synthetic ribosome binding site and an *Asc*I cloning site) (*see* **Table 1**).
2. Purify the fragment from a 1.5% LMP gel.
3. Set up the following ligation reactions, using as vector an equimolar mixture of phagemid containing a precloned repertoire of human κ chain and phagemid containing a precloned repertoire of human λ chain: digested vector DNA (6 µg) X µL, digested fragment (5 µg) X µL, 10X ligase buffer 10 µL, H_2O to 95 µL.
4. Mix and spin briefly in a microfuge.
5. Add 5 µL T4 DNA ligase (400 U/µL).
6. Incubate overnight at 16°C.

3.7.2. Transformation

Perform exactly as described for the V_H repertoire in **Subheading 3.3.3.**

3.7.3. Rescue of Phage with Helper Phage

1. After 24 h add 5 mL of 2X TY to the square plates and loosen cells with a glass spreader; prepare glycerol stock as backup.
2. Add 100–500 µL (the inoculum should contain at least 10× the number of cells relative to the total library size to ensure that the diversity is not reduced) to 50 mL of 2X TY, containing 100 µg/mL ampicillin, 1% glucose and grow at 37°C to an OD_{600} of ~0. 5.
3. Add helper phage (e.g., M13 KO7, VCS-M13) and incubate at 37°C for 30 min without shaking and then for 30 min with shaking.
4. Centrifuge for 10 min at 3500 rpm and resuspend cells in 50 mL of 2X TY containing 100 µg/mL ampicillin and 50 µg/mL kanamycin but no glucose.
5. Incubate overnight at 30°C.
6. Centrifuge culture at 6000 rpm for 15 min.
7. Transfer supernatant to a fresh tube and add PEG/NaCl at 1:5 (vol:vol); mix well and incubate on ice for 1 h.
8. Centrifuge at 6000 rpm for 15 min. Discard supernatant and resuspend phage pellet in 1 mL of PBS.
9. Centrifuge at 13,000 rpm for 2 min to remove residual bacteria.
10. Transfer supernatant to a fresh tube and use X µL of phage for the next round of selection (the amount of phages used should be at least 10× the number of cells relative to the total library size to ensure that the diversity is not reduced).
11. Perform 3–4 rounds to enrich positive phage.
12. Analyze phage for enrichment by polyclonal phage-ELISA.

3.8. Characterization of Human Fab

The characterization of human Fab binders involves the sequencing and the biological/biochemical analysis of the selected Fab(s). Refer to **ref. 5** for detailed of the methods.

3.9. Conclusion

Selection of human antibodies from phage display libraries has given rise to Fab fragments. The relatively small size of these molecules makes them suitable for targeting radioisotopes in radioimmunolocalization and radioimmunotherapeutic approaches (*see* references in **Table 1**). Moreover, such molecules may serve as useful building blocks for the synthesis and engineering of different fusion proteins for therapeutic use *(14)* and may even be converted into fully human MAbs of each isotype *(15)*. A potential limitation of the method described for selection of human anti-tumor reagents is a loss in affinity, as we and others have observed *(5)* *(10)*. Such lower affinity of human antibodies might reflect the lack of precise homolog to the mouse templates in the human repertoire. However the availability of selected V genes in versatile and convenient phage vectors enables the use of powerful strategies, such as in vitro mutagenesis *(16,17)* and growth in bacterial mutator strains *(18)*, to improve affinity.

4. Notes

1. Human antibody repertoires can be amplified using human PBL as starting material. Most of the antigens listed in **Table 1** are self-antigens, so that very few natural antibodies are likely to be present in naïve repertoires. In cancer patients, tolerance is frequently broken, even if the level of specific antibody response is low and not sufficient to control the tumor.

2. For optimum transformation efficiency, purify the ligation reaction as follows: dilute the ligation mixture with 250 µL H_2O, extract the reaction once with P/C/I, once with C/I and precipitate with ethanol (−70°C for 15 min) in the presence of sodium acetate and 20 µg of glycogen. This greatly improves the recovery of precipitated ligation product.

3. Before proceeding to V_LC_L cloning, it is advisable to check whether the V_H alone is sufficient to determine the binding specificity to the target antigen, as reported for some MAb *(19)*, and to construct scFv from the hybridoma to ensure the identification of functional V_L (hybridomas frequently express mRNAs encoding abortive regions that can be amplified during PCR).

4. The repertoire must to be subjected to separate rounds of selection and infection to enrich the population for antigen binders. The first panning round is the most critical, because selection for any abnormalities or mistakes at this point will be amplified during further panning. Starting with 10^{12} phage, the first round of selection should yield at least 10^4 phage. Usually, the selection and reinfection must be carried out 2–3× to obtain a positive signal in polyclonal ELISA. If no enrichment is obtained after 4–6 pannings, change the conditions of panning (temperature, incubation time, fixation of cells), use an alternative cell line if possible, and/or carry out a new selection from the beginning.

5. When applicable parameters such as antigen expression level, local density of antigen, and local environment that controls antigen/determinant accessibility should be optimized or at least considered for their potential relevance in determining the final outcome of selection. When soluble antigen is available for selection, panning can be performed on immobilized or biotinylated antigens; several human reagents against antigens of nontumor or tumor origin have been successfully selected. However, as recently noted in a study specifically aimed at defining the parameters that determine the success of phage antibody selection on complex antigens, selection on intact cells sometimes compares favorably to selection on purified antigen *(20)*.

6. Stringency conditions should be fine-tuned according to the biology of the target antigen. Use low stringency (selecting cells with high antigen density and minimize the number and duration of washes), in the initial rounds of selection so as not to lose rare binders; use more stringent conditions in later rounds.

7. For cells growing in suspension, each wash step can be done using centrifugation (select speed to balance the risk of cell loss due to flotation vs cell damage due to squashing). Alternatively, attach cells to the plastic by polylysine.

8. Infection of bound phages by direct addition of the *E. coli* strain containing the V_LC_L to the cells generally leads to an increased number of rescued phage without an increase in background. Alternatively, bound phages can be eluted from the with 100 mM triethylamine or 50 mM glycine-HCl, pH 2.7, and 150 mM NaCl.

9. Since aeration is very important at this stage of growth, yields can be increased by placing the 96-well plate in a box without a lid.

10. In the procedure described, the light chain of a murine MAb was used to guide heavy chain pairings from a repertoire of human heavy chains; however either heavy or light chain can be used. In the case of selection of rare binders from naïve libraries, it was recently reported that even selection guided by one of the two chains is not sufficient to retrieve specific binding clones, and sequential shuffling of each chain was suggested in order to make full use of each chain repertoire *(21)*.

Acknowledgments

Partially supported by AIRC/FIRC. We thank A. Cipollina for editing the manuscript.

References

1. Glennie, M. J. and Johnson, P. W. (2000) Clinical trials of antibody therapy. *Immunol. Today* **21,** 403–410.
2. Clark, M. (2000) Antibody humanization: a case of the 'Emperor's new clothes'? *Immunol. Today* **21,** 397–402.
3. Cai, X. and Garen, A. (1995) Anti-melanoma antibodies from melanoma patients immunized with genetically modified autologous tumor cells: Selection of specific antibodies from single-chain Fv fusion phage libraries. *Proc. Natl. Acad. Sci. USA* **92,** 6537–6541.
4. Siegel, D. L., Chang, T. Y., Russell, S. L., and Bunya, V. Y. (1997) Isolation of cell surface-specific human monoclonal antibodies using phage display and magnetically-activated cell sorting: applications in immunohematology. *J. Immunol. Methods* **206,** 73–85.
5. Figini, M., Obici, L., Mezzanzanica, D., Griffiths, A. D., Colnaghi, M. I., Winter, G., and Canevari, S. (1998) Panning phage antibody libraries on cells: isolation of human Fab fragments against ovarian carcinoma using guided selection. *Cancer Res.* **58,** 991–996.
6. Noronha, E. J., Wang, X., Desai, S. A., Kageshita, T., and Ferrone, S. (1998) Limited diversity of human scFv fragments isolated by panning a synthetic phage-display scFv library with cultured human melanoma cells. *J. Immunol.* **161,** 2968–2976.
7. Yip, Y. L., Hawkins, N. J., Smith, G., and Ward, R. L. (1999) Biodistribution of filamentous phage-Fab in nude mice. *J. Immunol. Methods* **225,** 171–178.
8. Figini, M., Marks, J. D., Winter, G., and Griffiths, A. D. (1994) In vitro assembly of repertoires of antibody chains on the surface of phage by renaturation. *J. Mol. Biol.* **239,** 68–78.
9. Jespers, L. S., Roberts, A., Mahler, S. M., Winter, G., and Hoogenboom, H. R. (1994) Guiding the selection of human antibodies from phage display repertoires to a single epitope of an antigen. *BioTechnology* **12,** 899–903.

10. Klimka, A., Matthey, B., Roovers, R. C., Barth, S., Arends, J. W., Engert, A., and Hoogenboom, H. R. (2000) Human anti-CD30 recombinant antibodies by guided phage antibody selection using cell panning. *Br. J. Cancer* **83,** 252–260.

11. Marks, J. D., Hoogenboom, H. R., Bonnert, T. P., McCafferty, J., Griffiths, A. D., and Winter, G. (1991) By-passing immunization: human antibodies from V-gene libraries displayed on phage. *J. Mol. Biol.* **222,** 581–197.

12. Griffiths, A. D., Williams, S. C., and Hartley, O. (1994) Isolation of high affinity human antibodies directly from large synthetic repertoires. *EMBO J.* **13,** 3245–3260.

13. Hoogenboom, H. R., Griffiths, A. D., Johnson, K. S., Chiswell, D. J., Hudson, P., and Winter, G. (1991) Multi-subunit proteins on the surface of filamentous phage: methodologies for displaying antibody (Fab) heavy and light chains. *Nucleic Acids Res.* **19,** 4133–4137.

14. Winter, G. and Milstein, C. (1991) Man-made antibodies. *Nature* **349,** 293–299.

15. Boel, E., Verlaan, S., Poppelier, M. J., Westerdaal, N. A., Van Strijp, J. A., and Logtenberg, T. (2000) Functional human monoclonal antibodies of all isotypes constructed from phage display library-derived single-chain Fv antibody fragments. *J. Immunol. Methods* **239,** 153–166.

16. Hawkins, R. E., Russell, S. J., and Winter, G. (1992) Selection of phage antibodies by binding affinity: mimicking affinity maturation. *J. Mol. Biol.* **226,** 889–896.

17. Chowdhury, P. S. and Pastan, I. (1999) Improving antibody affinity by mimicking somatic hypermutation in vitro. *Nature Biotechnol.* **17,** 568–572.

18. Low, N., Holliger, P., and Winter, G. (1996) Mimicking somatic hypermutation: affinity maturation of antibodies displayed on bacteriophage using a bacterial mutator strain. *J. Mol. Biol.* **260,** 359–368.

19. Ward, E. S., Gussow, D. H., Griffiths, A. D., Jones, P. T., and Winter, G. (1989) Binding activities of a repertoire of single immunoglobulin variable domains secreted for *Escherichia coli. Nature* **341,** 544–546.

20. Mutuberria, R., Hoogenboom, H. R., van der Linden, E., de Bruine, A. P., and Roovers, R. C. (1999) Model systems to study the parameters determining the success of phage antibody selections on complex antigens. *J. Immunol. Methods* **231,** 65–81.

21. Wang, Z., Wang, Y., Li, Z., Li, J., and Dong, Z. (2000) Humanization of a mouse monoclonal antibody neutralizing TNF-alpha by guided selection. *J. Immunol. Methods* **241,** 171–184.

22. Crippa, F., Bolis, G., Seregni, E., Gavoni, N., Bombardieri, E., Scarfone, G., et al. (1995) Single dose intraperitoneal radioimmunotherapy with the murine monoclonal antibody 131I-MOv18: clinical results in patients with minimal residual disease of ovarian cancer. *Eur. J. Cancer* **31A,** 686–690.

23. Canevari, S., Stoter, G., Arienti, F., Bolis, G., Colnaghi, M. I., Di Re, E., et al. (1995) Regression of advanced ovarian carcinoma by intraperitoneal treatment with autologous T-lymphocytes retargeted by a bispecific monoclonal antibody. *J. Natl. Cancer Inst.* **87,** 1463–1469.

24. van Zanten-Przybysz, I., Molthoff, C. F., Roos, J. C., Plaizier, M. A., Visser, G. W., Pijpers, R., et al. (2000) Radioimmunotherapy with intravenously administered 131I-labeled chimeric monoclonal antibody MOv18 in patients with ovarian cancer. *J. Nucl. Med.* **41,** 1168–1176.

25. Madiyalakan, R., Yang, R., Schultes, B. C., Baum, R. P., and Noujaim, A. A. (1997) OVAREX MAb-B43. 13:IFN-gamma could improve the ovarian tumor cell sensitivity to CA125-specific allogenic cytotoxic T cells. *Hybridoma* **16,** 41–45.

26. Mahe, M. A., Fumoleau, P., Fabbro, M., Guastalla, J. P., Faurous, P., Chauvot, P., et al. (1999) A phase II study of intraperitoneal radioimmunotherapy with iodine-131-labeled monoclonal antibody OC-125 in patients with residual ovarian carcinoma. *Clin. Cancer Res.* **5,** 3249S–3253S.

27. Burris, H. A. (2000) Docetaxel (Taxotere) in HER-2-positive patients and in combination with trastuzumab (Herceptin). *Semin. Oncol.* **27,** 19–23.

28. Hird, V., Maraveyas, A., Snook, D., Dhokia, B., Soutter, W. P., Meares, C., et al. (1993) Adjuvant therapy of ovarian cancer with radioactive monoclonal antibody. *Br. J. Cancer* **68,** 403–406.

29. Prinssen, H. M., Molthoff, C. F., Verheijen, R. H., Broadhead, T. J., Kenemans, P., Roos, J. C., et al. (1998) Biodistribution of 111In-labelled engineered human antibody CTM01 (hCTM01) in ovarian cancer patients: influence of prior administration of unlabelled hCTM01. *Cancer. Immunol. Immunother.* **47,** 39–46.

30. Juweid, M., Sharkey, R. M., and Alavi, A. (1997) Regression of advanced refractory ovarian cancer treated with 131I-labeled anti-CEA monoclonal antibody. *J. Nucl. Med.* **38,** 257–260.

31. Juweid, M., Swayne, L. C., Sharkey, R. M., Dunn, R., Rubin, A. D., Herskovic, T., and Goldenberg, D. M. (1997) Prospects of radioimmunotherapy in epithelial ovarian cancer: results with iodine-131-labeled murine and humanized MN-14 anti- carcinoembryonic antigen monoclonal antibodies. *Gynecol. Oncol.* **67,** 259–271.

32. Rosenblum, M. G., Verschraegen, C. F., Murray, J. L., Kudelka, A. P., Gano, J., Cheung, L., and Kavanagh, J. J. (1999) Phase I study of 90Y-labeled B72. 3 intraperitoneal administration in patients with ovarian cancer: effect of dose and EDTA coadministration on pharmacokinetics and toxicity. *Clin. Cancer Res.* **5,** 953–961.

33. Alvarez, R. D., Partridge, E. E., Khazaeli, M. B., Plott, G., Austin, M., Kilgore, L., et al. (1997) and Meredith, R. F., Intraperitoneal radioimmunotherapy of ovarian cancer with 177Lu-CC49: a phase I/II study. *Gynecol. Oncol.* **65,** 94–101.

10

Human Recombinant Fab Antibodies with T-Cell Receptor-Like Specificities Generated from Phage Display Libraries

Jan Engberg, Ali F. Yenidunya,
Rikke Clausen, Liselotte B. Jensen,
Peter Sørensen, Pernille Kops, and Erik Riise

1. Introduction

In this chapter we describe efficient procedures for the construction, expression and screening of comprehensive libraries of human Fab antibody fragments displayed on the surface of filamentous phage. Phagemid vectors are used for placing randomly paired light (L) and heavy (H) chain coding regions under transcriptional control of P*lac*. The H chain coding region is fused in-frame with the phage gene, *ΔgIII*, coding for a truncated version of the phage surface protein pIII (ΔpIII). After superinfection with helper phage and induction of P*lac*, Fd (composed of V_H and C_H1 domains) and κ- or λ- L chains assemble into Fab fragments in the periplasm of the *Escherichia coli* host strain, and the Fab-ΔpIII protein complex is displayed at one end of the phage by displacing one (or more) of the wild-type pIII proteins. Enrichment of Fab phages with affinity for a selected "antigen" is then carried out by successive rounds of affinity purification using "antigen"-coated immunotubes or plastic beads followed by reinfection of *E. coli* cells with the eluted bound phages (*see* **refs. *1–10***). An outline of the method is illustrated in **Fig. 1**.

Using this technology, we have generated antibodies with a large range of different specificities including such that have specificities similar to that of T cell receptors, that is, antibodies that recognize MHC/peptide complexes in a peptide specific and MHC-restricted manner *(11,12)*. Furthermore, this type of antibodies have been used for specific targeting of toxin to antigen presenting cells and we have observed peptide specific cell killing *(13)* which suggests novel approaches for immunotherapeutic settings *(14)*. Here we present protocols for generating human Fab libraries of the IgG isotype and their use in search for binders recognizing MHC/peptide complexes in a

From: *Methods in Molecular Biology, vol. 207: Recombinant Antibodies for Cancer Therapy: Methods and Protocols*
Edited by: M. Welschof and J. Krauss © Humana Press Inc., Totowa, NJ

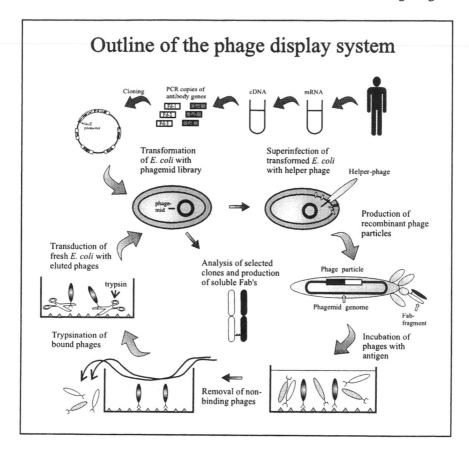

Fig. 1. Overview of the steps involved in the generation of human antibody Fab libraries. Messenger RNA is isolated from peripheral blood of donors and copied into cDNA. This material is then used as template for PCR amplification of immunoglobulin gene fragments, which in turn are cloned and expressed as functional Fab molecules in fusion with a phage surface protein (pIII) as mentioned in the text. The entire mixture of phage-displayed Fab molecules are then submitted to affinity purification methods to obtain specific binders to a selected "antigen."

peptide specific manner. Protocols for generating a selected MHC/peptide complex are also described, but it should be noted that such protocols vary depending on the individual nature of the MHC molecule in question.

The present protocols for phage display human Fab libraries describe the cloning of κ (or λ) and VH DNA in two steps into a specially developed vector that already contains human CH1γ1 fused to ΔgIII. Following the cloning in a bacterial expression vector, the relevant sequences encoding the Fab region can be transferred to a mammalian expression vector and transfected into mammalian cells for expression of correctly processed antibodies of full size.

2. Materials

2.1. Isolation of Lymphocytes, Preparation of Total RNA, cDNA, and Cloning in pFAB74H.TT

1. Anticoagulant buffer (ACD from Baxter Health Care Ltd., Thetford, UK).
2. Lymphoprep from Nycomed Pharma A/S (Oslo, Norway).
3. Commercial kits for total RNA preparation and cDNA synthesis.
4. AmpliTaq Gold polymerase, 10X Taq buffers I and II (Perkin-Elmer Cetus, Norwalk, CT).
5. Qiagen DNA purification columns (Qiagen GmbH, Hilden, Germany).
6. Restriction enzymes *Sfi*I, *Asc*I, *Nhe*I, *Mlu*I, *Eag*I, and *Not*I (New England Biolabs, Beverly, MA).
7. Endonuclease buffers: 10X NEB2, 3, and 4 (New England Biolabs).100X BSA (New England Biolabs).
8. T4 DNA ligase (1 U/µL) and 5X T4 ligase buffer (Gibco-BRL).
9. Glycogen (20 mg/mL from Boehringer Mannheim).
10. The phagemid vector pFAB74H.TT is depicted in **Fig. 2B**.
11. LB (per liter: 10 g Tryptone, 5 g yeast extract and 5 g NaCl); 2X YT (per liter: 16 g Tryptone, 10 g yeast extract [Gibco] and 5 g NaCl); SOC media (per liter: 20 g Bacto-Tryptone, 5 g yeast extract, 0.5 g NaCl, and 0.19 g KCl). TE buffer (10 m*M* Tris-HCl, pH 8.0; 1 m*M* EDTA). These solutions are prepared as described in **ref. 15**.
12. Antibiotics: ampicillin is used at a concentration of 50 µg/mL and tetracycline at 10 µg/mL.
13. *E. coli* strains: TOP10F': *mcrA*, Δ(*mrr-hsdRMS-mcrBC*), θ80, *lacZΔM15*, Δ*lacX74*, *deoR*, *recA1*, *araD139*, Δ(*ara-leu*)7697, *galU*, *galK*, *rpsL*(StrR), *endA1*, *nupG*, F'(*lacIq Tn10* [TetR]) (Invitrogen). TG1: F' (*traD36,lacIq,*Δ[*lacZ*]*M15, proA+B+*)/Δ(*lac-proAB*), *thi-1*, *supE*, Δ(*hsdM-mcrB5*(rk⁻, mk⁺, *McrB⁻*).

2.2. PCR-Primers for Cloning in pFab74H.TT

The direct cloning method for making human antibody Fab libraries involves five steps as described in **Subheading 3.2.** For illustrative purposes, the principal components involved in these steps are shown in **Fig. 2A**.

1. Human H-chain V-Region Back Primers. The aggregate concentration of all PCR primer mixes is 20 m*M*.

   HVH-1: CAG CCA GCA ATG GCA **CAG GTN CAG CTG GTR CAG TCT GG**
   HVH-2: CAG CCA GCA ATG GCA **CAG GTC CAG CTK GTR CAG TCT GGG G**
   HVH-3: CAG CCA GCA ATG GCA **CAG GTK CAG CTG GTG SAG TCT GGG**
   HVH-4: CAG CCA GCA ATG GCA **CAG GTC ACC TTG ARG GAG TCT GGT CC**
   HVH-5: CAG CCA GCA ATG GCA **CAG GTG CAG CTG GTG GAG WCT GG**
   HVH-6: CAG CCA GCA ATG GCA **CAG GTG CAG CTG GTG SAG TCY GG**
   HVH-7: CAG CCA GCA ATG GCA **CAG GTG CAG CTG CAG GAG TCG G**
   HVH-8: CAG CCA GCA ATG GCA **CAG GTG CAG CTG TTG SAG TCT G**
   HVH-9: CAG CCA GCA ATG GCA **CAG GTG CAG CTG GTG CAA TCT G**
   HVH-10: CAG CCA GCA ATG GCA **CAG GTG CAG CTG CAG GAG TCC GG**
   HVH-11: CAG CCA GCA ATG GCA **CAG GTG CAG CTA CAG CAG TGG G**
   HVH-12: CAG CCA GCA ATG GCA **CAG GTA CAG CTG CAG CAG TCA G**

A   **B**

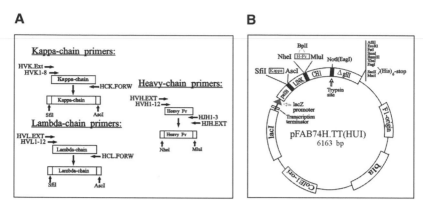

Fig. 2. (**A**) Overview of the PCR primers involved in the cloning of human light chain gene and the heavy Fv fragments. Primers depicted below boxes are forward primers and complementary to mRNA. Primers above boxes are complementary to first-strand cDNA. (**B**) Map of the expression vector pFab74H.TT. This vector contains several improvements to the pFab73H vector described by us previously *(9)*. In the polylinker region downstream of Δg*III*, an adaptor was introduced that contained an *Eag*I site followed by six histidine codons and a stop codon. This makes it possible to delete Δg*III* by digestion with *Eag*I, (*Eag*I recognizes a subset of the *Not*I recognition sequence present upstream of Δg*III*) and religation, which also regenerates a *Not*I site. Additionally, (CAT)$_6$TGA is in reading frame with C$_K$, and the (His)$_6$ tail facilitates easy purification of free Fab molecules on metal affinity columns. Finally a transcription terminator region *(16)* was introduced in front of the *LacZ* promoter to reduce read-through transcription of the Fab encoding regions. The depicted vector has stuffer fragments inserted between cloning sites for H- and L-chain gene fragments.

Symbol	Meaning	Symbol	Meaning
A	Adenine	W	A or T/U
C	Cytosine	S	C or G
G	Guanine	K	G or T/U
T	Thymine	D	A, G or T/U
U	Uracil	H	A, C or T/U
R	puRine(A or G)	V	A, C or G
Y	pYrimidine(C or T/U)	B	C, G or T/U
M	A or C	N	A, C, G or T/U

(The one-letter nucleotide symbols are used according to IUB nomenclature).

These primers consist of 12 individually synthesized oligonucleotides representing 31 variants. The nucleotides in bold correspond to the 5'-sequences of the V$_H$ region starting with the codon for amino acid number one. Primers are invariant for the first five nucleotides from position +1 of the V region. The first 15 nucleotides at the 5'-end of the primers correspond to the 3'-part of the *pel*B leader. This gives a unique template for HVH.Ext, used in the extension PCR (*see* **step 6**). The concentration of each variant in the solution used for PCR is 0.65 pmol/µL.

2. Human H-Chain J-Region Forward Primers.

HJH1: GGC TGA GGA GAC RGT GAC CAG GGT

HJH2: GGC TGA AGA GAC GGT GAC CAT TGT

HJH3: GGC TGA GGA GAC GGT GAC CGT GGT

The J-region primers consist of three individually synthesized oligonucleotides representing a total of 4 variants. All nucleotides are complementary to the J-region and the first codon at the 5'-end corresponds to amino acid residue 114 of C_H1 acc. to the Kabat nomenclature. The concentration of each variant in the mixture used for PCR is 5 pmol/µL.

3. Human H-Chain Extension Primers.

HVH.Ext:GCA GCC GCT GGA TTG TTA TTG <u>CTA GC</u>A GCA **CAG CCA GCA ATG GCA CAG GT**

HJH.Ext.*MluI*:GCG AAT TGG GCC <u>ACG CGT</u> GGA **GGC TGA RGA GAC RGT GAC C**

Nucleotides in HVH.Ext corresponding to sequences in HVH1-12 are in bold, and the *Nhe*I site is underlined. Nucleotides in HJH.Ext corresponding to sequences in HJH1-3 are in bold, and the *Mlu*I site is underlined. The concentration of each variant in the HJH.Ext mixture used for PCR is 5 pmol/µL.

4. Human κ-Chain V-Region Back Primers.

HVK-1: G CCG GCC ATG GCC **GAC ATC CAR WTG ACC CAG TCT CC**

HVK-2: G CCG GCC ATG GCC **GAC ATC CRG ATG ACC CAG TCT CCW TC**

HVK-3: G CCG GCC ATG GCC **GAC ATC GTG MTG ACC CAG TCT CC**

HVK-4: G CCG GCC ATG GCC **GAC ATC GTG TTG ACS CAG TCT CCR GG**

HVK-5: G CCG GCC ATG GCC **GAC ATC GTG ATG ACY CAG WCT CCA C**

HVK-6: G CCG GCC ATG GCC **GAC ATC GTG ATG AYR CAG TCT CCA GC**

HVK-7: G CCG GCC ATG GCC **GAC ATC GTG MTG ACW CAG TCT CCA GA**

HVK-8: G CCG GCC ATG GCC **GAC ATC GTA ATG ACA CAG TCT CCA CC**

These primers consist of eight individually synthesized oligonucleotides representing 27 variants. Nucleotides in bold correspond to the 5'-sequence of the V_κ gene starting with the codon for amino acid number one. The N-terminal two amino acids of the V region are invariant. The sequences upstream of the V region represent the 3'-part of the *pel*B leader gene (located between the *Asc*I and *Nhe*I sites). This constitutes a unique template for the primers used in the extension PCR (*see* **step 6** below). The concentration of each variant in the solution used for PCR is 0.74 pmol/µL.

5. Human $_\kappa$-Chain Constant-Region Forward Primer, HCK.For.

HCK.For: GTC TCC TTC TCG A<u>GG CGC GCC TCA CTA</u> **ACA CTC TCC CCT GTT GAA GCT**

HCK.For is complementary to codons for the seven carboxy-terminal amino acid residues of the C_κ domain, indicated by bold letters. The tandem stop codons and the *Asc*I site are underlined

6. Human$_\kappa$-Chain Extension Primers, HVK.Ext.

HVK.Ext: CA GTC ACA GAT CCT CGC GAA TTG <u>GCC CA</u>**G CCG GCC ATG GCC GAC ATC**

The boldfaced part of HVK.Ext overlaps with the 5'-end of the primary PCR primers. The *Sfi*I site introduced into the extended V_κ PCR products is underlined. HCK.For is used for both primary and secondary amplifications.

7. Human λ-Chain V-Region Back Primers.

HVL-1:   G CCG GCC ATG GCC **CAG TCT GYC CTG ACT CAG CCT G**

HVL-2:   G CCG GCC ATG GCC **CAG TCT GCC CTG ACT CAG CCT C**

HVL-3:   G CCG GCC ATG GCC **CAG TCT GTG CTG ACT CAG CCG TC**

HVL-4:   G CCG GCC ATG GCC **CAG TCT ATG CTG ACT CAG CCC CAC TC**

HVL-5:   G CCG GCC ATG GCC **CAG TCT GTG CTG ACT CAG CCA CCC TC**

HVL-6:   G CCG GCC ATG GCC **CAG TCT GAG CTG ACT CAG GAC CCT GC**

HVL-7:   G CCG GCC ATG GCC **CAG TCT GAG GTG ACT CAG GAG CC**

HVL-8:   G CCG GCC ATG GCC **CAG TCT GTG ATG ACY CAG TCT CMA**

HVL-9:   G CCG GCC ATG GCC **CAG TCT GTG CTG ACT CAG CCA CC**

HVL-10: G CCG GCC ATG GCC **CAG TCT GTS BTG ACG CAG CCG CC**

HVL-11: G CCG GCC ATG GCC **CAG TCT CAG CTG ACG CAG CCT GC**

HVL-12: G CCG GCC ATG GCC **CAG TCT TTA YTG ACT CAA YCG CCC TC**

These primers consist of 12 individually synthesized oligonucleotides representing 24 variants. Nucleotides in bold correspond to the 5'-sequences of the Vλ genes starting with the codon for amino acid number one. The remaining nucleotides are identical to the similarly positioned nucleotides in the κ primers. The concentration of each variant in the solution used for PCR is 0.83 pmol/μL.

8. Human λ-Chain Constant-Region Forward Primer, HCL.For.

HCL.For: GTC TCC TTC TCG A<u>GG CGC GCC TCA CTA</u> **TGA ACA TTC YGT AAG GGC MAC**

HCL.For contains four variants and is complementary to codons for the seven carboxy-terminal amino acid residues of the λ constant domain, indicated by bold letters. The tandem stop codons and the *Asc*I site are underlined. The concentration of each variant in the solution used for PCR is 5 pmol/μL.

9. Human λ-Chain Extension Primers, HVL.Ext.

HVL.Ext: CA GTC ACA GAT CCT CGC GAA TT<u>G GCC CA</u>G CCG GCC ATG GCC CAG TCT

The features of HVL.Ext are analogous to those of the κ-chain extension primer, HVK.Ext. HCL.For is used for both primary and secondary amplifications.

2.3. Preparation of Ultracompetent Cells

1. *E. coli* Pulser, 0.2- and 0.1 cm electroporation cuvets (Bio-Rad, Hercules, CA).
2. pUC18 DNA (Stratagene).
3. *E. coli* strains: TG1 or Top10F'.

2.4. Electroporation of Library DNA, Cell Growth, and Storage

1. Glycerol solution: 10% glycerol in water.
2. Nunclon Δ Square Dishes (500 cm^2) from NUNC (Roskilde, Denmark).

2.5. Production and Titration of Fab Phages from Libraries

1. Phage-precipitation buffer: 20% polyethylene glycol (PEG$_{6000}$), 2.5 M NaCl.
2. Helper phage R408 (Stratagene).
3. IPTG stock solution: 100 mM isopropyl-β-D-thiogalactopyranoside in sterile water.

2.6. Selection of Antigen Binders by Panning

1. Bovine serum albumin (BSA) from KEBO Lab (Denmark).
2. Washing buffer: 0.5% Tween 20 in PBS buffer.

3. Blocking buffer: 2% skimmed milk powder (Difco, Detroit, MI) in PBS buffer.
4. Trypsin elution buffer: 1 mg Trypsin (Worthington, Freehold, NJ)/mL PBS buffer.
5. Glycin elution buffer: 0.1 M glycin-HCl, pH 2.2, containing 1 mg/mL BSA.
6. Maxisorp microtiter plates and immunotubes (NUNC). Sulfated latex beads (diameter 5 μm from Interfacial Dynamics Corporation)
7. Peroxidase-conjugated anti-M13 (Pharmacia Biotech, Sollentuna, Sweden).

2.7. Generation of HLA-A2 in the Form of Inclusion Body Material

1. Glycerol stocks of BL21(DE3) cells transformed with recombinant plasmids containing relevant MHC sequences under transcriptional control of inducible T7 RNA polymerase expression (pET, pGEMEX, etc).
2. Superbroth-medium per liter: 32 g tryptone, 20 g yeast extract, 5 g NaCl, 5 mL 1 N NaOH. Add 100 μg/mL ampicillin, 12 mL/L magnesium sulphate (stock of 4%, sterile filtered) and 20 mL/L sucrose (stock of 20%, sterile-filtered).
3. TE50/20-buffer: 50 mM Tris-HCl, pH 7.4, 20 mM EDTA (autoclaved).
4. TE50/20-buffer + 1% Triton X-100 (made from TE50/20-buffer and 25% Triton X-100 stock soln.).
5. 25% Triton X-100 soln. in H$_2$O. Prepare in advance.
6. Lysozyme stock solution (5 mg/mL) in H$_2$O. Store at –20°C.
7. 100 mM IPTG in H$_2$O. Store at –20°C.
8. 5 M NaCl. Sterile-filter. Store in the cold.
9. Sorvall centrifuge with GSA and SS34 rotors and corresponding tubes.

2.8. Refolding of HLA-A2 with Peptide and Purification of Complex

1. Kit for measuring protein concentration (Pierce).
2. Refolding buffer: 0.1 M Tris-HCl, pH 8.0, 0.5 M L-arginine, 0.9 mM GSSG (gluthatione, oxidized), 2 mM EDTA, pH 8.0. pH must be 8.0–8.5. Chill buffer to 10°C in the cold room.
3. Minitan Acrylic Ultrafiltration System (Millipore).
4. Centricon Plus-20 Concentrator, Biomax-8 (Millipore).
5. Sephadex G-100 (Pharmacia).
6. NaN$_3$ stock solution (1%) in PBS buffer.
7. Reagents for silver staining of polyacrylamide gels *(15)*.

3. Methods

3.1. Extraction of Total RNA from Human Blood Lymphocytes and Preparation of cDNA

1. Lymphocyte isolation: Bleed 100 mL human blood into 14 mL anticoagulant (ACD) buffer, mix with an equal vol of PBS containing the same concentration of anticoagulant as the diluted blood, and layer on Lymphoprep placed in clear centrifuge tubes. Centrifuge at 400g for 30 min at room temperature. Collect the lymphocytes at the interphase between plasma and Lymphoprep, pellet cells by centrifugation at 800g for 10 min.
2. Isolation of total RNA and preparation of cDNA can be done as previously described *(10)* or by applying commercially available kits. The resulting cDNA is resuspended in sterile water at a concentration of 0.1 to 1 μg/μL.

3.2. Methods for PCR Amplification and Cloning

The direct cloning method for constructing human antibody Fab libraries consists of five steps:

1. Primary PCR amplifications of V_H H-chain and κ and λ L-chains (*see* **Note 1**).
2. "Tagging" the primary amplification products with restriction enzyme sites.
3. Separate cloning of κ and λ L-chain genes into the pFAB74H.TT vector.
4. Cloning of V_H gene fragments in pFAB74H.TT-Light chain libraries.
5. Electroporation, growth, and storage of the libraries (*see* **Subheading 3.4.**).

All PCR reactions (100 μL) are carried out in PCR tubes and covered with paraffin oil except when performed in PCR machines with hot-lids.

1. Primary amplifications of V_H gene fragments: 5 μL cDNA (*see* **Subheading 3.1.**, **step 2**), 10 μL 10X Buffer I, 10 μL 10X dNTP (2 mM each), 1 μL HVH1-12 (20 μM mix), 1 μL HJH1-3 (20 μM mix), 73 μL sterile water,
2. Primary amplification of κ genes: 5 μL cDNA (*see* **Subheading 3.1.**, **step 2**), 10 μL 10X Buffer I, 10 μL 10X dNTP (2 mM each), 1 μL HVK1-8 (20 mM mix), 1 μL HCK.For (20 mM), 73 μL sterile water.
3. Primary amplification of λ genes: 5 μL cDNA (*see* **Subheading 3.1.**, **step 2**), 10 μL 10X buffer I, 10 μL 10X dNTP (2 mM each), 1 μL HVL1-12 (20 mM mix), 1 μL HCL.For (20 mM), 73 μL sterile water.
4. PCR program: 94°C, 5 min, suspend, add 0.3 μL AmpliTaq Gold Polymerase (5 U/μL); 94°C, 1 min, 55°C, 1 min, 72°C, 1 min; 30 cycles, 72°C, 10 min, refrigerate.
5. Gel-purify the primary amplification products by standard agarose gel electrophoresis followed by Qiagen extraction of the relevant fragments. V_H gene fragments are about 430 bp and κ- and λ-gene fragments are about 700 bp.
6. For PCR extension of the primary PCR products, proceed as described above using about 1 ng purified template DNA and 1 μL of 20 μM solutions of the following primers:
   For V_H extension: HVH.Ext and HJH.Ext.*Mlu*I
   For κ extension: HVK.Ext and HCK.For
   For λ extension: HVL.Ext and HCL.For
   PCR program: 94°C, 5 min, suspend, add 0.3 μL AmpliTaq Gold polymerase (5 U/μL); 94°C, 1 min, 55°C, 1 min, 72°C, 1 min; 15 cycles, 72°C, 10 min, refrigerate.
7. Gel-purify the secondary amplification products as in **step 5** above. Extended V_H gene fragments are about 450 bp and extended κ and λ genes about 720 bp.
8. Digest the pFab74H.TT(HUI) vector and the extended κ and λ DNA with *Asc*I in NEB4, then with *Sfi*I in NEB2 + BSA at 50°C and gel-purify relevant fragments as in **step 5** above.
9. For ligation of insert to vector, mix in a microfuge tube and incubate overnight at 16°C: insert 6.0 μL DNA from **step 8** above (50 ng/μL), 6.0 μL vector DNA from **step 8** above (50 ng/μL), 10.0 μL 5 × T_4 ligase buffer, 25.5 μL sterile water, 2.5 μL T_4 DNA ligase (2.5 U).
10. Add 100 μL TE buffer to the ligation mixture and extract once with phenol/chloroform/isoamyl alcohol (25:24:1). Add 0.1 vol 3 M NaOAc, pH 5.2, and 1 μL glycogen (*see* **Note 2**), mix, precipitate with 2–2.5 vol ethanol, and, depending on DNA concentration, centrifuge for 10–30 min at 15,000g in a microfuge. Rinse pellet with 70% alcohol 3–4× to remove as much salt as possible, dry lightly in a SpeedVac centrifuge, and dissolve the DNA in water at a concentration of 10–20 ng/μL.

11. Proceed with **Subheading 3.4.** to produce the human κ and λ libraries. Make DNA maxi-preps of the two libraries.
12. Digest aliquots representing the pFAB74H.TT κ and λ libraries and the extended V_H DNA with *Mlu*I at 37°C, and then with *Nhe*I at 37°C and gel-purify as in **step 5** above.
13. Ligate and extract and precipitate the ligation products as described in **steps 9–10**, above. Proceed with **Subheading 3.4.** to produce the final human κ and λ Fab library (*see* **Note 3**).

3.3. Preparation of Ultracompetent Cells

High efficiency of electroporation is important for producing large libraries. Using cells prepared by the following protocol and taking heed of the stated precautions, we routinely obtain efficiencies of $2–6 \times 10^{10}$ colony-forming units (cfu)/µg supercoiled pUC18 test DNA (Stratagene) with Top10F' and TG1 cells. These strains give the highest efficiencies using 0.1 cm electroporation cuvets, 25 µL cells at a density of $5–6 \times 10^{10}$/mL, a field strength of 20 kV/cm, and amounts of DNA that give a time constant between 5.0 and 5.5 ms. (For other *E. coli* strains, electroporation conditions should be optimized by varying field strength and cell density. The optimal field strength for most strains is between 16 and 19 kV/cm *[17]*.)

1. Inoculate 1 L rich medium (LB or 2X YT) + tetracycline with newly grown Top10F' cells (*see* **Note 4**) at an OD_{600} of maximum 0.020. Divide the culture between two baffled 2L flasks, and shake at 37°C at a minimum of 300 rpm to ensure good aeration (*see* **Note 5**).
2. Transfer cells to four detergent-free 500 mL centrifuge flasks at an OD_{600} of 0.8–1.0, and chill by swirling in an ice/water bath for 5 min. Cells, buffer, and *all* equipment are kept ice-cold throughout the remaining procedure.
3. Pellet cells for 6–8 min at 5000*g* in a GS-3 rotor (*see* **Note 6**). Decant as much supernatant as possible, resuspend each cell pellet carefully and completely in 5–10 mL 10% glycerol solution using an ice-cold 10 mL glass pipet. Add 300 mL glycerol buffer to each flask and mix.
4. Repeat **step 3** above, but reduce the number of centrifuge flasks to two. Add 300 mL glycerol solution to each of the two flasks and mix.
5. Repeat the previous step twice.
6. Resuspend the final pellets from **step 5** above in 5–10 mL glycerol solution, transfer cells to a 50 mL centrifuge tube, add glycerol solution to a total of 40 mL, mix, and centrifuge cells at 4000–5000 rpm for 6–8 min (*see* **Note 6**).
7. Resuspend pellet in the remaining supernatant and add buffer to a total of 1.25 mL. Assuming 2×10^8 cells/mL at $OD_{600} = 1$, this corresponds to $6–12 \times 10^{10}$ cells/mL, depending on strain, cell loss, and so forth.
8. Dispense 25–200 µL of cells in chilled microfuge tubes, quick-freeze the tubes in ethanol at –80°C (or a dry ice/ethanol bath), and store at this temperature.
9. Test that cells are free of contaminant plasmids, phagemids, or phages.

3.4. Electroporation of Library DNA, Cell Growth, and Storage

This protocol is dimensioned to obtain libraries containing up to 5×10^8 independent cfu.

1. Set the *E. coli* Pulser at 2000 V and thaw ultracompetent Top10F' cells on ice (*see* **Subheading 3.3.**). Place electroporation cuvets, cuvet holder, cells, and DNA on ice. Dilute cells to $5–6 \times 10^{10}$ cell/mL with ice-cold sterile water.

2. Carefully mix 10–40 ng purified, salt-free DNA from **Subheading 3.2., steps 11** and **13** with 25 µL cells.
3. Place the mixture in a 0.1 cm electroporation cuvet, taking care not to leave air bubbles. Tap the cuvet gently to get all liquid to cover all of the bottom. Make sure that the cuvet is dry on the outside.
4. Pulse and add instantly 0.5–1.0 mL of SOC medium supplemented with 10 mM $MgCl_2$, and mix. The time constant should be in the 5–5.5 ms range. Transfer the mixture, or pools of mixtures to a capped tube and allow phenotypic expression by shaking at 250 rpm for 1 h at 37°C.
5. Withdraw 1 µL, make dilutions and spread on LB-ampicillin plates to obtain an estimate of the number of cfu for each electroporation or pool of electroporations.
6. For each individual transformation, use 40 mL LB-ampicillin/tetracycline medium supplemented with 1% glucose, which act as catabolite repressor of Plac. We usually do 25–50 electroporations at a time.
7. Propagate cells in liquid culture (a) or on plates (b):
   a. Shake cells at 37°C until an OD_{600} of 1–2 is reached. This takes about 10 h. To increase the effectiveness of the ampicillin selection, cells can be pelleted and resuspended in fresh prewarmed LB-ampicillin/tetracycline medium after 6–8 h of growth.
   b. Alternatively, spread cells from five electroporations on an air-dried Nunclon Δ Square Dish (500 cm^2), and incubate overnight at 37°C. For each D Square Dish, scrape off cells using 10 mL LB, transfer to a shake flask, add 100 mL LB-ampicillin/ tetracycline medium, shake for 2 h, and combine cells.
8. Pellet two portions of 10^{11} cells (equivalent to 250–500 mL from **step 7a** above). Resuspend one portion in LB at 10^{10} cells/mL, and make 10 individual glycerol stocks *(15)*. Prepare Qiagen maxiprep DNA from the other.

3.5. Production and Titration of Fab Phages from Libraries

This protocol is dimensioned to libraries that contain about 10^8 independent cfu. If a differently sized library is used, scale up or down correspondingly. Tetracycline is added to ensure that all growing cells have sex pili.

1. Inoculate 400 mL prewarmed LB-ampicillin/tetracycline medium with 2×10^9 cells (200 µL of a glycerol stock from **Subheading 3.4., step 8**). Grow cells about four generations at 37°C with shaking until OD_{600} reaches 0.5.
2. Add 2×10^{12} R408 helper phages (*see* **Note 7**) to the 400 mL culture. This high multiplicity (about 50) increases the chance that all cells become infected.
3. Shake gently for 20 min at 37°C and add IPTG to a final concentration of 100 mM (*see* **Note 8**).
4. Transfer the culture flask to a shaker at room temperature (*see* **Note 9**), and continue shaking at 300 rpm for a minimum of 10 and a maximum of 16 h (cell lysis occur after 16 h).
5. Pellet the cells by centrifugation at 15,000g for 10 min.
6. Transfer supernatant and repeat centrifugation as in **step 5** above.
7. Transfer supernatant to a fresh centrifuge flask and add 1 vol of phage-precipitation buffer to 4 vol of phage supernatant. Mix the solution by shaking and incubate at 0 or 4°C for 1 h or longer.
8. Pellet the phage particles by centrifugation at 15,000g for 30 min. Resuspend pellet in 8 mL of PBS buffer, transfer to a 10 mL centrifuge tube, and make a clearing spin at 15,000g for 10 min.

9. Transfer supernatant to a fresh tube, precipitate phages as in **step 7** above, and centrifuge at 15,000*g* for 30 min.

10. Resuspend pellet in 1 mL PBS buffer, transfer to a microfuge tube, make a clearing spin, transfer supernatant to a fresh tube, and precipitate phages as above. Resuspend pellet in 1 mL PBS buffer and filtrate through a 0.2- or 0.45-μm filter. Store the phage stock at 4°C or −20°C.

11. Mix 125 μL exponentially growing Top10/F' cells (or other male *E. coli* cells) at an OD_{600} of 0.8–1.0 with an equal volume of a series of diluted Fab phages. Include controls with phage dilutions alone and titration cells alone. Place the mixtures at 37°C for 10 min, and then chill on ice.

12. Spread 20 and 200 μL from each mixture on LB-ampicillin/tetracycline plates and incubate overnight at 37°C. Also spread 50 mL cells on an LB plate to make sure that the titration cells were free of wild-type phage.

13. Count colonies, correct for background and calculate cfu/mL. A titer of about 10^{13} cfu/mL of the concentrated phage stock is typical.

3.6. Selection of Antigen Binders by Panning on Antigen-Coated Plastic (see Note 10)

1. Coat microtiter wells with 100 μL of a 0.5 μ*M* HLA-A2/peptide solution in PBS overnight at 4°C followed by two to three short rinses with washing buffer and block for 2 h at room temperature with blocking buffer using 200 μL/well.

2. Rinse the wells briefly 2–3 times in washing buffer, and add about 10^{11} Fab phages diluted in 100 μL blocking solution per well.

3. Incubate for 2–3 h with rocking at room temperature. After incubation, the wells are washed and rinsed briefly 10–15× with washing buffer (*see* **Note 11**). Bound phages are eluted by one of two methods: glycine-buffer treatment (**steps 4** and **5** below) or digestion with trypsin (**step 6** below).

4. Add 100 μL 0.1 *M* glycine elution buffer per well and incubate for 15 min at room temperature.

5. Transfer eluates to fresh microtiter wells containing 8 μL 2 *M* Tris-base to neutralize the acid.

6. Add 100 μL trypsin elution buffer and incubate for 30 min at room temperature.

7. The eluates from **steps 5** or **6** above are transferred to vials containing 400 μL exponentially growing Top10F' cells with an OD_{600} of 0.8–1.0.

8. Incubate at 37°C for 20 min with gentle shaking.

9. Withdraw 5 μL from each culture, make serial dilutions, and spread on ampicillin plates to determine the number of ampicillin-transducing phages in the eluate.

10. Transfer each culture to 40 mL 2X TY-medium supplemented with 1% glucose, ampicillin and tetracycline, and incubate at 37°C with shaking overnight. Alternatively, plate each culture on a Nunclon Δ Square Dish, continue as in **Subheading 3.4., step 7b**, and proceed with **step 11** below.

11. Prepare 1-mL glycerol stocks and make plasmid Qiagen miniprep DNA.

12. For preparation of phages for the next round of panning, use 200 μL of the glycerol stock (about 2×10^8 cells) to inoculate 30 mL 2X TY medium containing ampicillin and tetracycline.

13. When the culture reaches an OD_{600} of 0.5–0.8, add 2.5×10^{11} R408 helper phages and incubate at 37°C with gentle shaking for 20 min.

14. Add IPTG, grow cells, and prepare and titrate Fab phages for the next panning round as described in **Subheading 3.5., steps 3–13**.

15. Between each round of panning, determine the number of eluted bound phages relative to the amount of phages added to the wells. Likewise, the ELISA signal generated from a fixed amount of eluted bound phages should be monitored between each round of panning (we use peroxidase-conjugated anti-M13 as secondary antibody). An increase in these two parameters by a factor of 10 or more should be observed between each round of panning.
16. After three or four rounds of panning, isolate individual clones, and characterize their binding characteristics by ELISA assays.

3.7. Generation of HLA-A2 as Inclusion Body Material

Day 1: Streak out the desired clone on a selective plate.

Day 2: Inoculate an Erlenmeyer flask cont. 100 mL LB + antibiotics with a loopfull from 10 randomly picked colonies. Incubate overnight with shaking at 37°C.

Day 3: Measure OD_{600} of a ×10 diluted sample.

1. Calculate the volume needed to inoculate one liter of Superbroth (+ antibiotics, sucrose and Mg_2SO_4) to generate a culture with an initial OD_{600} of 0.05.
2. Inoculate and divide the culture into two 2-L flasks with baffles.
3. Start growth by incubation at 37°C with shaking (300 rpm).
4. Measure OD_{600} of the culture at every 20 min.
5. At $OD_{600} = 3.0$ (after about 3 h) add IPTG to a final conc of 2 mM.
6. Further incubation for 2 h. Measure OD_{600} after 2 h. Expect an increase in OD of about 30%.
7. Transfer culture to precooled 500 mL GS-3 tubes. Max 330 mL per tube.
8. Centrifuge at 4500 rpm, 4°C for 30 min. Discard supernatant into waste flask. Resuspend individual pellets in 15 mL TE50/20-buffer (Whirlmix).
9. Collect resuspended cells from 1 L culture + a 5 mL TE50/20 wash of all three tubes (that is, a total of 50 mL) into a single 250 mL GSA tube.
10. Cap the tube and freeze at –80°C.

Day 4:

1. Add 130 mL TE50/20-buffer to the 50 mL frozen inclusion body solution and let it thaw.
2. Add 8 mL lysozome stock solution, shake well and incubate for 60 min at room temperature with intermittent shaking.
3. Add 20 mL 5 M NaCl and shake well.
4. Add 20 mL 25% Triton X-100 and shake well.
5. Incubate the mixture for 30 min at room temperature. Shake well and often during incubation.
6. Centrifuge 13,000g for 50 min at 4°C (GSA).
7. Resuspend the pellet completely in 200 mL TE50/20-buffer + 1 % Triton X-100.
8. Repeat **step 6**.
9. Resuspend the pellet completely in 200 mL TE50/20-buffer.
10. Repeat **step 6**.
11. Repeat **steps 9–10** above 3× (that is, a total of 6 centrifugations).
12. Before the last centrifugation, transfer 1 mL of the resuspended inclusion body material to an eppendorf vial, centrifuge at 4°C at 13,000g for 50 min using a microtube centrifuge. Freeze and store inclusion body pellets in their centrifugation tubes at –80°C.
13. Resuspend the pellet from the microtube-centrifugation in 200 μL PBS-buffer and test for protein concentration (Pierce) and for purity by analyzing 1, 5, and 15 μL on 15%

SDS gels. This purity check is done before solubilization of the main portion of the inclusion body material as the solubilization buffer prevents analysis by SDS gel electrophoresis. Also it permits an estimate of the yield of the expected protein material. Expect a 90% purity of a total of 100–200 mg of the relevant protein.

3.8. Refolding of HLA-A2 with Peptide and Purification of Complex

The protocol below describes the refolding of a mono-chain construct composed of human β_2-microglobulin (located at the N-terminus) in fusion with the HLA-A2 heavy chain via a 15 amino acid peptide linker (Gly$_4$Ser)$_3$. Refolding is performed in the presence of the selected peptide. Individually prepared β2-microglobulin and HLA-A2 heavy chain can be refolded according to the same protocol but gives lower yield of correctly refolded HLA/peptide complex. Purified complexes are tested for positive reaction in ELISA assays using antibodies recognizing HLA-A2/peptide complexes in a peptide dependent (not peptide specific) manner such as W6/32 or Tü155 (*see* **ref. 21**).

3.8.1. Solubilization of Inclusion Bodies

1. Dissolve inclusion body pellet purified from 1 L bacterial culture in 10 mL solubilization buffer using tissuemizer; this gives about 8 mg protein/mL.
2. Measure protein concentration (pierce). Dilute a sample of the stock solution to 4 mg/mL with solubilization buffer to obtain a total volume of 5 mL. Freeze and store the remainder of the denatured protein at –80°C.
3. Weigh out 50 mg of dry DTE and add to the 5 mL solubilization solution. The final DTE concentration is 65 mM (10 mg/mL).
4. Check pH using pH strips. The pH must be 8.0–8.5.
5. Incubate the solution for at least 2 h.

3.8.2. Renaturation

1. Weigh out 6 mg of peptide and dissolve in 1 mL refolding buffer.
2. Add the dissolved peptide to the refolding buffer (500 mL) while it is rapidly stirring and then add the solubilized single-chain scβ_2-A$_2$ protein at 5 mL/10 s.
3. Incubate the refolding solution in the cold room for 36–48 h without stirring.

3.8.3. Purification

1. The refolding solution is concentrated initially to approx 50 mL using a Minitan Acrylic Ultrafiltration System from Millipore with a filter membrane plate retaining proteins larger than 10 kD. Then further to 1–2 mL by an Centricon Plus-20 concentrator (Biomax-8, 8 kD from Millipore). Do the concentration at 4°C. Centrifuge the concentrated solution for 10 min at 4000g.
2. The concentrated protein is then applied on a G-100 sephadex column prepared from a 150 mL, 75% slurry solution of G-100 sephadex in PBS loaded on a XK 16/70 column from Pharmacia. The protein is eluted by PBS, 0.5 mL/min. Collect fractions of 5 mL.
3. 15 µL of the protein containing fractions are analyzed by 15% SDS PAGE to determine the MHC/peptide profile of the eluate. Analyze under reduced as well as nonreduced conditions. The gels are silver stained.
4. Fractions corresponding to the monomer complex are pooled and concentrated to 1 mL using a Centricon Plus-20 concentrator. Determine the protein concentration by the Pierce

assay. Add azide to 0.05% and store at 4°C or freeze at –20°C (freeze and defreeze only once otherwise the protein will denature).

4. Notes

1. Ideally, separate PCR reactions should be performed with each individual V_H primer and the MJH1-3 mix as well as with each individual Vκ- or Vλ primers and MCK1 followed by mixing of the individual reaction products in equimolar amounts before proceeding with the subsequent PCR extention reactions and cloning. It is important that only high quality oligonucleotide preparations (predominantly containing full-size oligonucleotides) should be used. The rationale behind the design of our rather extensive series of PCR primers for the variable H and L chains has been reported previously *(4)*. In short, we believe that the primer sets used should match all available sequence data for these regions and we argued that highly degenerate primers for the variable regions are likely to generate biased libraries and to introduce amino acids not normally found in the variable regions.

2. Addition of (inert) glycogen to a standard ethanol precipitation, ensures quantitative recovery and that the pellet is always visible

3. To avoid reduction in diversity of the first-step library, it is necessary that the number of transformants in the second cloning step is several-fold higher than in the first.

4. The protocols presented here assume the use of Top10F' cells. We generally prefer this strain because it produces Fab phages that give high antigen-binding capacity per unit number of Fab phages *(7)*, electrocompetent cells that give extraordinarily high electroporation efficiencies, and DNA of high quality.

5. Some strains are many-fold more competent, if cells are grown at room temperature *(18)*. For Top10F', we see a twofold increase in competency. For growth at room temperature, it is convenient to start the culture the day (evening) before at an OD_{600} of 0.002–0.005 (strain-dependent), and shake vigorously overnight. For Top10F', freshly prepared LB that is not autoclaved, increases competency by a factor of two and LB and 2XYT gives similar results.

6. Centrifuge cells as slowly as possibly, so as to make it easy to resuspend them *gently and completely*. A recovery of only 50–75% of the start cells (corresponding to 90–95% recovery in each centrifugation step) ensures very gentle treatment of the cells. The optimal centrifugation speed is strain dependent.

7. R408 helper phage production: Infect log-phase Top10F' cells at $OD_{600} = 0.5$ in baffled culture flasks with a 20-fold excess of R408, and shake at 200 rpm overnight at 37°C. Prepare and titrate phages as described in **ref.** *(15)* by mixing phage/cell dilutions with 3 mL of molten topagar and spread on LB-tetracycline plates. Expect more than 10^{14} plaque forming units (pfu)/L supernatant.

8. We have varied the IPTG concentration used for induction of P*lac* during superinfection between 0 and 2 m*M* and found no increase in Fab phage production with IPTG concentrations above 100 μ*M*.

9. It is important to incubate between 22° and 30°C following superinfection for two reasons: a) folding of active Fab molecules proceeds more successfully at room temperature than at 37°C *(19)*, and b) Fab-phages will not be lost as a result of reinfection because sex pili are not generated at temperatures below 30°C *(20)*.

10. Binders to HLA-A2/peptide complexes are selected by panning on microtiter plates or beads coated with HLA-A2-peptide complexes. Alternatively, panning can be

performed using HLA-A2 transfected RMA.S cells pulsed with selected peptides. We have argued about the benefit of alternating between these two panning matrices (*see ref. 11*).

Panning on beads: 1.5×10^7 sulfated latex beads are incubated with $0.5 \ \mu M$ HLA-A2-peptide complexes in a total volume of 150 μL over night at 4°C with end-over-end rotation. The beads are spun down for 4 min at 4000g, blocked with 150 μL 2% BSA in PBS buffer and rotated end-over-end for 2 h at 4°C. Following two washings in ice-cold 2% BSA in PBS buffer, a 300 μL mixture containing 10^{10}–10^{11} phages and 5% BSA in PBS buffer is added. During some rounds of panning, β_2-microglobulin and/or HLA-A2-β_2m in complex with an irrelevant peptide, can be added as competitors in a concentration of 1 μM. The final mixture is rotated end-over-end for 3 h at 4°C followed by precipitation of the beads by centrifugation. Beads are then washed 3× in ice-cold 2% BSA. Bound phages are eluted by adding 100 μL glycine elution buffer (0.1 M Tris-HCL, pH = 2.2.) and incubation for 15 min at room temperature. Beads are spun down and the supernatant neutralized with 6 μL 2 M Tris-base (not pH-adjusted). 400 μL exponentially growing TOP10F' or TG1 cells are added and the mixture incubated at 37°C for 20 min. 5 μL are withdrawn form the culture, diluted serially, and a suitable volume plated on selective plates to determine the number of ampicillin-transducing phages in the eluate. The rest of the culture is transferred to 40 mL 2X YT media containing the relevant antibiotics and 1% glucose and incubated overnight at 37°C with shaking (250 rpm). Glycerol stocks are made at a concentration of about 10^9 cells/mL. A small volume of the overnight culture is used for preparation of plasmid DNA.

Panning on cells: 4×10^6 HLA-A2 transfected RMA.S cells in 2 mL RPMI media are cultured in the presence of the relevant peptide in a concentration of 0.1 mM over night at 26°C. The cells are spun down (5 min at 2000 rpm) and washed once in media before resuspension in 200 μL PBS. 100 μL cells are mixed with 10^{10}–10^{11} phages making a total volume of 200 μL. The mixture is incubated for 3 h at room temperature, with gentle shaking. The suspension is subsequently centrifuged for 5 min at 2000 rpm, the supernatant removed and the cells washed 3× in RPMI media. Bound phages are eluted with 100 μL Trypsin elution buffer for 30 min at 37°C following pelleting of the cells by centrifugation. The supernatant is added to 400 μL exponentially growing TOP10F' or TG1 cells and the culture is incubated at 37°C for 20 min. From here on, follow the same procedure as described for phages eluted from beads.

11. The outlined washing procedure has been used successfully when screening for high-affinity binders (apparent K_d of about 10^{-9} M) normally present in libraries generated from immunized animals. When dealing with low-affinity binders (apparent K_d of about 10^{-6} M), the number of washes is reduced to three brief washes in washing buffer.

References

1. Hoogenboom, R. H., Griffiths, A. D., Johnson, K. S., Chiswell, D. J., Hudson, P., and Winter, G. (1991) Multi-subunit proteins on the surface of filamentous phage: methodologies for displaying antibody (Fab) heavy and light chains. *Nucleic Acids Res.* **19**, 4133–4137.
2. Kang, A. K., Barbas, C. F., Janda, K. D., Benkovic, S. J., and Lerner, R. A. (1991) Linkage of recognition and replication functions by assembling combinatorial antibody Fab libraries along phage surfaces. *Proc. Natl. Acad. Sci. USA* **88**, 4363–4366.

3. Breitling, F., Dübel, S., Seehaus, T., Klewinghaus, I., and Little, M. (1991) A surface expression vector for antibody screening. *Gene* **104,** 147–153.
4. Ørum, H., Andersen, P. S., Riise, E., Øster, A., Johansen, L. K., Bjørnvad, M., et al. (1993) Efficient method for constructing comprehensive murine Fab antibody libraries displayed on phage. *Nucleic Acids Res.* **21(19),** 4491–4498.
5. Hoogenboom, H. R., Marks, J. D., Griffiths, A. D., and Winter, G. (1992) Building antibodies from their genes. *Immunol. Rev.* **130,** 41–68.
6. Winter, G., Griffiths, A. D., Hawkins, R. E., and Hoogenboom, H. R. (1994) Making antibodies by phage display technology. *Ann. Rev. Immunol.* **12,** 433–455.
7. Johansen, L. K., Albrechtsen, B., Andersen, H. W., and Engberg, J. (1995) pFab60: a new efficient vector for expression of antibody Fab fragments displayed on phage. *Protein Eng.* **8(10),** 1063–1067.
8. Jespersen, L.K., Kuusinen, A., Orellana, A., Keinänen, K., and Engberg, J. (2000) Novel use of proteoliposomes and phage display to obtain glutamate receptor specific antibodies *Eur. J. Biochem.* **257,** 1382–1389. **14(1),** 53–69.
9. Dziegiel, M., Nielsen, L., Andersen, P. S., Blancher, A., Dickmeiss, E., and Engberg, J. (1995) Phage display used for gene cloning of human recombinant antibody against the erythrocyte surface antigen, rhesus D. *J. Immunolog. Methods* **182,** 7–19.
10. Engberg, J., Johansen, L.K., Westengaard-Hildinge, M., Riise, E. S., and Albrechtsen, B. (1999) Phage-display libraries of murine and human antibody Fab fragments, in *Nucleic Acid Protocols Handbook* (Rapley, R., ed.), Humana Press Inc., Totowa, NJ, pp. 449–478.
11. Andersen, P. S., Stryhn, A., Hansen, B. A., Fugger, L., Engberg, J., and Buus, S. (1996) A recombinant antibody with the antigen-specific, MHC-restricted specificity of T cells. *Proc. Natl. Acad. Sci. USA* **93(3),** 1820–1825.
12. Krogsgaard, M., Wucherpfennig, K. W., Andersen, C.B ., Hansen, B. E., Svejgaard, A., Pyrdol, J., et al. (2000) Visualization of myelin basic protein T-cell epitopes in multiple sclerosis lesions using a monoclonal antibody specific for the HLA-DR2-MBP 85-99 complex. *J. Exp. Med.* **101(108),** 1395–1412.
13. Reiter, Y., Di Carlo, A., Fugger, L., Engberg, J., and Pastan, I. (1997) Peptide-specific killing of antigen-presenting cells by a recombinant antibody-toxin fusion protein targeted to MHC/peptide class I complexes with T cell receptor-like specificity. *Proc. Natl. Acad. Sci. USA* **94(10),** 4631–4636.
14. Engberg, J., Krogsgaard, M., and Fugger, L. (1999) Recombinant antibodies with the antigen-specific, MHC restricted specificity of T cells: novel reagents for basic and clinical investigations and immunotherapy. *Immunotechnology* **4,** 273–278.
15. Sambrook, J., Fritsch, E. F., and Maniatis, T. (1989) *Molecular Cloning. A Laboratory Manual*, 2nd ed. Cold Spring Harbor Laboratory Press, Cold Spring Harbor, NY.
16. Krebber, A., Burmester, J., and Plückthun, A (1996) Inclusion of an upstream transcriptional terminator in phage display vectors abolishes background expression of toxic fusions with coat protein g3p. *Gene* **178,** 71–74.
17. Zoller, P. (1994) How optimal electroporation efficiency varies for different strains of *E. coli. BIO-RADiations* **90,** 5.
18. Chuang, S.-E., Chen, A.-L., and Chao, C.-C. (1995) Growth of *E. coli* at low temperature increases the transformation frequency by electroporation. *Nucleic Acids Res.* **23(9),** 1641.
19. Dower, W. J., Miller, J. F., and Ragsdale, C. W. (1988) High efficiency transformation of E. coli by high voltage electroporation. *Nucleic Acids Res.* **16(13),** 6127–6145.

20. Plückthun, A. and Skerra, A. (1989) Expression of functional antibody Fv and Fab fragments in *Escherichia coli. Methods Enzymol.* **178,** 497–515.
21. Barnstable, C. J., Bodmer, W. F., Brown, G., Galfrè, G., Milstein, C., Williams, A. F., and Ziegler, A. (1978) Production of monoclonal antibodies to group A erythrocytes, HLA and other human cell surfaceantigens: new tools for genetic analysis. *Cell* **14,** 9–20.

11

Engineering Hot Spots
for Affinity Enhancement of Antibodies

Partha S. Chowdhury

1. Introduction

The potential of antibodies as magic bullets for targeting therapeutic drugs or imaging agents has been well-documented and is now an emerging area of molecular medicine. Because antibodies act first by binding to their specific antigens it is easy to envisage that the specific activity of antibody-based drugs depends to a large extent on the antigen-binding affinity of antibodies. For a variety of reasons under many circumstances instead of whole antibodies, smaller antigen-binding units of antibodies such as Fabs and Fvs are better suited to perform the job of the magic bullet. The conversion of whole antibodies into Fabs and Fvs (scFvs or dsFvs) is often associated with a drastic reduction in the antigen-binding affinity. It is therefore pertinent that for efficient use of Fvs as targeting agents their binding affinities need to be improved. Until the recent past there had been two different approaches to improve binding affinity of antibodies (whole IgGs, Fabs, and Fvs). One approach relied on the high-resolution crystal structure of antibody-antigen complex followed by engineering of key contact residues in the Fv portion to enhance the interaction. Although this approach is very logical and has greater chances of success, it is not readily feasible. The other approach that has been used to improve affinities of antibodies involved mutating the CDRs randomly or semi-randomly and create large expression libraries (for example, scFv or Fab phage-display libraries), which served as a potential source of high-affinity variants. This approach has been used successfully several times and in fact has become the method of choice to improve antibody affinity. However, it requires the construction, maintenance, and handling of large and/or multiple phage-display libraries. These tasks require technical expertise and at times they can be time-consuming and expensive.

The method described herein is a new approach that also uses the scFv phage antibody-display technology but aims at creating small libraries that can be a rich source of

From: *Methods in Molecular Biology, vol. 207: Recombinant Antibodies for Cancer Therapy: Methods and Protocols*
Edited by: M. Welschof and J. Krauss © Humana Press Inc., Totowa, NJ

higher-affinity variants. Although described here for scFvs, the approach can be employed to dsFvs, Fabs, and whole antibodies too. Because Fvs are the smallest antigen-binding units of antibodies, it is easier to work and engineer the Fvs for affinity improvements and then convert them to whole immunoglobulins at the end. Therefore the whole discussion on affinity improvement in this chapter will be based on affinity improvement of Fvs. The essence of the approach described here is to mimic in vitro the natural somatic hypermutation process that underlies affinity maturation of antibodies in vivo. It is based on results published by the groups of Caesar Milstein and Michael Neuberger, which indicate that during somatic hypermutation, the mutations in the antibody variable region genes are not randomly distributed but are preferentially focused in certain regions *(1–3)*. These regions have been termed "hot spots." Although the exact features of hot spots are yet to be understood, there seems to exist certain consensus nucleotide sequence and codons to define them. The consensus sequence is a tetranucleotide that can be defined as RGYW (where R can be a purine, Y can be a pyrimidine, and W can be an A or a T). The codons that seem to constitute a hot spot in many cases are the AGY serine codons (where Y is a pyrimidine). It is to be noted that the AGY codon may or may not be part of the RGYW consensus sequence. The existence of antibody-variable region hot spots is not restricted to mammals but has also been identified in birds, and it is not known if they exist in the lower vertebrates too.

One of the important lessons we learn from biology is that mother nature executes her actions in a very efficient manner. Thinking of the widely occurring natural process of antibody affinity maturation during an immune response, it is not surprising to assume or think that the existence of hot spots in antibody-variable region genes may be nature's way to efficiently improve the affinities of antibodies by localizing mutations to certain regions for directed evolution of better binding variants. However, it is important to realize based on the existing literature that although *de novo* affinity maturation of antibodies has been found to be associated with a mutation in hot spots, hot spot mutations have not always been found to be associated with improvement in affinity of an antibody *(1–3)*.

If one looks into the nucleotide sequence of V_H and V_L of any antibody, one would be overwhelmed by the existence of a large number of hot spots localized all over the V-domain. The location and number of these hot spots varies depending on the germ line origin of the V-domain. So how does one decide which hot spot to manipulate for in vitro affinity improvements of a given Fv? To make this decision, one needs to keep in mind certain basic principles of the Fv region. These are (1) conserved residues in variable regions play important structural roles; (2) complementarity-determining regions (CDRs) contribute mainly to antigen binding; (3) buried residues in CDRs are not likely to interact with the antigen and (4) junctional residues in the V_HS undergo natural selection inside the body (important particularly when the Fv being studied is obtained from an immunized animal or person). The current method takes into consideration the concept of hot-spot mutation for *de novo* affinity maturation of antibodies as mentioned earlier and couples it to the existing knowledge of Fv structures. This enables one to eliminate a large number of hot spots that code for residues that fall into the FRs and also those CDR residues that are either conserved, buried, or occupy junctional positions between FR3 and CDR3 and/or CDR3 and FR4 (in case of V$_H$s). The shortlisted hot spots are then randomly mutated to generate small sized phage display libraries. These libraries are then panned on the relevant antigen to enrich the binders. Randomly picked clones from among the binders are then studied in detail to identify binders that are better than the parental type. Because analysis of phage clones is affected by the number of scFvs on the phage surface monomeric scFvs or monomeric scFv-fusion proteins are purified to make a final assessment about affinity of the Fv for its antigen. The method described here has been found to work in several systems (*see* **refs. *4* and *5*).

2. Materials
2.1. Bacterial Strains and Bacteriophages
1. *Escherichia coli* TG1: *K12 Δ(lac-pro), supE, thi, hsdΔ5/F'*[traD36, proAB, lacI^q, lacZΔM15].
2. *E. coli* CJ236: F' *cat* (= pCJ105; M13^s*Cm^r*)/*dut ung 1, thi-1 relA1, spoT1* mcrA.
3. M13KO7 (available from Pharmacia, Invitrogen) and R408 (available from Stratagene) helper phage.

2.2. Recombinant DNA
1. A phagemid with the scFv of interest fused in frame with the gIII of M13 or a related filamentous phage (for example, pCANTAB5E from Pharmacia). It is important to know the antibiotic resistance marker, the *E. coli* origin of replication, and the direction of the phage origin of replication.
2. A plasmid that has the lacI^q gene and a different antibiotic resistance marker and a different *E. coli* origin of replication than the phagemid.

2.3. Reagents
2.3.1. Enzymes
1. T7 DNA Polymerase (included in the in vitro mutagenesis refill kit from Bio-Rad).
2. T4 DNA Ligase (included in the in vitro mutagenesis refill kit from Bio-Rad).
3. Polynucleotide kinase (3' phosphatase free) (Roche).
4. A high fidelity thermostable DNA polymerase (for example, Pwo, Pfu, or *Vent.*).
5. Restriction enzymes flanking the scFv coding region in the phagemid and enzymes for two other unique and mutually incompatible restriction sites that lie outside the scFv-gIIIp coding region (these enzymes would vary depending upon the phage display vector being used).

2.3.2. Buffers and Chemicals
1. 10X Buffers for all enzymes (usually provided with the enzymes).
2. 10X Annealing buffer: 200 mM Tris-HCl, pH 7.4 (at 37°C), 20 mM MgCl$_2$, 500 mM NaCl (included in the in vitro mutagenesis refill kit from Bio-Rad).
3. 10X Synthesis buffer: 5 mM each dATP, dCTP, dGTP, dTTP, 10 mM ATP, 100 mM Tris-HCl, pH 7.4 (at 37°C), 50 mM MgCl$_2$, 20 mM dithiothreitol (DTT) (included in the in vitro mutagenesis refill kit from Bio-Rad).
4. T7 DNA Polymerase dilution buffer: 20 mM potassium phosphate, pH 7.4, 1 mM DTT, 0.1 mM EDTA, 50% glycerol (included in the in vitro mutagenesis refill kit from Bio-Rad).
5. 50 mM sodium bicarbonate buffer, pH 9.4–9.6.

6. 20% PEG 8000-2.5 *M* NaCl (Store at 4°C on bringing to room temperature after autoclaving).
7. 1X NET: 100 m*M* NaCl, 1 m*M* EDTA, 10 m*M* Tris-HCl, pH 7.5.
8. Agarose for analytical gels and low melting-point agarose for preparative gels.
9. Buffer saturated phenol (*see* **Note 1**).
10. Phenol:chloroform:iso-amyl alcohol, 25:24:1 (*see* **Note 2**).
11. Chloroform (*see* **Note 2**).
12. Chilled ethanol 100% (*see* **Note 3**).
13. 8 *M* Lithium chloride.

2.3.3. Antibodies, Antibody Enzyme Conjugates, and Accessories

1. Anti-tag antibody (the tag is a peptide between the scFv and the gIIIp. It can vary depending on the phage display vector used).
2. Anti-M13 gVIIIp monoclonal antibody.
3. Secondary antibody against the anti-tag antibody and anti-gVIIIp antibody coupled to alkaline phosphatase or horseradish peroxidase (for example, if the anti-tag antibody is a mouse IgG then the secondary antibody will be anti-mouse IgG-AP or anti-mouse IgG-HRP).
4. Substrate for the enzyme attached to the secondary antibody (for example, DAB for HRP).

2.3.4. Oligonucleotides

Oligonucleotides for doing the mutagenesis and polymerase chain reactions (PCRs) should be of high-quality purified preferably by HPLC or at least through a reverse phase cartridge.

2.4. Special Apparatuses and Accessories

1. Dot-blot apparatus.
2. Enzyme-linked immunosorbent assay (ELISA) reader.
3. Densitometric scanner (optional).
4. Heat blocks at 15–18°C, 65°C and 72°C.
5. Nitrocellulose or polyvinylidene fluoride (PVDF) membranes.
6. Nonfat dry milk.
7. Tween-20.
8. LB medium: To 950 mL of deionized water add: 10 g Bacto-tryptone, 5 g Bacto-yeast extract, 10 g NaCl. Dissolve the solutes and adjust pH to 7.0 with 5 *N* NaOH. Add deionized water to a final volume of 1 L. Sterilize by autoclaving for 20 min at 15 lb/sq. in on liquid cycle. To make LB plates, add agar to a final concentration of 1.5% before autoclaving. After the medium is cooled to about 45°C add the ampicillin to a final concentration of 100 μg/mL. For glucose plates add a 20% sterile solution of glucose to a final concentration of 2% after autoclaving and cooling the LB medium to 37°C.
9. 2X YT medium: To 900 mL of deionized water add: 16 g Bacto-tryptone, 10 g Bacto-yeast extract, 5 g NaCl. Dissolve the solutes and adjust pH to 7.0 with 5 *N* NaOH. Adjust the volume to 1 L with deionized water. Sterilize by autoclaving for 20 min at 15 lb/sq. in on liquid cycle.
10. S.O.C. medium: To 80 mL water add 2 g Bacto-tryptone, 0.5 g Bacto-yeast extract, 54.5. mg NaCl, 18.64 mg Potassium chloride, 95.2 mg Magnesium chloride, 120 mg Magnesium sulphate. Dissolve solutes. Adjust pH to 7.0 with 5 *N* NaOH. Adjust volume to 98 mL with deionized water. Sterilize by autoclaving for 20 min at 15 lb/sq. in on liquid cycle. Add 2 mL of a 1 *M* solution of sterile glucose to make to volume to 100 mL.

11. M63 Glucose-BI plates.
    a. Solution A: 12 g potassium dihydrogen phosphate, 28 g dipotassium hydrogen phosphate, 8 g ammonium sulphate. Adjust volume to 2 L with distilled water. Autoclave. Cool.
    b. Solution B: 60 g agar, 1.6 L distilled water. Autoclave. Cool.
    c. Solution C: 2 mL 0.1% ferrous sulphate solution, 0.98 g magnesium sulphate hepta hydrate, 332 mL distilled water. Autoclave. Cool.
    d. Solution D: 8 g glucose, 40 mL distilled water. Autoclave. Cool.
    e. Solution E: 8 mL sterile stock solution of 0.5% thiamine.
    Mix solutions A–E. Dispense 40 mL per plate.

3. Methods

The methods to randomize hot spots for in vitro affinity improvement of scFvs consists of several steps, which are as follows:

1. Identification of hot spots in the V_H and V_L.
2. Rational selection of hot spots for mutations.
3. Randomly mutating the residues covered by the selected hot spots.
4. Constructing and panning phage-display library/libraries.
5. Analysis of selected clones.

Each of these steps is described below in **Subheadings 3.1.–3.5.**

3.1. Identification of Hot Spots in the V_H and V_L

Hot spots in antibody variable region can be identified either manually or with the help of a computer. All that one needs to do is identify the tetranucleotide A/G-G-C/T-A/T (RGYW) and identify serine codons which are either AGC or AGT (AGY). Mark each tetranucleotide hot spot with a rectangle and each AGY serine codon with a circle. One would frequently find many hot spots spread over a V_H and V_L. One might also see that many of the AGY serine codons also form part of the tetranucleotide hot spots.

3.2. Rational Selection of Hot Spots for Mutations

Once the hot spots are identified one needs to select only a few of these to target random mutations to. To do this we need to put to use our existing knowledge on antibody structure. The way to do this is shown schematically in **Fig. 1** and consists essentially of the following steps:

1. Eliminate the hot spots that fall onto the FRs. This is because FR residues do not usually contribute directly to antigen binding.
2. Eliminate hot spots that code for conserved and buried residues in CDRs: The hot spots in the CDRs may code for residues that are either highly conserved or are buried. These are residues that one should not change. To determine if any particular residue(s) is (are) conserved and/or buried one would have to look into the variability and exposure state of that particular residue. The variability of a residue can be determined by looking into the Kabat database (maintained by Johnson and Wu: http://immuno.

Step 1:   Remove hotspots from FRs.

Step 2:   Remove hotspot that code for
          conserved and buried residues in CDRs.

Step 3:   Keep aside CDR1 and CDR2 hotspots
          (low priority).

Step 4:   Seggregate VH and VL CDR3 hotspots.

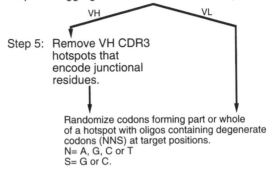

Step 5:   Remove VH CDR3
          hotspots that
          encode junctional
          residues.

          Randomize codons forming part or whole
          of a hotspot with oligos containing degenerate
          codons (NNS) at target positions.
          N= A, G, C or T
          S= G or C.

Fig. 1. Steps involved in the selection of hot spots in antibody V genes for targeting random mutations for in vitro affinity improvement.

bme.nwu.edu). The details of the exposure state of different CDR residues can be determined by referring to Fig. 1A and 1B in **ref. 6** and Tables 1 and 2 in Chapter 14. For most antibodies generally the following holds true. Residues 25, 29, 33 in V_L CDR1; 51 in V_L CDR2; 89, 90, and 97 in V_L CDR3 are buried residues. In the V_H, residues 32 and 34 in CDR1; and residues 51, 52, and 63 in CDR2 are buried. V_H CDR3 usually do not have any buried residue. For example if there is a hot spot covering residues 89 and 90 in V_L then by looking at the Kabat database one will find that position 90 has a fairly conserved glutamine and as mentioned earlier residue 90 is buried. Therefore this hot spot should not be targeted for random mutations (*see* **Note 4**).

3. For the first experiment keep aside hot spots that fall into the CDR1 and 2. Because it is usually CDR3s that contribute mostly to antigen binding, modification of these regions are usually preferred for in vitro affinity maturation. Once the CDR3 hot spots have been worked on one can go back to those in CDR1 and 2 for more engineering.

4. At this point one would be left with hot spots coding only for exposed residues in the CDR3 of V_H and V_L. The exposed residues for V_L CDR3 are good candidates for mutations.

5. Eliminate VHCDR3 hot spot(s) if it (they) code for residues formed by N addition. If the antibody being studied originated from an immunized animal then hot spots covering exposed residues in VH CDR3 should go through another round of consideration. If a hot spot in V_H CDR3 codes for junctional residues, then these should be carefully evaluated. By comparing the V_H CDR3 sequence with the different germline D and J minigenes (available in the Kabat database) one can make out whether the junctional residues were formed by N addition. If they are found to be formed by N addition then do not touch these residues. Because residues formed by N addition already went through a natural selection process in the immunized animal, it is preferred to leave them unchanged. Therefore for the V_H CDR3, only those hot spots should be selected for targeting mutations that

code for residues that are not formed by N addition.

3.3. Random Mutations of Codons Covered by the Selected Hot Spots

This section will describe the steps to randomize the codons that fall within one or more hot spots. A problem that is frequently faced when using one clone as a template to make a randomized library is the overrepresentation of the parental clone from template carry over (background). A good way to overcome this problem is to first insert in the parental clone a stop codon in the region where the randomization is intended to be targeted and then use this as a template to make the library. This eliminates the background contamination by the parental clone. The procedure to do this is described below.

3.3.1. Preparation of the Template for Introducing the Stop Codon by Kunkel's Mutagenesis

Day 1:

1. Cotransform CJ236 cells (electro-competent cells are available from Bio-Rad) with 5 ng of the scFv encoding phagemid and 5 ng of a lac I^q encoding plasmid (*see* **Note 5**).
2. Plate 10–100 μL onto LB $Cm_{30\mu g/mL}$ plates containing 2% glucose for selecting the transformants (*see* **Note 6**).
3. Incubate overnight at 37°C.
4. Streak CJ236 onto a LB $Cm_{30\mu g/mL}$ plate and TG1 onto M63 glucose, B1 plate (*see* **Note 7**).
5. Incubate overnight at 37°C.

Day 2:

1. Inoculate a bacterial loop full of transformants from d 1 plates into 150 mL of LB $Cm_{15\mu g/mL}$ $Glc_{2\%}$ $Uridine_{50\mu g/mL}$ plus the appropriate antibiotics to an initial OD_{600nm} of about 0.1. Use a 2 L baffle flask (*see* **Note 8**). The culture volume can be scaled up or down.
2. Incubate at 37°C with shaking at 250 rpm. Check OD_{600nm} every 30 min.
3. When OD_{600nm} reaches about 0.3, add helper phage, to a multiplicity of infection (m.o.i.) of 3–5 (*see* **Note 9**).
4. Incubate at 37°C with shaking at 100 rpm for 1 h.
5. Incubate at 37°C with shaking at 300 rpm for 6 h. At the end of 4 h, start a 10–15 mL culture of CJ236 in LB $Cm_{15\mu g/mL}$ and a TG1 culture in LB medium (*see* **Note 7**). Incubate at 37°C with shaking at 250 rpm till OD_{600nm} is about 0.3–0.4. Keep ready plates containing LB agar and the antibiotic for the selection of the scFv encoding phagemid (*see* **Note 6**). These plates will be needed for titration.
6. Chill culture.
7. Pellet the cells by centrifuging the chilled culture at 3000g for 15 min at 4°C in a Sorvall RC4B centrifuge or an equivalent.
8. Centrifuge the supernatant from the above step at 17,000g for 15 min at 4°C.
9. Collect supernatant. Save 1 mL in a properly labeled sterile Eppendorf tube.
10. Measure the volume of the rest of the supernatant and add to it one-fifth its volume of cold 20% PEG-2.5 M NaCl. Mix thoroughly but gently (*see* **Note 10**).
11. Store overnight at 4°C.
12. Titrate phage in TG1 (*see* **Note 7**) and CJ236 cells as described in the following **steps 13–25**.
13. Take 8 × 1.5 mL Eppendorf tubes. Mark them 1 to 8.

14. Take 450 µL of 2X YT or LB medium into each tube.

15. Add 50 µL of the culture supernatant to tube 1 (10-fold dilution).

16. Vortex to mix thoroughly.

17. Take 50 µL from this tube and add to the next (tube 2, 100-fold dilution).

18. Likewise continue up to the eighth tube.

19. Take 9×1.8 mL autoclaved Eppendorf tubes and mark them as follows: TG1-10^{-1}, TG1-10^{-2}, TG1-10^{-3}, TG1-10^{-4}, CJ236-10^{-4}, CJ236-10^{-5}, CJ236-10^{-6}, CJ236-10^{-7} and CJ236-10^{-8} (*see* **Note 7**).

20. Pipet 300 µL of fresh TG1 culture (OD_{600nm} of about 0.3) into tubes 1–4 (*see* **Note 7**) and 300 µL of fresh CJ236 culture (OD_{600nm} of about 0.3) into tubes 5–8.

21. Add 100 µL from tubes 1–4 to TG1 tubes (*see* **Note 7**) and 100 µL from tubes 4–8 into CJ236 tubes.

22. Mix by tapping.

23. Incubate at 37°C for 30 min. At the end of 15 min, mix by tapping the contents of the tube again.

24. At the end of incubation, plate 40 µL onto LB plates containing the appropriate antibiotic for the selection of the scFv-gIIIp encoding phagemid (*see* **Note 6**).

25. Incubate overnight at 37°C.

Day 3:

1. Count colonies in plates. Determine titer. The difference in phage titer between TG1 (*see* **Note 5**) and CJ236 cells should typically be between 10,000–100,000-fold. Extract single-stranded uracil containing DNA (ssuDNA) from the phage as described in the following **steps 2–33**:

2. Centrifuge the PEG-NaCl treated culture supernatant from d 2 at 27,000*g* for 30 min at 4°C (*see* **Note 11**).

3. Look for the pellet. Mark the outside of the tube to locate the translucent pellet. Discard supernatant.

4. Invert the centrifuge bottle over an impermeable diaper. Let the trace amount of solution adhering to the centrifuge tube or bottle drain out.

5. Add 10 mL of NET buffer to the pellet. Let it stand for 10–15 min at RT. The pellet will become loose. Resuspend pellet completely by pipetting repeatedly but gently. Transfer the resuspended pellet to a clear (polycarbonate) SS-34 tube (*see* **Note 11**).

6. Centrifuge at 3000*g* for 15 min at 4°C.

7. Collect the supernatant very carefully. Discard pellet (if any) (*see* **Note 12**).

8. Add 2 mL of PEG-NaCl solution to the supernatant. Mix.

9. Keep in ice for 20 min.

10. Centrifuge at 27,000*g* for 30 min at 4°C.

11. Look for the pellet. Discard supernatant.

12. Invert the centrifuge bottle over an impermeable diaper. Let the trace amount of solution adhering to the centrifuge tube or bottle drain out.

13. Add 10 mL of NET buffer to the pellet. Let it stand for 10–15 min at RT. Resuspend pellet completely by pipetting repeatedly but gently. Transfer the resuspended pellet to a clear (polycarbonate) SS-34 tube (*see* **Note 11**).

14. Centrifuge at 3000*g* for 15 min at 4°C. Carefully collect the supernatant into an opaque (polypropylene) SS-34 tube (*see* **Note 13**). Discard pellet (*see* **Note 12**).

15. Add equal volume of buffer saturated phenol (*see* **Note 1**).

16. Vortex for 1 min.
17. Mix/shake at RT for 20 min.
18. Centrifuge at 27,000*g* for 15 min at 4°C.
19. Collect the upper aqueous layer into another polypropylene SS-34 tube. Add equal volume of Phenol: Chloroform: Isoamyl alcohol mixture and vortex for 1 min (*see* **Note 13**).
20. Mix/shake at RT for 15 min.
21. Centrifuge at 27,000*g* for 15 min at 4°C.
22. Collect the upper aqueous layer into another polypropylene SS-34 tube (*see* **Note 13**).
23. Add equal volume of Chloroform and vortex for 1 min.
24. Mix/shake at RT for 15 min.
25. Centrifuge at 27,000*g* for 15 min at 4°C.
26. Measure the volume of the upper aqueous layer and collect into a clear SS-34 clear (polycarbonate) tube (*see* **Note 11**).
27. Add one-tenth the volume of sterile 8 *M* lithium chloride and 3 vol of 100% chilled ethanol. Mix thoroughly (*see* **Note 14**).
28. Keep in dry ice for 20 min.
29. Centrifuge at 27,000*g* for 20 min at 4°C.
30. The pellet will be very light and off-white in color. Carefully decant the supernatant. Invert tube on an impermeable diaper to drain out the remaining solution from the tube.
31. Air-dry sample.
32. Dissolve the pellet in 100–200 µL of 10 m*M* Tris-HCl, pH 7.4.
33. Run a 1.2% agarose gel with 1 and 2 µL sample. The sample should show a distinct and clean band. Although the ssuDNA will be half the size of the scFv-gIIIp encoding phagemid, in the gel it might run with an apparent lower molecular weight because of secondary structure formation.

3.3.2. Designing the Oligonucleotide for Inserting the Stop Codon (see **Note 15**)

The design of the oligonucleotide for Kunkel's mutagenesis depends on the orientation of the gene of interest and the direction of the F' origin of replication. Follow the following rules.

1. If the gene of interest and the F' ori are in the clockwise direction then the oligo should be made complementary to the coding strand of the gene.
2. If the gene of interest is in the clockwise direction and the F' ori in the anti-clockwise direction then the oligo should be complementary to the noncoding strand of the gene.
3. If the gene of interest is in the anti-clockwise direction and the F' ori is in the clockwise direction then the oligo should be complementary to the noncoding strand and
4. If the gene of interest and the F' ori are both in the anti-clockwise direction then oligo should be complementary to the coding strand of the gene. The oligo should be designed in such a way that it introduces a TAA stop codon at or near the site where random mutations will be targeted. Keeping 12–15 nucleotides at either side of the mutagenic region (which introduces the TAA codon) that anneals perfectly with the ssuDNA is sufficient.

3.3.3. Phosphorylation of Oligo

The volume of the reaction components listed here can be scaled up or down as desired.

Add:

Water	25 μL
10X Ligase buffer	~~03 μL~~
Oligo (250 pmol/μL)	01 μL
Polynucleotide kinase (10U/μL)	01 μL
	30 μL

1. Mix by tapping. Gerntly vortex. Spin briefly (5 s).
2. Incubate at 37°C for 30 min.
3. Heat at 65°C for 10 min.
4. Store in ice temporarily. (For long term, store at –20°C.)

3.3.4. Annealing of the Template and Oligo

1. The amount of phosphorylated oligo is typically kept between 8–10 pmol. 5–10 ng of template is sufficient. Before starting the annealing step keep ready one heat block at 72–75°C and another at around 15–18°C. Prepare the following tubes

	Tube no.	
	1(expt.)	2 (cont.)
Water	7 μL	8 μL
10X Annealing buffer	1 μL	1 μL
Template (diluted in water)	1 μL	1 μL
Phosphorylated oligo(s)	1 μL	0
	10 μL	10 μL

(If more than one oligo is being used, then it is important to use them at equimolar amount. The volume can be adjusted by reducing the amount of water used.)

2. Mix by tapping. Vortex. Spin briefly.
3. Put the tubes in 72°C heat block for 2 min.
4. Take another heat block kept at around 15–18°C. Put it on the table.
5. At the end of 2 min put the 72°C heat block with the annealing tubes in it over the colder heat block on the table.
6. Leave it there for 1 h or until the temperature of the top block gets down to <30°C.
7. Store the tubes in ice or at 4°C.

3.3.5. Extension

1. Add the following to the annealing tubes.

	Tube no.	
	1(expt.)	2 (cont.)
10X Synthesis buffer	1.3 μL	1.3 μL
T4 DNA Ligase (3 U/μL)	1.0 μL	1.0 μL
T7 DNA Polymerase		

(1 U/μL diluted 1:1 in	1.0 μL	
T7 Pol dilution buffer)	———	———
	13.3 μL	13.3 μL

2. Mix by tapping. Vortex gently. Spin briefly.
3. Incubate in ice for 10 min.
4. Incubate at RT for 10 min.
5. Incubate at 37°C for 2 h.
6. Store in ice.
7. Transform competent TG1 cells (*see* **Notes 7** and **16**).
8. Plate 10, 25, 50, and 100 μL onto LB agar plates containing $Glc_{2\%}$ and the appropriate antibiotic for selecting the scFv-gIIIp encoding phagemid.
9. Incubate overnight at 37°C.
10. Analyze clones for the introduction of the TAA mutation.

3.3.6. Mutagenesis for Introducing Random Mutations into the Selected Hot spots

The construction of the randomized library can be done in two different ways: One is by Kunkel's mutagenesis and the other is by "splicing by overlap extension" (SOE) PCR. For both of these methods the scFv-gIIIp encoding phagemid with a TAA stop codon is used as the template.

3.3.7. Randomization of Hot Spots by Kunkel's Mutagenesis

This involves the same steps of making ssuDNA as in **Subheading 3.3.1.** The only difference is that the ssuDNA is made for the TAA containing phagemid instead of the original parental phagemid.

3.3.8. Designing of the Oligonucleotides for Randomized Library

The basic rules for designing the oligos will be the same as in **Subheading 3.3.2.** except for the following. One has to keep in mind the following points. 1) The codons falling into the hot spot regions has to be randomized and 2) if the TAA stop codon was inserted outside the hot spot region then it has to be reverted back to the original codon or one that encodes the wild-type amino acid. Thus, the oligos to be used for the randomization step should have degenerate codons. A good degenerate codon is NNS (N = A, G, C OR T and S = G or C). This codes for all the amino acids but not the TAA and TGA stop codons. Although it codes for TAG stop codon, this is not a serious drawback because TG1 is a supE strain and can read through TAG codons. Therefore while designing the oligo one should substitute all the codons falling either wholly or partly into the hot spot with NNS codons.

3.3.9. Mutagenesis (see **Note 17**)

This step is essentially the same as **Subheadings 3.3.3.–3.3.5.** But in this step one should be particularly careful about the amount of template to be used. The results of the titration experiment described in d 2, **steps 14–25** in **Subheading 3.3.1.** would indicate the approximate number of phage particles that were used for extracting the ssuDNA. For example one may have a total volume of 200 μL of the ssuDNA obtained from 10^{11} phage particles. Now if one tries to randomize 4 codons the minimum library size would be 20^4 or 1.6×10^5. To get a complete representation of all clones one would have to make a library of about 1.6×10^6. To achieve this one should typically take enough ssuDNA that would have about 10^7 to 10^8 copies of the template. In other words, one should take between 0.02–0.2 µL stock solution of the ssuDNA. This is important since in Kunkel's mutagenesis the complexity of the library being made would dependent directly on the number of template molecules that are being used in addition to the diversity in the oligos employed for mutagenesis. The other thing that one should do while making a library is ethanol precipitate the DNA after the extension reaction and resuspend it in 5–10 µL of water. This is important for good transformation efficiency.

3.3.10. Randomization of Hot Spots by "Splicing by Overlap Extension" (SOE) PCR (see **Note 18**)

SOE PCR is a well-established method of introducing mutations in a given gene. Therefore it is not being discussed in detail here. The important steps are shown in **Fig. 2** and are listed below.

1. Take the scFv containing phagemid with the TAA stop codon introduced in or near the hot spot region.
2. Linearize the phagemid with two unique restriction enzymes that are outside the scFv and that do not form compatible ends.
3. Purify the phagemid fragment that contains the scFv-gIIIp gene.
4. Use this fragment to set up two PCR reactions using sets of two primers (primers 1 and 2 in one tube and primers 3 and 4 in the other tube) to get two different fragments of the scFv gene, which overlap partially in the region where mutation is being targeted.
5. Purify the fragments and splice them together using only the outer primers (1 and 4).
6. Purify the full-length product.
7. Digest the fragment with unique restriction enzymes flanking the scFv gene and purify the fragment.
8. Also digest the TAA containing phagemid with the same restriction enzymes used for the scFv and purify the backbone fragment.
9. Ligate the two using about 300–400 ng of the insert and about 75 ng of the vector (maintaining an approximate molar ratio of about 1:1–1:3).
10. Purify the ligation product by ethanol precipitation and resuspend in 5–10 µL of distilled water. Use this to transform TG1 cells (number of transformation will depend on the library size desired).

3.4. Construction and Panning of the Phage Library (see **Note 19**)

This is described elsewhere in this book and therefore will not be discussed in detail. An important point to be noted here is that during panning one should be able to see enrichment of binders. Typically for libraries made by targeting random mutations to hot spots an enrichment of about 200 fold occurs by the end of round 2. This becomes about 2000 by round 3 and then plateaus off. However, these values can vary.

3.5. Analysis of the Binders (see Note 20)

Analysis of binders following panning is also discussed elsewhere in this volume and therefore will not be discussed here. However, after analysis one should be able to see a number of phage clones that will have better binding characteristics than the parental clone. A prototypical ELISA result is shown in **Fig. 3**. A drawback of the phage system for affinity maturation of scFvs (and also for panning out binders from an immunized or naive library) is that it is not free from interference due to avidity effects. In other words analysis of phage binding can be misleading because some phage clones may have more copies of the scFvs displayed per particle than others or some clones may have greater percentage of particles displaying the scFv than other clones. Therefore before choosing any particular phage clone (for downstream application of the scFv) based on initial analysis, it is important to compare the relative levels of scFv molecules displayed on the various selected mutants and the parental type. This can be done in a dot-blot format. This experiment is dependent on the presence of a peptide tag between the scFv and the gIIIp. A peptide tag is usually present in all phage-display constructs that are commonly used. The protocol for this method is described below:

1. Purify recombinant phage particles (wild-type and mutants) by PEG-NaCl precipitation and titrate them.
2. On two separate nitrocellulose or PVDF membranes spot different number of phage ranging from 10^8–10^{11} or more. Include M13KO7 helper phage as a control.
3. Probe one membrane with anti-gVIIIp antibody and the other with the anti-tag antibody. Since the scFv-gIIIp is expressed in low amount the anti-tag antibody should be used at low dilution (1:500 to 1:1000) and since gVIIIp is expressed at very high amount the anti-gVIIIp antibody should be used at higher dilution (1:5000 to 1:10,000). The details of doing a dot-blot experiment is not included here. The method for spotting the sample would depend on the apparatus used and treatment of the membranes will be like any Western-blot experiment described elsewhere in this volume.

Figure 4 is a hypothetical figure provided to help explain what one should expect to see in this type of dot-blot experiment. One should see in the membrane probed with anti-gVIIIp a similar degree of staining intensity for each dilution for all samples including M13KO7. This intensity should decrease with decrease in number of the phage particles applied to the membrane. But in the membrane probed with anti-tag antibody, the intensity of staining may vary across a given dilution for different samples and this would indicate the relative expression of the scFv on the surface of the phage particles. Typically one should focus on those mutants that give the same or less signal compared to the wild-type clone for a given dilution (e.g., Mut 2 in the the **Fig. 4**). In this blot one should not see any signal for M13KO7.

Based on the results of the dot-blot experiment the scFvs from the promising clones should be purified and the affinity of the purified sample should be compared to the wild-type scFv. Details for this is described elsewhere in this volume. Alternatively, one can make fusion proteins with the wild-type and the selected mutant scFvs and compare their affinity and other biological activity. A typical example of this type of study can be found in **refs. 4** and **5**.

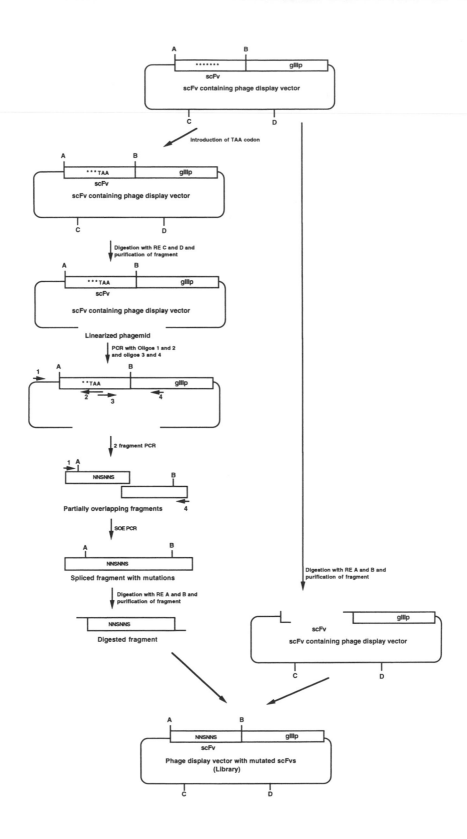

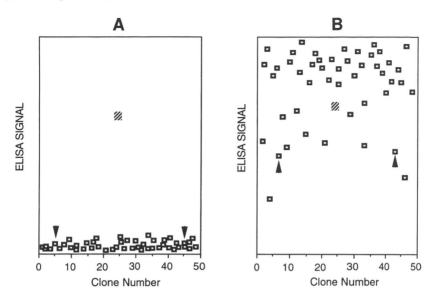

Fig. 3. A prototypical illustration of what one is likely to see in an ELISA assay of culture supernatants containing phage particles recovered from clones obtained after panning a hot spot randomized library. Each square symbol represents phage particles from one single clone. Panel **A** represents ELISA of the phage clones on an irrelevant antigen (e.g., BSA) and panel **B** represent ELISA done on the relevant antigen. The phage particles should specifically bind only to the antigen on which they were selected. Occasionally one may come across clones (hatched square) that bind to both the antigens. These represent nonspecific binders. During these assays, it is important to include the wild type parental clone during phage rescue and ELISA to compare the difference in antigen binding between the mutated clones and the parental clone. In the diagram parental clone is shown twice, represented by open square and marked with an arrow. From a hot spot randomized library one would see a number of clones that show better binding than the parental clone and few that could have lower or comparable binding. The titer of phage for randomly picked samples should be done to verify whether they are comparable.

Fig. 2. *(opposite page)* Flow diagram to illustrate the steps involved in PCR mediated construction of a randomized library starting from a single template. Introduction of a TAA stop codon and linearizing the phagemid eliminates template carry over and background contamination of the library by the wild type clone. Restriction enzymes A and B represent the cloning sites for the scFv. Restriction enzymes C and D are unique sites in the phagemid and are uncompatible with each other. * Represents the hot spots to be randomized. Primers 1 and 4 anneal to sites about 50 to 100 nucleotides away from the scFv. This creates a fragment that can be efficiently cleaved by enzymes A and B. Primers 2 and 3 are degenerate mutagenic primers. These primers have complementary 5' ends which helps to splice the fragments they generate in a "splicing by overlap extension" PCR. Digestion of the spliced fragment is followed by its ligation into the parental phagemid backbone obtained by digestion with the same enzymes, A and B.

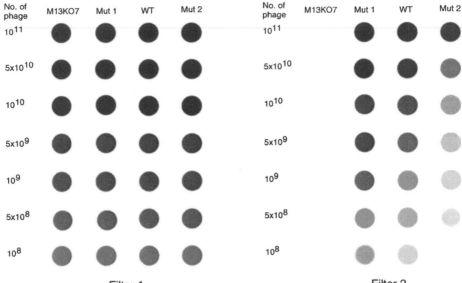

Fig. 4. A prototypic illustration of how one can make an estimate of the relative level of scFv expression on the surface of phage particles from different clones. M13KO7 should be used as a control. Mut 1 and 2 represent two mutant clones with greater antigen binding by ELISA in a preliminary screening assay. Different number of purified phage particles are to be spotted onto two different nitrocellulose or PVDF membranes. One should be developed with anti-gVIIIp antibody while the other should be developed with an anti-tag antibody. The relative intensity of the mutants with respect to each other and to the parental clone would give an indication of the expression of the scFv on each clone. If the intensities are same or lower and ELISA signals are different then the one with lower intensity in the dot blot but comparable or higher signal in ELISA is likely to have greater affinity and vice versa.

4. Notes

1. Phenol should be distilled, buffer saturated and stored in amber colored bottles at 4°C.
2. Should be stored in amber colored bottles at 4°C.
3. Ethanol (100% and 70%) can be chilled in –20°C freezers. Do not use a self-defrosting freezer to store any volatile or flammable material.
4. Residues are numbered based on the Kabat numbering scheme.
5. CJ236 does not have a lacI^q gene. Therefore, lacI^q containing plasmid is required to stop any leaky expression of the scFv-gIIIp fusion protein that affects bacterial growth. The other important point to remember is that the scFv-gIIIp containing phagemid, the lacI^q containing plasmid and the helper phage should have different *E. coli* origin of replication and/or selection markers to co-exists together in the CJ236 cells.
6. If using a phage-display vector include 2% glucose to the medium.
7. DH5αF' cells can be used instead of TG1. DH5αF' will grow on LB plates.
8. One can scale up or down the volume of culture for preparing ssuDNA.

9. Do not use helper phage at a multiplicity of infection (m.o.i.) of greater than 3–5.

10. This can be done either in autoclaved glass bottles or polycarbonate centrifuge bottles or tubes.

11. Use a polycarbonate tube whenever there is a need to see and collect the phage or DNA pellet.

12. This pellet represents trace amount of contaminating bacterial cells.

13. Use polypropylene centrifuge tubes when using organic solvents like phenol, phenol:chloroform:isoamyl alcohol and chloroform for extraction of ssuDNA.

14. Lithium chloride should be used for precipitating the ssuDNA because it does not precipitate with DNA during ethanol precipitation and therefore the ssuDNA obtained is relatively free of salts.

15. Introduction of the TAA stop codon is a crucial step. Although TGA is known to be a good stop codon, it can be leaky under some circumstances and therefore would not serve the purpose of eliminating the background representation of wild-type phage in a library.

16. Getting good-quality plasmid DNA from TG1 is sometimes difficult. If using any of the commercial plasmid purification kits wash the colums 2–3× before eluting the plasmid DNA.

17. If one makes a library by Kunkel's mutagenesis the quality of the ssuDNA should be very good. Any bacterial chromosomal DNA, helper phage DNA and small molecular-weight DNA and RNA fragments that runs with the bromophenol blue in an agarose gel can be very deleterious. Tricks to get a good-quality ssuDNA involves the following:

    a. Do not use helper phage at a multiplicity of infection (m.o.i.) of greater than 3–5.

    b. Using helper phage R408 is useful because it is packaging deficient and therefore is not produced very efficiently in the presence of a phagemid with normal phage origin of replication (such as the scFv containing phagemid). To calculate the m.o.i. one may note that 1 OD_{600nm} unit of CJ236 contains about 5×10^8 bacteria.

    c. When recovering the phage for making ssuDNA do not let the culture age for more than 7 h post-helper-phage addition.

    d. When harvesting the ssuDNA containing phage, as mentioned in **Subheading 3.3.1.**, do at least two rounds of centrifugation to get rid of any bacteria remaining in suspension. Also when the phage particles are PEG purified additional centrifugation steps between PEG precipitation (as mentioned in **Subheading 3.3.1.**) helps to get rid of trace contaminants of bacteria.

18. When making a PCR based library it is important to purify the fragments at each step. Commercial PCR purification kits are good but they do not completely get rid of the primers. Gel purification is a better way to purify PCR products. Recovery of the fragment from agarose gels can be done by electroelution or by using gel purification kits. There are several commercial kits available in the market and all of them have good performance. An important point to note is that some of these kits involve a isopropanol washing step. The author has found that this greatly reduces the recovery of DNA without any improvement in quality of the recovered fragment. Bypassing the isopropanol step increases the recovery greatly.

19. Rescued phage samples as well as the phage samples eluted after panning should be treated like proteins. Unless required for the purpose of experiment these samples should always be kept at 4°C.

20. Success of the analysis step depends upon (a) accurate titration of the phage samples and (b) identification of false positive signals. Like most other screening systems false positive signal is of common occurrence with the phage display system. What it means is a particular phage clone may show very good antigen binding property, but the scFv on its surface may have a much lower affinity or be nonspecific. Therefore, preliminary screening should be done on both the actual antigen and on a negative control antigen. Also,

chances for a false positive clone should be addressed immediately after a preliminary screening identifies the specific binders. The dot blot analysis is helpful before selecting a particular scFv for downstream application.

References

1. Betz, A. G., Neuberger, M. S., and Milstein, C. (1993) Discriminating intrinsic and antigen-selected mutational hot spots in immunoglobulin V genes. *Immunol. Today* **14,** 405–411.
2. Neuberger M. S. and Milstein C. (1995) Somatic Hypermutation. *Curr. Opi. Immunol.* **7,** 248–254.
3. Jolly, C. J., Wagner, S. D., Rada, C., Klix, N., Milstein, C., and Neuberger, M. S. (1996) The targeting of somatic hypermutation. *Semimars Immunol.* **8,** 159–168.
4. Chowdhury, P. S. and Pastan, I. (1999) Improving antibody affinity by mimicking somatic hypermutation in vitro. *Nat. Biotechnol.* **17,** 568–572.
5. Beers, R., Chowdhury, P. Bigner, D., and Pastan, I. (2000) Immunotoxins with increased activity against epidermal growth factor receptor vIII-expressing cell lines produced by antibody phage display. *Clin. Can. Res.* **6,** 2835–2843.
6. Chowdhury, P. S., Vasmatzis, G., Beers, R., Lee, B.-K., and Pastan, I. (1998) Improved stability and yields of a Fv-toxin fusion protein by computer design and protein engineering of the Fv. *J. Mol. Biol.* **281,** 917–928.

12

Simultaneous Humanization and Affinity Optimization of Monoclonal Antibodies

Herren Wu

1. Introduction

Monoclonal antibodies (MAbs) have broad therapeutic applications in cancer therapy, prevention and treatment of viral infection, immune suppression, etc. However, many well-characterized MAbs are derived from murine sources, and these antibodies have been shown to induce strong immunogenicity when administered into the human body. The ensuring human anti-mouse antibody (HAMA) response consequently can induce fast clearance of administered antibodies from serum resulting in significantly reduced efficacy. In addition, murine MAbs also have weak effector function in human, which is important for certain clinical applications. To overcome these shortcomings, humanization techniques are used to modify nonhuman MAbs for therapeutic use. Humanization can reduce and potentially eliminate the human immune response to administered foreign antibodies. It is a critical step in maximizing the usage of MAbs as therapeutic agents.

The principle of humanization is to convert nonhuman MAbs into human-like antibodies while maintaining their designated function. Two methodologies have allowed the development of humanization techniques. The first development is the construction of chimeric antibodies (1–2). Chimeric antibodies are produced by combining the V regions of murine MAbs with the constant regions of human antibodies. The modified antibodies usually retain full function. Yet in most cases, this modification can only reduce, not eliminate, the human immune response because the chimeric antibodies are only partially human-like (about 67%) (3,4). As a result, chimeric antibodies have limited therapeutic use and are often used for acute or short-term treatments.

The second development enabling humanization is complementarity-determining regions "CDR" grafting (5). In this method, antibodies are constructed by transplanting murine CDR loops, which are the antigen binding site, onto a human antibody framework. The resulting antibodies are ≈ 92% human-like, thus reducing the

From: Methods in Molecular Biology, vol. 207: Recombinant Antibodies for Cancer Therapy: Methods and Protocols
Edited by: M. Welschof and J. Krauss © Humana Press Inc., Totowa, NJ

potential for human immune response significantly. The remaining ≈8% difference is found within CDR loops, which naturally are highly diversified, and thus, are less likely to elicit immunogenicity. However, CDR-grafted antibodies often do not retain full antigen-binding ability *(6,7)*. Certain mouse framework residues have been shown to be involved in supporting the conformation of CDR loops, and some are even involved in contacting the antigen. Therefore, in order to maintain the binding affinity, these key mouse residues need to be retained. Although assessment of the contribution of framework residues specific to antibody affinity can be complicated, structural modeling has been used in humanization with success. However, the complexity that arises from the large number of framework residues that are potentially involved in binding ability has slowed the rate of success. Furthermore, in many cases, enhancement in antibody affinity becomes desirable so that potency may increase while material costs may decrease. The affinity maturation focused on CDR mutagenesis is usually performed after the antibody is humanized *(8)*. This stepwise approach consumes considerable time and potentially obscures the beneficial combinations of framework and CDR residues.

Therefore, a one-step approach for the humanization and affinity optimization of nonhuman MAbs would be beneficial. Such an approach as described herein results in the identification of humanized antibodies that have higher affinity than the parent MAb. Although this process was first developed for the humanization and optimization of a murine MAb against the human CD40 receptor *(9)*, the method can be applied to any nonhuman MAb. The underlying principle of this approach entails the construction of a combinatorial library that contains human/murine wobble residues in key framework positions for humanization, along with single mutations in CDR regions for affinity optimization. The constructed library is screened for humanized clones that display higher affinity than the parental antibody.

For humanization, the most homologous human germline sequence is used. Human CDR regions are replaced with murine CDR counterparts. The framework residues that differ between murine sequence and the human template are assessed for their effect on antigen binding, antibody folding, and immunogenicity. Residues that are likely to affect affinity are rated as "high-risk" residues. The high-risk residues include canonical residues, which determine the main chain conformation of the CDRs *(10)*, and contact residues, which interact with the opposite domain in the V_H-V_L interface. Other "high-risk" factors to be aware of are: (1) proximity to CDRs; (2) potential glycosylation site; (3) rare residues; and (4) residues within the "Vernier" zone, which forms a layer underlying the CDRs, and are positioned to support and adjust the CDR conformation for antigen binding *(11)*. Both surface-exposed *(12)* and buried murine residues are changed to the corresponding human amino acids if the residues are not rated at high risk. Predicted importance of framework residues in modulating CDR activity *(13)*, and the relatedness of amino acids are also incorporated into the assessment. Framework residues that are at high risk are constructed as human/murine wobble residues in the combinatorial library for characterization.

For affinity optimization, single mutations rather than total randomization are introduced in the CDR regions for the following reasons: (1) single mutations mimic the in vivo affinity maturation as antibodies acquire improved affinity through the accumulation of beneficial single mutations in vivo; (2) total randomization of CDR regions destroys the in vivo selected binding sites; and (3) single mutations result in a focused small-size library that facilitates quicker screening. Since the affinity and specificity of antibodies are often determined predominantly by the heavy-chain CDR3 (HCDR3) and secondarily by the light chain CDR3 (LCDR3), the single mutation library is made to encompass changes in both HCDR3 and LCDR3, or HCDR3 alone.

There are three key steps in this approach: (1) assay development for screening; (2) construction of a combinatorial library; and (3) screening and characterization. A M13-based phage-expression vector containing backbones for human IgG1 CH1 and Cκ is used in this approach (**Fig. 1**) *(14,15)*. However, common phage display vectors and panning technology can also be adapted for this system. Hybridization mutagenesis *(16)* is used for the construction of combinatorial libraries. In the case of simultaneous humanization and affinity optimization of the anti-CD40 antibody *(9)*, exhaustive screening of the combinatorial framework-HCDR3 (FR-H3) library $(2.0 \times 10^6$ clones screened) resulted in the identification of a humanized antibody with 10-fold higher affinity than the parent antibody. Conversely, only the partial screening of the combinatorial framework-HCDR3-LCDR3 (FR-H3-L3) library led to the identification of a humanized antibody with 200-fold higher affinity than the parent antibody. Interestingly, even though less than 2% of the FR-H3-L3 library was screened $(5.5 \times 10^5$ clones), the affinity of the best clone identified was better than that of the best clone identified from the exhaustive screening of the FR-H3 library. This may be owing to the fact that partial screening had sampled enough clones to identify certain beneficial mutations in HCDR3 and LCDR3, and the combinatorial effect of the beneficial mutations leads to higher affinity than a single mutation alone. If the key framework residues affecting the affinity are less than the number of selected wobble framework positions characterized in the library, the number of clones needed to be screened will be lowered significantly. In the optimization of the anti-CD40 antibody, the redundant clones and the consensus beneficial CDR mutations were identified in the FR-H3-L3 library, suggesting that the library was screened thoroughly enough. The combinatorial FR-H3 library is used as an example in this chapter to illustrate the methodology.

2. Materials

2.1. Escherichia coli *Strains*

1. CJ236 (Bio-Rad).
2. DH10B (Gibco-BRL).
3. XL-I-Blue (Stratagene).

2.2. Enzymes

1. *pfu* DNA polymerase (2.5 U/μL) (Strategene).
2. T4 polynucleotide kinase (10 U/μL) (Roche).
3. T4 DNA ligase (1 U/μL) (Roche).
4. T4 DNA polymerase (1 U/μL) (Roche).
5. *Eco*RI (10 U/μL) (Roche).

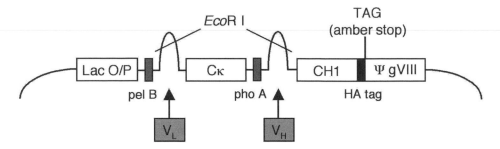

Fig. 1. The partial region of the phage vector involved in Fab expression. The M13-based phage vector contains the constant region of human kappa chain (Cκ) and the first constant region of the human γ1 chain (CH1). Single-stranded DNA of V_H and V_L chain is annealed simultaneously to the distinct cloning site containing a palindromic loop. Each palindromic loop contains a unique EcoRI site which enables the removal of the vectors that do not incorporate both V_H and V_L chains. A decapeptide tag (HA tag) fused at the end of CH1 region is for the detection of heavy chain expression.

2.3. Antibodies

1. Goat anti-human kappa antibody (mouse adsorbed) (Southern Biotechnology Associates Inc., cat. no. 2060-01, 1 mg/mL).
2. Goat anti-human kappa-alkaline phosphatase conjugate (mouse adsorbed) (Southern Biotechnology Associates Inc., cat. no. 2060-04).
3. Goat anti-mouse IgG_{2b} (γ_{2b} chain specific)-alkaline phosphatase conjugate (Southern Biotechnology Associates Inc., cat. no. 1090-04).

2.4. Buffers and Solutions

2.4.1. Capture Lift, Filter Lift, and SPE

1. Carbonate coating buffer, pH 9.3: 0.015 M Na_2CO_3 (1.86 g/L) and 0.035 M $NaHCO_3$ (2.94 g/L).
2. Phosphate-buffered saline (PBS), pH 7.2: 0.14 M NaCl, 2.7 mM KCl, 1.5 mM KH_2PO_4, and 8.1 mM Na_2HPO_4.
3. PBS/0.1% Tween 20: PBS containing 0.1% Tween-20.
4. 1% Bovine serum albumin (BSA)/PBS: PBS containing 1% (w/v) BSA.
5. 3% BSA/PBS: PBS containing 3% (w/v) BSA.
6. Blotto blocking solution: 5% nonfat powdered milk, 0.2 % Tween 20, 0.01% antifoam A emulsion (Sigma, cat. no. A-5758), and 0.01% thimerosal (Sigma, cat. no. T-5125) in PBS.
7. Reagents for alkaline phosphatase-based capture lifts or filter lifts:
   a. AP buffer (substrate buffer): 0.1 M Tris-HCl, pH 9.5.
   b. Substrate A (NBT): 40 mM nitro blue tetrazolium (2,2'-di-p-nitrophenyl-5,5'-diphenyl-3,3'-[3,3'-dimethoxy-4,4'-diphenylene]ditetrazolium chloride (Sigma, cat. no. N-6876) in 70% N,N-dimethyl formamide).
   c. Substrate B (BCIP): 38 mM 5-bromo-4-chloro-3-indoxyl phosphate mono-(p-toluidinium) salt (JBL scientific, Inc., cat. no. 1280C) in 100% N,N-dimethyl formamide.
   d. AP substrate: Add substrate A and B both at 1:100 dilution in AP buffer.

8. Reagents for alkaline phosphatase-based ELISAs:
   a. Substrate buffer (store in the dark): 0.2 M AMP (2-amino-2-methyl-1-propanol) (JBL Scientific, Inc., cat. no. 1250B), 0.5 M Tris-HCl, pH 10.2, 0.1% sodium azide. To make 1 L of substrate buffer: 19.8 g AMP (stock AMP is 9.59 M and has a density of 0.950 g/mL), 60.55 g Trizma base, 1 g sodium azide. Adjust pH to 10.2 with concentrated HCl.
   b. PMP substrate (phenolphthalein monophosphate) (JBL Scientific, Inc., cat. no. 1270D): Dissolve 0.3 g of substrate in 50 mL of substrate buffer. Add 50 μL per well to develop. Solution is stable for 1–2 wk when stored at 25°C in the dark.
   c. Stop buffer: 30 mM Tris-HCl, pH 10.2, 15 mM EDTA. *Note:* Reactions are terminated with equal volume of stop buffer. Absorbance at 560 nm is measured.

2.4.2. Others

1. 2X B&W buffer: 10 mM Tris-HCl, pH 7.5, 1 mM EDTA, 2 M NaCl, and 0.1% Tween-20.
2. 10X Annealing buffer: 200 mM Tris-HCl, pH 7.0, 500 mM NaCl, and 20 mM MgCl$_2$.
3. 10X Synthesis buffer: 5 mM dNTP, 10 mM ATP, 100 mM Tris-HCl, pH 7.4, 50 mM MgCl$_2$, and 20 mM DTT. Store at –20°C.
4. Top agar: 0.75% agar in LB medium. Maintain at 50–55°C in an incubator.
5. Phage elution buffer: 10 mM Tris-HCl, pH 7.4, and 100 mM NaCl.
6. Resuspension buffer for extracting Fab from periplasmic space: 50 mM Tris-HCl, pH 8.0, 1 mM EDTA, and 500 mM sucrose.

2.5. Miscellaneous Materials

1. Streptavidin-coated magnetic beads (Roche).
2. Nitrocellulose filter (82 mm) (Schleicher & Schuell Protran, cat. no. 20440).

3. Methods
3.1. Construction of Chimeric Fab

For assay development, chimeric Fab is expressed using an appropriate phage-expression vector (*see* **Fig. 1**). Murine V_H and V_L genes are amplified by polymerase chain reaction (PCR) using *pfu* DNA polymerase. To clone both genes into a M13-based vector by hybridization mutagenesis *(16)*, single-stranded DNA (ssDNA) encoding V_H and V_L, respectively, is prepared by using streptavidin-coated magnetic beads (*see* **Note 1**). Purified minus-strand ssDNA of V_H and V_L chain is annealed simultaneously to the distinct cloning site containing a palindromic loop in the phage vector, and the annealed DNA is elongated by DNA polymerase, and linked by DNA ligase. The synthesized DNA is then electroporated into DH 10B cells for phage packaging. The resultant phage can be used to infect XL-1-Blue cells for the production of chimeric Fab. Each palindromic loop contains a unique *Eco*RI site, which enables the removal of the vectors that do not incorporate both V_H and V_L chains (*see* **Subheading 3.1.2.**, step 4.

3.1.1. Preparation of Single-Stranded DNA

1. PCR amplification of V_L and V_H gene: Biotinylated forward primer containing sequence specific to the framework 1 region and an overhanging sequence annealed to the end of leader sequence (pel B or pho A), and reverse primer from the conserved constant region

(Cκ or CH1) are used to amplify the V gene under standard PCR conditions. Reverse primer for Cκ is 5'-CTC TGT GAC ACT CTC CTG GGA-3' (153 bp downstream from the beginning of Cκ). Reverse primer for CH1 is 5'-GTA GTC CTT GAC CAG GCA-3' (78 bp downstream from the beginning of CH1). The right size for heavy (H) chain is 489 bp, and for light (L) chain is 525 bp.

2. Purify PCR products from agarose gel, or by using commercial PCR purification kit. The removal of unincorporated biotinylated primers and nonspecific PCR products is important so as not to interfere with the latter steps.

3. 5'-Phosphorylation of PCR product: 2 μg PCR product, 1 μL of T4 polynucleotide kinase (10 U/μL), 2 μL of 10X PNK buffer, 1 μL of 10 mM ATP in a total volume of 20 μL adjusted by ddH$_2$O. Incubate at 37°C for 45 min, and heat inactivate at 65°C for 10 min. Bring reaction volume to 200 μL by adding ddH$_2$O for the next step.

4. Wash 100 μL of streptavidin-coated magnetic beads twice with 200 μL 2X B&W buffer (100 μL beads, equal to 1 mg, can bind more than 3.3 μg 500 bp-PCR product). Resuspend beads in 200 μL 2X B&W buffer.

5. Mix phosphorylated PCR product with beads, and incubate at room temperature (RT) for 16 min with mild shaking.

6. Sediment beads, and wash twice with 200 μL 2X B&W buffer.

7. Elute non-biotinylated ssDNA (minus strand) with 300 μL freshly prepared 0.15 M NaOH at RT for 10 min with mild shaking. A second NaOH elution can increase the yield slightly (optional). Centrifuge the eluant to remove any trace of beads.

8. Precipitate ssDNA from the supernatant by adding 1 μL glycogen (20 mg/mL), 1/10 vol of 3 M NaOAc, pH 5.2, and 2.5 vol of EtOH. Wash precipitated ssDNA with 70% EtOH. Lyophilize for 3 min and dissolve in 20 μL dd H$_2$O (*see* **Note 2**). Quantitate the ssDNA by spotting on ethidium bromide (EtBr) agarose plate with DNA standards, or by measuring OD$_{260}$. The sample is ready for cloning.

3.1.2. Cloning of V_H and V_L into the Phage-Expression Vector

V_H and V_L are cloned into the phage-expression vector by hybridization mutagenesis *(16)* using reagents described in the Mut-Gene M13 In Vitro Mutagenesis Kit (Bio-Rad).

1. Prepare uridinylated templates by infecting CJ236 *E. coli* strain (*dut⁻ ung⁻*) with M13-based phage (phage-expression vector).

2. Set up an annealing reaction using ≈8-fold molar ratio increase of insert to vector: 200 ng of uridinylated phage vector (8.49 kb), 92 ng phosphorylated single-stranded H chain (489 bases), 100 ng phosphorylated single-stranded L chain (525 bases), 1 μL 10X annealing buffer. Adjust total volume with ddH$_2$O to 10 μL. Carry out the annealing reaction in the PCR machine: 85°C hold for 5 min (denaturation). Ramp to 55°C over 1 h. Chill on ice.

3. Minus strand synthesis: To the annealed product add: 1.4 μL 10X synthesis buffer, 1 μL T4 DNA ligase (1 U/μL), 1 μL T4 DNA polymerase (1 U/μL). Incubate on ice for 5 min, RT for 5 min, and 37°C for 1.5 h. Ethanol precipitate, and dissolve DNA pellet in 10 μL of ddH$_2$O.

4. Digest DNA with 1 μL *Eco*RI (10 U/μL) for 2 h at 37°C, and heat inactivate at 65°C for 20 min. Transfect 1 μL of digested DNA into 30 μL of electrocompetent DH10B cells by electroporation. Titer the produced phage by growing on an XL-I-Blue bacterial lawn at 37°C overnight. Sequence to validate the anticipated cloning.

3.2. Assay Developments

3.2.1. Capture Lift Assay

The capture lift assay (*see* **Fig. 2**) was developed for the initial high throughput screening of large libraries *(9,17)*. This assay is semiquantitative, and by using this procedure up to 10^5 clones can be screened from one 82-mm filter. Normally, one million clones can be screened in a day. Phage-expressed chimeric Fab is used for establishing the screening conditions, such as the concentration of antigen and capturing antibody (*see* **Note 3**), incubation time, washing, and the choice of secondary antibody (or NeutrAvidin-alkaline phosphatase if biotinylated antigen is used). Once a strong specific signal is easily reproduced (shown as clear deep-color spots), the concentration of antigen is gradually reduced until the signal is barely detectable (very faint spots). Under such conditions, during the screening of the combinatorial library, only those spots that have a deeper color than chimeric Fab are eventually isolated. These clones should have higher affinity than chimeric Fab. The established conditions and steps used in the selection of high affinity humanized anti-CD40 antibodies *(9)* are listed below:

1. Place 10 mL of 10 µg/mL goat anti-human kappa antibody in PBS into a 100-mm Petri dish.
2. Label an 82-mm nitrocellulose filter with nonwater-soluble ink. Using tweezers, carefully float the filter, label side up, above antibody solution for at least 2 h at RT. Then, flip the filter, submerge it in the solution, and shake for 20–30 min.
3. Remove the filter, blot excess buffer lightly off the edge of the filter, and lay the filter with label side down on a sheet of Saran Wrap in a tissue culture hood until dry (approx 30 min).
4. Block the filter (label side down) in 10 mL of 1% BSA/PBS on a shaker for 2 h at RT.
5. Remove the filter from blocking solution, and rinse 3× with PBS.
6. Blot excess buffer as in **step 3**.
7. Overlay the filter on plaque lawn (Fab library), and incubate overnight at 22°C in an incubator. The filter should be laid with the label side up on the agar. Mark the filter position by poking holes in the filter with a needle and mark the holes on the bottom of plate with a felt pen.
8. Prepare 5 ng/ mL human CD40-Fc (murine γ_{2b}) in PBS/1%BSA (4 mL/filter) and keep on ice.
9. Peel the filter off agar and rinse 3× with PBS.
10. Immerse filter, label side down, in 4 mL antigen solution (CD40-Fc) and place on a shaker for 3 h at RT.
11. Wash filter on vacuum washer apparatus 4× with PBS/0.1%Tween-20.
12. Incubate filter (label side down) in 10 mL PBS/1%BSA containing goat anti-mouse IgG$_{2b}$ (γ_{2b} chain specific)-alkaline phosphatase conjugate diluted 1:3000. Shake for 1 h at RT.
13. Wash filter on vacuum washer apparatus 4× with PBS/0.1% Tween-20.
14. Develop with alkaline phosphatase substrate (NBT-BCIP) for 1 h on a shaker.
15. Isolate plaques that develop as darker spots on filters compared to chimeric Fab phage. Elute the phage in phage elution buffer.
16. Since up to 10^5 phages are plated on a bacterial lawn (the plate looks confluent), the isolated phages are further purified by titering on a bacterial lawn, and the capture lift assay is repeated.

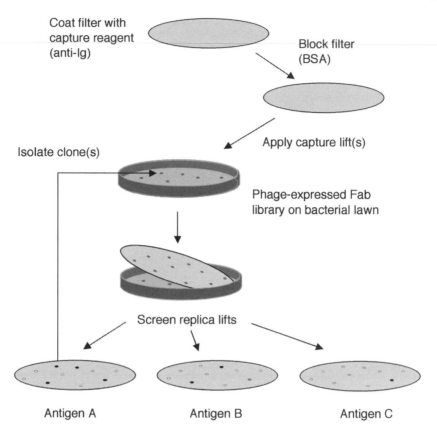

Fig. 2. Schematic for capture lift assay used in screening the combinatorial Fab library. Nitrocellulose membrane is coated with anti-kappa chain capturing antibody, blocked by BSA and laid on a phage plate to capture the expressed Fab fragments. The captured Fab variants can be screened against different antigens by applying replica lifts on the same plate followed by incubating the filters with different antigens. Only clones that show specific binding to desired antigen are isolated for further confirmation.

3.2.2. Single Point ELISA (SPE)

SPE is employed for the secondary screening *(18)*, as such, to confirm the clones identified by capture lift assay. It can also be used for initial screening if the size of the library is $\leq 1 \times 10^4$. The capturing antibody, antigen and secondary antibody are used in a manner similar to that of the capture lift. SPE is quantitative, in that an OD signal is obtained, which correlates with the affinity of clones (compare **Fig. 3A,B**) (*see* **Note 3**). The throughput is about 10^2 clones per plate. One person can screen about 500 clones/d.

1. Coat Immulon 2 U-bottom plate with goat anti-human kappa antibody at 5 μg/mL in carbonate coating buffer at 4°C overnight.

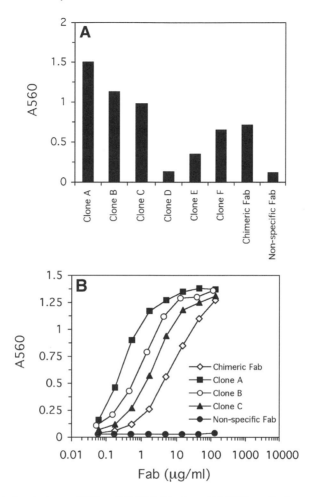

Fig. 3. Correlation between SPE and ELISA titration. (**A**) SPE results from an initial library screening. Clones (A, B, and C) with higher SPE signal are isolated for ELISA titration. (**B**) ELISA titration using crude Fab extracts on immobilized antigen shows strong correlation between the SPE signal and affinity improvement (compare clones A, B, C, and chimeric Fab).

2. Tap out coating solution. Block with 3% BSA/PBS (200 μL/well) for 1 h at 37°C.
3. Wash 3× with PBS/0.1% Tween-20.
4. Add 50 μL Fab extract from periplasmic preparation (*see* **Subheading 3.2.2.1.**) (*see* **Note 4**). Incubate for 1 h at RT.
5. Wash 3× with PBS/0.1% Tween-20.
6. Add 50 μL/well human CD40-Fc (murine γ_{2b}) at 0.1 μg/mL in PBS/1% BSA. Incubate for 2 h at RT.
7. Wash 3× in PBS/0.1% Tween-20.
8. Add 50 μL/well goat anti-mouse IgG_{2b}-alkaline phosphatase diluted 1:3000 in PBS/1% BSA. Incubate for 1 h at RT.

9. Wash 3× with PBS/0.1% Tween-20.
10. Add 50 µL/well AMP-PMP substrate. Develop in the dark for 25 min or until appropriate signals appear.

3.2.2.1. ISOLATION OF SOLUBLE FAB FROM PERIPLASMIC SPACE (15 ML-PREP)

1. Grow XL-I-Blue cells in 2X YT medium containing 10 µg/mL of tetracycline at 37°C in a shaker at 250 rpm until OD$_{600}$ reaches 0.9–1.2.
2. Add 0.5 mM IPTG to XL-I-Blue cells, and aliquot 15 mL each into 50-mL polypropylene conical tubes for each phage clone to be characterized.
3. Infect bacteria with 10 µL of high titer phage (titer = ≈5 × 10^{11} pfu/mL), and incubate for 1 h at 37°C (*see* **Note 5**). Switch the temperature to RT, and grow overnight.
4. Spin down the cells at 3000 rpm for 25 min (≈2000g).
5. Aspirate and discard the supernatant. Remove as much culture medium as possible.
6. Resuspend the pellet in 640 µL of resuspension buffer, vortex, and place the sample on ice for 1 h with occasional gentle shaking.
7. Pellet the cellular debris in a microcentrifuge by spinning at 9000 rpm for 10 min at 4°C.
8. Isolate the supernatant, and store at 4°C.

3.3. Construction of Combinatorial Framework-HCDR3 Phage Library

The most homologous human germline templates for both murine V$_H$ and V$_L$ are identified by comparing the sequences with the human germline data bank. The V$_H$ framework sequence has 74% homology to human germline VH7/JH4, and V$_L$ framework sequence has 75% homology to human germline VKIII/JK4 (*see* **Fig. 4** for sequence alignment). Residues that differ between the murine and human sequences are evaluated for their importance for maintaining the activity of the antibody. Several common rules are described in **Subheading 1.** Detailed analysis has been described in an earlier publication (*9*). Overall, seven V$_H$ and one V$_L$ residues have been determined to be potentially critical for antigen binding, and these positions are characterized in a combinatorial library expressing all possible combinations of murine and human amino acids at these positions (marked with an asterisk in **Fig. 4**). For CDR optimization, single mutations are introduced into HCDR3. Codon-based mutagenesis is used to synthesize the oligonucleotides that encode single mutations within HCDR3 (*19*).

To construct a library for simultaneous framework and CDR optimization, an overlapping PCR method is used for the total synthesis of V$_H$ and V$_L$ gene (*see* **Fig. 5**). The combinatorial library is composed of murine CDRs grafted onto the human templates. In addition, there are eight murine/human wobble residues within framework, and single mutations at HCDR3. The combination yields 1.1×10^5 variants. The procedure for library construction is described below:

1. Synthesize overlapping oligonucleotide encoding partial sequences of V$_H$ and V$_L$ to a size of around 63–76 nucleotides (nt) with 18–21 nt overlapping. Purify oligonucleotides from an 8% polyacrylamide gel.
2. Overlapping PCR:

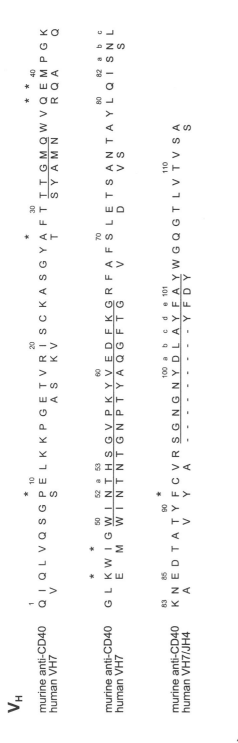

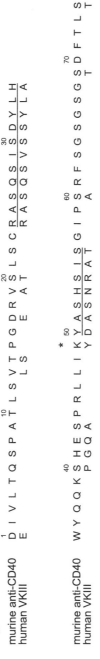

Fig. 4. Amino-acid alignments of V regions. The murine anti-CD40 sequences are aligned with the most homologous human germline sequences (*9*). The entire murine sequences are shown. For human sequences, only framework residues that are different from murine sequences are shown. The underlined areas are CDR regions defined by Kabat et al. (*20*). Framework positions marked with an asterisk are expressed as human/mouse wobble residues in the combinatorial library.

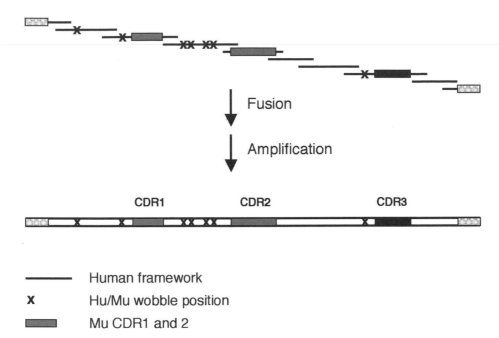

- ―――――― Human framework
- **x** Hu/Mu wobble position
- ▨▨▨ Mu CDR1 and 2
- ▬▬▬ Mu CDR3 with single mutations
- ▨▨▨ Phage vector sequence

Fig. 5. Overlapping PCR for library construction. V_H gene is synthesized by PCR fusion and amplification of oligonucleotides as shown. V_L gene is synthesized similarly. Human/murine wobble residues and single mutations within HCDR3 are incorporated by oligo synthesis. Both genes are then cloned into M13-based expression vector to form a combinatorial Fab library.

    a. Fusion: 50 pmol each oligonucleotides, 2 µL *pfu* DNA polymerase, 10 µL 10X *pfu* buffer, 2 µL dNTP (10 m*M* each). Add up to 100 µL total volume with ddH₂O. PCR program: 95°C, 1 min. 94°C, 20 s; 50°C, 30 s; ramp 1 min to 72°C; 72°C, 30 s; 5 cycles. 94°C, 20 s; 55°C, 30 s; ramp 1 min to 72°C; 72°C, 30 s; 25 cycles. 72°C, 7 min.

    b. Amplification: 2 µL (*see* **Note 6**) fusion product, 100 pmol biotinylated forward primer, 100 pmol reverse primer, 10 µL 10X *pfu* buffer, 2 µL *pfu* DNA polymerase, 2 µL dNTP (10 m*M* each). Add up to 100 µL total volume with ddH₂O. PCR program: Same as the program used in the fusion reaction except 30 cycles are run instead of 25 cycles.

3. Resolve the amplified PCR product on an agarose gel. Extract DNA from the gel by electroelution.
4. Perform the following steps such as the phosphorylation of the PCR product, purification of the single-stranded DNA, and cloning into phage-expression vector according to **Sub-headings 3.1.1.** and **3.1.2.** with a minor modification. After the *Eco*RI digestion (**Sub-heading 3.1.2., step 4**), and heat inactivation, precipitate DNA by ethanol, and resuspend in 10 µL of ddH₂O. Electroporate all of the DNA into DH10B cells (*see* **Note 7**), and amplify the phage on an XL-I-Blue bacterial lawn for 6 h at 37°C. Flush the plates with a

solution containing 10 mM Tris-HCl, pH 7.4, 1 mM EDTA, and 100 mM NaCl. Centrifuge at 3000 rpm for 30 min to remove cell debris. Add glycerol to 10%, NaN3 to 0.02%, and store the phage library at –80°C. The phage titer of the library is about 3×10^{11} pfu/mL.

3.3.1. Characterization of Phage Library

Characterize the constructed phage library by replicate filter assay *(15)* and DNA sequencing (*see* **Note 8**). Use the replicate filter assay to determine the co-expression rate of heavy chain (HC) and light chain (LC) of Fab fragments in the library as described in the following protocol:

1. Plate the phage library on the bacterial lawn by diluting the library to yield about 300 plaques per 100-mm plate. Add diluted phage to 200 µL of overnight culture of XL-I-Blue in 14-mL disposal cell culture tubes. Add IPTG to 1 mM, then add 3 mL of top agar, and pour the mixture onto LB plates. Wait for 10 min at RT, then incubate the plates upside down at 37°C overnight.
2. Take out plates from 37°C incubator, and store at RT for 15 min to cool. Place nitrocellulose filter on top of agar. Once filter is completely wet, make orientation marks with needle. Incubate at least 3 h or overnight at RT.
3. Remove filters and block with Blotto for 1–2 h at RT in an orbital shaker.
4. Add alkaline phosphatase-conjugated antibody diluted in Blotto, and incubate for minimum of 2 h at RT with shaking. For LC detection, use goat anti-human kappa-alkaline phosphatase conjugate at 1:2000 dilution. For HC detection, use mouse anti-decapeptide (HA) MAb-alkaline phosphatase conjugate at 1:5000 dilution.
5. Wash with PBS/0.1% Tween-20 5× with shaking in between washes. Incubate at RT for 5 min for each wash.
6. Transfer filters to a new container. Add 50 mL of AP substrate.
7. After the first filter lift, phage growth is resumed by incubating the plate for an additional 2 h at 37°C. The second filter is then applied. Repeat **steps 2–6** for the detection of HC (assuming the first filter is for LC detection).

3.3.2. Screening of Phage Library and Characterization of the Selected Clones

The scheme for the library screening and characterization of selected clones is as following: (1) capture lift; (2) plaque purification; (3) confirmation by SPE; (4) ELISA titration; (5) DNA sequencing; and (6) kinetic analysis by Biacore and other assays. The phage library is first screened by capture lift assay (*see* **Subheading 3.2.1.**). Screen 20 plates containing 10^5 phages. Pick and plate phages corresponding to darker spots than chimeric Fab at lower density for another capture lift (plaque purification). After plaque purification, SPE (*see* **Subheading 3.2.2.**) is used to confirm that the clones identified by capture lifts have higher affinity than the chimeric clone. Use an ELISA titration on immobilized antigen by using Fab prepared from a 15-mL prep (*see* **Subheading 3.2.2.1.**) to estimate the degree of increased affinity of the isolated Fab variants (*see* **Fig. 3B**). After ELISA, perform DNA sequencing of the Fab variants. Fab is then purified for further characterization, such as Biacore analysis for kinetic information, ligand inhibition assay, and so on (not described here).

4. Notes

1. Two methods for the preparation of ssDNA were compared. One is by using streptavidin-coated magnetic beads as described in this chapter, and the other is by asymmetric PCR. We found that method using streptavidin-coated beads was robust and easy.

2. It is usually not necessary to check the eluted ssDNA. However, if desired, load 1.5 μL of ssDNA on 2% agarose gel using formamide loading dye (heat 5 min at 85–90°C to denature the secondary structure, and chill on ice before loading). Sometimes dye will comigrate with the ssDNA, and mask the EtBr-staining. To overcome this problem, load samples containing 50% formamide without dye.

3. The reason for using capturing antibodies is to increase the sensitivity and specificity of the assay *(17)*. In theory, by using constant amount of capturing reagent, the same amount of expressed Fab can be captured onto the nitrocellulose membrane (capture lift), or microtiter well (single point ELISA to be described later). This setup will circumvent the signal effect caused by different expression level of Fab variants. As a result, the signal on filters or plates reflects directly the affinity of the Fabs. However, owing to the difference in signal readout, single point ELISA is a more quantitative assay than capture lift (OD signal vs intensity of spot on filters).

4. For confirmation purpose, Fab extracts are generally prepared from 15 mL-bacterial culture. For initial screening, Fab extracts are prepared from 1 mL-bacterial culture grown in 96 deep-well plates.

5. If there is no high titer phage stock, one can infect bacteria with 50 μL of eluted phage. Phage plaques picked from a bacterial lawn and eluted into 200 μL of phage elution buffer usually yield a titer about 2×10^8 pfu/mL. However, this procedure sometimes results in about 3–10-fold lower Fab yield than the procedure using high-titer phage.

6. A 25 μL-PCR amplification is run first to determine the optimal amount of fusion product to be used as a template. Volumes ranging from 0.5–10 μL is tested, and in this case, the minimal volume required for the efficient amplification of the synthesized gene was found to be 2 μL.

7. To cover the size of the library, 500 ng of phage vector is used. After the mutagenesis, DNA is aliquoted into two portions, and each portion is electroporated into 150 μL of electrocompetent DH10B cells. The number of independent clones is 2.3×10^6, which is large enough to cover the size of the library (1.1×10^5) even after taking into the consideration of the rate of coexpression and unwanted mutagenesis (*see* **Note 8**). The transfection efficiency is about 4.6×10^6 pfu/μg of phage vector.

8. The co-expression rate for HC and LC of the combinatorial FR-H3 library is ≈40% as determined by replica filter lift (for FR-H3-L3 library, the co-expression rate is ≈60%). PCR screening can be used to examine the co-expression rate, too. The co-expression rate determined by PCR is usually significantly higher than that determined by replicate filter lift. The possible reason is that certain clones that contain both HC and LC genes as determined by PCR may not express functional HC or LC due to unwanted deletion within the genes, which results in frameshift and leads to negative signal on filter lift. In the instance of FR-H3 library, DNA sequencing of 20 coexpressors reveals that the appropriate mutation ratio is incorporated in both the framework and the HCDR3 regions. However, there are unwanted mutations or deletions (1–3 nt deletions and point mutations) that occurred at a frequency of 9 out of 20 clones (45%). The unwanted mutations or deletions can result from the oligo synthesis and PCR amplification.

Acknowledgments

I would like to thank Sanjaya Singh and Catherine M. Falcon for their critical review of the manuscript.

References

1. Morrison, S. L., Johnson, M. J., Herzenberg, L. A., and Oi, V. T. (1984) Chimeric human antibody molecules: mouse antigen-binding domains with human constant region domain. *Proc. Natl. Acad. Sci. USA* **81,** 6851–6855.
2. Boulianne, G. L., Hozumi, N., and Shulman, M. J. (1984) Production of functional chimaeric mouse/human antibody. *Nature* **312,** 643–646.
3. Hale, G., Clark, M. R., Marcus, R., Winter, G., Dyer, M. J. S., Philips, J. M., et al. (1988) Remission induction in non-Hodgkin lymphoma with reshaped human monoclonal antibody Campath-1H. *Lancet* **2,** 1394–1399.
4. Khazaeli, M. B., Conry, R. M., and LoBuglio, A. F. (1994) Human immune response to monoclonal antibodies. *J. Immunother.* **15,** 42–52.
5. Jones, P. T., Dear, P. H., Foote, J., Neuberger, M. S., and Winter, G. (1986) Replacing the complementarity-determining regions in a human antibody with those from a mouse. *Nature* **321,** 522–525.
6. Riechmann, L., Clark, M., Waldmann, H., and Winter, G. (1988) Reshaping human antibodies for therapy. *Nature* **332,** 323–327.
7. Foote, J. and Winter, G. (1992) Antibody framework residues affecting the conformation of the hypervariable loops. *J. Mol. Biol.* **224,** 487–499.
8. Wu, H., Beuerlein, G., Nie, Y., Smith, H., Lee, B. A., Hensler, M., et al. (1998) Stepwise *in vitro* affinity maturation of Vitaxin, an $\alpha_v\beta_3$-specific humanized mAb. *Proc. Natl. Acad. Sci. USA* **95,** 6037–6042.
9. Wu, H., Nie, Y., Huse, W. D., and Watkins, J. D. (1999) Humanization of a murine monoclonal antibody by simultaneous optimization of framework and CDR residues. *J. Mol. Biol.* **294,** 151–162.
10. Chothia, C., Lesk, A. M., Tramontano, A., Levitt, M., Smith-Gill, S. J., Air, G., et al. (1989) Conformations of immunoglobulin hypervariable regions. *Nature* **342,** 877–883.
11. Foote, J. and Winter, G. (1992) Antibody framework residues affecting the conformation of the hypervaribale loops. *J. Mol. Biol.* **224,** 487–499.
12. Padlan, E. A. (1991) A possible procedure for reducing the immunogenicity of antibody variable domains while preserving their ligand-binding properties. *Mol. Immunol.* **28,** 489–498.
13. Harris, L. and Bajorath, J. (1995) Profiles for the analysis of immunoglobulin sequences: Comparison of V gene subgroups. *Protein Sci.* **4,** 306–310.
14. Glaser, S., Kristensson, K., Chilton, T., and Huse, W. D. (1995) Engineering the antibody combining site by codon-based mutagenesis in a filamentous phage display system, in *Antibody Engineering*, 2nd ed. (Borrebaeck, C. A. K., ed.), Oxford University Press, Oxford, pp. 117–131.
15. Huse, W. D., Stinchcombe, T., J., Glaser, S. M., Starr, L., Maclean, M., et al. (1992) Application of a filamentous phage pVIII fusion protein system suitable for efficient production, screening, and mutagenesis of F(ab) antibody fragments. *J. Immunol.* **149,** 3914–3920.

16. Kunkel, T. A. (1985) Rapid and efficient site-specific mutagenesis without phenotypic selection. *Proc. Natl. Acad. Sci. USA* **82,** 488–492.

17. Watkins, J. D., Beuerlein, G., Wu, H., McFadden, P. R., Pancook, J. D., and Huse, W. D. (1998) Discovery of human antibodies to cell surface antigens by capture lift screening of phage-expressed antibody libraries. *Anal. Biochem.* **256,** 169–177.

18. Watkins, J. D., Beuerlein, G., Pecht, G., McFadden, P. R., Glaser, S. M., and Huse, W. D. (1997) Determination of the relative affinities of antibody fragments expressed in *Escherichia coli* by enzyme-linked immunosorbent assay. *Anal. Biochem.* **253,** 37–45.

19. Glaser, S. M., Yelton, D. E., and Huse, W. D. (1992) Antibody engineering by codon-based mutagenesis in a filamentous phage vector system. *J. Immunol.* **149,** 3903–3913.

20. Kabat, E. A., Wu, T. T., and Bilofsky, H. (1977) Unusual distributions of amino acids in complementarity-determining (hypervariable) segments of heavy and light chains of immunoglobulins and their possible roles in specificity of antibody-combining sites. *J. Biol. Chem.* **252,** 6609–6616.

13

Tailoring Kinetics of Antibodies
Using Focused Combinatorial Libraries

Herren Wu and Ling-Ling An

1. Introduction

Antibodies have been used extensively for diagnostic applications for decades. Antibodies also can be used to target specific cells or specific molecules to produce agonist, antagonist, or neutralizing activity. Antibody therapies have been applied successfully in the treatment of several human diseases *(1)*. The advantages of antibodies over other molecules are that they have high affinity for their targets and they bind to targets with high specificity. Antibodies, with six highly diversified complementarity-determining regions (CDRs) supported by stable β-sheet framework regions, are capable of binding virtually any molecule including proteins, carbohydrates, nucleic acids, and haptens. The intrinsic features of specificity and affinity when combined offer a great advantage in the discovery of a wide-range of lead drug candidates.

For more than 20 years, hybridoma technology has been used routinely to generate monoclonal antibodies (MAbs) with reasonable affinity and defined antigen specificity. However, this technology is time consuming and labor intensive. To increase the speed and efficiency for antibody discovery, phage display technology *(2)* emerged about 10 years ago *(3–6)*. Although this technology enables the selection and amplification of desired clones from pools of millions, generating a large diverse antibody library containing the desired rare clones becomes the rate-limiting step. Combinatorial libraries derived from "immunized" B-cell repertoires isolated from infected *(7)* or vaccinated people *(8)* have been made, and high-affinity human antibodies ($K_d < 10$ nM) have been successfully identified from such libraries. However, human "immunization" is unrealistic for most antigens, and particularly for self-antigens. In addition, new libraries may be required for each antigen. To bypass immunization and to make a single antibody library suitable for any antigen, naïve *(9,10)* as well as synthetic libraries *(11,12)* were constructed with size $\leq 10^8$ complexity. Early results with such libraries were not encouraging. Most antibodies isolated were at affinities in the 0.1–1 μM

From: *Methods in Molecular Biology, vol. 207: Recombinant Antibodies for Cancer Therapy: Methods and Protocols*
Edited by: M. Welschof and J. Krauss © Humana Press Inc., Totowa, NJ

range, typical for antibodies generated from the primary immune response *(13)*. Since MAbs with these low affinities would require administration of huge amount of antibodies, they are not practical for most therapeutic applications. Since the diversity of the antibody repertoire influences the identification of tight binders *(14)*, great efforts have been made to create very large naïve *(15–18)* and synthetic libraries *(19,20)*. The size of these libraries ranged from 2×10^9 to 3×10^{11} complexity; antibodies isolated from these libraries had affinities within the 10–100 nM range. Many antibodies with nanomolar and sub-nanomolar affinities that are comparable to those from secondary immune response were also successfully isolated.

The current development of a "single pot" large antibody library has clearly accelerated the identification of lead antibodies for therapeutic applications. However, fine-tuning of the lead antibodies is still necessary to ensure that optimal antibodies are selected for clinical development. Although high-affinity clones ($K_d < 10$ nM) were readily isolated in a single step for some antigens, only modest-affinity antibodies ($K_d = 10$–100 nM) could be obtained for other antigens *(16,18–20)*. Enriching rare high-affinity clones from a large library can be problematic *(21)*. When the frequency of a rare clone is lower than the nonspecific binding to the antigen, it becomes difficult to isolate such a clone. Furthermore, when a panel of antibodies is identified against a particular antigen, affinity is not the only factor that determines the therapeutic efficacy. The epitope that is recognized by the antibody is usually crucial for the function of the antibody. The most potent antibody within the isolated panel may be an antibody that binds to the critical epitope with low affinity. For such antibodies, affinity maturation offers the chance to further increase the potency and thereby reduce the amount of the antibody administered to a patient.

Affinity maturation is often the first step for antibody optimization because affinity of an antibody is an important factor in determining its biological activity *(22–25)*. Many successful examples of improving affinities using phage display and other technologies have been reported *(26–35)*. In tumor targeting, increased affinity has resulted in better biodistribution and tumor retention of the antibody *(36–38)*. Beyond affinity maturation, the specificity of the antibodies can be modified or fine-tuned using designed screening or selection conditions *(39–42)*. Likewise the stability of an antibody can be improved by grafting the antigen-binding residues from a less stable antibody onto the framework of a highly stable and well-folded antibody *(43)*. In this instance, the improvement enhanced the tumor targeting ability of the antibody significantly.

Presented here is a simple, efficient and robust approach toward antibody optimization, which includes affinity maturation, kinetics manipulation, and specificity fine-tuning while not requiring detailed structural information of the antibody of interest. This approach involves: (1) constructing antibody libraries focused on CDR regions; (2) screening for beneficial mutations; and (3) combining beneficial mutations. This procedure follows the iterative process seen in nature for functional improvement of proteins, including affinity maturation of antibody *(44)*. Individual mutations can be combined to further improve antibody affinity *(27)*, protein stability *(45)*, and enzyme activity *(46)*, or to manipulate the substrate specificity of an enzyme *(47–49)*. The distinguishing feature of the current approach for antibody optimization is that the size of the constructed libraries is extremely small. Typically, libraries contain less than 400 variants, can be constructed easily, and allow various functional screening that may not be suitable to the affinity enrichment strategy. The small size of the library obviates the need for phage affinity selection.

The first step of this combinatorial approach is to construct focused antibody libraries. Because the antigen-binding site of an antibody is formed by six CDR loops, six CDR mutation libraries are constructed simultaneously. The codon-based mutagenesis approach *(39)* with modification is used to synthesize the oligonucleotides, which will introduce mutations within each CDR *(33)*. This modified approach segregates the diversity into pools based on the degree of mutagenesis, permitting the synthesis of oligonucleotides that encode single, double, triple, or more mutations. The parental antibody to be optimized is cloned into an M13-based phage vector *(50,51)* containing leader sequences and IgG1 CH1/kappa constant regions. Each CDR region is deleted respectively by hybridization mutagenesis *(52)*, then a synthesized oligonucleotide encoding the corresponding CDR region with mutations is annealed back to the vector for the construction of the CDR mutation library. Variants of Fab fragments are expressed by infecting *E. coli* XL-1 Blue with the phage library, and Fab fragments accumulated in both the periplasmic space and the culture medium (through leakage) are subjected to screening.

For affinity maturation, it was observed that single-mutation CDR libraries are preferable and sufficient since limited mutagenesis allows the maintenance of the original binding domain, and results in a small-size library *(33)*. Furthermore, this process mimics in vivo affinity maturation of antibody *(44)*. Typically, a beneficial single mutation can improve the antibody affinity 2–13 fold (*see* **Table 1**) *(33)*. As the size of each CDR library is normally less than 400 variants, the screening for beneficial mutations can be easily completed in a short time. The final step is to combine the beneficial single mutations from each CDR loop. Multiple-site hybridization mutagenesis is used for the construction of the combinatorial library *(53)*. The accumulative effect can enhance the affinity dramatically *(27,28,33)*. For example, in the affinity maturation of Vitaxin, an anti-$\alpha_v\beta_3$ humanized MAb, up to 92-fold enhancement was achieved by combining three mutations of which two were from the heavy chain CDR3 (H3) and one was from the light chain CDR3 (L3) (clone 37 in **Table 1**) *(33)*. As a result, the affinity was improved from 27.6 nM to 0.3 nM. For the optimization of an anti-CD40 antibody, the affinity was increased from 48.3 nM to 0.1 nM, a 483-fold enhancement by the combination of one mutation from H3 and two mutations from L3 *(54)*. In another case, the affinity of a humanized antibody against respiratory syncytial virus (RSV) was improved from 5.2 nM to 2.5 pM (>2000-fold increase) resulting from the combination of four mutations, one each from H3, L3, heavy chain CDR1 (H1), and light chain CDR2 (L2) (unpublished results).

Although in many cases, mutations affecting substrate binding, protein–protein interaction, protein–DNA interaction, or protein stability can be combined and exhibit a simple additive effect *(55)*, many combinations of CDR mutations demonstrate complex additivity as seen in the optimization of Vitaxin *(33)*, and an anti-HIV antibody *(28)*. Selected data from Vitaxin optimization is shown in **Table 1**. The only simple

Table 1
Representative Beneficial Mutations from Viaxin Primary
and Combinatorial Libraries (33)

| Library | Clone | Sequence | | | | | | | K_d, nM | K_d (wt)/K_d |
		L1 32	L3 92	L3 96	H2 60	H3 97	H3 101	H3 102		
	Wild-type	H	G	H	L	Y	A	Y	27.6	1.0
Primary										
L1	F32	F							2.5	11.0
L3	N92		N						5.7	4.8
	L96			L					9.2	3.0
H2	P60				P				5.8	4.8
H3	H97					H			13.8	2.0
	Y101						Y		2.2	12.5
	S102							S	6.0	4.6
	D102							D	3.5	7.9
	E102							E	n.d.	n.d.
Combinatorial										
	17	F						S	0.5	55.2
	56	F			P			S	0.5	55.2
	7	F			P	H		S	1.2	23.0
	V357D	F						D	0.5	55.2
	C59	F			P			D	0.5	55.2
	2G4			L				S	0.4	69.0
	6H6			L		H		S	0.4	69.0
	6G1			L	P			S	0.7	39.4
	C37			L			Y	E	0.3	92.0
	C29			L	P	H	Y	S	0.5	55.2

additivity effect observed was by the combination of the F32 mutation from light-chain CDR1 (L1) (11-fold improvement) with the S102 mutation from H3 loop (4.6-fold improvement) resulting in clone 17 with a 55-fold improvement. Other additional mutations resulted in complex additivity (compare clones 17, 56, and 7). One favorable cooperative interaction was observed in clone 2G4. Clone 2G4 contains the L96 mutation from L3 loop (3-fold improvement) and the S102 mutation from H3 loop (4.6-fold improvement), and its affinity is increased 69-fold over Vitaxin. Simple additivity would have produced a 13.8-fold increase in affinity. As shown for Vitaxin, the combinatorial effect of affinity improvement is complex and is difficult to predict. One plausible explanation is that simple additivity is usually observed from the combinations of noninteracting distant mutations at rigid molecular interfaces where the structure or binding mechanism is less likely to be altered significantly by mutations (55). In the case of CDRs, the loops are fairly flexible, and their conformations are easily perturbed by mutations.

Affinity maturation of antibodies can be governed by two factors: association rate constant (k_{on}) and dissociation rate constant (k_{off}). The equilibrium dissociation constant (K_d) is calculated from $K_d = k_{off}/k_{on}$. In most instances of in vitro affinity maturation, the affinity is improved predominantly through the decrease of k_{off} (*27,28,30,33–35,54*). One possible explanation for the observed results is that there may be structural constraints inherent in the geometry of the binding site that limit the level of k_{on} improvement as implicated by Foote and Milstein (*13*). In their observation of the maturation of an anti-hapten antibody repertoire, the k_{on} values of the antibodies studied were determined predominantly by the V gene families they belong to. The k_{on} value of the low-k_{on} group was increased fourfold by somatic mutations, but rarely went beyond 10^7 $M^{-1}s^{-1}$, which is one-tenth of that of the high-k_{on} group. On the contrary, the k_{off} value for both groups can be reduced by somatic mutations up to 100-fold (*13*). Another explanation is that the selection or screening conditions used for in vitro affinity maturation favors the selection of k_{off} improvement (*27,28,30,33–35,54*). Long contact time between antigen and antibody is the key cause. The kinetic interaction between antigen and antibody can be simulated by a BIAcore simulation program. The surface plasmon resonance reflects the amount of antigen bound to the immobilized antibody in real time. As illustrated by the simulation in **Fig. 1A**, one antibody and its three variants with different k_{on} and k_{off} values (**Table 2**) are captured on the sensor chip in the same amount and allowed to interact with the antigen in solution for 60 min, then dissociate for 20 min. Variants 3 and 2, both with improved k_{off} appear as good binders. To be able to direct the screening toward the k_{on} improvement, very short association and dissociation time is necessary. When the association time is shortened to 6 min and the dissociation time is shortened to 1 min, variants 1 and 3, both with improved k_{on} appear as good binders (simulation shown in **Fig. 1B**). The k_{on} and k_{off} values (**Table 2**) were artificially created for simulations based on prior experience with antibody optimization. It was observed that single mutations in CDRs could decrease k_{off} up to 10-fold (*33*), while they could only increase k_{on} from 50 to 100% (*33*; unpublished results). In the current approach, the focused CDR libraries are amenable to a wide variety of assays at the primary screen, such as the ones that incorporate the simulation parameters for the selection of high k_{on} variants (*see* **Subheading 3.**). Through iterative CDR mutagenesis, the k_{on} of an antibody was improved more than sevenfold (data unpublished).

Depending on the mechanism of disease, different kinetic characteristics of therapeutic antibodies may be needed. For example, for prophylaxis of viral infection, antibodies with high k_{on} value (fast association) to viral particles may be more desirable because theoretically such antibodies can neutralize the virus before it has the chance to infect cells. Likewise, if antibodies are designed to block certain activation cascades, high k_{on} antibodies also will be more suitable because antibodies can neutralize the activated target before it triggers the activation cascade. For tumor therapy, antibodies with high k_{on} may penetrate the tumor more effectively and distribute more thoroughly than antibodies with low k_{off} since very slow dissociation of antibodies from tumor cells can render antibodies trapped in the peripheral area of the tumor (*38*). For antibodies that neutralize and/or eliminate certain secreted proteins in the body, high affinity is usually desired because it will lower the dose of antibody required. In such cases, k_{off}-driven engineering is favorable because k_{off} is much easier to improve than k_{on}.

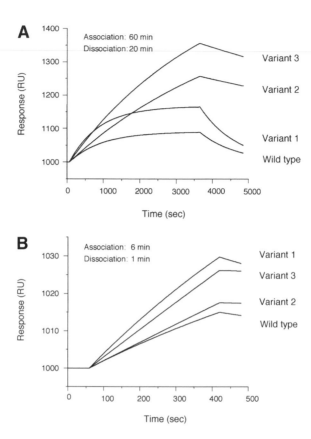

Fig. 1. Kinetic simulation of antibody-antigen interaction. A BIAcore simulation program is used for the simulation of the kinetic interaction between antibody and antigen. One antibody and its three variants with different k_{on} and k_{off} values are captured on the sensor chip, and interact with the antigen in solution under different conditions. (**A**) Antigen concentration is 10 nM, and the association time between antibody and antigen is long (60 min). The best clones isolated are variant 3 and 2, both with decreased k_{off}. (**B**) Antigen concentration is 5 nM. The association and dissociation time between antibody and antigen are short, 6 min and 1 min, respectively. The best clones isolated are variant 1 and 3, which correlates with increased k_{on}.

Table 2
Clones Used for Kinetic Simulation

Clone	k_{on} ($\times 10^4$), $M^{-1} s^{-1}$	k_{off} ($\times 10^{-3}$), s^{-1}	K_d ($\times 10^{-7}$), M
Wild-type	1.0	1.0	1.0
Variant 1	2.0	1.0	0.5
Variant 2	1.0	0.1	0.1
Variant 3	1.5	0.1	0.07

Affinity maturation and kinetics manipulation of antibodies can extend the application potentials of antibodies by producing high performance therapeutic antibodies suitable for prophylactic, acute, and chronic treatment of human diseases. The combinatorial approach presented here results in rapid antibody optimization, including affinity maturation and kinetics tailoring, in the absence of detailed structural information of antibodies. This approach facilitates quick identification of optimal antibodies for clinical development.

2. Materials

2.1. Escherichia coli *Strains*

1. CJ236 (Bio-Rad).
2. DH10B (Gibco-BRL).
3. XL-1Blue (Strategene).

2.2. *Enzymes*

1. *pfu* DNA polymerase (2.5 U/µL) (Strategene).
2. T4 polynucleotide kinase (10 U/µL) (Roche).
3. T4 DNA ligase (1 U/µL) (Roche).
4. T4 DNA polymerase (1 U/µL) (Roche).
5. *Eco*RI (10 U/µL) (Roche).
6. RNase A.

2.3. *Antibodies and Enzyme Conjugates*

1. Goat anti-human kappa antibody (mouse adsorbed) (1 mg/mL) (Southern Biotechnology Associates Inc., cat. no. 2060-01).
2. Goat anti-human Fab antibody (≈8 mg/mL) (ICN-Cappel, cat. no. 55010).
3. Goat anti-human kappa-alkaline phosphatase conjugate (mouse adsorbed) (Southern Biotechnology Associates Inc., cat. no. 2060-04).
4. NeutrAvidin-alkaline phosphatase (1.8 mg/mL) (Pierce, cat. no. 31002).
5. Streptavidin-alkaline phosphatase (1000 U/mL) (Roche, cat. no. 1089161).

2.4. *Buffers and Solutions*

Capture lifts and ELISAs.

1. Carbonate coating buffer: 0.015 M Na_2CO_3, 0.035 M $NaHCO_3$, pH 9.3.
2. Phosphate-buffered saline (PBS): 0.14 M NaCl, 2.7 mM KCl, 1.5 mM KH_2PO_4, 8.1 mM Na_2HPO_4, pH 7.2.
3. PBS/0.1% Tween-20: PBS containing 0.1% Tween-20.
4. PBS/0.05% Tween-20: PBS containing 0.05% Tween-20.
5. 1% BSA/PBS: PBS containing 1% (w/v) bovine serum albumin (BSA).
6. 3% BSA/PBS: PBS containing 3% (w/v) BSA.
7. HEPES/NP40 buffer: 50 mM HEPES, 150 mM NaCl, 1 mM $CaCl_2$, and 0.1% NP40.
8. Reagents for alkaline phosphatase-based capture lifts:

   a. AP buffer (substrate buffer): 0.1 M Tris-HCl, pH 9.5.
   b. Substrate A (NBT): 40 mM nitro blue tetrazolium (2,2'-di-p-nitrophenyl-5,5'-diphenyl-3,3'-[3,3'-dimethoxy-4,4'-diphenylene]ditetrazolium chloride (Sigma, cat. no. N-6876) in 70% *N,N*-dimethyl formamide).

c. Substrate B (BCIP): 38 mM 5-bromo-4-chloro-3-indoxyl phosphate mono-(*p*-toluidinium) salt (JBL scientific, Inc., cat. no. 1280C) in 100% *N,N*-dimethyl formamide.

d. AP substrate: Add substrate A and B both at 1:100 dilution in AP buffer.

9. Reagents for alkaline phosphatase-based ELISAs:

a. Substrate buffer (store in the dark): 0.2 M AMP (2-amino-2-methyl-1-propanol) (JBL Scientific, Inc., cat. no. 1250B), 0.5 M Tris-HCl, pH 10.2, and 0.1% sodium azide. To make 1 L of substrate buffer: 19.8 g AMP (stock AMP is 9.59 M and has a density of 0.950 g/mL), 60.55 g Trizma base, 1 g sodium azide, and adjust pH to 10.2 with concentrated HCl.

b. PMP substrate (phenolphthalein monophosphate) (JBL Scientific, Inc., cat. no. 1270D): Dissolve 0.3 g of substrate in 50 mL of substrate buffer. Add 50 µL per well to develop. Solution is stable for 1–2 wk when stored at 25°C in the dark.

c. Stop buffer: 30 mM Tris-HCl, pH 10.2, and 15 mM EDTA. Reactions are terminated with equal volume of stop buffer. Absorbance is measured at 560 nm.

10. Reagents for horseradish peroxidase-based ELISAs:

a. TMB substrate: 0.01% (w/v) 3,3',5,5'-tetramethylbenzidine, 0.003% H_2O_2, and 20 mM NaOAc, pH 6.0.

b. Stop solution: Add H_2SO_4 to the final concentration of 0.5 M.

11. 2X B&W buffer: 10 mM Tris-HCl, pH 7.5, 1 mM EDTA, 2 M NaCl, and 0.1% Tween-20.

12. 10X Annealing buffer: 200 mM Tris-HCl, pH 7.0, 500 mM NaCl, and 20 mM $MgCl_2$.

13. 10X Synthesis buffer: 5 mM dNTP, 10 mM ATP, 100 mM Tris-HCl, pH 7.4, 50 mM $MgCl_2$, and 20 mM DTT. Store at –20°C.

14. Top agar: 0.75% agar in LB medium. Maintain at 50–55°C in an incubator.

15. Phage elution buffer: 10 mM Tris-HCl, pH 7.4, and 100 mM NaCl.

16. TES buffer: 30 mM Tris-HCl, pH 8.0, 2 mM EDTA and 20% sucrose.

17. Resuspension buffer for extracting Fab from periplasmic space: 50 mM Tris-HCl, pH 8.0, 1 mM EDTA, and 500 mM sucrose.

2.5. Miscellaneous

1. Streptavidin-coated magnetic beads (Roche, cat. no. 1641786).
2. Nitrocellulose filter (82-mm) (Schleicher & Schuell Protran, cat. no. 20440).
3. Silent screen plate (Nalge Nunc International, cat. no. 256065) (96 microwell plate with low protein binding nylon 66 membrane, loprodyne, 1.2 µm).
4. Lysozyme (Sigma, cat. no. L-6876).
5. IgG Fab standard (purified human IgG Fab) (ICN-Cappel, cat. no. 55909).

3. Methods

3.1. Cloning of Parental Antibody into Phage Vector

The V_L and V_H genes of the parental antibody are cloned into one M13-based phage vector *(50,51)* under the control of the *lacZ* promoter by hybridization mutagenesis *(52)*. The vector contains the backbone of the human kappa constant region (Cκ), the first constant region of the human γ1 chain (CH1), and two annealing sites for the cloning of V_L and V_H genes. The vector also contains a pel B leader sequence for the light chain and a pho A leader sequence for the heavy chain to target the expressed Fab fragments into periplasmic space in *E. coli.*

3.1.1. PCR Amplification of V_L and V_H Gene

The forward primers for both V_L and V_H gene are biotinylated to facilitate the purification of minus-strand V genes at the later step for annealing into phage vector. The forward primers contain sequence specific to the framework 1 region and an overhanging sequence annealed to the end of the leader sequence (pel B or pho A). Similarly, the reverse primers contain sequence specific to the framework 4 region and an overhanging sequence annealed to the beginning of the constant region (Cκ or C_H1).

1. PCR conditions: 10 ng V gene template (DNA), 100 pmol biotinylated forward primer, 100 pmol reverse primer, 2 μL *pfu* DNA polymerase, 10 μL 10X *pfu* buffer, 2 μL dNTP (10 m*M* each). Add up to 100 μL in total volume with ddH$_2$O.
   PCR program: 95°C, 1 min. 94°C, 30 s; 55°C, 30 s; 72°C, 1.5 min; 35 cycles. 72°C, 7 min. 4°C.
2. The expected size of the amplified product is 360 bp for the V_L gene and 408 bp for the V_H gene. Size will vary slightly depending on the antibody of choice.
3. PCR products are purified from an agarose gel to remove unincorporated biotinylated primers and nonspecific PCR products.

3.1.2. Isolation of Single-Stranded DNA

The minus single-stranded DNA (ssDNA) is isolated by the dissociation of the double-stranded PCR product with sodium hydroxide while the plus biotinylated strand is captured by streptavidin-coated magnetic beads.

1. 5'-Phosphorylation of double stranded PCR product: 2 μg PCR product, 1 μL of T4 polynucleotide kinase (10 U/μL), 2 μL of 10X PNK buffer, 1 μL of 10 m*M* ATP in a total volume of 20 μL adjusted by ddH$_2$O. Incubate for 45 min at 37°C, and denature for 10 min by heat at 65°C. Bring reaction volume to 200 μL by adding ddH$_2$O for the next step.
2. Wash 100 μL of streptavidin-coated magnetic beads twice with 200 μL 2X B&W buffer (100 μL beads, equal to 1 mg, can bind more than 3.3 μg 500 bp-PCR product). Resuspend beads in 200 μL 2X B&W buffer.
3. Mix phosphorylated PCR product with beads, and incubate for 16 min at room temperature (RT) with moderate shaking.
4. Sediment beads by a magnet, and wash twice with 200 μL 2X B&W buffer.
5. Elute nonbiotinylated ssDNA (minus strand) with 300 μL freshly prepared 0.15 *M* NaOH for 10 min at RT with mild shaking. A second NaOH elution can increase the yield slightly (optional). Centrifuge the eluant to remove any trace of beads.
6. Precipitate ssDNA from the supernatant by adding 1 μL glycogen (20 mg/mL), 1/10 vol of 3 *M* NaOAc, pH 5.2, and 2.5 vol of EtOH. Wash precipitated ssDNA with 70% EtOH. Lyophilize for 3 min and dissolve into 20 μL ddH$_2$O. Quantitate the ssDNA by spotting on an ethidium bromide (EtBr) agarose plate with DNA standards, or by measuring OD$_{260}$.

3.1.3. Preparation of Uridinylated Template (U-template)

1. Grow CJ236 cells: A single colony is grown in 50 mL of 2X YT medium with 30 μg/mL chloremphenicol at 37°C in the shaker overnight. Inoculate 1 mL of overnight CJ236

culture into 50 mL of 2X YT (no chloremphenicol) and grow for 2 h at 37°C. Infect bacteria with 10 μL of 100-fold diluted high-titer phage stock, and incubate for 6 h at 37°C in a shaker. The titer of high-titer phage stock is usually about 5×10^{11} pfu/mL.

2. Precipitate U-phage: Spin down cells at 5000 rpm for 15 min (supernatant containing U-phage can be stored overnight, but it should be clarified again by centrifugation). Take 40 mL of supernatant, add 10 mL of 20% PEG/3.5 M NH$_4$OAc, mix well, and incubate on ice for 0.5–1 h or at 4°C overnight. Take 1 mL of supernatant for titration.

3. Titration of U-phage: Serially dilute U-phage 10× with 2X YT. Infect 200 μL of CJ236 and XL-1 Blue cells respectively with diluted U-phage, mix with 3 mL of top agar, and pour the mixture onto LB plates. Wait for 10 min at RT, then incubate the plate upside down at 37°C overnight. Next morning, if the U-phage population grown on the CJ236 lawn is more than 10^4 times higher than that grown on the XL-1 Blue lawn, the U-phage are of high quality.

4. Digest U-template with RNase A: Centrifuge overnight precipitated supernatant at 12,000 rpm for 20 min. Pour off the supernatant carefully, and resuspend the phage pellet by pipetting up and down and gentle vortex in 1 mL of residual PEG supernatant. Transfer the suspension to a 1.5 mL tube, add 50 μL of 10 mg/mL RNase A, incubate for 30 min at RT, and chill on ice. Spin down the phage at 12,000 rpm in a micro-centrifuge for 10 min at 4°C, and remove the supernatant. Spin again to remove the residual supernatant. Resuspend the pellet in 400 μL of high salt buffer (300 mM NaCl, 100 mM Tris-HCl, pH 8.0, 1 mM EDTA). Incubate on ice for 5 min, centrifuge for 2 min at 12,000 rpm to precipitate residual debris. Transfer the supernatant to a fresh tube and keep at 4°C.

5. Purification of U-template with phenol/chloroform extraction: Add 150 μL of phenol into 300 μL of U-phage, vortex vigorously for 15 s. Add 150 μL of chloroform into the mixture and vortex vigorously for 15 s. Centrifuge for 5 min in a microcentrifuge, carefully take the top portion out and transfer to a new tube. Repeat the phenol/choroform extraction. Take the top portion and add equal volume of chloroform. Vortex, centrifuge, and transfer the top portion to a new tube.

6. Ethanol precipitation of U-template: Add 1/50 vol of 5 M NaCl and 2 vol of 100% EtOH. Incubate for 15 min at –70°C. Centrifuge for 25 min at 4°C. Carefully remove the supernatant, and resuspend the pellet in 80 μL of TE buffer, pH 8.0. Add 20 μL of 7.5 M NH$_4$OAc, and 200 μL of 100% EtOH. Incubate for 15 min at –70°C. Centrifuge for 15 min at 4°C. Wash the pellet with 70% EtOH once, vacuum dry for 3 min, and resuspend in 40 μL of TE buffer. Apply 1 μL of U-template to 0.7% agarose gel to check the purity. Measure OD$_{260}$ for the concentration.

3.1.4. Hybridization Mutagenesis

1. Set up an annealing reaction using approx eightfold molar ratio increase of insert to vector: 200 ng of uridinylated phage vector (8.49 kb), 77 ng phosphorylated single-stranded H chain (408 bases), 68 ng phosphorylated single-stranded L chain (360 bases), 1 μL 10X annealing buffer. Adjust total volume with ddH$_2$O to 10 μL. Carry out the annealing reaction in the PCR machine: 85°C hold for 5 min (denaturation). Ramp to 55°C over 1 h. Chill on ice.

2. Minus strand synthesis: To the annealed product add: 1.4 μL 10X synthesis buffer, 1 μL T4 DNA ligase (1 U/μL), 1 μL T4 DNA polymerase (1 U/μL). Incubate on ice for 5 min, RT for 5 min, and 37°C for 1.5 h. Ethanol precipitate, and dissolve DNA pellet in 10 μL of ddH$_2$O.

3. Digest DNA with 1 μL *Eco*RI (10 U/μL) for 2 h at 37°C (*see* **Note 1**), and heat-inactivate at 65°C for 20 min. Transfect 1 μL of digested DNA into 30 μL of electrocompetent DH10B cells by electroporation. Titer the produced phage by growing on an XL-1Blue bacterial lawn at 37°C overnight.

4. PCR can be used to screen for the phage that incorporates both V_L and V_H chain. The selected clones are further confirmed by DNA sequencing.

3.2. Construction of Focused CDR Libraries

For CDR library construction, the parental CDR region needs to be deleted first to avoid the domination of the library by the parental clone. In a successful single-site hybridization mutagenesis, the mutagenesis rate is usually between 50–80%. If the parental antibody is used as a template for the library construction, there will be 20 to 50% of the library population that is parent, and this will increase the difficulty of screening. The CDR region can be deleted by mutagenesis as described in **Subheading 3.1.4**. The oligonucleotide for mutagenesis is designed to replace the CDR region with a stop codon (TAA) and an extra nucleotide (A) to cause the frameshift. After the clone (ΔCDR) is made, it is used as a template for the construction of its corresponding CDR library. Altogether six CDR-deleted templates corresponding to individual CDR library need to be prepared. To construct focused CDR libraries, the codon-based mutagenesis approach *(39)* is used to synthesize the oligonucleotides coding for CDR mutations. With modification, one can synthesize oligonucleotides containing single, double, triple mutations, etc., respectively. The oligonucleotides are then used for library construction by hybridization mutagenesis *(52)*. For affinity maturation, single-mutation libraries are sufficient. If significant characteristic change is desired for the antibody, double and more mutations may be needed.

3.2.1. Modified Codon-Based Mutagenesis

The modified codon-based mutagenesis approach is used to synthesize oligonucleotides to introduce mutations into CDR regions. By using this synthesis approach, the mutations are segregated into pools of oligonucleotides (*see* **Fig. 2**). Taking an eight-residue CDR as an example, the synthesis starts with one DNA synthesizer column for the synthesis of 18-nucleotide (nt) CDR flanking region. When the synthesis reaches the CDR region, the synthesis reaction is paused. The beads from the column are split, then repacked into two new columns for the synthesis of the eighth codon of the CDR (*see* **Note 2**). On one column a parental DNA sequence is synthesized, and on the other column a random (C/A)NN sequence encoding all 20 amino acids is synthesized. The only stop codon that appears in this doping strategy is UAG, which can be suppressed in *supE E. coli* strains such as XL-1 Blue. After the synthesis of the eighth codon, the beads are split and repacked into four new columns for the synthesis of the seventh codon. In the same manner, on two columns a parental DNA sequence is synthesized (as indicated by dotted arrows in **Fig. 2**), and on the other columns a random (C/A)NN sequence is synthesized (as indicated by filed arrows). The beads from the columns coding for the same degree of mutagenesis are pooled, then split into new columns for the synthesis of the sixth codon (at this time, six columns are used). The synthesis-pool-split cycle is repeated for each CDR codon as

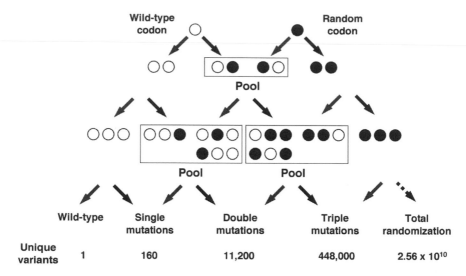

Fig. 2. Modified codon-based mutagenesis. This approach allows the segregation of diversity into pools based on the degree of mutagenesis. The open circles represent wild-type codons, and the filled circles represent random codons. The dotted arrows indicate the synthesis of the wild-type codon, and the filled arrows indicate the synthesis of the random codon. Unique variants shown underneath of each oligonucleotide are based on the protein level.

shown in **Fig. 2**. After the CDR region is synthesized, the reaction continues for the synthesis of the other end of the CDR flanking region. In the end, nine oligonucleotides will be synthesized coding for different degree of mutagenesis (including wild-type). As the mutation number increases, the number of unique variants (based on protein level) increases dramatically (**Fig, 2**). For example, there are 160 variants coded by the single-mutation oligonucleotide, 11,200 variants by double-mutation oligonucleotide, and 448,000 variants by triple-mutation oligonucleotide. In most cases, only single- and double-mutation oligonucleotide are needed (*see* **Note 3**). It is therefore not necessary to do the full-scale synthesis for all the nine oligonucleotides.

3.2.2. Construction and Characterization of Single-Mutation CDR Libraries

Single-mutation CDR libraries are particularly useful for affinity maturation. The oligonucleotides coding for single CDR mutations are synthesized by the modified codon-based mutagenesis approach, and are purified by polyacrylamide gel electrophoresis (PAGE). Uridinylated template for each ΔCDR clone is prepared according to **Subheading 3.1.3.** Each CDR library is constructed and characterized as following:

1. Phosphorylation of oligonucleotide: 200 pmol oligonucleotide, 2 µL 10X PNK buffer, 1 µL 10 m*M* ATP, 1 µL T4 polynucleotide kinase (10 U/µL). Add up to 20 µL in total volume with ddH$_2$O. Incubate for 45 min at 37°C, and denature for 10 min by heat at 65°C. Keep at 4°C for the next step. The concentration of the phosphorylated oligonucleotide is 10 pmol/µL.

2. Annealing: The molar ratio of oligonucleotide to template is 20. 200 ng (= 0.069 pmol) Uridinylated ΔCDR template (8.8 kb), 1.4 pmol phosphorylated oligonucleotide, 1 μL 10X annealing buffer. Add up to 10 μL in total volume with ddH$_2$O. Incubate the mixture for 5 min at 85°C, and cool for 10 min at RT.
3. Minus strand synthesis: To the annealed product add: 1.4 μL 10X synthesis buffer, 1 μL T4 DNA ligase (1 U/μL), 1 μL T4 DNA polymerase (1 U/μL). Incubate at RT for 5 min, and 37°C for 1.5 h. Keep at 4°C for the next step.
4. Electroporation: Electroporate 1 μL of the above mutagenesis mixture into 30 μL of electrocompetent DH10B cells. Add 200 μL of LB medium to the cuvet. Titer the produced phage on XL-1 Blue bacterial lawn at 37°C overnight.
5. Library characterization: Randomly sequence some phage to examine the distribution of the mutations in the CDR region. This information can also be used to estimate the mutagenesis rate, which will affect the number of the clones needed to be screened for the library.

3.3. Screening of Focused CDR Libraries

The screening strategy can affect what kind of antibody variants are selected from the library. One can mimic the conditions used in the kinetic simulation to select the higher affinity variants either driven by k_{off} (**Fig. 1A**) or by k_{on} (**Fig. 1B**). First, a capturing reagent is used to capture a constant amount of antibody variants for the assay. Antigen concentration should be lower than the K$_d$ value to favor high affinity clones. For k_{off}-driven screening, improved variants are isolated under conditions allowing the interaction between antibody and antigen for at least 1 h; then the dissociation is carried out by frequent wash and incubation with wash buffer (*see* **Subheadings 3.3.1.1.** and **3.3.1.2.**). To select for variants with improved k_{on} value, both the association and dissociation time need to be as short as possible (preferably ≤10 min total). Usually this process will result in a weak signal output. A signal amplification step may be added to increase the signal/noise ratio (*see* **Subheading 3.3.2.**).

To screen a library exhaustively with high confidence, three times the size of the library is screened. Typical mutagenesis rates for library construction are ≥50%, thus a twofold factor needs to be adjusted for the mutagenesis background. Since each single-mutation CDR library normally contains less than 400 variants, approx 2400 clones (= 400 × 3 × 2) need to be screened per library.

3.3.1. k_{off}-Driven Screening

Two assays can be used for k_{off}-driven screening. One is the capture lift assay (*56*), and the other is the single-point ELISA assay (SPE) (*57*). The capture lift assay was developed for the initial high-throughput screening of large libraries (*33,54,56*). This procedure is semi-quantitative, and up to 10^5 clones can be screened from one 82-mm filter. The phage-expressed parental Fab is used as a control. Only the variants that show a stronger signal, that indicates higher affinity, than the parental phage will be isolated. It is usually necessary to confirm the selected variants by the second screening assay, SPE to eliminate certain false positive clones. Alternatively, SPE can be used for primary screening when the size of the libraries is small. SPE is a quantitative procedure, in that an OD signal is obtained, which correlates to the affinity of the clones. In addition, SPE has better signal/noise ratio than capture lift. As an example, the established conditions and steps for capture lift and SPE assays used in the selection of high-affinity humanized anti-$\alpha_v\beta_3$ antibodies *(33)* are listed below.

3.3.1.1. CAPTURE LIFT ASSAY

1. Place 10 mL of 10 μg/mL goat anti-human kappa antibody in PBS into a 100-mm Petri dish.
2. Label an 82-mm nitrocellulose filter with nonwater-soluble ink. Using tweezers, carefully float the filter, labeled side up, on antibody solution for at least 2 h at RT. Flip the filter, submerge it in the solution, and incubate for 20–30 min with shaking.
3. Remove the filter, blot excess buffer lightly off the edge of the filter, and lay the filter with the labeled side down on a sheet of Saran Wrap in a tissue culture hood until dry (approx 30 min).
4. Block the filter (labeled side down) in 10 mL of 1% BSA/PBS on a shaker for 2 h at RT.
5. Remove the filter from blocking solution, and rinse 3× with PBS.
6. Blot excess buffer as in **step 3**.
7. Overlay the filter onto the plaque lawn, and incubate overnight at 22°C in an incubator. The filter should be laid with the labeled side up on the agar. Mark the filter position by poking holes in the filter with a needle and mark the holes on the bottom of plate with a felt pen.
8. Prepare 1.0 μg/mL ($\approx$4.2 n*M*) of biotinylated $\alpha_v\beta_3$ in HEPES/NP40 buffer (4 mL/filter) and keep on ice.
9. Peel the filter off agar and rinse 3× with PBS.
10. Immerse filter, labeled side down, in 4 mL antigen solution (biotinylated $\alpha_v\beta_3$) and place on a shaker for 3 h at 4°C.
11. Wash filter on vacuum washer apparatus 4× with HEPES/NP40 buffer.
12. Incubate filter (labeled side down) in 10 mL HEPES/NP40 buffer containing 4.5 μg/mL of NeutrAvidin-alkaline phosphatase. Shake for 15 min at RT.
13. Wash filter on vacuum washer apparatus 4× with HEPES/NP40 buffer.
14. Develop with alkaline phosphatase substrate (NBT-BCIP) for 10–15 min at RT on a shaker.
15. Isolate plaques that develop as darker spots on filters compared to parental Fab phage. Elute the phage in 200 μL phage elution buffer for ≥1 h at 37°C or overnight at 4°C. The titer of eluted phage is usually $\approx$2 × 10^8 pfu/mL.

3.3.1.2. SINGLE POINT ELISA (SPE)

1. Coat Immulon 2 plate with an anti-decapeptide MAb at 10 μg/mL in PBS at 4°C overnight. The MAb recognizes a peptide tag on the carboxy-terminus of the Fab heavy chains in the library.
2. Tap out coating solution. Block with 3% BSA/PBS (200 μL/well) for 1.5 h at 37°C.
3. Wash 3× with HEPES/NP40 buffer.
4. Add 50 μL of Fab extract from periplasmic preparation (*see* **Subheading 3.3.1.2.1.**) (*see* **Note 4**). Incubate for 2 h at RT.
5. Wash 7× with HEPES/NP40 buffer.
6. Add 0.5–1.0 μg/mL of biotinylated $\alpha_v\beta_3$ in HEPES/NP40 buffer, and incubate for 1 h at RT. Biotinylated a_vb_3 should be prepared and used in 10 d.
7. Wash 7× with HEPES/NP40 buffer.
8. Add 50 μL/well of streptavidin-alkaline phosphatase at 0.5 U/mL in HEPES/NP40 buffer for 15 min at RT.

9. Wash 7× with HEPES/NP40 buffer.
10. Add 50 μL/well AMP-PMP substrate. Develop in the dark for 25 min or until appropriate signals appear.

3.3.1.2.1. Isolation of Soluble Fab from Periplasmic Space (0.36 mL-Prep)

1. Grow XL-1 Blue cells in 2X YT medium containing 10 μg/mL of tetracycline at 37°C in a shaker at 250 rpm until OD_{600} reaches 0.9–1.2.
2. Add 0.5 mM IPTG to XL-1 Blue cells, and transfer 0.75 mL of bacteria to each well of a 96-well deep-well plate.
3. Infect bacteria in each well with 5–25 μL of the eluted phage stock (for phage elution, *see* **Subheading 3.3.1.1., step 15**), and incubate for 1 h at 37°C. Switch the temperature to RT, and grow overnight.
4. Filter 360 μL of phage-infected bacteria through a "silent screen plate" using a vacuum-filtration manifold.
5. Place a 96-well microtiter plate under the filtration device. To lyse cells, add 200 μL of TES buffer containing 2 mg/mL of lysozyme to each well of "silent screen plate". Incubate for 10 min at RT.
6. Apply vacuum for 1 h to collect filtrate into the microtiter plate. The filtrate is used for assays.

3.3.2. k_{on}-Driven Screening

Developing a reliable assay to screen for the variants with improved k_{on} values is more difficult than developing an assay to screen k_{off}-based improved clones. In the current example, only the ELISA assay, k_{on}SPE is established.

1. Coat Immulon 1B plate with goat anti-human kappa antibody at 1 μg/mL in carbonate coating buffer at 4°C overnight.
2. Tap out coating solution. Block with of 1% BSA/PBS (200 μL/well) for 1 h at RT.
3. Remove BSA, and add 200 μL of Fab extract from periplasmic preparation to each well (*see* **Subheading 3.3.1.2.1.**) (*see* **Note 4**). Incubate for 2 h at RT.
4. Wash 3× with PBS/0.1% Tween-20.
5. Add 50 μL/well of antigen-horseradish peroxidase (HRP) complex, and incubate for 10 min at RT (*see* **Note 5**).
6. Wash 3× with PBS/0.1% Tween-20 quickly.
7. Add TMB substrate, and incubate for 15 min at RT. Stop the reaction with 0.5 M H_2SO_4 (final concentration).

3.4. Confirmation of Isolated Fab Variants

The k_{off}-driven high affinity clones are confirmed by ELISA titration on immobilized antigen. The variants with increased k_{on} values are confirmed by kinetic analysis using BIAcore biosensor. Fab extracts isolated from a 15-mL culture periplasmic preparation are used for the confirmation. BIAcore analysis of parental Fab and several variants with different degrees of k_{on} improvement based on the k_{on}SPE assay is shown in **Fig. 3**. Background binding to a nonspecific antigen and the chip matrix was subtracted before the kinetic analysis was performed. Three repeats were performed, and every sample was prepared independently. BIAcore measurements confirmed that the variants isolated indeed have higher k_{on} value than that of the parental antibody.

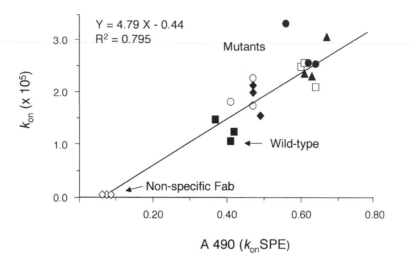

Fig. 3. Correlation between k_{on}SPE and k_{on} determined by BIAcore. Parental Fab (■) and five variants (other symbols) identified by k_{on}SPE assay were analyzed by BIAcore biosensor. Straight line is the linear regression fit of the data. BIAcore analysis not only confirmed the k_{on} improvement, but also validated the reliability of the k_{on}SPE assay. Three repeats were performed using Fab samples from 15-mL periplasmic preparation, and every sample was prepared independently.

The protocols for 15 mL-periplasmic preparation, and Fab quantitation are provided below:

3.4.1. Isolation of Soluble Fab from Periplasmic Space (15 mL-Prep)

1. Grow XL-1 Blue cells in 2X YT medium containing 10 µg/mL of tetracycline at 37°C in a shaker at 250 rpm until OD_{600} reaches 0.9–1.2.
2. Add 0.5 mM IPTG to XL-1 Blue cells, and aliquot 15 mL each into 50-mL polypropylene conical tubes for each phage clone to be characterized.
3. Infect bacteria with 10 µL of high titer phage (titer = ≈5 × 10^{11} pfu/mL), and incubate for 1 h at 37°C. Switch the temperature to RT, and grow overnight.
4. Spin down the cells at 3000 rpm for 25 min (≈2000g).
5. Aspirate and discard the supernatant. Remove as much culture medium as possible.
6. Resuspend the pellet in 640 µL of resuspension buffer, vortex, and place the sample on ice for 1 h with occasional gentle shaking.
7. Pellet the cellular debris in microcentrifuge at 9000 rpm for 10 min at 4°C.
8. Isolate the supernatant, and store at 4°C.

3.4.2. Fab Quantitation Assay

1. Coat Immulon 1 microtiter plates with goat anti-human Fab capture antibody (ICN-Cappel, cat. no. 55010) (≈8 mg/mL) diluted 4000-fold in carbonate coating buffer overnight at 4°C.
2. Wash 3× in PBS/0.1% Tween-20.
3. Dilute IgG Fab standard in PBS/0.05% Tween-20. The standard curve starts at 50 ng/mL

and is diluted serially, twofold to 0.391 ng/mL (50, 25, 12.5, 6.25, 3.125, 1.563, 0.781, and 0.391 ng/mL).

4. Dilute the Fab samples. For 15 mL-prep, the initial dilution should be 50-fold into PBS/0.05% Tween-20. Dilute serially, 2-fold to a 6400-fold dilution (8 dilutions total).
5. Incubate the serially diluted Fab samples with the capture antibody for 1 h at 37°C.
6. Wash 3× in PBS/0.1% Tween-20.
7. Add goat anti-human kappa-alkaline phosphatase conjugate diluted 1000-fold in PBS/0.05% Tween-20, and incubate for 1 h at 37°C.
8. Wash 3× in PBS/0.1% Tween-20.
9. Add alkaline phosphatase substrates (AMP-PMP) for 1 h.
10. The Fab standard curve is plotted and used to estimate the concentrations of Fab samples.

3.5. Construction, Screening, and Characterization of Combinatorial Mutations

Single-mutation clones, isolated with confirmed desired affinity improvements, are DNA sequenced. Beneficial mutations from six focused CDR libraries are tabulated. A combinatorial library is constructed by multiple-site hybridization mutagenesis *(53)* using degenerate oligonucleotides encoding beneficial mutations and the parental uridinylated template. Because not all mutations are compatible with each other, the wild-type residue should always be included at each combinatorial CDR position in each degenerate oligonucleotide. The library is randomly sequenced to analyze the distribution of combined mutations. Assays described previously are used to screen the combinatorial library. Once the improvement of the identified combinatorial clones are confirmed, the clones are DNA sequenced. Finally, Fab fragments are purified or intact antibodies are generated for subsequent functional characterizations.

4. Notes

1. The annealing sites for V_L and V_H gene contain a palindromic loop, and each loop contains a unique *Eco*RI site. By digesting the mutagenesis mixture with *Eco*RI, the vectors that did not incorporate both V_L and V_H chains are fragmented; as a result, the co-expression rate of V_L and V_H chains is increased.
2. Since the oligonucleotide is intended for the mutagenesis purpose, the complementary strand is synthesized. Thus, for the CDR region, the complementary strand starts with the last residue (in the current example, the eighth residue).
3. The modified codon-based mutagenesis approach uses a hierarchical molecular design (*see* **Fig. 2**). The mathematical basis of hierarchical molecular design is:

$$R = n!/(n - m)!m! \times p^{n-m} \times q^m$$

R: % yield of each oligonucleotide. n: number of codons in the CDR region (residue number). m: number of mutations in the oligonucleotide. p: % of parental codon. q: % of random codon (= 1 − p). Using this equation, one can calculate the yield of each oligonucleotide at the end of synthesis. Since the yield is determined by n, m, p and q, one can maximize the yield toward the oligonucleotides desired by adjusting the percentage of beads during the "split" step. For example, with an eight-residue CDR, if single- and double-mutation oligonucleotides are desired, to obtain optimal yields 80% (p) of the beads should be split for the synthesis of the parental sequence at each cycle, and 20% (q) for the random sequence. This would result in 33.6% (= $8!/(8 − 1)!1! \times 0.8^7 \times 0.2^1$) of the yield for the single-mutation oligonucleotide, and 29.4% ($= 8!/(8-2)!2! \times 0.8^6 \times 0.2^2$) for the double-mutation oligonucleotide. Other p values will result in lower combined yield and disproportional yield distribution of both oligonucleotides.

4. Alternatively, a culture supernatant can be used instead of the periplasmic preparation for assays. Although Fab fragments expressed by bacteria are assembled and accumulated in periplasmic space, significant amounts of Fabs leak into culture medium. The concentrations of the Fab fragments for 0.36 mL-periplasmic preparation and culture medium are similar, mostly ranging from 1–3 µg/mL depending on the clones. To prepare culture medium containing Fab for screening, follow **Subheading 3.3.1.2.1., steps 1–3**, then centrifuge the deep-well plate at 2000 rpm for 20 min. Use 50 µL of supernatant from each well for assays.

5. The antigen-HRP complex is used to skip one incubation step (for the detection of bound antigen), resulting in decreased dissociation time. It is also used to increase the sensitivity of the assay (signal amplification). The complex is formed by mixing biotinylated antigen (0.5 nM), streptavidin-HRP, and biotinylated HRP with a molar ratio of 1:4:9 for 30 min at 37°C. The antigen is biotinylated at a ratio of 20:1 of biotin to antigen. The ratio of the three components is determined by serial dilutions, and the optimal ratio is selected based on the degree of signal amplification. For different antigen-antibody interactions, the parameters should be always determined by experiments.

Acknowledgments

We would like to thank Patrice O. Yarbough, Catherine M. Falcon, and Sanjaya Singh for their critical review of the manuscript.

References

1. Glennie, M. J. and Johnson, P. W. M. (2000) Clinical trials of antibody therapy. *Immunol. Today* **21,** 403–410.
2. Smith, G. P (1985) Filamentous fusion phage: novel expression vectors that display cloned antigens on the virion surface. *Science* **228,** 1315–1317.
3. McCafferty, J., Griffiths, A. D., Winter, G., and Chiswell, D. J. (1990) Phage antibodies: filamentous phage displaying antibody variable domains. *Nature* **348,** 552–554.
4. Barbas, C. F., Kang, A. S., Lerner, R. A., and Benkovic, S. J. (1991) Assembly of combinatorial libraries on phage surfaces: The gene III site. *Proc. Natl. Acad. Sci. USA* **88,** 7978–7982.
5. Chang, C. N., Landolfi, N. F., and Queen, C. (1991) Expression of antibody Fab domains on bacteriophage surfaces. Potential use for antibody selection. *J. Immunol.* **147,** 3610–3614.
6. Hoogenboom, H. R., Griffiths, A. D., Johnson, K. S., Chiswell, D. J., Hudson, P., and Winter, G. (1991) Multi-subunit proteins on the surface of filamentous phage: methodologies for displaying antibody (Fab) heavy and light chains. *Nucleic Acids Res.* **19,** 4133–4137.
7. Burton, D. R., Barbas, C. F., Persson, M. A. A., Koenig, S., Chanock, R. M., and Lerner, R. A. (1991) A large array of human monoclonal antibodies to type 1 human immunodeficiency virus from combinatorial libraries of asymptomatic seropositive individuals. *Proc. Natl. Acad. Sci. USA* **88,** 10,134–10,137.
8. Zebedee, S. L., Barbas, C. F., Hom, Y.-L., Caothien, R. H., Graff, R., DeGraw, J., et al. (1992) Human combinatorial antibody libraries to hepatitis B surface antigen. *Proc. Natl. Acad. Sci. USA* **89,** 3175–3179.
9. Marks, J. D., Hoogenboom, H. R., Bonnert, T. P., McCafferty, J., Griffiths, A. D., and

Winter, G. (1991). By-passing immunization. Human antibodies from V-gene libraries displayed on phage. *J. Mol. Biol.* **222**, 581–597.

10. Griffiths, A. D., Malmqvist, M., Marks, J. D., Bye, J. M., Embleton, M. J., McCafferty, J., et al. (1993) Human anti-self antibodies with high specificity from phage display libraries. *EMBO J.* **12**, 725–734.

11. Barbas, C. F., Bain, J. D., Hoesktra, D. M., and Lerner, R. A. (1992). Semisynthetic combinatorial antibody libraries: a chemical solution to the diversity problem. *Proc. Natl. Acad. Sci. USA* **89**, 4457–4461.

12. Hoogenboom, H. R. and Winter, G. (1992). By-passing immunisation. Human antibodies from synthetic repertoires of germline V_H gene segments rearranged in vitro. *J. Mol. Biol.* **227**, 381–388.

13. Foote, J. and Milstein, C. (1991) Kinetic maturation of an immune response. *Nature* **352**, 530–523.

14. Perelson, A. S. and Oster, G. F. (1979) Theoretical studies of clonal selection: minimal antibody repertoire size and reliability of self-non-self discrimination. *J. Theor. Biol.* **81**, 645–670.

15. Vaughan, T. J., Williams, A. J., Pritchard, K., Osbourn, J. K., Pope, A. R., Earnshaw, J. C., et al. (1996) Human antibodies with sub-nanomolar affinities isolated from a large non-immunized phage display library. *Nat. Biotechnol.* **14**, 309–314.

16. Sheets, M. D., Amersdorfer, P., Finnern, R., Sargent, P., Lindovist, E., Schier, R., et al. (1998) Efficient construction of a large nonimmune phage antibody library: the production of high-affinity human single-chain antibodies to protein antigens. *Proc. Natl. Acad. Sci. USA* **95**, 6157–6162.

17. de Haard, H. J., van Neer, N., Reurs, A., Hufton, S. E., Roovers, R. C., Henderikx, P., et al. (1999) A large non-immunized human Fab fragment phage library that permits rapid isolation and kinetic analysis of high affinity antibodies. *J. Biol. Chem.* **274**, 18,218–18,230.

18. Sblattero, D. and Bradbury, A. (2000) Exploiting recombination in single bacteria to make large phage antibody libraries. *Nat. Biotechnol.* **18**, 75–80.

19. Griffiths, A. D., Williams, S. C., Hartley, O., Tomlinson, I. M., Waterhouse, P., Crosby, W. L., et al. (1994) Isolation of high affinity human antibodies directly from large synthetic repertoires. *EMBO J.* **13**, 3245–3260.

20. Knappik, A., Ge, L., Honegger, A., Pack, P., Fischer, M., Wellnhofer, G., et al. (2000) Fully synthetic human combinatorial antibody libraries (HuCAL) based on modular consensus frameworks and CDRs randomized with trinucleotides. *J. Mol. Biol.* **296**, 57–86.

21. de Bruin, R., Spelt, K., Mol, J., Koes, R., and Quattrocchio, F. (1999) Selection of high-affinity phage antibodies from phage display libraries. *Nature Biotechnol.* **17**, 397–399.

22. Usinger, W. R. and Lucas, A. H. (1999) Avidity as a determinant of the protective efficacy of human antibodies to pneumococcal capsular polysaccharides. *Infect. Immun.* **67**, 2366–2370.

23. Johnson, S., Griego, S. D., Pfarr, D. S., Doyle, M. L., Woods, R., Carlin, D., et al. (1999) A direct comparison of the activities of two humanized respiratory syncytial virus monoclonal antibodies: MEDI-493 and RSHZl9. *J. Infect. Dis.* **180**, 35–40.

24. Mita, H., Yasueda, H., and Akiyama, K. (2000) Affinity of IgE antibody to antigen influences allergen-induced histamine release. *Clin. Exp. Allergy* **30**, 1583–1589.

25. Parren, P. W. H. I., Mondor, I., Naniche, D., Ditzel, H. J., Klasse, P. J., Burton, D. R., and Sattentau, Q. J. (1998) Neutralization of human immunodeficiency virus type 1 by anti-

body to gp120 is determined primarily by occupancy of sites on the virion irrespective of epitope specificity. *J. Virol.* **72,** 3512–3519.

26. Gram, H., Marconi, L. A., Barbas, C. F., Collet, T. A., Lerner, R. A., and Kang, A. S. (1992) In vitro selection and affinity maturation of antibodies from a naive combinatorial immunoglobulin library. *Proc. Natl. Acad. Sci. USA* **89,** 3576–3580.

27. Yelton, D. E., Rosok, M. J., Cruz, G., Cosand, W. L., Bajorath, J., et al. (1995) Affinity maturation of the BR96 anti-carcinoma antibody by codon-based mutagenesis. *J. Immunol.* **155,** 1994–2004.

28. Yang, W. P., Green, K., Pinz-Sweeney, S., Briones, A. T., Burton, D. R., and Barbas, C. F. (1995) CDR walking mutagenesis for the affinity maturation of a potent human anti-HIV-1 antibody into the picomolar range. *J. Mol. Biol.* **254,** 392–403.

29. Schier, R., Bye, J., Apell, G., McCall, A., Adams, G. P., Malmqvist, M., et al. (1996) Isolation of high-affinity monomeric human anti-c-erbB-2 single chain Fv using affinity-driven selection. *J. Mol. Biol.* **255,** 28–43.

30. Schier, R., McCall, A., Adams, G. P., Marshall, K. W., Merritt, H., Yim, M., et al. (1996) Isolation of picomolar affinity anti-c-erbB-2 single-chain Fv by molecular evolution of the complementarity determining regions in the center of the antibody binding site. *J. Mol. Biol.* **263,** 551–567.

31. Thompson, J., Pope, T., Tung, J. S., Chan, C., Hollis, G., Mark, G., and Johnson, K. S. (1996) Affinity maturation of a high-affinity human monoclonal antibody against the third hypervariable loop of human immunodeficiency virus: use of phage display to improve affinity and broaden strain reactivity. *J. Mol. Biol.* **256,** 77–88.

32. Schier, R., Balint, R. F., McCall, A., Apell, G., Larrick, J. W., and Marks, J. D. (1996) Identification of functional and structural amino-acid residues by parsimonious mutagenesis. *Gene* **169,** 147–155.

33. Wu, H., Beuerlein, G., Nie, Y., Smith, H., Lee, B. A., Hensler, M., et al. (1998) Stepwise in vitro affinity maturation of Vitaxin, an alphav beta3- specific humanized MAb. *Proc. Natl. Acad. Sci. USA* **95,** 6037–6042.

34. Chowdhury, P. S. and Pastan, I. (1999) Improving antibody affinity by mimicking somatic hypermutation in vitro. *Nature Biotechnol.* **17,** 568–572.

35. Boder, E. T., Midelfort, K. S., and Wittrup, K. D.(2000) Directed evolution of antibody fragments with monovalent femtomolar antigen-binding affinity. *Proc. Natl. Acad. Sci. USA* **97,** 10,701–10,705.

36. Adams, G. P., Schier, R., Marshall, K., Wolf, E. J., McCall, A. M., Marks, J. D., and Weiner, L. M. (1998) Increased affinity leads to improved selective tumor delivery of single-chain Fv antibodies. *Cancer Res.* **58,** 485–490.

37. Viti, F., Tarli, L., Giovannoni, L., Zardi, L., and Neri, D. (1999) Increased binding affinity and valence of recombinant antibody fragments lead to improved targeting of tumoral angiogenesis. *Cancer Res.* **59,** 347–352.

38. Adams, G. P. and Schier, R. (1999) Generating improved single-chain Fv molecules for tumor targeting. *J. Immunol. Methods* **231,** 249–260.

39. Glaser, S. M., Yelton, D. E., and Huse, W. D. (1992) Antibody engineering by codon-based mutagenesis in a filamentous phage vector system. *J. Immunol.* **149,** 3903–3913.

40. Martin, F., Toniatti, C., Salvati, A. L., Ciliberto, G., Cortese, R., and Sollazzo, M. (1996) Coupling protein design and in vitro selection strategies: improving specificity and affinity of a designed beta-protein IL-6 antagonist. *J. Mol. Biol.* **255,** 86–97.

41. Hemminki, A., Niemi, S., Hoffren, A. M., Hakalahti, L., Soderlund, H., and Takkinen, K. (1998) Specificity improvement of a recombinant anti-testosterone Fab fragment by

CDRIII mutagenesis and phage display selection. *Protein Eng.* **11,** 311–319.

42. Chames, P. and Baty, D. (1998) Engineering of an anti-steroid antibody: amino acid substitutions change antibody fine specificity from cortisol to estradiol. *Clin. Chem. Lab Med.* **36,** 355–359.

43. Willuda, J., Honegger, A., Waibel, R., Schubiger, P. A., Stahel, R., Zangemeister-Wittke, U., and Pluckthun, A. (1999) High thermal stability is essential for tumor targeting of antibody fragments: engineering of a humanized anti-epithelial glycoprotein-2 (epithelial cell adhesion molecule) single-chain Fv fragment. *Cancer Res.* **59,** 5758–5767.

44. Griffiths, G. M., Berek, C., Kaartinen, M., and Milstein, C. (1984) Somatic mutation and the maturation of immune response to 2-phenyl oxazolone. *Nature* **312,** 271–275.

45. Sandberg, W. S. and Terwilliger, T. C. (1993) Engineering multiple properties of a protein by combinatorial mutagenesis. *Proc. Natl. Acad. Sci. USA* **90,** 8367–8371.

46. Moore, J. C. and Arnold, F. H. (1996) Directed evolution of a para-nitrobenzyl esterase for aqueous-organic solvents. *Nature Biotechnol.* **14,** 458–467.

47. Wells, J. A., Cunningham, B. C., Graycar, T. P., and Estell, D. A. (1987) Recruitment of substrate-specificity properties from one enzyme into a related one by protein engineering. *Proc. Natl. Acad. Sci. USA* **84,** 5167–5171.

48. Wells, J. A., Powers, D. B., Bott, R. R., Graycar, T. P., and Estell, D. A. (1987) Designing substrate specificity by protein engineering of electrostatic interactions. *Proc. Natl. Acad. Sci. USA* **84,** 1219–1223.

49. Russell, A. J. and Fersht, A. R. (1987) Rational modification of enzyme catalysis by engineering surface charge. *Nature* **328,** 496–500.

50. Huse, W. D., Stinchcombe, T., J., Glaser, S. M., Starr, L., Maclean, M., et al. (1992) Application of a filamentous phage pVIII fusion protein system suitable for efficient production, screening, and mutagenesis of F(ab) antibody fragments. *J. Immunol.* **149,** 3914–3920.

51. Glaser, S., Kristensson, K., Chilton, T., and Huse, W. D. (1995) Engineering the antibody combining site by codon-based mutagenesis in a filamentous phage display system, in *Antibody Engineering*, 2nd ed. (Borrebaeck, C. A. K., ed.), Oxford University Press, Oxford, pp. 117–131.

52. Kunkel, T. A. (1985) Rapid and efficient site-specific mutagenesis without phenotypic selection. *Proc. Natl. Acad. Sci. USA* **82,** 488–492.

53. Perlak, F. J. (1990) Single step large scale site-directed in vitro mutagenesis using multiple oligonucleotides. *Nucleic Acids Res.* **18,** 7457–7458.

54. Wu, H., Nie, Y., Huse, W. D., and Watkins, J. D. (1999) Humanization of a murine monoclonal antibody by simultaneous optimization of framework and CDR residues. *J. Mol. Biol.* **294,** 151–162.

55. Wells, J. A. (1990) Additivity of mutational effects in proteins. *Biochemsitry* **29,** 8509–8517.

56. Watkins, J. D., Beuerlein, G., Wu, H., McFadden, P. R., Pancook, J. D., and Huse, W. D. (1998) Discovery of human antibodies to cell surface antigens by capture lift screening of phage-expressed antibody libraries. *Anal. Biochem.* **256,** 169–177.

57. Watkins, J. D., Beuerlein, G., Pecht, G., McFadden, P. R., Glaser, S. M., and Huse, W. D. (1997) Determination of the relative affinities of antibody fragments expressed in *Escherichia coli* by enzyme-linked immunosorbent assay. *Anal. Biochem.* **253,** 37–45.

IV

ANTIBODY FRAGMENTS WITH ADDITIONAL PROPERTIES

14

Engineering scFvs for Improved Stability

Partha S. Chowdhury and George Vasmatzis

1. Introduction

1.1. Antibodies as Drug Carriers

The high binding specificity and affinity of antibody molecules is a biological wonder. Because of these properties they have been used as prophylactic, diagnostic, and analytical reagents for almost a century now. Their use as "magic bullets" for targeted therapy was conceived by Ehrlich in the late 19th century. With the advent first of the hybridoma technology *(1)* and then of recombinant DNA technology dawned the era of antibody-based therapies. Not long after the beginning of this new field of medicine, the hurdles associated with the pharmakokinetic properties of antibodies became clear. It was realized that the large size of the antibody molecules precluded their proper penetration into masses of biological tissues such as solid tumors *(2)*. It was also realized that additional effector functions can be hooked on to antibody molecules. There was the urge to widen the spectrum of effector functions of antibodies by substituting the constant domains with enzymes (to make prodrug), toxins (immunotoxins) and radionucleides *(3)*. These requirements led to the development of the recombinant Fab and the Fv technology. The Fv technology greatly aided in solving not only the problems associated with the large size of the antibody but also in reducing the immunogenecity of mouse monoclonal antibodies (MAbs) in humans. However, it had its own drawbacks, one of which was the loss of stability of many Fvs as compared to the corresponding IgGs *(4)*. This is a serious drawback in view of the fact that for a molecule to be therapeutically successful it has to be stable at 37°C. It is therefore conceivable that some Fvs that have the potential for therapeutic use because of their antigen binding specificity can face the severe limitations arising out of their inherent instability. It is generally believed that the hydrophobic interaction between the V_H and V_L strongly contribute to the stability of a Fv. But in many Fvs this interaction is not strong enough. Because of this Fvs are modified into scFvs where a flexible peptide linker, typically a $(Gly4Ser)_3$ repeat is used to hold the two V domains together

From: *Methods in Molecular Biology, vol. 207: Recombinant Antibodies for Cancer Therapy: Methods and Protocols*
Edited by: M. Welschof and J. Krauss © Humana Press Inc., Totowa, NJ

(5). With the application of the scFv technology to many different Fvs, it was realized that although the linker was effective in covalently holding the two V-domains together, it was not always effective in keeping a scFv active. In other words the chains could still unfold and lead to aggregation. This had led to the hypothesis that increasing the interaction between the two V-domains may be important to enhancing the stability of a biologically active Fv (being capable of remaining as a monomer and bind antigen). Several approaches trying to increase the stability of Fvs have been described. One of the earlier approaches involved engineering disulphide bonds into the framework regions of Fvs such that they are covalently held together *(6).* Other technologies involve either decreasing hydrophobic patches on scFvs to minimize aggregation *(7,8)* and to increase the strength of non-covalent interaction between the V domains *(8).* This involves identifying the potentially "problematic" residues that either reduce the interdomain interaction and/or causes aggregation. This chapter is meant to help the reader in identifying the potentially problematic residues and in making a judgement call on substitution(s) that is (are) likely to stabilize the Fv. The discussion that follows and the strategy that is presented is largely based on information that was gathered from the Kabat database (Kabat database maintained by Johnson and Wu, http://immuno.bme.nwu.edu). Similar types of information is also available in the Martin database (http://www.biochem.ucl.ac.uk/~martin/abs/abs.info). But what follows below is a simple way to help molecular biologists to identify with reasonable accuracy in the absence of crystal structures amino acids in Fvs that can be mutated to other residues in order to make the Fv more stable. In the discussion to follow we will cite as an example the scFv derived from a MAb called K1. K1 scFv was very unstable, with a half life of only 4 h at 37°C. By following the strategy discussed here, K1 scFv was found to remain fully stable even after 48 h of incubation at 37°C.

1.2. Features of Fvs and Issues About Their Instability

A Fv is composed of the heavy-chain variable domain (V_H) in noncovalent interactions with the light-chain variable domain (V_L). Each chain in a Fv is composed of three complementarity-determining regions (CDRs) and four framework regions (FRs). The CDRs form loops that together build the antigen-binding pocket while the FRs appear as beta-sheets. The beta sheet of each domain has residues that are buried to varying degree and they also have residues that occur on the surface of the sheet. Many of these surface residues form hydrophobic patches and participate in the strong hydrophobic interaction between the beta sheets of the two variable domains, which juxtapose against each other to form the scaffold on which the CDRs rest. The interactions between the V_H and V_L is therefore mostly hydrophobic in nature and is mostly confined to the interface between the V_H and V_L. Because the CDRs are mostly involved with antigen binding specificity and to a great extent determine the affinity for the antigen and are minimally involved in V_H-V_L pairing, it is best not to alter them in an effort to improve the stability of the Fv. One is therefore left with the framework residues to engineer for altering the stability of the Fvs.

An engineered Fv that is devoid of the rest of the Ig molecule is usually less stable than the whole Ig or even a Fab. In a Fab and in a whole Ig the Fv domain rests on a relatively stable platform that is created by the constant domains. Therefore, in the natural state, the Fv presumably gains from at least two sources of stability, first through a decrease in its degrees of freedom and second from favorable hydrophobic interactions with the constant domains. This is probably the reason that the Fvs can afford to acquire naturally occurring somatic mutations that could improve affinity in the expense of stability making the antibody more useful. In an engineered Fv, the V_L and the V_H are without the constant domains and can come apart much easily and are therefore less stable. The somatic mutations that were acquired to improve affinity as Igs could at this time be detrimental for the stability. Fvs or scFvs with such mutations are unstable and therefore cannot be used as parts of therapeutic agents.

At times the somatic mutations are conservative substitutions that have little effect in destabilizing the molecule. Such mutations to unusual residues can be tolerated if they are at exposed positions and are hydrophilic or buried and hydrophobic. Likely, such mutations in spite of being unusual are potentially unproblematic. However, sometimes mutations occur in the interface of the V_L and V_H to promote induced fitting of the antigen. If, in such cases, the mutation is nonconservative it is likely to destabilize the Fv. Most often these mutations are unusual and are potentially problematic.

In the present chapter a scheme is presented to identify the unusual and potentially problematic residues in antibodies taking into account their frequency of occurrence in the antibody database and their exposure state to render them as possible factors of Fv instability. Fvs are known to be unstable because of several factors. There might be other factors involved that are not completely understood currently. The known factors of Fv instability include:

1. Exposure of hydrophobic residues that in an whole Ig molecule is hidden at the interface with the constant domain.
2. Exposure of hydrophobic residues on the surface of the Fv that can lead to intermolecular aggregation.
3. Presence of a hydrophilic residue in the interior of the Fv beta sheet.
4. Presence of hydrophilic residues at the normally hydrophobic interface between V_H and V_L.

It is unusual to have hydrophilic amino acids in the core of a protein and to have hydrophobic residues exposed on the surface. Hydrophilic residues in the core of Fvs may cause the chains to unfold. As a result more hydrophobic patches are likely to be exposed, which can ultimately lead to aggregation. Similarly hydrophobic surface residues tend to cause intermolecular aggregation in an effort to get away from the aqueous environment. As a result, these unusual residues can therefore be potentially problematic with respect to the stability of the Fv proteins. One can therefore envisage that one way to make scFvs more stable would be to identify the unusual and potentially problematic residues in the structure of the Fv.

1.3. What Are Unusual and Problematic Residues?

There is no hard and fast definition of unusual residues in the Fv. We have found it useful to consider a residue to be unusual if it occurs in a particular position with less than 5% frequency in the Kabat database. Antibody sequences, especially framework sequences, are conserved not only within the same subgroups and family but also between different subgroups and families. Usually in every Fv one would come across a number of residues that are very poorly represented for their respective positions. Because the framework forms the scaffold of the Fv and largely dictates its folding and stability, and since Fvs differ in their stability it is logical to suspect these rare residues that are not conserved among different Fvs as playing a role in the instability of the Fvs. However, not all the unusual residues are responsible for the instability of Fvs. Only one or few of them may be responsible. These are what we call the problematic residues. We define an unusual residue as problematic if its hydrophobicity is incompatible with its solvent exposure state. In other words, buried hydrophilic residues and exposed hydrophobic residues are likely to be potentially problematic.

2. Materials

2.1. Bacterial Strains and Bacteriophages

1. *E. coli* TG1: *K12* Δ*(lac-pro)*, *supE*, *thi*, *hsd*Δ5*/F'*[traD36, proAB, lacI^q , lacZΔM15].
2. *E. coli* DH5αF': F'/endA1 hsdR17 (r_k-m_k-) supE44 thi-1 recA1 gyrA (Nal^r) relA1 Δ(laciZYA-argF)U169 deoR(p80dlacΔ (lacZ)M15).
3. *E. coli* CJ236: F' cat (=pCJ105; M13^sCm^r)/*dut ung 1, thi-1 relA1, spoT1 mcrA*.
4. M13KO7 (available from Pharmacia Invitrogen). If one is using a phage display vector then one should also have helper phage R408 (from Stratagene).

2.2. Recombinant DNA

1. A phagemid with the scFv of interest. It is important to know the antibiotic resistance marker, the *E. coli* origin of replication, and the direction of the phage origin of replication.
2. If one is using a phage-display vector, then one should also have a plasmid that has the lacI^q gene and a different antibiotic resistance marker and a different *E. coli* origin of replication than the phagemid.

2.3. Enzymes

1. T7 DNA Polymerase: (Bio-Rad Invitro Mutagenesis kit).
2. T4 DNA Ligase: (Bio-Rad Invitro Mutagenesis kit).
3. Polynucleotide kinase: (3' phosphatase free) (Roche).
4. Taq Polymerase (Promega).
5. Thermostable ligase (New England Biolabs).

2.4. Buffers and Chemicals

1. 10X Buffers for all enzymes (usually provided with the enzymes) (Roche).
2. 10X Annealing buffer: 200 m*M* Tris-HCl, pH 7.4 (at 37°C), 20 m*M* MgCl$_2$, 500 m*M* NaCl (Bio-Rad in vitro mutagenesis refill kit).
3. 10X synthesis buffer: 5 m*M* each dATP,dCTP, dGTP, dTTP, 10 m*M* ATP, 100 m*M* Tris-HCl, pH 7.4 (at 37°C), 50 m*M* MgCl$_2$, 20 m*M* dithiothreitol (DTT) (Bio-Rad in vitro mutagenesis refill kit).
4. 10X Thermostable ligase buffer: 25 m*M* potassium acetate, 20 m*M* Tris-HCl, pH 7.6, 10 m*M* magnesium acetate, 0.1% Triton X-100, 10 m*M* DTT, 1 m*M* NAD^+.
5. T7 DNA Polymerase dilution buffer: 20 m*M* potassium phosphate, pH 7.4, 1 m*M* DTT, 0.1 m*M* EDTA, 50% glycerol.

6. 20% PEG 8000-2.5 *M* NaCl (autoclve and store at 4°C).
7. 1X NET: 100 m*M* NaCl, 1 m*M* EDTA, 10 m*M* Tris-HCl, pH 7.5.
8. Agarose for anlytical gels and low melting point agarose for preparative gel.
9. Buffer-saturated phenol (store at 4°C in amber-colored bottle).
10. Phenol:chloroform:isoamyl alcohol, 25:24:1 (store at 4°C in amber-colored bottle).
12. Chilled ethanol.
12. 8 *M* Lithium chloride in water.

2.5. Oligonucleotides for Mutagenesis and PCRs

These should be high quality oligos purified preferably by HPLC or at least through a reverse phase cartridge.

2.6. Other Apparatus and Accessories

1. Heat blocks at 15–18°C, 65°C, and 72°C.
2. Water bath.
3. Thermocycler.
4. LB Medium: To 950 mL of deionized water add 10 g Bacto-tryptone, 5 g Bacto-yeast extract, 10 g NaCl. Dissolve the solutes and adjust pH to 7.0 with 5 *N* NaOH. Add deionized water to a final volume of 1 L. Sterilize by autoclaving for 20 min at 15 lb/sq. in on liquid cycle. To make LB plates add agar to a final concentration of 1.5% before autoclaving. After the medium is cooled to about 45°C add the ampicillin to a final concentration of 100 µg/mL. For glucose plates add a 20% sterile solution of glucose to a final concentration of 2% after autoclaving and cooling the LB medium to 37°C.
5. 2X YT medium: To 900 mL of deionized water add 16 g Bacto-tryptone, 10 g Bacto-yeast extract, 5 g NaCl. Dissolve the solutes and adjust pH to 7 with 5 *N* NaOH. Adjust the volume to 1 L with deionized water. Sterilize by autoclaving for 20 min at 15 lb/sq. in on liquid cycle.
6. S.O.C. medium: To 80 mL water add 2 g Bacto-tryptone, 0.5 g Bacto-yeast extract, 54.5 mg NaCl, 18.64 mg Potassium chloride, 95.2 mg Magnesium chloride, 120 mg Magnesium sulphate. Dissolve solutes. Adjust pH to 7.0 with 5 *N* NaOH. Adjust volume to 98 mL with deionized water. Sterilize by autoclaving for 20 min at 15 lb/sq. in on liquid cycle. Add 2 mL of a 1 *M* solution of sterile glucose and deionized water to make to volume to 100 mL.
7. M63 Glucose-BI Plates:

    a. Solution A: 12 g Potassium dihydrogen phosphate, 28 g Dipotassium hydrogen phosphate, 8 g Ammonium sulphate. Adjust volume to 2 L with distilled water. Autoclave.
    b. Solution B: 60 g Agar, 1.6 L distilled water. Autoclave.
    c. Solution C: 2 mL 0.1% ferrous sulphate solution, 0.98 g Magnesium sulphate hepta hydrate, 332 mL distilled water. Autoclave.
    d. Solution D: 8 g Glucose, 40 mL distilled water. Autoclave.
    e. Solution E: 8 mL Sterile stock solution of 0.5% thiamine.

    Mix solutions A, B, C, D, and E. Dispense 40 mL per plate.

3. Methods

3.1. How to Identify the Unusual and Potentially Problematic Residues?

As discussed earlier, the unusual residues can be identified by comparing every residue in the framework regions of an Fv with the frequency of different amino acids that occur at that position based on antibody databases. For identifying problematic residues, one would have to resort to the three-dimensional structures of antibodies. To make it easy for the experimentalists to identify unusual and potentially problematic residues three tables, one for the V_Hs (**Table 1**) and the other two for the V_Ls (**Tables 2A,B**) are provided. **Table 2A** is for the kappa light chains and **Table 2B** for the lambda light chains. For the light chains, two different tables are shown because the amino acid sequence for the variable domain of the kappa and the lambda chains are different. These tables are meant to help the reader in identifying the unusual and problematic residues in any given mouse or human Fv.

3.1.1. Description of Tables 1, 2A, and 2B

There are four parts to the tables. The top part of each table shows the primary sequence of the V_H or V_L underlain by single-letter codes that indicate the exposure state for the amino acid at each position. (For details please, *see* ref. *3*.) In **Table 1**, the top part shows the primary sequence of the V_Hs of three antibodies whose crystal structures are known. The 2fb4 is a human V_H segment from the crystal structure of a Fab, 1fvc is the V_H of a humanized Fv, and 1igc is the V_H of a mouse Fab. The top part of **Table 2A** contains the primary sequence of the Vκ of 2fvc and 1igc and the top part of **Table 2B** shows the primary sequence of Vλ of 2fb4. Therefore these three antibodies would serve as good representatives of the vast majority of variable domain that are usually worked with.

The first part of each table is followed by an empty row. This row is provided for the reader to use in determining the potentially problematic residue(s) of the V_H/V_L in use. This is followed by the sequence of an antibody called K1. This is an antibody on which the authors have worked on and is shown as an example of how to use the table.

The bottom part of each table helps the reader to identify the unusual residues in their V_H/V_L sequence. It will also help them to make a selection on what residue to mutate any potentially problematic residue that they may identify. This part of the table shows the frequency of occurrence of different amino acids for each position of the V_H and V_L. The percent frequency of different amino acids have been sorted into bins. In cases where one bin has more than one amino acid, the amino acids have been ranked in the order of descending frequency.

3.1.2. How to Use the Table

Efforts have been made to make the tables easy and simple to use. If you have a Fv that is inherently unstable and would like to generate a more stable variant then try to follow the **steps 1–7** listed below.

1. Determine whether the light chain is a kappa or lambda type. (Note that most mouse light chains are of the kappa type but in humans kappa and lambda occur with almost equal frequencies.) Usually it is easy to determine whether a light chain is kappa or lambda by looking at the sequence of the V-domain. A useful tip is to look at the end of the V-domain. Kappa chains usually end with KLEIK or KLELK or KVELK or KVEVK or sequences close to these. Lambdas end with TVLG or TVLR or TVLS or variants of these. Even by looking at the N-terminus of the V_Ls one can make out whether it is a kappa or a lambda chain. If for any reason one is not able to identify the type of light

Table 1
Exposure State and Frequency of Occurrence of Different Amino Acids for each Position of the Framework Region of V_H

```
VHs  <--------FR1-------><--CDR1--><---FR2---><--CDR2--><---FR3---><--CDR3---><--FR4-->
            1    2    3          4    5        6    7    8    9    10        11
     12345678901234567890123456789012345678901234567890123456789012345678901234567890ABCDEFGHIJK123456789012

2fb4 EVQLVQSGGGVVQPGRSLRLSCSSSGFTFSSYAMY WVRQAPGKGLEWVAIMD DGSTDQHYADSVKGRFTISRNDSKNTLFLQMDSLRPETGVYFCARDGHGFCSSASCFGP DYWGQGTPVTV
     ebebebegggcCcgeebebebebegbebeepbbL  blbLpegegLlelbblbbp egeepLlblpbegbebebepeeebbpbpeebecebbglblbbbbgegeLllellLgL 1eLglgbebcC
1igc DVQLVESGGGLVQPGSRKLSCAASGFTFSSFGMH  WRQAPEKGLEWVAYISS GSSTLHYADTVKGRFTISRDNPKNTLFLQMTSLRSEDTGMYYCARWGNYPYYAM   DYWGQGTNVTVSS
     ebebebegggCbepgegepbpbebegbebeebgbL blbLeellgLlelbblbbp geeepllllebegbbebebpepeeepbbbebeeeebpgpblbbbLgelllLL      LllglgbCbcbcc
1fvc EVQLVESGGGLVQPGSLRLSCAASGFNIKDTYIH  WRQAPGKGLEWVARIYP TNGYTRYADSVKGRFTISADTSKNTAYLQMNSLRAEDTAVYYCSRWGGDGFYAM   DYWGQGTLVTVSS
     epebebegggebeegggebeebgpqbeeebpbL   blbLpegegLlelbblbpb epgeplblepbegbebebepeeebbbpbeeebbbpblbbbLggegLlLL        LllglgbebebeeE
```

```
K1   QVKLQQSGGGLVKVSCAASGFDFSRYWMS WVRQAPGKGLEWIGEINP DSSTIVYTPSLKDFTMSRDNAKNTLYLQTSKVRSADTALYCARRGSHYYGYRTGYF DVWGAGTVTVSS
```

Percent Frequency			
50–100	EVQLQQSG ELVKPG SVKLSCKASGYTF	WVKQAPGKGLEWIG GLEWIG	K TLT D SSSTAYMQLSSLTSEDSAVYYCAR	WGQGT VTVSS
30–50	Q E AG A L F / P	WKQ PG GLEMIG	RA ISV K L M T	TL
20–30	K V G Q G I A	Q A	F R T K N L N	L A / S
10–20	P R SQ SMT TV S	S ERR V / P S L	S A P QVF ER RT T F / N A A / I	A
5–10	DI K AST R STT L I / L I	I TH A	TI K QI K NVK D L T / L A Q	T
3–5	A T M N	F NK HA	I V ED A IT F R	VS / T
2–3	TS A SE V / VD K D / M	KKS KL	D Y A	A L SF S / K N G K G	MT S G / T
1–2	TET SVIL LRR V EF DI / H TD G / M	M D Y A	TNVHFVHT D A R R / G	K G

The top three sequences in this table are the V_Hs of the Fv portions of two Fabs (PDB id: 2fb4 and 1igc) and one Fv (PDB id: 1fvc) with their residues numbered according to their Kabat scheme. The structure of these molecules has been solved by X-ray crystallography. The single letter code under each sequence is the exposure profile as defined in **ref. 8**: [(e) exposed, (p) partially exposed, (b) buried, (C)/(c) partial/full interface with heavy chain constant domain; (L)/(l):partial/full interface V_H residue with V_L domain]. The empty row in the table is for the reader to paste in their V_H sequence for identifying the unusual and problematic residues in their V_Hs. The sequence of K1 is shown as an example. The bottom part of the table has amino acids sorted in bins according to their frequency in the Kabat database for each position (amino acids in CDR segments and of lower than 1% frequency are not shown).

243

Table 2

Exposure State and Frequency of Occurrence of Different Amino Acids for each Position of the Framework Regions of (A) V_κ and (B) V_λ

A

VLs (kappa)	<------FR1------> <-----CDR1-----> <---FR2---> <--CDR2> <---------FR3---------> <--CDR3--> <--FR4-->
	1 2 3 4 5 6 7 8 9 10
	1234567890123456789012345ABCDEF67890123456789012345678901234567890123456789012345ABCDEF67890123456789012345ABCDEF67890123456 7
1igc	NIVMTQSPKSMSMSVGERVTLTCKASE NVVTYVSWYQQKPEQSPKLLIYGASNRYTGVPDRFTGSGSATDFTLTISSVQAEDLADYHCGQGNSYP YTFGGGTKLEIK
	hbebebephebebeeegeeebepbebbe ebeeHbHbHDHcceeHHeHbbHgbeepfhgbeebbeegegeeebpbpbeebeCpbCbpbHbgbgpeHH HbHgggbcbcCc
1fvc	DIQMTQSPSSLSASVGDRVTITCRASQ DVNTAVAWYQQKPGKAPKLLIYSASFLYSGVPSRFSGSRSGTDFTLTISSLQPEDFATYYCQQHYTTP PTFGQGTKVEIK
	ebebebeeebbebpegeeebpbebee ebeebbHbHbHeegeHHeHbbhhbeepHegbpebbeegepgpbbgpbbbeebeeebbpbHbHbHeeHH HbHgegbebeee

K1	SVSYMWH QQKPGSSPRLLIYDTSNLASGVPVRFSGSGSGTSYSLTISRMEAEDAATYCQQWSSYP PTFGGGTKLELK
	DVVLTQSPAIMSASPGEKVTMTCSASS

Percent Frequency		
50-100	DIVMTQSP SLS S G VTISC	WYQQKPG SPKLLIY GVP RFSGSGSGTDFSLTISS EAED A YYC	TFGGGTKLEIK
30-50	L A M V L EK T	Q A YT V AT	L
20-30	T SI A P ASM	L S RW S S K RMQ GV F	Y A LG
		L	
10-20	QVQ L P TV QQ	TP Q T N V	W S
	K	P	
5-10	E L TKF A T L	F R DGTVR V I NN SDI D	R
	T S	S H P F	F
		E	P
3-5	S AT T I	L QE P K RQ FS Q S	P
		M	
		I	
2-3	NNEI AH NYM ISKP	H E T S V R Q R T KT T	I T
	K T	S M	H
1-2	L VI DEPLV S G VN	KE WAAI A H SK IS Y RA T V TH	I T
	QFYT T F	E HFG F G Y VE	H
		N D	

244

B

Table 2.

VL (Lambda)	FR1	CDR1	FR2	CDR2	FR3	CDR3	FR4
position	1 — 2	3	4 — 5	5	6 — 7 — 8 — 9	9	10
numbering	123456789012345678901	234567ABCDEF8901234567	89012345678	901234567	89012345678901234567890123456789012345	ABCDEF67890	1234567
2fb4	QSVLTQPP	SASGTPGQRVTISCSGTSSN	IGSSTVNWYQQLPGMAPKLLIY	RDAMRPSG	VPDRFSGSKSGASASLAIGGLQSEDETDYYCAAWDVSLNA		YVFGGTGTKVTVL
(exposure)	ehebebpe	ebegegeebebebegeepb	bghHhbHbHbHeegeHHeHbbhhpeep	pegbpeb	begebegeeepbbbggbecebcbbbHbbbHbhehHH		HbHgegbebcCc

Percent Frequency

```
            FR1                         FR2             FR3                              FR4
50-100:  Q VLTQPPSSVS SPGQ VTITC   WYQQ PG AP L IY   GVP RFSGS SG TA LTISGLQAEDEADYC   VFGGGTKLTVLGQP
30-50:   S                         K  KL             ID  K  N  T                       V
                  G  T  S              V                 S
20-30:   SAA  S  VAL  SA  L         Q  VT            TS      V                          W          V
              A   R                    S                                              
10-20:   YEV  A  A   IS              H TG R M        SE     S    K    A    A    SA SG   VI   T      S
              L      R                L                     N    T                      G   A
                                                           L                               Y
5-10:    P  E A TTT EK K             F ER DHLFTYILG   A    RI  S  RY    RTEPD   I        A   S   T
            N G                        V V  SLG  MF     N  DG  R  V                      L   R
              A                        H      P            A                            F
3-5:     F  SH  E  K                 HQS QV VR        RFSG D LA AVI GV N VM  E          RL    Q    TRES
         L  D                        I   K                 SE S                   
         T                                                 A
2-3:     NPM L  S  I                 FE  L  H         NT  AA GD F LL  K   S              P
         E                           S               DS  KI                            S
         A                           T               W   N  T
                                                         G
1-2:     GDGES RV F KG R  E P        LRLYQARV IF SS   E V L T D MN  I A I  DGM H         QA  R  IIVLGA
         DVQ  M                      PA  A            S          N      N  I            IG     NL P
         D                                                       C                      M         S
```

Table 2. (**A**) (*Opposite page*) The top two sequences in this table are the V$_\kappa$s of the Fv portions of one mouse Fabs (PDB id: 1igc) and one humanized Fv (PDB id: 1fvc) with their residues numbered according to their Kabat scheme.

(**B**) The top sequence in this table is of a V$_\lambda$ of the Fv portions of one human Fab (PDB id: 2fb4).

The structure of these molecules has been solved by X-ray crystallography. The single-letter code under each sequence is the exposure profile as defined in **ref. 8**: [(e) exposed, (p) partially exposed, (b) buried, (C)/(c):partial/full interface with light chain constant domain; (H)/(h):partial/full interface V$_H$ residue with V$_L$ domain]. The empty row in the table is for the reader to paste in their V$_L\kappa$ sequence for identifying the unusual and problematic residues in their V$_L$s. The sequence of K1 is shown as an example. The bottom part of the table has amino acids sorted in bins according to their frequency in the Kabat database for each position (amino acids in CDR segments and of lower than 1% frequency are not shown).

245

chain of the antibody they are working with, then another easy way to do so is to make use of Andrew Martin's home page. Go to http://www.bioinf.org.uk/abs/, then click on Sequences and then click on human subgroups. Paste the amino acid sequence of the light chain in the box provided and click on submit. Once the light chain type has been determined, proceed as follows.

2. Put in the primary sequence of the V_H in the empty row in **Table 1**. If the V_L is kappa then paste the primary sequence of V_L in the empty row in **Table 2A**. If it is lambda then use **Table 2B**. Make sure that your sequence is aligned to the reference sequences in the tables according to the Kabat numbering scheme (*see* **Note 1**).

3. Once this is done look for unusual residues in the V_H and V_L. Remember that this is done only for the framework residues. Using the lower part of the tables (the frequency bins) look for residues in your sequence that occur with less than 5% frequency in the database. For example if you look at the K1 sequence in you will find five underlined residues in **Table 1** and two in **Table 2A**. Note that all these residues are represented at less than 5% frequency in the Kabat database.

4. Once you have found the unusual residues use the upper part of the tables, which show the exposure state of the different positions. Verify whether the hydrophobicity of the unusual residues in your sequence is compatible with the exposure state of residues in the corresponding positions in sequences shown. For example in each of **Tables 1** and **2A** you will see two unusual residues, which are shown in bold. If you note carefully you will realize that the hydrophobicity of these residues do not match with their exposure state. In other words in **Table 1** there is a threonine at position 82. This is a position occupied by a buried residue. Threonine is quite hydrophilic and therefore not a very good residue to be buried in a protein. Likewise in **Table 2A**, there is a histidine at position 36. This position is at the interface with the V_H and therefore a hydrophobic residue is better suited for this position. These residues are therefore considered potentially problematic. In contrast if you look at V20 or D28 in **Table 1** you will note that they are compatible with the exposure state of residues occurring in the corresponding positions in the reference sequences shown at the top of the table. Thus, position 20 is buried in nature and therefore a hydrophobic residues is best for that position. Because in K1 position 20 is occupied by valine, which is hydrophobic it is not considered a problematic residue.

5. Once you have narrowed down your list of unusual amino acids to the ones that are potentially problematic, you need to mutate them to something that is likely to make the Fv more stable. The decision about which residues into which to mutate the potentially problematic residues is made by looking again at the frequency bins in the lower part of the table. Usually one can choose the amino acid that is most frequently represented at that position. For example in case of K1 Threonine82 in V_H was mutated to a Leucine. Similarly Histidine36 in V_L was mutated to a tyrosine because these are the most frequently used residues for their corresponding positions.

6. Occasionally some potentially problematic residues may require special consideration. In some cases two or more residues in the V_H or V_L may be coupled. For example in the V_L it is usually seen that an aspartate at position 60 is usually accompanied by an arginine at position 54. Crystal structure shows that these residues interact through a salt bridge. In these cases the choice of the mutation to be introduced should be based on the type of residue that is present on the other position. For example in K1 we decided to mutate Valine 60 not to the most frequently occurring aspartate for that position, but to mutate it into a serine because the residue at position 54 in K1 was not an arginine but a leucine. And as can be seen from the table and from the database V_H leucine 54 is usually accom-

panied by serine at position 60. These are very special cases and it is not possible to cover all these situations within the scope of the present chapter.

3.2. Mutagenesis of the Problematic Residues

The problematic residues can be mutated by either Kunkel's method or by PCR. For Kunkel's method one must have the scFv in a phagemid vector. It involves making a single stranded circular DNA of the scFv phagemid. The advantage is that one can use the same template to make separate as well as combined mutants of the different problematic residues. If the scFv is not in a phagemid vector then one has to do the mutagenesis by PCR, either SOE-PCR or ligase PCR. SOE-PCR will be covered else where in this book and therefore will not be described in detail here. We will touch base only with ligase-PCR, which is less frequently used.

3.2.1. Preparation of the Template for Introducing Mutation by Kunkel's Method (see **Notes 2** and **3**).

Day 1:

1. Transform CJ236 cells (electro-competent cells are available from Bio-Rad) with 5 ng of the scFv encoding phagemid. If the scFv is in a phage display vector then co-transform with 5 ng of a lac I^q encoding plasmid.
2. Plate 10–100 µL onto LB Cm$_{30\mu g/mL}$ plates containing the appropriate antibiotics for selecting the transformants. If using a phage display vector add 2% glucose to the selecting plates in addition to the antibiotics (*see* **Note 4**).
3. Incubate overnight at 37°C.
4. Streak CJ236 onto a LB Cm$_{30\mu g/mL}$ plate and TG1 onto M63 glucose, B1 plate (*see* **Note 5**).
5. Incubate overnight at 37°C.

Day 2:

1. Inoculate a bacterial loop full of transformants from day 1 plates into 150 mL of LB Cm$_{15\mu g/mL}$ Glc$_{2\%}$ Uridine $_{50\mu g/mL}$ plus the appropriate antibiotics to an initial OD$_{600nm}$ of about 0.1. Use a 2 L Baffle flask (*see* **Note 6**).
2. Incubate at 37°C with shaking at 250 rpm. Check OD$_{600nm}$ every 30 min.
3. When OD$_{600nm}$ reaches about 0.3 add helper phage, to a multiplicity of infection (m.o.i.) of 3–5.
4. Incubate at 37°C with shaking at 100 rpm for 1 h.
5. Incubate at 37°C with shaking at 300 rpm for 6 h. (At the end of 4 h start a 10–15 mL culture of CJ236 in LB Cm$_{15\mu g/mL}$ and a TG1 or DH5α culture in LB medium. Incubate at 37°C with shaking at 250 rpm till OD$_{600nm}$ is about 0.3–0.4. Keep ready plates containing LB agar with the antibiotic for the selection of the scFv encoding phagemid. These plates will be needed for titration (*see* **Note 6**).
6. Chill culture.
7. Pellet the cells by centrifuging the chilled culture at 3000g for 15 min at 4°C in a Sorvall RC4B centrifuge or an equivalent.
8. Centrifuge the supernatant from the above step at 17,000g for 15 min at 4°C.
9. Collect supernatant. Save 1 mL in a properly labeled sterile Eppendorf tube.
10. Measure the volume of the rest of the supernatant and add to it one-fifth its volume of cold 20% PEG-2.5 M NaCl. Mix thoroughly but gently (*see* **Note 7**).
11. Store overnight at 4°C.

12. Titrate phage in TG1 (*see* **Note 5**) and CJ236 cells as described in the following **steps 13–25.**
13. Take 8×1.5 mL Eppendorf tubes. Mark them 1 to 8.
14. Take 450 µL of 2X YT or LB medium into each tube.
15. Add 50 µL of the culture supernatant to tube 1 (10-fold dilution).
16. Vortex to mix thoroughly.
17. Take 50 µL from this tube and add to the next (tube 2, 100-fold dilution).
18. Likewise continue up to the eighth tube.
19. Take 9×1.8 mL autoclaved Eppendorf tubes and mark them as follows: TG1-10^{-1}, TG1-10^{-2}, TG1-10^{-3}, TG1-10^{-4}, CJ236-10^{-4}, CJ236-10^{-5}, CJ236-10^{-6}, CJ236-10^{-7}, and CJ236-10^{-8} (*see* **Note 5**).
20. Pipet 300 µL of fresh TG1 culture (OD_{600nm} of about 0.3) into tubes 1–4 and 300 µL of fresh CJ236 culture (OD_{600nm} of about 0.3) into tubes 5–8 (*see* **Note 5**).
21. Add 100 µL from tubes 1–4 to TG1 tubes and 100 µL from tubes 4–8 into CJ236 tubes.
22. Mix by tapping.
23. Incubate at 37°C for 30 min. (At the end of 15 min mix by tapping the contents of the tube again.)
24. At the end of incubation, plate 40 µL onto LB plates containing the appropriate antibiotic for the selection of the scFv encoding phagemid (*see* **Note 6**).
25. Incubate overnight at 37°C.

Day 3:

1. Count colonies in plates. Determine titer. The difference in phage titer between TG1 (*see* **Note 5**) and CJ236 cells should typically be between 10,000–100,000 fold.
    Extract single-stranded uracil containing DNA (ssuDNA) from the phage as described in the following steps:
2. Centrifuge the PEG-NaCl treated culture supernatant from the d 2 at $27,000g$ for 30 min at 4°C.
3. Look for the pellet. Mark the outside of the tube to locate the translucent pellet. Discard supernatant.
4. Invert the centrifuge bottle over an impermeable diaper. Let the trace amount of solution adhering to the centrifuge tube or bottle drain out.
5. Add 10 mL of NET buffer to the pellet. Let it stand for 10–15 min at RT. The pellet will become loose. Resuspend pellet completely by pipetting repeatedly but gently. Transfer the resuspended pellet to a clear (polycarbonate) SS-34 tube (*see* **Note 8**).
6. Centrifuge at $3000g$ for 15 min at 4°C.
7. Collect the supernatant very carefully. Discard pellet (if any) (*see* **Note 8**).
8. Add 2 mL of PEG-NaCl solution to the supernatant and mix.
9. Keep in ice for 20 min.
10. Centrifuge at $27,000g$ for 30 min at 4°C.
11. Look for the pellet. Discard supernatant.
12. Invert the centrifuge bottle over an impermeable diaper. Let the trace amount of solution adhering to the centrifuge tube or bottle drain out.
13. Add 10 mL of NET buffer to the pellet. Let it stand for 10–15 min at room temperature. Resuspend pellet completely by pipetting repeatedly but gently. Transfer the resuspended pellet to a clear (polycarbonate) SS-34 tube (*see* **Note 8**).
14. Centrifuge at $3000g$ for 15 min at 4°C. Carefully collect the supernatant into an opaque (polypropylene) SS-34 tube (*see* **Note 9**).
15. Add equal volume of buffer saturated phenol (*see* **Note 10**).

16. Vortex for 1 min.
17. Mix/shake at room temperature for 20 min.
18. Centrifuge at 27,000*g* for 15 min at 4°C.
19. Collect the upper aqueous layer into another polypropylene SS-34 tube. Add equal volume of Phenol: Chloroform: Isoamyl alcohol mixture and vortex for 1 min (*see* **Note 11**).
20. Mix/shake at RT for 15 min.
21. Centrifuge at 27,000*g* for 15 min at 4°C.
22. Collect the upper aqueous layer into another polypropylene SS-34 tube (*see* **Note 9**).
23. Add equal volume of Chloroform and vortex for 1 min (*see* **Note 11**).
24. Mix/shake at RT for 15 min.
25. Centrifuge at 27,000*g* for 15 min at 4°C.
26. Measure the volume of the upper aqueous layer and collect into a clear SS-34 clear (polycarbonate) tube (*see* **Note 8**).
27. Add one-tenth the volume of sterile 8 *M* lithium chloride and 3 vol of 100% chilled ethanol. Mix thoroughly (*see* **Note 12**).
28. Keep in dry ice for 20 min.
29. Centrifuge at 27,000*g* for 20 min at 4°C.
30. The pellet will be very light and off white in color. Carefully decant the supernatant. Invert tube on an impermeable diaper to drain out the remaining solution from the tube.
31. Air-dry sample.
32. Dissolve the pellet in 100–200 mL of 10 m*M* Tris, pH 7.4.
33. Run a 1.2% agarose gel with 1 and 2 µL sample. The sample should show a distinct and clean band. Although the ssuDNA will be half the size of the scFv encoding phagemid, in the gel it might run with an apparent lower molecular weight because of secondary structure formation.

3.2.2. Design of Oligonucleotides for Introducing the Mutations

The design of the oligonucleotide for Kunkel's mutagenesis depends on the orientation of the gene of interest and the direction of the F' origin of replication. Follow the following rules:

1. If the gene of interest and the F' ori are in the clockwise direction then the oligo should be made complementary to the coding strand of the gene.
2. If the gene of interest is in the clockwise direction and the F' ori in the anti-clockwise direction then the oligo should be complementary to the noncoding strand of the gene.
3. If the gene of interest is in the anti-clockwise direction and the F' ori is in the clockwise direction then the oligo should be complementary to the noncoding strand and
4. If the gene of interest and the F'ori are both in the anti-clockwise direction then oligo should be complementary to the coding strand of the gene.

The oligo should be designed in such a way that there are 12–15 nucleotides at either side of the mutagenic region that anneal perfectly with the ssuDNA. If there are more than one site that needs to be mutated and if these sites are placed at a distance of about 20 nucleotides, then more than one oligo can be used simultaneously to introduce all the mutations together. It is helpful to have diagnostic restriction enzyme site in each oligo. If bases are changed to introduce the diagnostic restriction sites, then it is important to have 12–15 perfectly matching residues on either side of any mismatch between the template and the oligo.

3.2.3. Phosphorylation of Oligo

The volume of the reaction components shown below can be scaled up or down as desired. This is for the phosphorylation of each oligo used for mutagenesis (if there is a need to use more than one).

Water	25 µL
10X Ligase buffer	03 µL
Oligo (250 pmol/µL)	01 µL
Polynucleotide kinase (10U/µL)	01 µL
	30 µL

1. Mix by tapping. Gently vortex. Spin briefly (5 s).
2. Incubate at 37°C for 30 min.
3. Heat at 65°C for 10 min.
4. Store in ice temporarily. (For long term, store at –20°C.)

3.2.4. Annealing of the Template and Oligo

1. The amount of phosphorylated oligo is typically kept between 8–10 pmol. The amount of template to be used depends on the type of experiment. For an experiment in which a single clone is sufficient 5–10 pg of the ssuDNA is sufficient. If more than one mutants is desired, the amount of template can be doubled. Before starting the annealing step keep ready one heat block at 72–75°C and another at around 15–18°C. Prepare the following tubes:

	Tube No.	
	1 (expt.)	2 (cont.)
Water	7 µL	8 µL
10X Annealing buffer	1 µL	1 µL
Template (diluted in water)	1 µL	1 µL
Phosphorylated oligo(s)	1 µL	0
	10 µL	10 µL

(If more than one oligo is being used, then it is important to use them at equimolar amount. The volume can be adjusted by reducing the amount of water used.)
2. Mix by tapping. Vortex. Spin briefly.
3. Put the tubes in 72°C heat block for 2 min.
4. Take another heat block kept at around 15–18°C. Put it on the table.
5. At the end of 2 min put the 72°C heat block with the annealing tubes in it over the colder heat block on the table.
6. Leave it there for 1 h or until the temperature of the top block gets down to <30°C.
7. Store the tubes in ice or at 4°C.

3.2.5. Extension

1. Add the following to the annealing tubes:

	Tube no.	
	1(expt.)	2 (cont.)
10X Synthesis buffer	1.3 µL	1.3 µL
T4 DNA Ligase (3 U/µL)	1.0 µL	1.0 µL
T7 DNA Polymerase (1U/µL diluted 1:1 in T7 Pol dilution buffer)	1.0 µL	1.0 µL

13.3 µL   13.3 µL

2. Mix by tapping. Vortex gently. Spin briefly.
3. Incubate in ice for 10 min.
4. Incubate at RT for 10 min.
5. Incubate at 37°C for 2 h.
6. Store in ice.
7. Transform competent TG1 cells (*see* **Note 5**).
8. Plate 10, 25, 50, and 100 µL onto LB agar plates containing Glc$_{2\%}$ and the appropriate antibiotic for selecting the scFv encoding phagemid (*see* **Note 6**).
9. Incubate overnight at 37°C.
10. Analyse clones for the introduction of the mutation(s). We have found that analyzing 24–30 clones usually gives all different combinations of the 3–4 single-site mutations.

3.2.6. Ligase-PCR (see **Notes 13 and 14**)

Kunkel's mutagenesis can be done on scFvs cloned in a phagemid vector. If a scFv is present in some other vector, then introduction of mutations in the middle of the Fv can be done by SOE-PCR. However, if there are more than one internal sites where mutations needs to be introduced then SOE-PCR becomes problematic because it would require the generation of several fragments of the gene being mutated and then splicing different fragments for the generation of different combination of mutants. We have found that ligase PCR works well under these circumstances. It is basically similar to any other PCR reaction with the exception of the fact that a thermostable ligase and a thermostable ligase buffer and phosphorylated internal (mutagenic) primers are included in the PCR mix. It is based on the method first described by Michael *(9)*. We have found the following conditions to work nicely for the incorporation of up to three different mutations spaced far apart to be covered by one oligo. A pictorial representation of the methods is shown in **Fig. 1**.

1. Mix 150 pmol pmol each Oligo 1 and 2 (external primers), mix 150 pmol each Oligos 3 and 4 (or more). (These oligos should be phosphorylated and preferably have diagnostic restriction sites.) 0.4 m*M* each dNTP, 1X Taq ligase buffer, 40 U Taq Ligase (NEB), 5U Taq DNA Polymerase (Promega). 10^{10} copies Template. 100 µL Total volume.
2. Run PCR: Reaction conditions: Cycle1: 94°C, 5 min; 50°C, 1 min; 65°C, 4 min. Cycle 2–24: 94°C, 1 min; 50°C, 1 min; 65°C, 4 min. Cycle 25: 94°C, 30 s; 50°C, 1 min; 65°C, 15 min.
3. After PCR run an aliquot in a 1.5% agarose gel. Usually more than one band is seen.
4. If a band of the desired length is seen then purify the PCR product through a PCR purification kit (Qiagen PCR purification kit works well) and then run a preparative low melting gel with the purified PCR product.
5. Excise out the band of the correct size and clone into the appropriate scFv vector.

3.3. Characterization of the Mutants

This will involve the expression and purification of the scFv mutant proteins and assays to determine their stability. Because the purification and bio-activity of scFvs are specific to each separate scFv, these parameters will be different from one laboratory to another. Typically one can incubate aliquots of the scFv proteins in a carrier protein such as 0.2% HSA or even in human plasma at 37°C for varying periods of time and then assay all the samples together for bioactivity. Plotting of the activity curve against incubation time at 37°C will show differences in the stability among the mutants and the wild-type. For K1, which has been used here as an example, the half life of the wild type scFv was 4 h, whereas the best mutants showed no loss of activity even after 48 h of incubation at 37°C *(8)*.

4. Notes

1. Identification of the unusual and potentially problematic residues by the method described in this chapter is largely dependant on the comparison between the antibody of interest (used by the reader) and the reference antibodies used in the tables. Therefore extreme caution must be maintained to align the sequences properly. Because the residues in the tables have been numbered by the Kabat scheme, all alignments must done in the Kabat numbering system. To do this, one can use one of several blasting tools. Alternatively one can keep in mind some of the most conserved residues such as cysteine 22 and 92, tryptophan 36 and 103 in the heavy chain and cysteine 23 and 88, tryptophan 36, phenylalanine 88 and glycine 89 in the light chain.

2. For Kunkel's mutagenesis one can scale up or down the volume of culture for preparing ssuDNA containing phage. The important point to remember is that if one is using a phage display vector for engineering the scFv then the scFv-gIIIp containing phagemid, the lacI^q containing plasmid and the helper phage should have different *E. coli* origin of replication and/or selection markers to co-exists together in the CJ236 cells. CJ236 does not have a lacI^q gene. Therefore lacIq containing plasmid is required to stop any leaky expression of the scFv-gIIIp fusion protein that affects bacterial growth.

3. The background in a good Kunkel's mutagenesis experiment can be as low as 1–2%. Typically it is about 15–20%. The background can be lowered by making good quality ssDNA. One can get this by doing the following:

    a. Do not use helper phage at a multiplicity of infection (m.o.i.) of greater than 3–5. To calculate the m.o.i. one may note that 1 O.D.$_{600nm}$ unit of CJ236 contains about 5×10^8 bacteria.

    b. Using helper phage R408 is useful because it is packaging deficient.

    c. When recovering the phage for making ssuDNA do not let the culture age for more than 7 h post-helper-phage addition.

    d. When harvesting the ssuDNA containing phage, as mentioned in **Subheading 3.** do at least two rounds of centrifugation to get rid of any bacteria remaining in suspension. Also when the phage particles are PEG-purified, additional centrifugation steps between PEG precipitation helps to get rid of trace contaminants of bacteria.

4. Instead of taking plates containing glucose, one can take plates containing the appropriate antibiotics and then spread 0.5 mL 20% glucose and let it dry in the hood. Although this does not give a exact final concentration of 2% for glucose it is good enough to suppress leaky expression of proteins from the lac promoter-operator. Use of 0.5 mL of 20% glucose is based on the assumption that each plate contains between 25–30 mL of LB agar.

5. One can also use a DH5α F' strain instead on TG1. Note that DH5α F' grows on LB and not on minimal plate.

6. 2% Glucose should also be included in the medium if a phage-display vector is being used.

7. This can be done either in autoclaved glass bottles or polycarbonate bottles or tubes.

8. Use a polycarbonate tube whenever there is a need to see and collect the phage or DNA pellet.

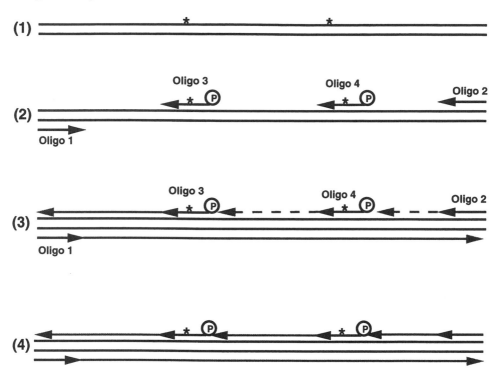

Fig.1. A schematic representation of ligase-PCR. (**A**) Shows a double-stranded DNA with the asterisks indicating regions to be mutagenized. (**B**) Four oligos used for ligase-PCR. Oligos 1 and 2 are like any other PCR primers. Oligo 3 and 4 encode the mutations to be introduced and are phosphorylated. 12–15 residues on either sides of the region of mutations anneal perfectly to the template. (**C**) During PCR the thermostable polymerase extends the primers in a 5'->3' direction (gray lines). The strands formed by the extension of the 3' primers (phosphorylated primers) ends where the primer upstream to it begins (gray dotted line). (**D**) the thermostable ligase acts to join these short stretches of the newly synthesized strands.

9. Use a polypropylene tube for phenol, phenol:chloroform:isoamyl alcohol and chloroform extraction.
10. The phenol used should be distilled, buffer-saturated, and colorless. It should be stored in amber-colored bottles at 4°C.
11. The Phenol:Chloroform:Isoamyl alcohol mixture and chloroform used should be stored in amber-colored bottles at 4°C.
12. Lithium chloride should be used for precipitating the ssuDNA because it does not precipitate with DNA during ethanol precipitation and therefore the ssuDNA obtained is relatively free of salts.
13. When doing ligase PCR, never expose the prep gel to UV light for any unnecessary time. The UV induced damage to DNA reduces efficiency of ligation.
14. After a full length DNA band from ligase-PCR is purified one can reamplify it with the external primers to have a back-up stock. Depending on the positions of the mutagenic

sites one can conduct a restriction digestion of the PCR product to analyze the efficiency of mutations.

References

1. Kohler, G. and Milstein, C. (1975) Continuous cultures of fused cells screeting antibody of predefined specificity. *Nature* **256**, 495–497.
2. Fujimori, K., Covell, D. G., Fletcher, J. E., and Weinstein, J. N. (1989) Modeling analysis of the global and microscopic distribution of immunoglobulin G, F(ab')2, and Fab in tumors. *Cancer Res.* **49**, 5656–5663.
3. Old, L. J. (1996) Immunotherapy of cancer. *Sci. Am.* **Sept.,** 136–143.
4. Glockshuber, R., Malia, M., Pfitzinger, I., and Pluckthun, A. (1990) Comparison of strategies to stabilize immunoglobulin Fv-fragments. *Biochemistry* **29**, 1362–1367.
5. Bird, R. E., Hardman, K. D., Jacobson, J. W., Johnson, S., Kaufman, B. M., Lee, S. M., et al. (1988) Single-chain antigen-binding proteins. *Science* **242**, 423–426.
6. Reiter, Y., Brinkmann, U., Lee, B., and Pastan,, I. (1996) Engineering antibody Fv fragments for cancer detection and therapy disulfide-stabilized Fv fragments. *Nature Biotechnol.* **14**, 1239–1245.
7. Nieba, L., Honegger, A., Krebber, C., and Pluckthun, A. (1997) Disrupting the hydrophobic patches at the antibody variable/constant domain interface: improved in vivo folding and physical characterization of an engineered scFv fragment. *Protein Eng.* **10,** 435–444.
8. Chowdhury, P. S., Vasmatzis, G., Beers, R., Lee, B., and Pastan, I. (1998) Improved stability and yield of a Fv-toxin fusion protein by computer design and protein engineering of the Fv. *J. Mol. Biol.* **281,** 917–928.
9. Michael, S. F. (1994) Mutagenesis by incorporation of a phosphorylated oligo during PCR amplification. *Biotechniques* **16**, 411–412.

15

Recombinant Single-Chain and Disulfide-Stabilized Fv Immunotoxins for Cancer Therapy

Revital Niv, Dina Segal, and Yoram Reiter

1. Introduction

The rapid progress in understanding the molecular biology of cancer cells has made a large impact on the design and development of novel therapeutic strategies.

The concept of targeted cancer therapy is thus an important mean to improve the therapeutic potential of anti-cancer agents and lead to the development of novel approaches such as immunotherapy.

The approach of cancer immunotherapy and targeted cancer therapy combines rational drug design with the progress in understanding cancer biology *(1–4)*. This approach takes advantage of some special properties of cancer cells: many of them contain mutant or overexpressed oncogenes on their surface, and these proteins are attractive antigens for targeted therapy. Example for these are overexpressed receptors such as epidermal growth factor receptor (EGFR), erbB2/HER2, interleukin-2 receptor (IL2R), differentiation antigens that are expressed on the surface of mature cells but not on the immature stem cells (CD19, CD20, and CD22 on B-cell lymphomas and leukemias and the interleukin-2 (IL-2) receptor on T-cell leukemias) *(9–11)*. Differentiation antigens have also been found on ovarian, breast, and prostate cancer *(12–15)*. It should be possible to use these molecular cell-surface markers as targets to eliminate the cancer cells while sparing the normal cells. For this approach to be successful, we must generate a targeting moiety that will bind very specifically the antigen or receptor expressed on the cancer cell surface and arm this targeting moiety with an effector cytotoxic moiety.

In the case of recombinant Fv immunotoxins the targeting moiety is a specific single-chain Fv antibody fragment (scFv) directed toward the cancer antigen. These are the variable domains (heavy and light chain) of monoclonal antibodies (MAbs) or phage-displayed derived antibody fragments *(16–19)*.

In the single-chain Fv, the variable domains are stabilized through a peptide linker *(16,18,19)*. In disulfide-stabilized Fv (dsFv) the two variable domains are connected

From: *Methods in Molecular Biology, vol. 207: Recombinant Antibodies for Cancer Therapy: Methods and Protocols*
Edited by: M. Welschof and J. Krauss © Humana Press Inc., Totowa, NJ

via an interchain disulfide bond engineered into framework residues *(20–22)*. The cyto-toxic arm in these engineered molecules are truncated forms of the very potent bacterial toxins derived from *Pseudomonas* exotoxin (PE) or diphtheria toxin (DT) *(1–4)*. The toxin moiety is fused to the single-chain Fv C-terminus or to either variable domains in the disulfide-stabilized form.

The Fv-immunotoxin therapy is based on the ability of these very potent cytotoxic agent to bind to cell-surface molecules, which will internalize the toxin moiety and result in cell death. One or a few molecules of either toxin is sufficient to kill cells if the toxin gains entry to the cytosol. We will describe here recombinant Fv immunotoxins based on a truncated form of PE, named PE38, which is composed of amino acids 253–364 and 381–613 of PE. In this form the cell-binding domain is deleted (*see* **Fig. 1**) and is replaced by the single-chain Fv antibody moiety. The Fv fragments carries domain II (translocation domain) and III (ADP-ribosylation domain) to the target cell surface.

PE kills cells by ADP-ribosylation of elongation factor 2, leading to inhibition of protein synthesis, apoptosis, and cell death. Many active recombinant scFv and dsFv-immunotoxins were developed so far and several of them already produce significant results in clinical trails *(22–42)*.

Thus, recombinant Fv immunotoxins are composed of two moieties: one is the targeting moiety (the Fv fragment), which delivers the molecule to its target. The second is the effector moiety, which mediates the biological toxic effect of the engineered molecule, i.e., killing the target via the toxin activity inside cells. Recombinant Fv immunotoxins are significantly improved molecules because of their tumor-penetration potential in vivo and improved pharmacokinetic and stability features. The development of advanced methods of recombinant-protein production enabled the large-scale production of recombinant immunotoxins of high purity and quality for clinical use in sufficient quantities to perform clinical trials.

This chapter will summarize the knowledge on the design and preparation of recombinant Fv immunotoxins, which utilize recombinant antibody fragments as the targeting moiety.

2. Materials

2.1. Plasmids

Plasmids for making recombinant Fv immunotoxins contain the DNA encoding the cloned Fv fragment originated from a hybridoma or a phage-display-derived recombinant fragment and the recombinant toxin gene (in this case the gene encoding the truncated form of PE, PE38) (*see* **Fig. 1**). These genes are under control of the T7 promoter *(43)* and contain usually ampicillin resistance gene.

These plasmids are stored at a concentration of 1 mg/mL in TE (0.01 M Tris-HCl, pH 7.4, 1 mM EDTA at 4°C (or –20°C for long periods of time).

The modification of Fv framework V_H and V_L residues to cysteine is performed by site-directed mutagenesis kits. These are available from various commercial sources (Bio-Rad, Promega, Pharmacia).

2.2. Transformation

1. Competent cells BL21/DE3 (Stratagene).
2. SOC medium.
3. Lauria Broth (LB) plates containing 100 µg/mL ampicillin.
4. Superbroth containing added glucose (0.5%), $MgSO_4$ (1.6 mM) and ampicillin (100 µg/mL).
5. Isopropyl-β-D-thiogalactopyranoside (IPTG) 100 mM in water.

2.3. Isolation of Inclusion Bodies

1. Triton X-100 (25%) in water (Sigma).
2. TE50/20 buffer: 50 mM Tris-HCl, pH 7.4, 20 mM EDTA.
3. Lysozyme 5 mg/mL in TE50/20 buffer (Sigma).
4. 5 M NaCl.

2.4. Solubilization of Inclusion Bodies and Refolding Buffer

1. Solubilization buffer: 6 M guanidine-HCl, 0.1 M Tris-HCl, pH 8.0, 5 mM EDTA (Sigma).
2. Dithioerythritol (DTE) (Sigma).
3. Coomassie Plus Protein Assay Reagent (Pierce, cat. no. 1856210).
4. Bovine serum albumin (BSA) standard (2 mg/mL).
5. Refolding buffer: 0.1 M Tris-HCl, pH 8.0, 0.5 M arginine-HCl, 2 mM EDTA, 0.9 mM oxidized glutathione (GSSG) (Sigma).
6. Dialysis buffer: 0.02 M Tris-HCl, pH 7.4, 0.1 M urea (Sigma).

2.5. Purification

1. Q-Sepharose Fast flow anion exchange resin (Pharmacia).
2. MonoQ anion exchange column (HR10/10, 8 mL) (Pharmacia).
3. TSK G3000SW column (TosoHaas).
4. Buffer A: 0.02 M Tris-HCl, pH 7.4.
5. Buffer B: 0.02 M Tris-HCl, pH 7.4, 1 M NaCl.
6. TSK equilibration and running buffer: PBS.

3. Methods

3.1. Plasmid Preparation: General Comments on the Construction of scFv and dsFv-Immunotoxin Expression Plasmids

Immunotoxin construction is initiated using a cloned scFv fragment derived from a phage-display library or a hybridoma. For cloning Fvs from hybridoma, specific primers for V_H and V_L variable domains are used that are designed in the 5'-end based on N-terminal amino-acid sequence analysis of the antibody and in the 3'-end on conserved constant region sequences. When N-terminal amino acid sequences of V_H or V_L are not available, 5'-end primers can be designed according to family-specific degenerate primer sets available from various databases, or alternatively a RACE (Rapid Amplification of cDNA Ends) reaction can be performed. This chapter will not focus on the cloning of Fv fragments from hybridoma MAb or phage-display. These are described in previous publications *(47,48)*. We will describe the modification of V_H and V_L residues for making disulfide-stabilized Fv fragments from scFv constructs

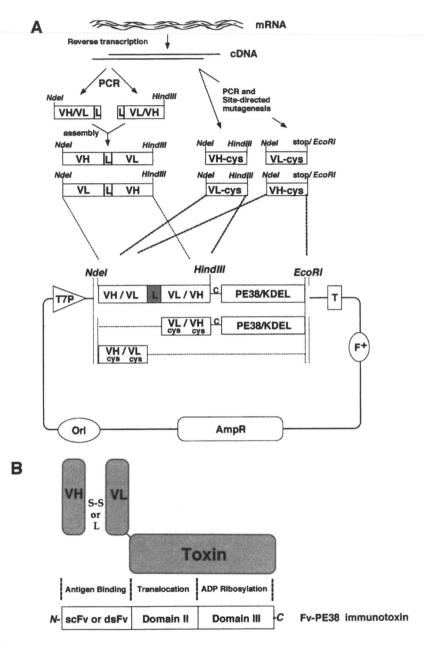

Fig. 1. Recombinant immunotoxins: design and engineering. Two types of recombinant Fv antibody fragments are used as the targeting moiety in recombinant Fv immunotoxins. ScFv fragments are stabilized by a peptide linker that connects the carboxyl-terminus of V_H or V_L with the amino terminus of the other domain. The V_H and V_L heterodimer in dsFvs are stabilized by the engineering of a disulfide bond between the two domains (*continued*).

(Continued from previous page)

(A) The targeting moiety: The genes encoding the V_H and V_L variable domains are cloned usually from hybridoma mRNA by reverse transcription, cDNA synthesis, and subsequent PCR amplification using degenerate primers that are complementary to the 5' or 3' end of the V_H and V_L genes or by primers, that are designed according to the amino-terminal amino acid sequence of the MAb to be cloned and conserved sequences at the N-terminal of the heavy and light constant regions. The variable genes can be also cloned by constant domains primers and using the RACE method (rapid amplification of cDNA ends). Restriction sites for assembling of the peptide linker sequence that connects the V_H and V_L domains, and for cloning into the expression vector are also introduced by PCR. Construction of dsFv involves the generation of two expression plasmids that encode the two components of the dsFv V_H-cys and V_L-cys. The cysteines are introduced in position 44 in FR2 of V_H and position 100 of FR4 of V_L or position 105 of FR4 in V_H and position 43 of FR2 in V_L (numbering system of Kabat et al.) by site-directed mutagenesis using as template a uracil-containing single-stranded DNA of the scFv construct from the F+ origin present in the expression plasmid and cotransfection with M13 helper phage. in addition to the cysteines, cloning sites, ATG translation-initiation codons, and stop codons are introduced at the 5' end and 5' end of the V_H and V_L genes as shown by site-directed mutagenesis or PCR. The antibody variable genes are subcloned into an expression vector which contains the gene for a truncated form of *Pseudomonas* exotoxin, PE38. (B) The effector (toxin) moiety. In PE-derived recombinant Fv-immunotoxins the Fv region of the targeting antibody (in a scFv or dsFv form) is fused to the N-terminus of a truncated form of PE, which contains the translocation domain (domain II) and enzymatically active ADP-ribosylation domain (domain III). The cell-binding domain of whole PE (domain I) is replaced by the Fv targeting moiety, thus preserving the relative position of the binding domain function to the other functional domains of PE. in the dsFv-immunotoxins there are two components. In one, the V_H or V_L domains are fused to the amino terminus of the truncated PE, and in the other, variable domain is covalently linked by the engineered disulfide bond.

---

and the production of recombinant scFv and dsFv- immunotoxins. The original positions for disulfide-stabilization of Fvs were identified using computer modeling. The positions identified are V_H-44 and V_L-100 according to Kabat numbering *(44)*. Because the locations for cysteine substitutions are located in structurally conserved regions, i.e., in the framework regions, they can be readily identified for any given Fv by simple sequence alignment using the assignment of the framework regions and complementary-determining regions (CDRs) according to the Kabat numbering system *(44)*. The disulfide stabilization approach is this designed to be generally applicable to any Fv from mouse as well as Fvs of other species including humans. Neither molecular modeling nor knowledge of the structures of the Fvs is necessary to identify these positions and many dsFv fragments and immunotoxins were constructed using this methodology *(20–22)*. The introduction of cysteine into the V_H and V_L positions is performed by site-directed mutagenesis.

The method of choice we use for mutagenesis are of Kunkel et al. *(45)* in which a uracil-containing single-stranded DNA from the F+ origin present in the expression plasmid is obtained by cotransfection of *Escherichia coli* CJ236 (Bio-Rad mutgenesis kit) with M13 helper phage and used as a template for site-directed mutagenesis (the cloning is described in **Fig. 1**).

The methods described here for plasmid expression in *E. coli* BL21/λDE3 cells are applicable for plasmids containing the T7 promoter and the ampicillin resistance gene.

Upon induction of the T7 RNA polymerase in *E. coli* BL21/λDE3 cells by IPTG, large amounts of recombinant protein are produced. The overexpressed Fv immunotoxin accumulate in insoluble intracellular inclusion bodies, which are subsequently isolated, purified, solubilized, and prepared for in vitro refolding.

To produce dsFv immunotoxins, two expression plasmids are required because the components of these molecule are expressed separately. One plasmid encodes the V_H and the other encodes the V_L domain. The toxin moiety can be fused to either V_H and V_L.

3.2. Transformation

1. Thaw competent *E. coli* BL21/λDE3 cells, stored in −70°C on ice (*see* **Notes 1–4**).
2. Mix 100 μL of bacteria with 4 μg of plasmid DNA on ice for 30–45 min.
3. Incubate the suspension at 42°C for 1 min and place back on ice.
4. Add SOC medium (0.9 mL) and shake the mixture at 37°C for 1 h.
5. Plate the bacterial mixture on 5 LB/Amp plates (200 μL/plate) and incubate at 37°C for 14–18 h. (for each liter of expression transform 100 μL *E. coli* BL21/λDE3 cells and plate on 5 LB/Amp plates).
6. Scrape bacteria from the 5 plates and resuspend in 1 L superbroth (with ampicillin, $MgSO_4$, and glucose) divided into two 2-L shake flasks (500 mL/flask). Shake vigorously at 250 rpm at 37°C to ensure good aeration. The OD_{600nm} of the initial culture should be 0.15–0.25.
7. Test the absorbance of culture sample at 600 nm (if OD_{600nm} is above 0.7–0.8 samples should be diluted 1:10 with superbroth and final OD should be calculated according to dilution factor).
8. At $OD_{600nm} \approx 2.4$, add IPTG (5 mL/500 mL culture of 100 mM) to a final concentration of 1 mM. Save 1 mL of culture before adding IPTG as a preinduction control sample.
9. Incubate the culture for 90 min by continued shaking at 37°C. Harvest the cells by centrifugation at 3000g for 30 min at 4°C. Save 1 mL aliquot of culture before centrifugation as a postinduction sample.
10. Discard supernatant. Cell pellet may be frozen at −70°C.
11. Analyze aliquots from **steps 8** and **9** by SDS-PAGE. Resuspend cell pellets in 1 mL TE buffer. Sonicate 20 s in bath sonicator and centrifuge in an Eppendorf centrifuge at maximal speed (5000g) for 10 min. Resuspend pellet in 0.1 mL TE. Sonicate 10–20 s and resuspend in 0.1 mL TE. Determine protein concentration and run equal amounts of protein on reduced SDS-PAGE to verify induction.

3.3. Isolation of Inclusion Body Protein

1. Resuspend cell paste from each liter of culture into 160 mL TE50/20 using a homogenizer. Transfer suspension to 250 mL sorvall centrifuge bottle (*see* **Note 5**).
2. Add 6.5 mL lysozyme at 5 mg/mL, mix well and incubate for 1 h at room temperature. Shake by hand frequently.
3. Add 20 mL of 25% Triton X-100, mix well, and incubate for 30 min at room temperature. Shake by hand frequently.
4. Centrifuge 27,500g (Sorvall, GSA rotor) for 60 min at 4°C in Sorvall GSA rotor.
5. Discard supernatant and resuspend pellet in 180 mL TE50/20 by using a homogenizer.
6. Repeat **steps 4** and **5** three to four times. Keep a small amount of inclusion bodies pellet after last wash for analyzing on SDS-PAGE as described in **Subheadings 3.2.–3.10** (*see* **Note 6**).

3.4. Solubilization and Reduction of Inclusion Bodies

1. Transfer the inclusion bodies pellet into 50 mL Oak Ridge Centrifuge Tubes (Nunc), using a spatula.
2. Resuspend the pellet in solubilization buffer (6 M guanidine HCl, 100 mM Tris-HCl, pH 8.0, 2 mM EDTA). 1.5–1.8 g Wet inclusion bodies solubilized into 10 mL solubilization buffer will give a protein concentration of ≈10 mg/mL.
3. Dissolve inclusion bodies in solubilization buffer (if required use homogenizer with a small probe) until completely dissolved.
4. Centrifuge solubilized inclusion bodies at 16,000g (Sorvall GSA rotor), 20 min, 4°C in Sorvall SS34 rotor.
5. Take supernatant, which is the solubilized inclusion bodies, determine protein concentration with Pierce Coomassie plus reagent. Dilute 10 µL of the denatured and solubilized protein 10–20-fold with denaturation buffer, and then add 5–10 µL to cuvets. Add 1 mL of 1:1 diluted reagent in water. The standard to be used is 2 mg/mL BSA (*see* **Notes 8–11**).
6. Dilute the protein to 10 mg/mL (if necessary) with solubilization buffer and add DTE (Dithioerithritol) to 10 mg/mL (65 mM final concentration), mix, and incubate for 4–24 h at room temperature (at least 4 h of incubation are required for complete reduction of disulfide bonds).
7. Prepare 100-fold more buffer then the volume of the denatured protein solution and chill to 10°C.

3.5. Refolding

1. Add 551 mg/L oxidized glutathione (GSSG) (final concentration 0f 0.9 mM) to the chilled refolding buffer.
2. To remove small amounts of undissolved material centrifuge the reduced, denatured, and solubilized recombinant protein at 40,000g for 20–40 min at 4°C.
3. Stir the chilled refolding buffer briskly, using a pipet add the denatured protein from **step 2** quickly over 20–30 s to a final protein concentration of 100 µg/mL. Dilute every 10 mL of solubilized recombinant protein at a concentration of 10 mg/mL (total 100 mg) is diluted 1:100 into 1 L of refolding solution to give a final protein concentration of 100 mg/mL).
4. Mix well for 2–3 min, stop stirring, and allow refolding at 10°C for 36–48 h (*see* **Note 7**).
5. For refolding of dsFv-immunotoxin the following steps should be taken: for dsFv immunotoxins two pools of reduced, denatured inclusion bodies exist: one for the V_H and one for the V_L-toxin fusion. For refolding the two components are mixed at 1:1 molar ratio keeping the final protein concentration in the refolding at 100 µg/mL. Thus, if preparing a dsFv-immunotoxin mix 6.67 mL (66.7 mg) of denatured V_L-toxin solution with 3.33 mL (33.3 mg) of denatured V_H solution and add to 1 L refolding buffer as in **Subheading 3**. The refolding buffer for making dsFv-immunotoxins is at pH 10.0.

3.6. Dialysis

1. To collect precipitated protein generated during refolding, centrifuged at 27,000g, Sorvall GSA rotor in 250 mL Sorvall centrifuge bottles for 30 min at 4°C.
2. Collect supernatant and dialyze at 4°C in 25-fold of the initial refolding volume against 20 mM Tris-HCl, pH 7.4, 100 mM urea. Change buffer 2–3 times until conductivity measures 3–4 mM HO (the ionic strength of the protein decreases below that of 55 mM NaCl).
3. The protein can be concentrated using large capacity concentrators, such as the CH2 system from Amicon, the TFF concentrator from Millipore or the MiniSet concentration system from Filtron. With these systems the buffer exchange is facilitated by ultrafiltration through a membrane having a 30-kDa cutoff. The protein is concentrated to 10–20%

of its original volume and dialysis buffer is added at the same rate as buffer is removed by ultrafiltration. After the ionic strength is reduced to appropriate level, the protein is removed from the ultrafiltration device.

3.7. Purification of Recombinant Protein

3.7.1. Ion Exchange Chromatography

All chromatography steps are performed at 4°C.

1. Load the dialyzed protein on a 5–8 mL Q-Sepharose column (Pharmacia) previously equilibrated and washed with 10 column volumes of buffer A, 10 column volumes of buffer B, and then 20 vol of buffer A. The protein is loaded at 2–4 mL/min.
2. After loading the protein (1–3 h), wash the column with buffer A until no protein is present in the flowthrough and elute in 5 mL fractions with 30% buffer B in buffer A (300 mM NaCl).
3. Pool the peak fractions, determined amount of protein by the Coomassie Plus Protein Assay Reagent and diluted fivefold with buffer A.
4. Load protein on a 8-mL high resolution MonoQ column (Pharmacia). This requires a high-pressure pump and is performed usually on an FPLC system. Protein is loaded at 2–4 mL/min.
5. Wash the column with 10–15 column volumes of buffer A until no protein is present in the flowthrough and elute with a linear gradient of 0–40% buffer B in buffer A at a flow rate of 2 mL/min over 10 column volumes. Collect 2 mL fractions. This will yield a gradient with a 1% increase in buffer B per 1 mL of elution.
6. Evaluate the peak fractions of protein, eluting typically at ~20% buffer B (0.2 M NaCl), are individually for protein concentration and for purity by sodium dodecyl sulfate poly-acrylamide gel electrophorese (SDS-PAGE) under reducing conditions.
7. Pooled fractions should be >90% pure and not be contaminated with proteins of similar molecular weight, otherwise these contaminants will still be present after the size exclusion chromatography step.

3.7.2. Size Exclusion Chromatography

1. Concentrate the pooled protein, purified on the MonoQ anion-exchange chromatography, by centricon 30 (Amicon) to a concentration of 2–3 mg/mL.
2. Load protein on a 7.5 × 60 cm TSK G3000SW column (equipped with a respective guard column), equilibrated with PBS. Elute the column with PBS. The protein usually elutes at 18–20 mL. The column can be previously calibrated with molecular-weight standard protein kit (Pharmacia) to verify the apparent elution size of the recombinant protein.
3. Analyze fractions from size exclusion chromatography, pooled, and stored at –70°C, by reducing conditions on SDS-PAGE. A typical yield of scFv or dsFv-immunotoxin is 5–10% and 10–15%, respectively, of total recombinant protein renatured.

3.8. Characterization of the Pure Recombinant Fv Immunotoxin

1. The protein concentration of the final pool is determined by the Pierce Coomassie Plus assay (Pierce) using BSA as a standard (*see* **Notes 10** and **11**).
2. Purity of the pooled purified protein can be determined by nonreducing and reducing SDS-PAGE.

3.8.1. Cytotoxicity Assays

1. The biological activity of recombinant Fv-immunotoxins is measured by the ability of the recombinant molecule to inhibit protein synthesis in target cells.
2. To test the biological cytotoxic activity of the purified Fv-immunotoxin on adherent cell-culture lines, plate 1.5×10^4 cells/well in 96-well plates and grow them for 24 h at 37°C, CO_2 incubator.
3. After 24 h add to the wells the Fv-immunotoxin and other control molecules and incubate for 16–24 hr at 37°C in a final culture medium (which varies with the cell type) volume of 200 μL.
4. Test Immunotoxin concentrations between 0.01–1000 ng/mL (final concentration in the assay). Make 1:10 serial dilutions. Performed the assay in triplicates and use wells without immunotoxins as controls for cell viability and maximal capability for protein synthesis.
5. After 24 h incubation with immunotoxin add 1–2 μCi/well of [^{3}H]-leucine for 4–6 h at 37°C.
6. To disintegrate the cells, freeze, and thaw the cells.
7. Harvest the cells using a cell harvester. Cell protein is bound onto glass-fiber filters and counted in a scintillation counter.
8. Calculate the extent of inhibition of protein synthesis as percent of control by comparing the incorporation of radioactive leucine in immunotoxin-containing wells and control wells without the toxin.
9. Determine the IC_{50} for each immunotoxin molecule, which is the concentration of immunotoxin necessary for 50% inhibition of protein synthesis.
10. To test cytotoxicity on nonadherent cell lines, plate $1–4 \times 10^4$ cells/well in 96-well plates in volume of 150 μL and add 50 μL aliquots of immunotoxin or control proteins. If the cells do not adhere to the plastic during the 16–24 h incubation prior to pulsing, they do not require freezing and thawing prior to harvesting.

3.8.2. Binding Assays: General Notes on Binding Assays

(Numerous protocols for binding assays on cells or purified antigens have been described and should be optimized for the experimental system that is being used.

1. To determine the binding affinity of the recombinant immunotoxin, label the ligand (antibody or antibody fragment not connected to the toxin) with ^{125}I.
2. Perform a standard displacement assay (also termed competition binding assay), in which increasing concentrations of either cold ligand or recombinant Fv-immunotoxin are added to a constant concentration of radiolabeled ligand, and the amount of bound radiolabeled ligand is determined.
3. Perform the binding assay on cell lines which overexpress the specific target molecule recognized by the ligand (antibody and Fv-immunotoxin).
4. The EC_{50} is the concentration of protein required to displace 50% of the radiolabeled ligand from binding to its receptor. This is the apparent Kd for the protein. The EC_{50} of the ligand (antibody) and the Fv-immunotoxin are compared to determine the binding affinity of the Fv and the extent to which fusion of the Fv fragment to the toxin influence its binding activity.

5. When performing binding assays of Fv-immunotoxins by competition with whole radio-labeled antibody one should take into consideration the effect of avidity, since the whole intact antibody is bivalent and the Fv fragment is monovalent. The displacement (competition) assay gives more accurate data than if the recombinant Fv immunotoxin is radiolabeled and its affinity determined directly by a Scatchard plot analysis, since radiolabeling of small proteins may damage them and decrease or abolish their binding capability.

6. Other binding assays for affinity measurements are possible such as using the BIAcore machine in which binding is determined by using real-time surface plasmon resonance (SPR) technology. In this method, the direct binding of the purified Fv-immunotoxin or Fv fragment is measured on chips to which the purified receptor or target molecule are immobilized (usually by using CM-5 carboxymethylated dextran chip). In these assays the kinetics of binding is determined by continuous flow and real-time conditions and the data are collected and analyzed with a special computer software (Biacore AB, Uppsala, Sweden).

4. Notes

1. For best expression results, fresh transformation of expression plasmids into Competent *E. coli* BL21/λDE3 cells should be performed. The transformation should not precede the expression by more then 18 h. The expression system has some leakines and can result in protein expression and in some cases bacterial lysis prior to induction by IPTG. This may result in reduced growth and viability of the bacteria during culture and poor expression after induction with IPTG.

2. In some cases premature protein expression occurs while bacteria are growing on the LB/Amp plates, leading to smaller than normal colonies. To decrease the leakiness of the expression system, an episome containing a repressor (*lac*Iq, *lac* repressor) can be added to the BL21/λDE3 cells.

3. In some cases protein expression may be poor because the eukaryotic DNA to be expressed in the bacteria contains codons that are rare for Gram-negative bacteria, such as AGA and AGG. This problem can be solved by using a plasmid encoding tRNA for these codons as well as a *lac* repressor *(46)*. The BL21/λDE3 cells are simply transformed with the episome, which contains a kanamycin resistance gene, and competent cells prepared for transformation with plasmid-encoding recombinant Fv-immunotoxin. The BL21-CodonPlus™ Competent Cells from Stratagene can be also used. They are designed for high-level expression of difficult heterologous proteins and eliminate additional procedures to express recombinant genes that encode rare codons. They contain extra copies of the genes that encode tRNAs for codons in *E. coli* that are rarely used. BL21-CodonPlus-RIL cells contain extra *argU, ileY*, and *leuW* tRNA genes and BL21-CodonPlus-RP cells contain extra *argU* and *proL* tRNA genes.

4. An alternative to transform DNA for producing a particular protein each time, is to prepare a master cell bank. To produce a master cell bank, a single colony obtained from a fresh transformation, is cultured in a shake flask with 200 mL of superbroth containing 100 μg/mL ampicillin. When the culture reaches an OD_{600nm} of ≈3, the cells are placed on ice, mixed with a 50% volume of 86% glycerol in water, and frozen at –70°C in 1.5 mL aliquots. Future fermentations can be started from a single aliquot.

5. A problem with some recombinant proteins is that their inclusion bodies often dissolve in detergents, such as the Triton X-100 that is being used to wash the inclusion bodies (**Subheading 3.3., step 3**). In these cases the number of washes with detergent must be minimized.

6. The protein concentration in the denaturing solution must be measured accurately because protein concentration in the final refolding is critical for successful renaturation of the recombinant protein. The protein in the denaturing solution (solubilization buffer) should be diluted 20-fold in solubilization buffer rather than water just prior to adding to the cuvet, since precipitation of protein will occur after dilution in water, leading to an inaccurate measurement of protein concentration. Measuring protein concentration in the refolding solution is difficult because of the presence of large concentration of L-arginine, but it can be measured accurately after the dialysis step of the refolding solution.

7. Stirring during the entire 36–48 h incubation of refolding at 10°C should not be done because it leads to increased and severe aggregation of the protein.

8. Isolated and purified inclusion bodies can be stored for prolonged periods at –70°C as a paste or in a solubilized form but without the reducing agent (DTE). After thawing, the inclusion bodies can be solubilized, then add DTE. Storage of solubilized inclusion bodies in the presence of DTE will cause a significant decrease in refolding efficiencies.

9. Recombinant proteins after the MonoQ column need to be evaluated by reducing conditions on SDS-PAGE to rule out contamination with disulfide-bonded impurities that might comigrate with the recombinant immunotoxin on a nonreducing gel but appear as lower molecular weight impurities on a reducing gel. The protein may be contaminated with dimeric or multimeric recombinant immunotoxin, which will not be apparent on a reducing gel, but these multimers can be removed subsequently by the size exclusion chromatography step.

10. The Coomassie reagent should be new; when the reagent becomes old, the absorbance is decreased and is no longer proportional to the amount of recombinant protein. Using old reagent will lead to inaccurate results even if a fresh standard is used.

11. The protein concentration can be also determined by measuring absorbance at 280 nm. The extinction coefficient should be determined for every new protein based on Coomassie assays.

References

1. Pastan, I., Chaudhary V., and FitzGerald, D. J. (1992) Recombinant toxins as novel therapeutic agents. *Ann. Rev. Biochem.* **61,** 331–354.
2. Vitteta, E. S. (1994) From the basic science of B cells to biological missiles at the bedside. *J. Immunol.* **153,** 1407–1420.
3. Kreitam, R. J. and Pastan, I (1998) Immunotoxins for targeted cancer therapy. *Ad. Drug Delivery Rev.* **31,** 53–88.
4. Kreitman, R. J. (1999) Immunotoxins in cancer therapy. *Curr. Opin. Immunol.* **11,** 570–578.
5. Veale, D., Kerr, N., Gibson, G. J., and Harris, A. L. (1989) Characterization of epidermal growth factor receptor in primary human non-small cell lung cancer. *Cancer Res.* **49,** 1313–1317.
6. Lau, J. L., Fowler, J., and Ghosh, L. (1988) Epidermal growth factor in normal and neoplastic kidney and bladder. *J. Urol.* **139,** 170–175.
7. Hung, M. C. and Lau, Y. K. (1999) Basic science of HER-2/neu, a review. *Semin. Oncol.* **26(4 Suppl 12),** 51–59.
8. Ross, J. S. and Fletcher, J. A. (1999) HER-2/neu (c-erb-B2) gene and protein in breast cancer. *Am. J. Clin. Pathol.* **112(1 Suppl 1),** S53–S67.
9. Vitteta, E. S., Sonte, M., AmLot, P., et al. (1991) Phase I immunotoxin trail in patients with B-cell lymphoma. *Cancer Res.* **51,** 4052–4058.

10. Grossbard, M. L., Lambert, J. M., Goldmacher, V. S., et al. (1993) Anti-B4-blocked ricine, a phase I trail of 7-day continuous infusion in patients with B-cell neoplasms. *J. Clin. Oncol.* **11,** 726–737.

11. Waldmann, T. A., Pastan, I, Gansow, O. A., et al. (1992) The multichain interleukin-2 receptor, a target for immunotherapy. *Ann. Intern. Med.* **116,** 148–160.

12. Chang, K., Pai, L. H., Batra, J. K., Pastan, I., and Willingham, M. C. (1992) Characterization of the antigen (CAK1) recognized by monoclonal antibody K1 present on ovarian cancers and normal mesothelium. *Cancer Res,* **52,** 181–186.

13. Chang, K. and Pastan, I. (1996) Molecular cloning of mesothelin, a differentiation antigen present on mesothelium, mesotheliomas, and ovarian cancers. *Proc. Natl. Acad. Sci. USA* **93,** 136–140.

14. Pastan, I., Lovelace, E., Rutherford, A. V., Kunwar, S., Willingham, M. C., and Peehl, D. M. (1993) PR1-a monoclonal antibody that reacts with an antigen on the surface of normal and malignant prostate cells. *J. Natl. Cancer Inst.* **85,** 1149–1154.

15. Pastan, I., Lovelace, E. T., Gallo, M. G., Rutherford, A. V., Magnani, J. L., and Willingham, M. C. (1991) Characterization of monoclonal antibodies B1 and B3 that react with mucinous adenocarcinomas. *Cancer Res,* **51,** 3781–3787.

16. Raag, R. and Whitlow, M. (1995) Single-chain Fvs. *FASEB J.* **9,** 73–80.

17. Winter, G. and Milstein, C. (1991) Man-made antibodies. *Nature* **349,** 293–299.

18. Huston, J. S., Levinson, D., Mudgett-Hunter, M., Tai, M. S., Novotny, J., Margolies, M. N., et al. (1988) Protein engineering of antibody binding sites, recovery of specific activity in an anti-digoxin single-chain Fv analogue produced in *Escherichia coli. Proc. Natl. Acad. Sci. USA* **85,** 5879–5883.

19. Bird, R. E., Hardman, K. D., Jacobson, J. W., Johnson, S., Kaufman, B. M., Lee, S. M., et al. (1988) Single-chain antigen-binding proteins. *Science* **242,** 423–426.

20. Brinkmann, U., Reiter, Y., Jung, S. H., Lee, B., and Pastan, I. (1993) A recombinant immunotoxin containing a disulfide-stabilized Fv fragment. *Proc. Natl. Acad. Sci. USA* **90,** 7538–7542.

21. Reiter, Y. and Pastan, I. (1996) Antibody engineering of recombinant Fv immunotoxins for improved targeting of cancer, disulfide-stabilized Fv immunotoxins. *Clin. Cancer Res.* **2,** 245–252.

22. Reiter, Y., Brinkmann, U., Lee, B., and Pastan, I. (1996) Engineering antibody Fv fragments for cancer detection and therapy, disulfide-stabilized Fv fragments. *Nature Biotechnol.* **14,** 1239–1245.

23. Batra, J. K., Jinno, Y., Chaudhary, V. K., Kondo, T., Willingham, M. C,. FitzGerald, D. J., and Pastan, I. (1989) Antitumor activity in mice of an immunotoxin made with anti-transferrin receptor and a recombinant form of Pseudomonas exotoxin. *Proc. Natl. Acad. Sci. USA* **86,** 8545–8549.

24. Chaudhary, V. K., Queen, C., Junghans, R. P., Waldmann, T. A., FitzGerald, D. J., and Pastan, I. (1989) A recombinant immunotoxin consisting of two antibody variable domains fused to Pseudomonas exotoxin. *Nature* **339,** 394–397.

25. Brinkmann, U., Pai, L. H., FitzGerald, D. J., Willingham, M., and Pastan, I. (1991) B3(Fv)-PE38KDEL, a single-chain immunotoxin that causes complete regression of a human carcinoma in mice. *Proc. Natl. Acad. Sci. USA* **88,** 8616–8620.

26. Batra, J. K., Kasprzyk, P. G., Bird, R. E., Pastan, I., and King, C. R. (1992) Recombinant anti-erbB2 immunotoxins containing Pseudomonas exotoxin. *Proc. Natl. Acad. Sci. USA* **89,** 5867–5871.

27. Kuan, C. T. and Pastan, I. (1996) Improved antitumor activity of a recombinant anti-Lewis(y) immunotoxin not requiring proteolytic activation. *Proc. Natl. Acad. Sci. USA* **93,** 974–978.

28. Reiter, Y., Wright, A. F., Tonge, D. W., and Pastan, I. (1996) Recombinant single-chain and disulfide-stabilized Fv-immunotoxins that cause complete regression of a human colon cancer xenograft in nude mice. *Int. J. Cancer* **67,** 113–123.

29. Reiter, Y., Pai, L. H., Brinkmann, U., Wang, Q. C., and Pastan, I. (1994) Antitumor activity and pharmacokinetics in mice of a recombinant immunotoxin containing a disulfide-stabilized Fv fragment. *Cancer Res.* **54,** 2714–2718.

30. Reiter, Y., Brinkmann, U., Jung, S. H., Lee, B., Kasprzyk, P. G., King, C. R., and Pastan, I. (1994) Improved binding and antitumor activity of a recombinant anti-erbB2 immunotoxin by disulfide stabilization of the Fv fragment. *J. Biol. Chem.* **269,** 18327–18331.

31. Mansfield, E., AmLot, P., Pastan, I., and FitzGerald, D. J. (1997) Recombinant RFB4 immunotoxins exhibit potent cytotoxic activity for CD22-bearing cells and tumors. *Blood* **90,** 2020–2026.

32. Kreitman, R. J., Chaudhary, V. K., Kozak, R. W., FitzGerald, D. J. P., Waldmann, T. A., Pastan, and I. (1992) Recombinant toxins containing the variable domains of the anti- Tac monoclonal antibody to the interleukin-2 receptor kill malignant cells from patients with chronic lymphocytic leukemia. *Blood* **80,** 2344–2352.

33. Kreitman, R. J., Chaudhary, V. K., Waldmann, T., Willingham, M. C., FitzGerald, D. J., and Pastan, I. (1990) The recombinant immunotoxin anti-Tac(Fv)-*Pseuodomonas* exotoxin 40 is cytotoxic toward peripheral blood malignant cells from patients with adult T-cell leukemia. *Proc. Natl. Acad. Sci. USA* **87,** 8291–8295.

34. Pai, L. H., Wittes, R., Setser, A., Willingham, M. C., and Pastan, I. (1996) Treatment of advanced solid tumors with immunotoxin LMB-1, an antibody linked to Pseudomonas exotoxin. *Nat. Med.* **2,** 350–353.

35. Pai, L. H. and Pastan, I. (1998) Clinical trials with Pseudomonas exotoxin immunotoxins. *Curr. Top. Microbiol. Immunol.* **234,** 83–96.

36. Pastan, I. H., Pai, L. H., Brinkmann, U., and Fitzgerald, D. J. (1995) Recombinant toxins, new therapeutic agents for cancer. *Ann. NY Acad. Sci.* **758,** 345–354.

37. Pastan, I. H., Archer, G. E., McLendon, R. E., Friedman, H. S., Fuchs, H. E., Wang, Q. C., et al. (1995) Intrathecal administration of single-chain immunotoxin, LMB-7 [B3(Fv)-PE38], produces cures of carcinomatous meningitis in a rat model. *Proc. Natl. Acad. Sci. USA* **92,** 2765–2769.

38. Reiter, Y., Pai, L. H., Brinkmann, U., Wang, Q. C., and Pastan, I. (1994) Antitumor activity and pharmacokinetics in mice of a recombinant immunotoxin containing a disulfide-stabilized Fv fragment. *Cancer Res.* **54,** 2714–2718.

39. Lorimer, I. A., Keppler-Hafkemeyer, A., Beers, R. A., Pegram, C. N., Bigner, D. D., and Pastan, I. (1996) Recombinant immunotoxins specific for a mutant epidermal growth factor receptor, targeting with a single chain antibody variable domain isolated by phage display. *Proc. Natl. Acad. Sci. USA* **93,** 14,815–14,820.

40. Chowdhury, P. S., Viner, J. L., Beers, R., and Pastan, I. (1998) Isolation of a high-affinity stable single-chain Fv specific for mesothelin from DNA-immunized mice by phage display and construction of a recombinant immunotoxin with anti-tumor activity. *Proc. Natl. Acad. Sci. USA* **95,** 669–674.

41. Kreitman, R. J., Wilson, W. H., Whie, J. D., Stetler-Stevenson, M., Jaffe, E. S., Giardina, S., et al. (2000) Phase I trail of recombinant immunotoxin anti-tac(Fv)-PE38 (LMB-2) in patients with hematological malignancies. *J. Clin. Oncol.* **18,** 1622–1636.

42. Kreitman, R. J., Wilson, W. H., Robbins, D., Margulies, I., Stetler-Stevenson, M., Waldmann, T. A., and Pastan, I. (1999) Responses in refractory hairy cell leukemia to a recombinant immunotoxin. *Blood* **94,** 3340–3348.

43. Studier, F. W. and Moffatt, B. A. (1986) Use of bacteriophage T7 polymerase to direct selective expression of cloned genes. *J. Mol. Biol.* **189,** 113–130.

44. Kabat, E. A., Wu, T. T., Perry, H. M., Gottesman, K. S., and Foeller, C. (1991) *Sequences of Proteins of Immunological Interest*, 5th ed., US Dept. of Health and Human Services, NIH Publication No. 91-3242, National Institutes of Health, Bethesda, MD.

45. Kunkel, T. A. (1985) Rapid and efficient site-specific mutagenesis without phenotypic selection. *Proc. Natl. Acad. Sci. USA* **82,** 488–492.

46. Brinkman, U., Mattes, R. E., and Buckel, P. (1989) High-level expression of recombinant genes in Escherichia coli is dependent on the availability of the *dna*Y gene product. *Gene* **85,** 109–114.

47. Hoogenboom, H. R. and Chames P. (2000) Natural and designer binding sites made by phage display technology. *Immunol. Today* **21,** 371–378.

48. Hoogenboom, H. R., Henderikx P., and de Haard H. (1998) Creating and engineering human antibodies for immunotherapy. *Adv. Drug Deliv. Rev.* **31,** 5–31.

16

Generation of Recombinant Immunotoxins
for Specific Targeting of Tumor-Related Peptides
Presented by MHC Molecules

Cyril J. Cohen, Galit Denkberg, Dina Segal, and Yoram Reiter

1. Introduction

Specificity in the immune system is dictated and regulated by specific recognition of peptide/major histocompatibility complex (MHC) complexes by the T cell receptor. Such peptide/MHC complexes are a desirable target for novel approaches in immunotherapy because of their highly restricted fine specificity. Expression of specific peptides in complex with MHC class I molecules on cells was shown to be associated with cancer and autoimmune disorders (1–8). For example, human melanomas express tumor-specific peptides that are presented to the immune
system in complex with class I HLA-A2 molecules (7,8). Specific targeting of drugs to these cells by using these specific peptide/MHC complexes will be a useful and promising therapeutic approach. To develop such a strategy, there is a need to isolate new targeting moieties such as recombinant antibodies that will recognize specifically peptide/MHC complexes.

Recently, phage display was used to isolate such antibodies that have T-cell receptor-like specificity. They recognizes mouse or human MHC class I molecules complexed with a haplotype-restricted peptide and do not cross-react with other MHC/peptide complexes nor with MHC without peptide or peptide alone (9–13). Example for such phage display-derived recombinant antibody is Fab 13.4.1 (9). This recombinant antibody recognizes mouse H2-K^k class I molecules complexed with the K^k-restricted influenza virus-derived peptide of hemagglutinin (peptide $_{Ha255\text{-}262}$) only and does not bind class I K^k molecules complexed with other peptides or class I molecules alone. Thus, this is a recombinant antibody with T-cell receptor-like specificity and restriction. This antibody can bind to soluble Ha/H-2K^k complexes as well as complexes expressed on cells and it can inhibit specifically peptide-dependent T-cell responses of T-cell hybridoma lines specific for the Ha$_{255\text{-}262}$/H-2K^k complex (9). It was also

From: *Methods in Molecular Biology, vol. 207: Recombinant Antibodies for Cancer Therapy: Methods and Protocols*
Edited by: M. Welschof and J. Krauss © Humana Press Inc., Totowa, NJ

demonstrated that Fab 13.4.1 shares a striking similarity to the specificity of T-cell hybridomas that recognize $Ha_{255-262}$ and most of the peptide residues, which were found to be recognized by the T cells, could also be recognized by the antibody *(14)*. To demonstrate that such an antibody can be used for specific targeting of a drug or toxin to antigen-presenting cells (APCs), a recombinant immunotoxin was constructed as a fusion protein composed of Fab 13.4.1 and a truncated form of *Pseudomonas* exotoxin (PE38), a very potent bacterial toxin, that contains the translocation and ADP ribosylation domains of whole PE but lacks the cell-binding domain *(10,15–17)* (*see* Chapter 15 for description of recombinant immunotoxins). The Fab 13.4.1-PE38 fusion protein kills specifically APCs that express the class I MHC/peptide complexes recognized by Fab 13.4.1. Moreover, the recombinant antibody-toxin fusion protein can kill specifically influenza virus-infected cells that present the MHC/peptide complex *(10)*.

The current results suggest that it should be possible to develop novel immunotherapeutic strategies against human cancer by making recombinant antibodies that will recognize cancer-related peptides complexed with MHC class I molecules on the surface of cancer cells, and using these to deliver toxins, radioisotopes, or cytotoxic drugs to the cancer cells. We will describe in this chapter the generation of immunotoxins against MHC-peptide complexes and the assays performed to characterize them. We will also describe the preparation of human class I recombinant MHC-peptide complexes for isolation of recombinant antibodies from phage-display libraries. The selection and isolation procedures of phage-display antibodies is beyond the scope of this chapter and are described in detail in reviews and in this series.

2. Materials

2.1. Plasmids

Plasmids for making recombinant immunotoxins that are specific for MHC-peptide complexes contain the DNA encoding the cloned Fv or Fab fragment originated from a phage display-derived recombinant fragment clone that was selected to a specific MHC-peptide complex and the recombinant toxin gene (in this case the gene encoding the truncated form of *Pseudomonas* Exotoxin PE, PE38) (*see* Chapter 15 for description of the truncated form of *Pseudomonas* Exotoxin and *see* **refs.** *15–17* for reviews).

These genes are under control of the T7 promoter *(18)* and contain usually ampicillin resistance gene (**Figs. 1** and **2**).

These plasmids are stored at a concentration of 1 mg/mL in TE (0.01 *M* Tris-HCl, pH 7.4, 1 m*M* EDTA at 4°C (or –20°C for long periods of time).

The plasmids for making human class I MHC HLA-A2 molecules are cloned from a human cell line *(19)* and introduced into a T7 promoter-based expression vector as described above. In the single-chain MHC molecule the β-2 microglobulin and the etracellular domain heavy chain HLA-A2 are fused into a single gene by a 15-amino acid long peptide linker connecting the C-terminus of β-2 microglobulin to the N-terminus of the HLA-A2 gene *(20)*.

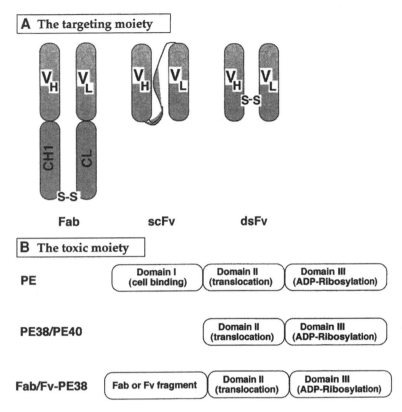

Fig. 1. Recombinant immunotoxins. (**A**) The targeting moiety. Three types of recombinant antibody fragments are used as the targeting moiety in recombinant immunotoxins. Fabs are composed of the light-chain and the heavy-chain Fd fragment (V_H and C_H1), connected to each other via the interchain disulfide bond between C_L and C_H1. ScFv fragments are stabilized by a peptide linker which connects the carboxyl-terminus of V_H or V_L with the amino terminus of the other domain. The V_H and V_L heterodimer in dsFv is stabilized by further engineering a disulfide bond between the two domains. (**B**) The toxic moiety. PE is a single-chain 66-kDa molecule composed of three major domains. The N-terminal domain Ia mediates cell binding to the *a2* macroglobulin receptor. Domain Ib is a small domain that lies between domain II and domain III and has no known function. Domain II mediates translocation of domain III, the carboxyl-terminal ADP-ribosylating domain, into the cytosol of target cells. When the whole toxin is used to make an immunotoxin, nonspecific toxicity occurs mainly due to binding of the toxin portion to cells, mediated domain Ia. The prototype molecule in which domain I has been deleted is PE40 (aa 253-613, MW 40 kDa). Because PE40 and its derivatives lack the binding domain (aa 1–252) they have very low nonspecific toxicity, but make very active and specific immunotoxins when conjugated to whole antibodies or fused to recombinant antibody fragments. Currently, almost all PE-derived recombinant immunotoxins are constructed with PE38 (MW 38 kDa), a PE40 derivative that has, in addition to the deletion of domain Ia, a second deletion encompassing a portion of domain Ib (aa 365–379).

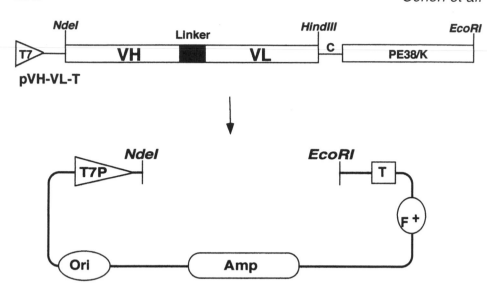

Fig. 2. Recombinant Fv Immunotoxins: design and engineering. The genes encoding the V_H and V_L variable domains are cloned usually from hybridoma mRNA by reverse transcription, cDNA synthesis, and subsequent PCR amplification using degenerate primers that are complementary to the 5' or 3' end of the V_H and V_L genes or by primers, which are designed according to the amino-terminal amino acid sequence of the MAb to be cloned and conserved sequences at the N-terminal of the heavy and light constant regions. The variable genes can be also cloned by constant domains primers and using the RACE method (rapid amplification of cDNA ends). Restriction sites for assembling of the peptide linker sequence which connects the V_H and V_L domains, and for cloning into the expression vector are also introduced by PCR. The antibody variable genes are subcloned into an expression vector that contains the gene for a truncated form of *Pseudomonas* exotoxin, PE38.

2.2. Transformation

1. Competent cells BL21/DE3 (Stratagene).
2. SOC medium.
3. Luria Broth (LB) plates containing 100 µg/mL ampicillin.
4. Superbroth containing added glucose (0.5%), $MgSO_4$ (1.6 mM) and ampicillin (100 µg/mL).
5. Isopropyl-β-D-thiogalactopyranoside (IPTG) 100 mM in water.

2.3. Isolation of Inclusion Bodies

1. Triton X-100 (25%) in water (Sigma).
2. TE50/20 buffer: 50 mM Tris-HCl, pH 7.4, 20 mM EDTA.
3. Lysozyme 5 mg/mL in TE50/20 buffer (Sigma).
4. 5 M NaCl.

2.4. Solubilization of Inclusion Bodies and Refolding Buffer

1. Solubilization buffer: 6 M Guanidine-HCl, 0.1 M Tris-HCl, pH 8.0, 5 mM EDTA (Sigma).
2. Dithioerythritol (DTE) (Sigma).

3. Bovine serum albumin (BSA) standard (2 mg/mL).
4. Refolding buffer: 0.1 *M* Tris-HCl, pH 8.0, 0.5 *M* Arginine-HCl, 2 m*M* EDTA, 0.9 m*M* oxidized glutathione (GSSG) (Sigma).
5. Dialysis buffer: 0.02 *M* Tris-HCl, pH 7.4, 0.1 *M* Urea (Sigma).

2.5. Purification

1. Q-Sepharose fast-flow anion exchange resin (Pharmacia).
2. MonoQ anion exchange column (HR10/10, 8 mL) (Pharmacia).
3. TSK G3000SW column (TosoHaas).
4. Buffer A: 0.02 *M* Tris-HCl, pH 7.4.
5. Buffer B: 0.02 *M* Tris-HCl, pH 7.4, 1M NaCl.
6. TSK equilibration and running buffer: PBS.

2.6. Characterization of Immunotoxin Activity

1. 96-Well microtiter plates.
2. Mutant antigen presenting cells (APCs) (transfected RMA-S for mouse MHC, T-2 for human).
3. Culture medium and serum depending on the cell type.
4. ^{3}H-Leucine (1 mCi/mL) (Amersham or NEN).
5. Cell Harvester.
6. Anti-MHC antibodies (class specific, human or mouse).
7. FITC-labeled goat anti-mouse IgG or Fab.
8. Rabbit anti-PE antibodies.
9. FITC-labeled goat anti-rabbit IgG.

3. Methods

3.1. Plasmid Preparation: Notes on Expression Plasmids

This chapter will not focus on the isolation and cloning of Fv or Fab fragments specific for MHC-peptide complexes from antibody phage-display. These are described in previous publications *(9–13,21,22)*.

We will describe the construction and production of the recombinant immunotoxins made with these constructs we will also describe the production of recombinant human MHC complexes using HLA-A2, the most frequent MHC haplotype to present cancer peptides. The expression and refolding procedures described for the recombinant immunotoxins and the MHC complexes are similar unless specifically stated. The methods described here for plasmid expression in *Escherichia coli* BL21/λDE3 cells is applicable for plasmids containing the T7 promoter and the ampicillin-resistance gene. Upon induction of the T7 RNA polymerase in *E. coli* BL21/λDE3 cells by IPTG, large amounts of recombinant protein are produced. The overexpressed Fv immunotoxin accumulate in insoluble intracellular inclusion bodies, which are subsequently isolated, purified, solubilized, and prepared for in vitro refolding.

3.2. Transformation

1. Thaw competent *E. coli* BL21/λDE3 cells, stored in –70°C on ice (*see* **Notes 1–4**).
2. Mix 100 μL of bacteria with 4 μg of plasmid DNA on ice for 30–45 min.

3. Incubate the suspension at 42°C for 1 min and place back on ice.
4. Add SOC medium (0.9 mL) and shake the mixture at 37°C for 1 h.
5. Plate the bacterial mixture on 5 LB/Amp plates (200 µL/plate) and incubate at 37°C for 14–18 h. (for each liter of expression transform 100 µL *E. coli* BL21/λDE3 cells and plate on 5 LB/Amp plates).
6. Scrape bacteria from the 5 plates and resuspend in 1-L superbroth (with ampicillin, MgSO$_4$, and glucose) divided into two 2-L shake flasks (500 mL/flask). Shake vigorously at 250 rpm at 37°C to ensure good aeration. The OD$_{600nm}$ of the initial culture should be 0.15–0.25.
7. Test the absorbance of culture sample at 600 nm (if OD$_{600nm}$ is above 0.7–0.8 samples should be diluted 1:10 with superbroth and final OD should be calculated according to dilution factor).
8. At OD600 nm ≈2.4, add IPTG (5 mL/500 mL culture of 100 m*M*) to a final concentration of 1 m*M*. Save 1 mL of culture before adding IPTG as a pre-induction control sample.
9. Incubate the culture for 90 min by continued shaking at 37°C. Harvest the cells by centrifugation at 3000*g* for 30 min at 4°C. Save 1 mL aliquot of culture before centrifugation as a post-induction sample.
10. Discard supernatant. Cell pellet may be frozen at –70°C.
11. Analyze aliquots from **steps 8** and **9** by sodium dodecyl sulfate polyacrylamide gel electrophoresis (SDS-PAGE). Resuspend cell pellets in 1 mL TE buffer. Sonicate 20 s in bath sonicator and centrifuge in an eppendorf centrifuge at maximal speed (5000*g*) for 10 min. Resuspend pellet in 0.1 mL TE. Sonicate 10–20 s and resuspend in 0.1 mL TE. Determine protein concentration and run equal amounts of protein on reduced SDS-PAGE to verify induction.

3.3. Isolation of Inclusion Body Protein

1. Resuspend cell paste from each liter of culture into 160 mL TE50/20 using a homogenizer. Transfer suspension to 250 mL sorvall centrifuge bottle (*see* **Note 5**).
2. Add 6.5 mL lysozyme at 5 mg/mL, mix well and incubate for 1 h at room temperature. Shake by hand frequently.
3. Add 20 mL of 25% Triton X-100, mix well, and incubate for 30 min at room temperature. Shake by hand frequently.
4. Centrifuge 27,500*g* (Sorvall, GSA rotor) for 60 min at 4°C in Sorvall GSA rotor.
5. Discard supernatant and resuspend pellet in 180 mL TE50/20 by using a homogenizer.
6. Repeat **steps 4** and **5** three to four times. Keep a small amount of inclusion bodies pellet after last wash for analyzing on SDS-PAGE as described in **Subheadings 3.2.–3.10**.

3.4. Solubilization and Reduction of Inclusion Bodies

1. Transfer the inclusion bodies pellet into 50 mL Oak Ridge Centrifuge Tubes (Nunc), (using a spatula).
2. Resuspend the pellet in solubilization buffer (6 *M* guanidine HCl, 100 m*M* Tris-HCl, pH 8.0, 2 m*M* EDTA). 1.5–1.8 g Wet inclusion bodies solubilized into 10 mL solubilization buffer will give a protein concentration of ~10 mg/mL.
3. Dissolve inclusion bodies in solubilization buffer (if required use homogenizer with a small probe) until completely dissolved.
4. Centrifuge solubilized inclusion bodies at 16,000*g* (Sorvall GSA rotor), 20 min, 4°C in Sorvall SS34 rotor.

5. Take supernatant which are the solubilized inclusion bodies, determine protein concentration with Pierce Coomassie plus reagent. Dilute 10 µL of the denatured and solubilized protein 10–20-fold with denaturation buffer, and then add 5–10 µL to cuvets. Add 1 mL of 1:1 diluted reagent in water. The standard to be used is 2 mg/mL BSA (*see* **Notes 6** and **8**).

6. Dilute the protein to 10 mg/mL (if necessary) with solubilization buffer and add DTE (Dithioerithritol) to 10 mg/mL (65 m*M* final concentration), mix, and incubate for 4–24 h at room temperature (at least 4 h of incubation are required for complete reduction of disulfide bonds).

7. Prepare 100-fold more buffer then the volume of the denatured protein solution and chill to 10°C.

3.5. Refolding

1. Add 551 mg/L oxidized glutathione (GSSG) (final concentration 0f 0.9 m*M*) to the chilled refolding buffer.

2. To remove small amounts of undissolved material centrifuge the reduced, denatured, and solubilized recombinant protein at 40,000*g* for 20–40 min at 4°C.

3. Stir the chilled refolding buffer briskly, using a pipet add the denatured protein from **step 2** quickly over 20–30 s to a final protein concentration of 100 µg/mL for the recombinant immunotoxin and 50 µg/mL for the recombinant MHC molecule. Dilute every 10 mL of solubilized recombinant protein at a concentration of 10 mg/mL (total 100 mg) for recombinant immunotoxin or 5 mg/mL (total 50 mg) for recombinant MHC is diluted 1:100 into 1 L of refolding solution to give a final protein concentration of 100 µg/mL for immunotoxin and 50 µg/mL for the recombinant MHC (*see* **Note 7**).

4. For refolding of MHC-peptide complex, add peptide immediately after the addition of the recombinant MHC in the previous step. Dissolve 10–15-fold molar excess of peptide in 0.5–1.0 mL refolding buffer and add immediately after the addition of the MHC protein. Insoluble peptides should be dissolved in dimethyl solfoxide (DMSO). The β2-microglobulin-HLA-A2 fusion MHC molecule (≈50 kDa) is refolded at 50 µg/mL which results at a concentration of 1 µ*M*. Therefore, a 10–15 molar excess of peptide would be 10–15 m*M* final concentration in the refolding solution. Assuming an average molecular weight of ≈1000 Dalton for a 8–9 amino acid peptide (the usual length of HLA-A2-restricted peptides) this means 10–15 mg of peptide per 1 L of refolding solution.

5. Mix well for 2–3 min, stop stirring and allow refolding at 10°C for 36–48 h.

3.6. Dialysis

1. To collect precipitated protein generated during refolding, centrifuged at 27,000g, Sorvall GSA rotor in 250 mL Sorvall centrifuge bottles for 30 min at 4°C.

2. Collect supernatant and dialyze at 4°C in 25-fold of the initial refolding volume against 20 m*M* Tris-HCl, pH 7.4 100 m*M* urea. Change 2–3 times buffer until conductivity measures 3–4 m*M* HO (the ionic strength of the protein decreases below that of 55 m*M* NaCl).

3. Concentrate the MHC-peptide complex by using the MiniSet concentration system from Filtron. With these system the buffer exchange is facilitated by ultrafiltration through a membrane having a 10-kDa cutoff. The protein is concentrated to 10–20% of its original volume and dialysis buffer is added at the same rate as buffer is removed by ultrafiltration. After the ionic strength is reduced to appropriate level, the protein is removed from the ultrafiltration device.

3.7. Purification of Recombinant Immunotoxin Protein

3.7.1. Ion Exchange Chromatography

All chromatography steps are performed at 4°C.

1. Load the dialyzed protein on a 5–8 mL Q-Sepharose column (Pharmacia) previously equilibrated and washed with 10 column volumes of buffer A, 10 column volumes of buffer B, and then 20 vol of buffer A. The protein is loaded at 2–4 mL/min.
2. After loading the protein (1–3 h), wash the column with buffer A until no protein is present in the flowthrough and elute in 5 mL fractions with 30% buffer B in buffer A (300 m*M* NaCl).
3. Pool the peak fractions, determine amount of protein by the Coomassie Plus Protein Assay Reagent and diluted fivefold with buffer A.
4. Load protein on a 8-mL high resolution MonoQ column (Pharmacia). This requires a high-pressure pump and is performed usually on an FPLC system. Protein is loaded at 2–4 mL/min.
5. Wash the column with 10–15 column volumes of buffer A until no protein is present in the flowthrough and elute with a linear gradient of 0–40% buffer B in buffer A at a flow rate of 2 mL/min over 10 column volumes. Collect 2 mL fractions. This will yield a gradient with a 1% increase in buffer B per 1 mL of elution.
6. Evaluate the peak fractions of protein, eluting typically at ≈20% buffer B (0.2 *M* NaCl), are individually for protein concentration and for purity by SDS-PAGE under reducing conditions (*see* **Note 9**).
7. Pooled fractions should be >90% pure and not be contaminated with proteins of similar molecular weight, otherwise these contaminants will still be present after the size-exclusion chromatography step.

3.7.2. Size-Exclusion Chromatography

1. Concentrate the pooled protein, purified on the MonoQ anion-exchange chromatography, by centricon 30 (Amicon) to a concentration of 2–3 mg/mL.
2. Load protein on a 7.5 × 60 cm TSK G3000SW column (equipped with a respective guard column), equilibrated with PBS. Elute the column with PBS. The protein usually elutes at 18–20 mL. The column can be previously calibrated with molecular-weight standard protein kit (Pharmacia) to verify the apparent elution size of the recombinant protein.
3. Analyze fractions from size-exclusion chromatography, pooled, and stored at –70°C, by reducing conditions on SDS-PAGE. A typical yield of scFv or dsFv-immunotoxin is 5–10% and 10–15%, respectively, of total recombinant protein renatured.

3.8. Purification of MHC-Peptide Complexes

1. Load the dialyzed and concentrated protein on a 8 mL Q-Sepharose or MonoQ column (Pharmacia), previously equilibrated and washed with 10 column volumes of buffer A, 10 column volumes of buffer B, and then 20 vol of buffer A. Load protein at 2–4 mL/min. This requires a high-pressure pump and is performed usually on an FPLC system.
2. After loading the protein, wash the column with buffer A until no protein is present in the flowthrough.
3. Elute the column with a linear gradient of 0–40% buffer B in buffer A at a flow rate of 2 mL/min over 10 column volumes collecting 2 mL fractions. This will yield a gradient with a 1% increase in buffer B per 1 mL of elution.
4. The peak fractions of correctly folded MHC-peptide protein elute typically between 6–12% buffer B (0.06–0.12 *M* NaCl). Evaluate samples individually for protein

concentration and for purity by SDS-PAGE under reducing conditions. The missfolded MHC-peptide complexes elute at higher ionic strength and are seen on nonreducing SDS-PAGE as larger aggregates.

5. Pooled fractions should be >90% pure and not be contaminated with proteins of similar molecular weight, otherwise these contaminants will still be present after the size exclusion chromatography step.
6. A size exclusion chromatography purification step is performed as described in **Subheading 3.7.2.**
7. After pooling of peak fractions of MHC-peptide complex from the TSK column, the specific peptide is added at a concentration of 1–5 μM to keep a constant presence of the peptide for complex stability.
8. Keep the purified MHC-peptide complexes at 4°C. For long periods the complexes can be frozen at –20°C or –70°C in the presence of peptide as described in **step 7**.

3.9. Characterization of the Pure Recombinant Fv Immunotoxin

1. Determine the protein concentration of the final pool by the Pierce Coomassie Plus assay (Pierce) using BSA as a standard (*see* **Notes 10–12**).
2. Determine the purity of the pooled purified protein by nonreducing and reducing SDS-PAGE.

3.10. Characterization of the Biological Activity of Recombinant Immunotoxin on Antigen Presenting Cells (APC)

3.10.1. Activity Cytotoxicity Assays on Mutant APCs

The biological activity of the recombinant immunotoxins is measured by the ability of the recombinant molecule to inhibit protein synthesis in target cells. This is performed first on the mouse mutant APCs RMA-S that are transfected with the corresponding class I MHC, in the case of Fab31.4.1 RMA-S are transfected with a mouse H2-K^k class I construct. RMA-S is a temperature-sensitive TAP (transporter-associated with antigen processing) mutant mouse cell *(23)*. The antigen-processing defective mutant RMA-S-K^k cells, when cultured at low temperature, express high amounts of MHC class I molecules that do not contain endogenously derived peptides. These empty MHC class I molecules can be stabilized by addition of MHC binding peptides. The activity of the immunotoxin is then tested on the peptide-loaded RMA-S MHC class I transfected cells. RMA-S can be also transfected with human MHC molecules such as HLA-A2 or the human T-B cell line T2 can be used to load endogenous peptide. This is a human line which has a mutant TAP and thus present empty HLA-A2 molecules on the cell surface. The protocol described here applies to the use of the temperature-sensitive mutant line RMA-S.

1. Incubate RMA-S-K^k cells (10^7) for 8–12 h with 0.1 mM peptides at 26°C in 5 mL medium without serum (*see* **Notes 13** and **14**).
2. Wash cells twice with medium and incubate for 24 h at 37°C, 5% CO_2 incubator with recombinant immunotoxin in a final volume of 200 μL in 96-well plates (10^5 cells/well).
3. Test Immunotoxin concentrations between 0.01–1000 ng/mL (final concentration in the assay). Make 1:10 serial dilutions. Performed the assay in triplicates and use wells without immunotoxins as controls for cell viability and maximal capability for protein synthesis.
4. Use cells loaded with control nonspecific peptides to determine the specificity of immunotoxin activity.

5. After 24 h incubation with immunotoxin add 1–2 µCi/well of [^{3}H]-leucine for 4–6 h at 37°C.
6. To disintegrate the cells, freeze and thaw the cells.
7. Harvest the cells using a cell harvester. Cell protein is bound onto glass-fiber filters and counted in a scintillation counter.
8. Calculate the extent of inhibition of protein synthesis as percent of control by comparing the incorporation of radioactive leucine in immunotoxin-containing wells and control wells without the toxin.
9. Determine the IC_{50} for each immunotoxin molecule, which is the concentration of immunotoxin necessary for 50% inhibition of protein synthesis.

3.10.2. Activity on Target APCs

1. To test the biological cytotoxic activity of the immunotoxin on adherent cell-culture lines, plate 1.5×10^4 cells/well in 96-well plates and let grow for 24 h at 37°C, 5% CO_2 incubator.
2. After 24 h add the specific and control immunotoxins and incubate for 16–24 h at 37°C in a final culture medium (which varies with the cell type) volume of 200 µL immunotoxin concentrations to be tested are usually between 0.01–1000 ng/mL (final concentration in the assay) with 1:10 serial dilutions. Assays are performed in triplicates and wells without immunotoxins are being used as controls for cell viability and maximal capability for protein synthesis.
3. Pulse the cells for 4–6 h at 37°C with 1–2 µCi/well of [^{3}H]-leucine.
4. To disintegrate the cells, freeze them on dry ice or at –70°C and then thaw them at 37°C. Harvest cells using a cell harvester in which cellular proteins bind onto glass-fiber filters and counte in a scintillation counter.
5. The extent of inhibition of protein synthesis is calculated as described in **Subheading 3.10.1., steps 8** and **9**.
6. To test cytotoxicity on nonadherent cell lines, plate $1–4 \times 10^4$ cells/well in 96-well plates in volume of 150 µL. Add 50 µL aliquots of immunotoxin or control proteins. If the cells do not adhere to the plastic during the 16–24 h incubation prior to pulsing, they do not require freezing and thawing prior to harvesting.

3.11. Binding Assay of Immunotoxin to APCs

To determine the binding affinity of the recombinant immunotoxin to mutant RMA-S-K^k cells the recombinant Fab antibody is radiolabeled with ^{125}I. In a standard displacement assay (also termed competition binding assay), increasing concentrations of either cold Fab fragment or recombinant immunotoxin are added to a constant concentration of radiolabeled ligand, and the amount of bound radiolabeled ligand is determined. The EC_{50} is the concentration of protein required to displace 50% of the radiolabeled ligand from binding to its receptor. This is the apparent K_d for the protein. The EC_{50} of the ligand (antibody) and the immunotoxin are compared to determine the binding affinity of the Fab and the extent to which fusion of the antibody fragment to the toxin influence its binding activity.

1. Load RMA-S-K^k cells with peptides as described in **Subheading 3.10.1., step 1** (*see* **Notes 13** and **14**).
2. Plate $1–4 \times 10^5$ cells/well in a 24-well culture plate in culture medium (usually RPMI-1640) without serum.

3. Wash cells three times with culture medium and incubated for 1 h at room temperature with a fixed amount of radiolabeled Fab antibody (usually 2×10^5 CPM/well) and increasing concentration of cold antibody or immunotoxin.
4. Wash cells three times with medium and lyse cells by adding culture medium + 2% SDS.
5. Collect cell extracts and determine cell-bound radioactivity by reading in a gamma counter.

3.12. FACS Analysis of Peptide Presentation by Mutant APCs and Staining with Recombinant Immunotoxin or Antibody

1. To determine the presentation of peptides on the mutant RMA-S-K^k cells, perform a FACS analysis using MAbs that recognize properly folded MHC-peptide complexes. The mutant APCs laoded with peptide can be subsequently stained with the recombinant immunotoxin or recombinant antibody itself.
2. Load RMA-S-K^k cells (10^7) with peptides as described in **Subheading 3.10.1.**
3. Wash cells twice with medium (centrifugation at $1500g$ for 10 min at 4°C) and incubate with fluorescein isothiocyante (FITC)-labeled anti-mouse H-2K^k (0.5 mg/10^6 cells) for 90 min on ice.
4. Wash cells twice with PBS and analyze by a FACS machine.
5. MHC-peptide complexes on APCs can be detected with purified recombinant Fab or immunotoxin and FITC-labeled goat anti-mouse IgG or Fab or rabbit anti-PE antibody and a second FITC-labeled anti-rabbit IgG.
6. Load RMA-S-K^k cells (10^7) with peptides as described in **Subheading 3.10.1.**
7. Wash cells twice with medium and incubate with recombinant antibody or immunotoxin for 1 h at room temeperature.
8. Wash cells twice with medium and incubate for 30 min at room temperature with Rabbit anti-PE antibody.
9. Wash cell twice with medium and incubate for 30 min at room temperature with FITC-labeled anti-rabbit IgG.

4. Notes

1. For best expression results, fresh transformation of expression plasmids into Competent *E. coli* BL21/λDE3 cells should be performed. The transformation should not precede the expression by more then 18 h. The expression system has some leakyness and can result in protein expression and in some cases bacterial lysis prior to induction by IPTG. This may result in reduced growth and viability of the bacteria during culture and poor expression after induction with IPTG.
2. In some cases premature protein expression occurs while bacteria are growing on the LB/Amp plates, leading to smaller than normal colonies. To decrease the leakiness of the expression system, an episome containing a repressor (*lac*Iq, *lac* repressor) can be added to the BL21/λDE3 cells.
3. In some cases protein expression may be poor because the eukaryotic DNA to be expressed in the bacteria contains codons that are rare for gram negative bacteria, such as AGA and AGG. This problem can be solved by using a plasmid encoding tRNA for these codons as well as a *lac* repressor *(46)*. The BL21/λDE3 cells are simply transformed with the episome, which contains a kanamycin-resistance gene, and competent cells prepared for transformation with plasmid-encoding recombinant immunotoxin. The BL21-CodonPlus™ Competent Cells from Stratagene can be also used. They are

designed for high-level expression of difficult heterologous proteins and eliminate additional procedures to express recombinant genes that encode rare codons. They contain extra copies of the genes that encode tRNAs for codons in *E. coli* that are rarely used. BL21-CodonPlus-RIL cells contain extra *argU*, *ileY*, and *leuW* tRNA genes and BL21-CodonPlus-RP cells contain extra *argU* and *proL* tRNA genes.

4. An alternative to transform DNA for producing a particular protein each time, is to prepare a master cell bank. To produce a master cell bank, a single colony obtained from a fresh transformation is cultured in a shake flask with 200 mL of superbroth containing 100 μg/mL ampicillin. When the culture reaches an OD_{600nm} of ~3, the cells are placed on ice, mixed with a 50% volume of 86% glycerol in water, and frozen at –70°C in 1.5 mL aliquots. Future fermentations can be started from a single aliquot.

5. A problem with some recombinant proteins is, that their inclusion bodies often dissolve in detergents, such as the Triton X-100 that is being used to wash the inclusion bodies (**Subheading 3.3., step 3**). In these cases the number of washes with detergent must be minimized.

6. The protein concentration in the denaturing solution must be measured accurately because protein concentration in the final refolding is critical for successful renaturation of the recombinant protein. The protein in the denaturing solution (solubilization buffer) should be diluted 20-fold in solubilization buffer rather than water just prior to adding to the cuvet, since precipitation of protein will occur after dilution in water, leading to an inaccurate measurement of protein concentration. Measuring protein concentration in the refolding solution is difficult because of the presence of large concentration of L-arginine, but it can be measured accurately after the dialysis step of the refolding solution.

7. Stirring during the entire 36–48 h incubation of refolding at 10°C should not be done because it leads to increased and severe aggregation of the protein.

8. Isolated and purified inclusion bodies can be stored for prolonged periods at –70°C as a paste or in a solubilized form but without the reducing agent (DTE). After thawing the inclusion bodies can be solubilized then add DTE. Storage of solubilized inclusion bodies in the presence of DTE will cause a significant decrease in refolding efficiencies.

9. Recombinant proteins after the MonoQ column need to be evaluated by reducing conditions on SDS-PAGE to rule out contamination with disulfide-bonded impurities that might comigrate with the recombinant immunotoxin on a nonreducing gel but appear as lower molecular weight impurities on a reducing gel. The protein may be contaminated with dimeric or multimeric recombinant immunotoxin, which will not be apparent on a reducing gel, but these multimers can be removed subsequently by the size exclusion chromatography step.

10. The Coomassie reagent should be new, when the reagent becomes old, the absorbance is decreased and is no longer proportional to the amount of recombinant protein. Using old reagent will lead to inaccurate results even if a fresh standard is used.

11. The protein concentration can be also determined by measuring absorbance at 280 nm. The extinction coefficient should be determined for every new protein based on Coomassie assays.

12. Purity of the pooled purified protein can be determined by nonreducing and reducing SDS-PAGE.

13. The affinity of each MHC-restricted peptide to the MHC is different and therefore peptide loading on the mutant APCs should be optimized. This can be determined by monitoring peptide presentation on the cell surface by FACS using specific mouse and human anti-MHC antibodies as described in **Subheading 3.12.**

14. When several peptides are being used in the biological assays on the mutant APCs, to verify the specificity or other biological properties of the recombinant immunotoxin or antibody, it should be considered that the results do not reflect differential binding of the peptides to the MHC, due to differences in binding affinity to MHC. Thus, the experimental results must be correlated with determination of peptide presentation by FACS analysis. The FACS profiles of all peptides used in an assay should be aligned (under the same FACS assay conditions) to determine the relative binding to the MHC molecule on the cell surface.

References

1. Rammensee, H. G., Falk, K., and Rotzschke, O. (1993) Peptides naturally presented by MHC class I molecules. *Ann. Rev. Immunol.* **11,** 213–244.
2. Germain, R. and Margulies, D. (1993) The biochemistry and cell biology of antigen processing and presentation. *Ann. Rev. Immunol.* **11,** 403–450.
3. Davis, M. M., Boniface, J. J., Reich, Z., Lyons, D., Hampl, J., Arden, B., and Chien, Y. (1998) Ligand recognition by alpha beta T cell receptors. *Ann. Rev. Immunol.* **16,** 523–544.
4. Lanzavecchia, A., Lezzi, G., and Viola, A. (1999) From TCR engagement to T cell activation: a kinetic view of T cell behaviour. *Cell* **96,** 1–4.
5. Rosenberg, S. A. (1997) Cancer vaccines based on the identification of genes encoding cancer regression antigens. *Immunol. Today* **18,** 175–182.
6. Van den Eynde, B. and Van der Bruggen, O. (1997) T-cell-defined tumor antigens. *Curr. Opin. Immunol.* **9,** 684–693.
7. Goodnow, C. C. (1996) Balancing immunity and tolerance: deleting and tuning lymphocyte repertoires. *Proc. Natl. Acad. Sci. USA* **93,** 2264–2271.
8. Steinman, L. (1996) A few autoreactive cells in an autoimmune infiltrate control a vast population of nonspecific cells: a tale of smart bombs and the infantry. *Proc. Natl. Acad. Sci. USA* **93,** 2253–2256.
9. Andersen, P. S., Stryhn, A., Hansen, B. E., Fugger, L., and Engberg, J. (1996) A recombinant antibody with the antigen specific, major histocompetibiby complex-restricted specificity of T cells. *Proc. Natl. Acad. Sci. USA* **93,** 1820–1824.
10. Reiter, Y., DiCarlo, A., Engberg, J., and Pastan, I. (1997) Peptide-specific killing of antigen-presenting cells by a recombinant antibody-toxin fusion protein targeted to MHC/peptide class I complexes with T-cell receptor-like specificity. *Proc. Natl. Acad. Sci. USA* **94,** 4631–4636.
11. Chames P., Hufton S. E., Coulie P. G., Uchanska-Ziegler B., and Hoogenboom H. R. (2000) Direct selection of a human antibody fragment directed against the tumor T-cell epitope HLA-A1-MAGE-A1 from a nonimmunized phage-Fab library. *Proc. Natl. Acad. Sci. USA* **97,** 7969–7974.
12. Krogsgaard, M., Wucherpfennig, K. W., Canella, B., Hansen, B. E., Svejgaard, A., Pyrdol, J., et al. (2000) Visualization of myelin basic protein (MBP) T cell epitopes in multiple sclerosis lesions using a monoclonal antibody specific for the human histocompatibility leukocyte antigen (HLA)-DR2-MBP 85-99 complex. *J. Exp. Med.* **191,** 1395–1412.
13. Engberg, J., Krogsgaard, M., and Fugger, L. (1999) Recombinant antibodies with the antigen-specific, MHC restricted specificity of T cells: novel reagents for basic and clinical investigations and immunotherapy. *Immunotechnology* **4,** 273–278.

14. Stryhn A., Andersen P. S., Pedersen L. O., Svejgaard A., Holm A., Thorpe C. J., et al. (1996) Shared fine specificity between T-cell receptors and an antibody recognizing a peptide/major histocompatibility class I complex. *Proc. Natl. Acad. Sci. USA* **93,** 10,338–10,342.

15. Pastan, I., Chaudhary V., and FitzGerald, D. J. (1992) Recombinant toxins as novel therapeutic agents. *Ann. Rev. Biochem.* **61,** 331–354.

16. Kreitam, R. J. and Pastan, I. (1998) Immunotoxins for targeted cancer therapy. *Adv. Drug Deliv. Rev.* **31,** 53–88.

17. Kreitman, R. J. (1999) Immunotoxins in cancer therapy. *Curr. Opin. Immunol.* **11,** 570–578.

18. Studier, F. W. and Moffatt, B. A. (1986) Use of bacteriophage T7 polymerase to direct selective expression of cloned genes. *J. Mol. Biol.* **189,** 113–130.

19. Salter, R. D., Howell, D., and Cresswell, P. (1985) Genes regulating HLA class I antigen expression in T-B lymphoblast hybrids. *Immunogenetics* **21,** 235–246.

20. Denkberg, G., Cohen, C. J., Segal, D., Kirkin, A. F., and Reiter, Y. (2000) Recombinant human single-chain MHC-peptide complexes made from *E. coli* by *in vitro* refolding: Functional single-chain MHC-peptide complexes and tetramers with tumor associated antigens. *Eur. J. Immunol.* **30,** 3522–3532.

21. Hoogenboom, H. R. and Chames, P. (2000) Natural and designer binding sites made by phage display technology. *Immunol. Today* **21,** 371–378.

22. Hoogenboom, H. R., Henderikx, P., and de Haard, H. (1998) Creating and engineering human antibodies for immunotherapy. *Adv. Drug. Deliv. Rev.* **31,** 5–31.

23. Schumacher, T. N., Heemels, M. T., Neefjes, J. J., Kast, W. M., Melief, C. J., and Ploegh, H. L. (1990) Direct binding of peptide to empty MHC class I molecules on intact cells and in vitro. *Cell* **62,** 563–567.

17

Construction and Characterization
of RNase-Based Targeted Therapeutics

Dianne L. Newton, Junichiro Futami,
Dale Ruby, and Susanna M. Rybak

1. Introduction

Cell targeting agents such as antibodies, antibody fragments (sFvs), or growth factors have been conjugated or genetically fused to a variety of plant and bacterial toxins. These targeted therapeutics, termed "immunotoxins," have been evaluated for their clinical efficacy in the treatment of cancer, AIDS, and immunological diseases *(1,2)*. Development of potentially promising clinical results, however, have been hampered by problems of toxicity and immunogenicity owing to the foreign proteins *(3–8)*. Although the development of humanized antibodies has alleviated some of these effects *(9,10)*, the toxins still remain a problem. In this regard the use of human proteins as components of the immunotoxin are highly desirable (reviewed in **ref. *11***). Human RNases such as EDN, angiogenin and pancreatic RNase A are not toxic to cells yet when linked chemically or fused genetically to cell surface-binding ligands have potent anti-tumor effects both in vitro and in vivo *(12–23)*. Furthermore in vivo experiments demonstrate that the RNase-based therapeutics cause fewer nonspecific toxic or immunogenic side effects than plant and bacterial toxins (*22,23* and reviewed in **ref. *11***).

This chapter describes the construction, expression, purification, and characterization of RNase fusion proteins. Briefly, the cell-targeting agent, e.g., the sFv or growth factor, and RNase are each modified separately by polymerase chain reaction (PCR). If no spacer is required to separate the RNase from the cell-targeting agent (such as with RNase growth factor fusion proteins *[17,18,21]*), each half of the fusion protein is modified to contain complementary sequences of the other half. If a spacer is required (such as with RNase-sFv fusion proteins *[19]*), each half is modified to contain the complementary spacer sequence of interest. The modified RNase and cell targeting agent genes are joined using the PCR technique of splicing

From: *Methods in Molecular Biology, vol. 207: Recombinant Antibodies for Cancer Therapy: Methods and Protocols*
Edited by: M. Welschof and J. Krauss © Humana Press Inc., Totowa, NJ

by overlap extension *(24)*. The DNA encoding the fusion protein is then transfected into bacteria specifically engineered for the expression of toxic proteins *(25)*. Following induction by isopropyl-β-D-thiogalactopyranoside (IPTG), fusion proteins are expressed as insoluble aggregates in inclusion bodies. Three methods to isolate and refold RNase fusion proteins are presented. The first method involves refolding the RNase fusion protein from purified inclusion bodies in which the fusion protein is the major component. The fusion protein is denatured and refolded in a buffer containing a redox system of oxidized and reduced glutathione to promote formation of disulfide bonds and 0.5 *M* arginine to enhance correct folding. While this method is laborious, it results in correctly refolded RNase fusion proteins. The second method is less tedious because the fusion protein is refolded from a crude preparation of inclusion bodies. High salt (0.4 *M*) in the folding buffer is included to prevent inhibition of folding by the nucleic acids, which contaminate the inclusion body preparation *(26)*. In addition, bacterial proteases present as contaminants may degrade the fusion protein during the refolding and purification process. These contaminants may decrease the yield of recombinant protein. In the third method, the crude preparation of inclusion bodies is treated with the novel S-alkylsulfidation reagent, TAPS-sulfonate, which introduces one positive charge per cysteine residue *(27–30)*. Treatment of crude inclusion bodies solubilized with 6 *M* guanidine-HCl with TAPS-sulfonate in the presence of dithiothreitol (DTT) allows all cysteine residues to be modified. This mixture is then dialyzed against acetic acid. Due to the positive charge of the RNase fusion protein, the TAPS-sulfonate modified RNase fusion protein remains soluble under acidic conditions in the absence of denaturant, whereas most of the TAPS-sulfonate modified bacterial proteins will precipitate. Following centrifugation to remove the bacterial impurities, the TAPS-modified fusion protein is refolded using a two step refolding scheme. Final purification of the RNase fusion protein obtained by any of the methods described earlier is accomplished with a two-step column procedure. Because RNases are basic proteins, a cationic exchanger resin is the recommended first column. A relatively pure protein can be obtained at this step because the majority of contaminating proteins do not adhere to this resin. The final column is an affinity resin such as Ni^{2+}-NTA agarose. Assays that characterize the activity of both components of the fusion protein, i.e., binding and ribonuclease activity, as well as activity of the entire fusion protein, i.e., in vitro cytotoxic activity, are described. Finally, the procedure for characterizing toxicity and efficacy of the fusion protein in vivo is included.

2. Materials

2.1. Construction of the RNase Fusion Gene

1. Genes encoding the cell targeting agent and the RNase.
2. Primers purified on oligonucleotide purification cartridges (OPC) (Annovis Inc., Ashton, PA) to remove any short failure sequences. Use of unpurified oligonucleotides can result in incorrect priming or introduction of a nucleotide deletion (*see* **Table 1** and **Subheading 3.1.**, **step 2** for discussion of the design of primers).
3. Vector, pET-11d or appropriate pET vector (Novagen, Madison, WI) (*see* **Note 1**).

Table1
Sequence of Junction and Primer Oligonucleotides Encoding PancsFv (16)

Primer	Sequence	Direction
A	5'-ATATAT**CTAGA**-*AATAATTTTGTTTAACTTTAAGAAGGAGATATACAT*-<u>ATG</u>aaggaatccgggccaagaaa-3'	Sense
B	5'-**ATCACTCTTCGGCGCCTGAGCCGTCGTTCAGTTTCTTGGC**-cacagttagcatcaaagtggac-3'	Antisense
C	5'-**GCCAAGAAACTGAACGACGCTCAGGCGCCGAAGAGTGAT**-gacatcaagatgaccagtct-3'	Sense
D	5'-TATAT**GGATCC**-<u>*CTATTA*</u>-*ATGGTGATG*-tgaggagactgtgagagtggt-3'	Antisense

Lower case sequence, gene sequence (A and B, human pancreatic ribonuclease, panc; C and D, single chain antibody against the human transferrin receptor, sFv); uppercase letters, clamp for later restriction enzyme digest; bold uppercase letters, restriction enzyme sites [*Xba*I (Primer A) and *Bam*HI (Primer D)]; italicized letters, modified cloning vector sequence; underlined uppercase letters, ATG start site; underlined italicized letters, two stop signals; underlined bold uppercase letters, spacer sequence (amino acid residues 48–60 of fragment B of staphylococcal protein A (**35**); italicized bold uppercase letters, histidine residues for affinity purification via Ni^{2+}-NTA agarose.

4. Appropriate restriction enzymes.
5. PCR thermocycler and reagents for performing PCR; GeneAmp PCR Reagent Kit (PE Biosystems, Foster City, CA).
6. Agarose and NuSieve 3:1 Agarose (Biowhittaker Molecular Applications, Rockland, ME) and appropriate gel electrophoresis apparatus.
7. GeneClean II (QBIOgene, Carlsbad, CA).
8. Rapid DNA ligation Kit (Roche Molecular Biochemicals, Indianapolis, IN).
9. DNA isolation kits: Wizard Plus Minipreps DNA Purification System (Promega, Madison, WI), Qiagen Plasmid Maxi Kit (Qiagen, Chatsworth, CA).
10. Competent bacteria for generating plasmid DNA: Any host that lacks the T7 RNA polymerase gene such as XL1-Blue , JM109 or HB101 (Stratagene, La Jolla, CA).
11. Luria broth (LB) and LB/ampicillin plates (100 μg/mL) prepared as described in **ref. *31***.
12. Ampicillin, 100 mg/mL in H_2O (Sigma, St. Louis, MO).

2.2. Analysis of Protein Expression

1. Competent bacteria for generating protein: BL21(DE3) (Novagen, Madison, WI) has been specifically engineered for the expression of toxic proteins. For extremely toxic proteins, BL21(DE3)pLysS or pLysE have been engineered.
2. Rifampicin, 20 mg/mL in methanol (Sigma, St. Louis, MO).
3. Isopropyl-β-ᴅ-thiogalactopyranoside (IPTG), 0.5 *M* in H_2O (Life Technologies, Inc., Grand Island, NY).
4. Sodium dodecyl (SDS)-polyacrylamide gels, 4–20% (Invitrogen, Carlsbad, CA) or equivalent.
5. Gel electrophoresis apparatus for running protein gels.

2.3. Purification of the Recombinant
RNase Fusion Protein from E. coli *Bacteria*

1. Terrific Broth (TB) prepared as described in *(31)*, add 4 mL of 100 mg/mL ampicillin.
2. Ampicillin, 100 mg/mL in H_2O.
3. Bacterial shaker, temperature 37°C.
4. Sucrose buffer #1 (ice-cold): 30 m*M* Tris-HCl, pH 7.5, containing 20% sucrose and 1 m*M* EDTA.
5. Sucrose buffer #2: 20 m*M* Tris-HCl, pH 7.5, containing 10% sucrose, 0.2 *M* NaCl and 10 m*M* $MgCl_2$.
6. Ice-cold H_2O.
7. Tris-EDTA buffer (TE): 50 m*M* Tris-HCl, pH 7.5, containing 20 m*M* EDTA.
8. Janke & Kunkel (Janke & Kunkel, GMBH, KG Staufen, West Germany) polytron tissuemizer or similar model equipped with a 100 mm long × 10 mm OD shaft.
9. Lysozyme (Sigma) 5 mg/mL in H_2O, prepare just before use.
10. 5 *M* NaCl: 292.2 g/L.
11. Triton X-100 (Sigma), 25% solution in H_2O, use low heat to solubilize.
12. Dithioerythritol (DTE) (Sigma).
13. 2-Mercaptoethanol (Sigma).
14. Dithothreitol (DTT) (Sigma).
15. BCA protein assay reagent (Pierce Chemical Co., Rockford, IL) or equivalent.
16. Solubilization buffer 1: 0.1 *M* Tris-HCl, pH 8.0, containing 6 *M* guanidine-HCl (573.2 g/L), and 2 m*M* EDTA.
17. Solubilization buffer 2: 0.1 *M* Tris-HCl, pH 8.0, containing 6 *M* guanidine-HCl (573.2 g/L).

18. Renaturation buffer 1 prechilled to 10°C: 0.1 M Tris-HCl, pH 8.0, containing 0.5 M L-arginine-HCl (105 g/L, Sigma), 4 mM oxidized glutathione (GSSG, 4.9 g/L, Roche Molecular Biochemicals, Indianapolis, IN), and 2 mM EDTA.

19. Renaturation buffer 2: 20 mM Tris-HCl, pH 8.0, containing 1.66 mM oxidized glutathione, and 50% glycerol.

20. Dialysis buffer (10X): 0.2 M Tris-HCl, pH 7.5, containing 1 M urea (60 g/L). Do not prepare more than 2–3 h in advance because cyanate ions form which can carbamylate amino groups. Dilute to 1X just before use.

21. 60 L Vat for dialysis equipped with a lower valve for easy emptying. The vat should contain a large stir bar, and sit on a large magnetic stirrer at 4°C.

22. DNase DN-25 (Sigma).

23. RNase A, Type II-A (Sigma).

24. Sonicator (Heat Systems Ultrasonics, Inc., Farmingdale, NY) or equivalent.

25. TAPS-sulfonate (Wako Chemicals USA, Inc., Richmond, VA).

26. Polyethleneimine, low molecular weight (Aldrich, Milwaukee, WI).

27. 10% Acetic acid.

28. Chromatography buffer A: 20 mM Tris-HCl, pH 7.5, containing 10% glycerol. All buffers that contain the RNase-sFv after the first chromatography column contain 10% glycerol to prevent the precipitation of the protein over time.

29. Chromatography buffer B: buffer A containing 0.5 M NaCl.

30. Chromatography buffer C: buffer A containing 1.0 M NaCl.

31. Chromatography buffer with varying imidazole: buffer A containing the following concentrations of imidazole; 40, 50, 60, 100, 200, 300, 400, and 500 mM.

32. Chromatography columns: CM-Sephadex C-50 (for angiogenin, pancreatic RNase, amphibian RNase fusion proteins), heparin Sepharose (for EDN fusion proteins) (both resins from Amersham Pharmacia Biotech, Inc., Piscataway, NJ), Ni^{2+}-NTA agarose (Qiagen).

33. FPLC system (optional) consisting of program controller, two pumps, a mixer, seven port M-7 valve, assorted sample loops, UV monitor, fraction collector, and appropriate columns such as cationic exchanger (Mono S HR 5/5) or anionic exchanger (Mono Q HR 5/5) (Amersham Pharmacia Biotech).

34. Millipore Millex-HV filters (Millipore Corporation, Bedford, MA).

2.4. Characterization of the Binding of the RNase-sFv

1. Ice-cold phosphate-buffered saline (PBS).

2. Ice-cold 1% bovine serum albumin (BSA) in PBS. (A squirt bottle containing this solution is very convenient.)

3. Unlabeled and [^{125}I] labeled antibody (*see* **ref. 32** for a discussion of the different methods of iodination).

4. Cells containing the appropriate antibody binding site.

5. Suction apparatus.

6. Gamma counter.

2.5. Characterization of Ribonuclease Activity of the RNase Fusion Protein

1. Disposable sterile 1.5 mL screw cap tubes and pipet tips.

2. Deionized H$_2$O autoclaved for 30 min (RNase-free H$_2$O).

3. tRNA (Sigma) in RNase-free H$_2$O.

4. Human serum albumin (HSA) (Sigma). HSA is a very good diluent for RNases and RNase fusion proteins. RNases maintain full activity even at very low concentrations *(33)*.
5. RNase assay buffer: for pH 7.5 or 8.0, 0.5 *M* Tris-HCl, pH 7.5 or 8.0, containing 5 m*M* EDTA and 0.5 mg/mL HSA; for pH 6.0, 30 m*M* MES, pH 6.0, containing 0.5 mg/mL HSA.
6. Dilution buffer, 0.5 mg/mL HSA in RNase-free H_2O.
7. Ice-cold perchloric acid, 3.4% (2.4 mL 70% perchloric acid diluted to 50 mL with H_2O).
8. H_2O bath or incubator at 37°C.
9. UV absorbance spectrophotometer.

2.6. Characterization of In Vitro Activity of the RNase Fusion Protein

1. 96-Well microtiter plates (Corning Inc., Corning, NY) or equivalent plates.
2. Serum- and leucine-free RPMI (Life Technologies, Inc., Grand Island, NY).
3. [^{14}C] leucine, 0.1 mCi in 10 µL phosphate-buffered saline (PBS) (NEN Life Science Products, Inc., Boston, MA) or WST-1 (Roche).
4. Glass-fiber filters (Brandel Inc., Gaithersburg, MD) (only if [^{14}C] leucine is used).
5. PHD cell harvester (Cambridge Technology Inc., Watertown, MA) (only if [^{14}C] leucine is used) or a microtiter plate reader (MR4000: Dynex Technologies, Chantilly, VA) or equivalent for WST-1 assay.
6. Scintillation fluid (only if [^{14}C] leucine is used).

2.7. Characterization of Toxicity of the RNase Fusion Protein In Vivo

1. Outbred male and female mice, 3/group, 6–8 wk of age, approx 20 g weight. Animal care procedures should be in accordance with standards described in the National Institutes of Health Guide for Care and Use of Laboratory Animals.
2. Dulbecco's phosphate-buffered saline (DPBS) or equivalent (Life Technologies).
3. 1 mL Syringes and 25-gauge needles.
4. Scale to weigh animals.

2.8. Characterization of the In Vivo Activity of the RNase Fusion Protein

1. Nude female mice, 8–10 wk old, approx 20 g weight (mice should be within a 5 g range), 8–10 animals/group. Use only one sex since the development of the tumor as well as the response to drug can vary between the sexes due to hormonal differences *(34)*.
2. Anti-asialo GM-1 (rabbit) (ASGM-1) (Wako Pure Chemical Industires, Ltd., Richmond VA). Prepare 1:20 dilution in H_2O.
3. Tumor cells.
4. Trypan blue stain, 0.4% (Life Technologies).
5. DPBS or equivalent (Life Technologies).
6. 1 mL Syringes and 25-gauge needles.
7. 1X Trypsin-EDTA (Life Technologies).
8. Falcon sterile cell strainer, 100-µm nylon (Becton Dickinson Labware, Franklin Lakes, NJ).
9. Mark I [^{137}]Cesium Irradiator (JL Shepherd and Associates, Glendale CA).
10. Fixatives; 10% formalin solution (Fisher Scientific, Pittsburgh, PA), Bouin's fixative solution (Ricca Chemical Co., Arlington, TX).

3. Methods

3.1. Construction of the RNase Fusion Gene

1. Determine the orientation of the RNase with respect to the cell targeting agent, i.e., should the cell targeting agent be attached to the 5' or 3' end of the RNase gene (*see* **Note 2**). The following protocol will describe the construction of an RNase-sFv fusion protein in which the RNase is fused at the C-terminus to the N-terminus of an sFv gene. Any differences in construction of the RNase fusion gene where the cell targeting agent is not an sFv will be described in the **Notes**.

2. Design four oligonucleotide primers to incorporate the following features into the RNase fusion protein (*see* **Table 1**):

   a. an appropriate enzyme restriction site at the 5' end of the RNase gene for insertion into the vector. Before designing this primer and the primer described in (d) below, analyze the DNA encoding the RNase and sFv for naturally occuring restriction enzyme sites contained within the genes. The use of two different restriction enzymes for cloning will facilitate the directional insertion of the gene into the vector. This primer will be in the sense direction (*see* **Table 1**, primer A).

   b. a spacer onto the 3' end of the RNase gene to separate the RNase and sFv genes. Amino acid residues 48–60 of fragment B of staphylococcal protein A *(35)* have been used successfully to separate the RNase and sFv *(16,19)*. RNase-sFv fusion proteins lacking such a spacer have lower enzymatic, receptor binding, and cytotoxic activities *(19)*. This primer will be in the antisense direction (*see* **Table 1**, primer B) (*see* **Note 3**).

   c. the same spacer described in b) above onto the 5' end of the sFv gene. This primer will be in the sense direction (*see* **Table 1**, primer C).

   d. residues for affinity purification (if not included in the vector), the termination signal and the appropriate restriction enzyme site at the 3' end of the sFv gene. This primer will be in the antisense direction (*see* **Table 1**, primer D).

3. Perform two separate PCR reactions in which the RNase gene is modified with primers A and B (PCR reaction 1) and the sFv gene is modified with primers C and D (PCR reaction 2) (*see* **Fig. 1**). Each reaction should contain the following for 100 µL: Final concentration: 10 mM Tris-HCl, pH 8.3, 50 mM KCl, 1.5 mM MgCl$_2$; 100 µM of each nucleotide; 0.5 µL AmpliTaq DNA polymerase to be added after the hot start; 0.5 µM primer A or C; 0.5 µM primer B or D; 500 ng/mL DNA.

   Program the PCR thermocycler as follows: 94°C, 5 min hot start before beginning the program; 94°C, 1 min (denaturation); 55°C, 2 min (annealing); 72°C, 2 min (extension); 20 cycles. Keep the number of cycles to a minimum to minimize the amplification of a PCR error. High concentrations of template DNA will also help minimize PCR error.

4. Analyze 10 µL of each reaction to determine the size of the product. Use NuSieve 3:1 agarose for PCR reaction 1 and a 1% agarose gel for PCR reaction 2. DNA <500 bp give faint bands on 1% agarose gels while NuSieve 3:1 agarose is capable of resolving DNA 30–1000 bp in length.

5. Purify the PCR product with GeneClean II following the manufacturer's instructions to remove primers and other components of the PCR reaction. Extract the resin with15 µL sterile H$_2$O.

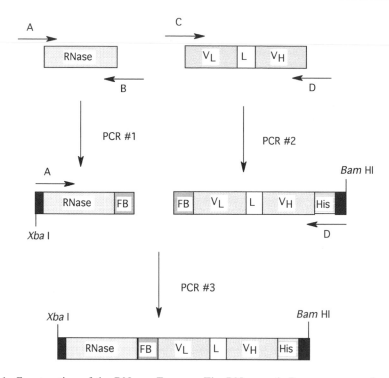

Fig. 1. Construction of the RNase-sFv gene. The RNase and sFv genes are each modified separately (PCR 1 and PCR 2) to contain restriction enzyme sites (*Xba*I and *Bam*HI) appropriate for cloning into the pET-11d vector (primers A and D for the 5' end of the RNase gene and 3' end of the sFv gene, respectively, *see* **Table 1**). In addition, Primer D encodes a His tag. Complementary sequences encoding the FB fragment of staphylococcal protein A is attached to the 3' end of the RNase gene (primer B) and the 5' end of the sFv gene (primer C). This allows the two genes to be spliced together using the technique of splicing by overlap extension *(24)*. After PCR, the two genes are purified as described in the text, mixed, and subjected to PCR #3 using primers A and D. The assembled gene is then cloned into the vector. V_L, light-chain variable region; V_H, heavy-chain variable region; L, peptide linker (GGGGS)$_3$; FB, fragment B of staphylococcal protein A (AKKLNDAQAPKSD) *(35)*.

6. The two genes now share a region of identical sequence (the spacer sequence or FB region) and can be spliced together using the technique of splicing by overlap extension *(24)* (*see* **Fig. 1**, PCR 3). The FB gene sequence will hybridize together allowing the two genes to be spliced together. Perform the PCR reaction as described above using 1–2 µL (50–100 ng) of each of the purified DNA from PCR 1 and PCR 2 as the DNA source and primers A (5' primer of the RNase gene) and D (3' primer of the sFv gene) (*see* **Notes 4** and **5**).

7. Repeat **steps 4** and **5** above using a 1% agarose gel for the analysis of the PCR reaction.

8. Restrict 7.5 µL of the isolated DNA from PCR 3 (approx 500 ng DNA) and 0.5 µg of the vector with the appropriate restriction enzymes. Adjust the final volume of the reaction to 100 µL with sterile H_2O and incubate at 37°C overnight.

9. Purify the restricted DNA and vector as described in **step 5**.
10. Ligate the two restricted DNAs (3 µL RNase-sFv [approx 100 ng] and 0.5 µL vector [15 ng]) together using the Rapid DNA Ligation Kit according to manufacturer's instructions. If the ligation reaction fails or if cloning into a single site, dephosphorylate the vector using calf intestinal phosphatase (CIP) (*see* **Note 6**).
11. Transform XL1-Blue competent bacteria with 1–2 µL (approx 5–10 ng) of the ligated DNA according to manufacturer's instructions. Streak 100 µL of the reaction mixture onto an LB/ampicillin plate and incubate overnight at 37°C (*see* **Note 7**).
12. Add 5 mL LB/ampicillin to each of 6 tubes. Inoculate each tube with a single colony picked from the overnight plate, and incubate overnight at 37°C with shaking (225 rpm). Place the plate containing the remaining colonies at 4°C for reuse if necessary.
13. Before beginning the mini prep procedure, streak a fresh LB/ampicillin plate with each of the overnight cultures (one plate can be divided into six sections, each section streaked with one overnight culture). This plate will serve as a record of the miniprep DNA and can be used to generate more DNA. Place this plate overnight at 37°C to allow growth of the colonies. The next day, seal the plate with parafilm to prevent drying out and store at 4°C. Isolate the plasmids containing the DNA inserts using the Wizard Plus Minipreps DNA Purification System or similar product following the manufacturer's instructions.
14. Restrict the miniprep DNA with the appropriate restriction enzymes and identify those clones containing an insert of the correct size by running the digests on 1% agarose gels. Occasionally the ligation reaction will result in destruction of a restriction enzyme site, thus if repeated ligation and transformation of a good PCR product fails to yield an insert, other restriction enzymes should be tried (*see* **Note 8**).

3.2. Analysis of Protein Expression

1. Transform BL21(DE3) competent bacteria with the plasmids that contained an insert of the appropriate size following the manufacturer's instructions (*see* **Note 9**).
2. Streak the reaction onto LB/ampicillin plates and incubate overnight at 37°C.
3. Place 1 colony from each transformation into 5 mL LB/ampicillin and incubate with shaking at 225 rpm at 37°C until the OD 600 nm reaches 0.5–0.6.
4. Remove 2.5 mL from each tube and place into a fresh tube. Each plasmid is now contained in two tubes. To one tube add 0.4 mM IPTG (final concentration). Add nothing to the second tube as this tube will serve as the uninduced control. Continue the incubation of all tubes for 30 min at 37°C with shaking.
5. Add 25 µL rifampicin (200 µg/mL final concentration) to all tubes and continue incubation for an additional 90 min (*see* **Note 10**).
6. Remove 100 µL from each tube, centrifuge, and aspirate the supernatant. Add 25 µL protein denaturing dye, resuspend the pellet, boil the samples for 5 min, and analyze the samples on a 4–20 % SDS polyacrylamide gel placing the uninduced and induced samples side by side for direct comparison.
7. Sequence the clone of interest to ensure that no PCR errors occurred.

3.3. Purification of the Recombinant RNase Fusion Protein from E. coli Bacteria

Three different methods for the isolation and folding of the crude RNase fusion protein from inclusion bodies are presented. The first method folds the fusion protein from purified inclusion bodies in which the fusion protein is the major protein present in the inclusion body, whereas the other two methods fold the fusion protein from an impure inclusion body preparation. The first method is more laborious than the other two, but active RNase fusion proteins are always obtained. The second method often results in proteolytic degradation of the fusion protein by contaminating bacterial proteases during the folding step. In addition, contaminating nucleic acids can inhibit the folding of the fusion protein reducing the final yield *(26)*. In the third method the inclusion body preparation is treated with TAPS-sulfonate in the denatured state before refolding *(27–30)*. TAPS-sulfonate reacts with cysteine residues forming mixed-disulfide bond products changing the net cationic charge of the protein. The positively charged TAPS-sulfonate modified RNase fusion proteins are soluble under acidic conditions in the absence of denaturant. Thus, dialysis of the TAPS-sulfonate treated inclusion body preparation against 10% acetic acid results in precipitation of most of the bacterial protein contaminants. The TAPS-sulfonate groups are then removed from the fusion protein by reduction with 2-mercaptoethanol and the fusion protein is refolded using a two step refolding procedure. All remaining purification steps are the same for the three different methods.

1. Transform competent bacteria [BL21(DE3)] with the vector containing the RNase fusion protein following the manufacturer's instructions.
2. Streak the reaction onto an LB/ampicillin plate and incubate overnight at 37°C.
3. Remove one colony from the overnight plate and resuspend it in 25 mL LB containing 400 µg/mL ampicillin. Remove 25 µL of the newly resuspended colony and place this into 25 mL fresh LB containing 400 µg/mL ampicillin. Grow the diluted suspension culture overnight at 37°C with shaking at 225 rpm.
4. The next morning place 5 mL of the overnight culture per liter of TB containing 400 µg/mL ampicillin and grow at 37°C with shaking at 225 rpm until the OD_{600nm} reaches 1.6–1.8. Since TB is an enriched medium, the OD_{600nm} should be >1.0. Induce with 0.5 mM IPTG for approx 2–4 h. The length of induction time should be optimized for each construct.
5. Centrifuge the bacteria at 4°C for 10–20 min at 7000 rpm (8000g). The bacteria can be frozen at –20°C until ready to be processed. Freezing times greater than 1 wk as well as frost-free freezers should be avoided. Follow **steps 6–18** from one of the folding methods listed below.

3.3.1. Method 1:
Folding the RNase-Fusion Protein from Purified Inclusion Bodies

Follow **steps 1–5** in **Subheading 3.3.**

6. Resuspend the pellet with ice-cold sucrose buffer. Use 200 mL sucrose buffer #1/L original bacterial culture. After 10 min incubation on ice, centrifuge the bacterial solution at 7000 rpm (8000g) for 20 min at 4°C.
7. Carefully pour off the supernatant and resuspend the pellet with ice-cold H_2O. Use 200 mL H_2O /L original bacterial culture. Place 25 mL bacterial solution into each of 8 polypropylene tubes, incubate on ice for 20 min, and centrifuge for 20 min at 4°C at 12,000 rpm (17,000g). Pour off supernatant. The pellet may be frozen at –70°C if not ready to process further.
8. Add 9 mL TE buffer to each tube and using a Janke & Kunkel polytron tissuemizer (or similar model) resuspend the pellet. Combine 2 tubes together such that each L of origi-

nal bacterial culture is now contained in four tubes. Allow the tubes to stand at room temperature for 30 min.

9. Add lysozyme (0.9 mL of 5 mg/mL) to each tube from **step 8** to a final concentration of 240 µg/mL. Continue incubation at room temperature for 60 min shaking the tubes occasionally.

10. Add 2.5 mL of both 5 *M* NaCl and 25% Triton X-100 to each tube. Continue incubation for 30 min again shaking occasionally.

11. Using the tissuemizer, homogenize the samples just before centrifugation at 12,000 rpm (17,000*g*) for 40 min at 4°C. The solution is very viscous and homogenization helps to produce a firmer pellet after centrifugation.

12. Pour off the supernatant carefully, add 15 mL TE, and resuspend the pellet using the tissuemizer. Centrifuge for 30 min as described in **step 11**. Repeat the washing steps 3 more times decreasing the centrifugation time to 20 min for the last two washes. The washed inclusion body may now be stored at –70°C until ready for solubilization. At this stage the RNase fusion protein should be the major protein found in the purified inclusion bodies.

13. Using the tissuemizer, resuspend the washed inclusion bodies in 10–20 mL solubilization buffer #1 and incubate for ≥2 h at room temperature. The solution should be free flowing and not too viscous. The final protein concentration will be adjusted to 8 mg/mL (*see* **step 15**).

14. Centrifuge 12,000 rpm (17,000*g*) for 20 min at 4°C. The supernatant can be stored at –70°C until ready for renaturation.

15. Determine the protein concentration of a 1:10 dilution of the supernatant. Use solubilization buffer #1 to make the dilution to avoid precipitation of the protein. Solubilization buffer affects the protein determination, thus should be included in the standard curve. Use the BCA protein assay reagent kit or similar protein determination kit following the manufacturer's instructions. Adjust the protein concentration to 8 mg/mL with solubilization buffer 1. Add dry DTE to a final concentration of 0.3 *M* and incubate at room temperature for ≥2 h. The final concentration of protein in the renaturation buffer affects the yield of the protein and should be determined for each fusion protein. We find that a final concentration of 80 µg/mL in the renaturation buffer works well for many RNase fusion proteins.

16. Renature the protein by diluting it 100-fold into renaturation buffer #1 that has been prechilled to 10°C. Add the denatured protein as a steady stream to the middle of the vortex of rapidly stirring renaturation buffer. Incubate for 2–3 d at 10°C. The DTE to GSSG ratio has been optimized to give a redox system of oxidized and reduced glutathione *(36)*. To maintain the proper redox system, the protein must be diluted exactly 100-fold. Temperature affects the yield of protein, therefore the buffer should be prechilled to 10°C before the addition of the protein. Precipitation due to aggregation and incorrect folding will occur during this step. The proper length of refolding time should be determined for each RNase fusion protein.

17. Dialyze the refolded protein against 10 volumes of dialysis buffer at 4°C with at least two changes over a 24-h period to decrease the L-arginine concentration. A large loss of protein may occur at this step due to improper folding and aggregation. The urea helps limit the precipitation *(36)*.

18. Centrifuge the dialyzed solution for 20 min at 4°C at 7000 rpm (8000*g*). Use care in decanting the supernatant as the pellet does not adhere tightly to the walls of the centrifuge cup. Proceed to **step 19**.

3.3.2. Method 2:
Folding the RNase-Fusion Protein from Crude Inclusion Bodies

Follow **steps 1–5** above in **Subheading 3.3.** with the following exception: freeze the bacterial pellet at –70°C until ready to be processed. The method described below is for 1 L of original bacterial culture.

6. Thaw the pellet at 37°C and with a tissuemizer, resuspend the pellet in 40 mL of sucrose buffer 2.
7. Freeze the solution at –70°C followed by thawing at 37°C.
8. Place 20 mL of solution per 50 mL tube, place on ice, and sonicate for 3 min.
9. Add 5 µg/mL each of DNase and RNase A and incubate for 15 min at 37°C.
10. Add Triton X-100 to a final concentration of 0.5%.
11. Centrifuge 5000 rpm (3800g) for 15 min at 4°C.
12. Using the tissuemizer, resuspend the pellet in 40 mL 0.5% Triton X-100 containing 0.2 M NaCl and 10 mM EDTA.
13. Repeat **step 11**.
14. Using the sonicator, resuspend the pellet in 10–20 mL of solubilization buffer 2. Add 2-mercaptoethanol to a final concentration of 30 mM and incubate for 60 min at 37°C.
15. Rapidly dilute the solubilized protein mixture into 6 vol of renaturation buffer 2 and incubate on ice for 60 min.
16. Rapidly dilute the mixture from **step 15** such that the final protein concentration is less than 150 µg/mL (determined as described in **Subheading 3.3.1.**, **step 15**). Adjust the buffer components to (final concentration) 20 mM Tris-HCl, pH 8.0, 0.4 M guanidine-HCl, 2 mM 2-mercaptoethanol, 0.66 mM oxidized glutathione, and 30% glycerol and incubate overnight at 4°C.
17. Remove the precipitate by centrifugation.
18. Dialyze the supernatant against 10 vol of H$_2$O before proceeding to **step 19**.

3.3.3. Method 3:
Modification of the Crude Inclusion Body Preparation
with TAPS-Sulfonate, Followed by Partial Purification
and Folding of the RNase Fusion Protein

Follow **steps 1–13** described in **Subheading 3.3.2.**

14. Using the sonicator, resuspend the pellet in 10–20 mL solubilization buffer #2. Add dry DTT to a final concentration of 50 mM and incubate for 60 min at 37°C.
15. Add TAPS-sulfonate to a final concentration of 150 mM and incubate at 37°C for 60 min. After the addition of excess TAPS-sulfonate, all –SH groups in DTT and in the protein react to form TAPS$_n$-SS-protein or TAPS$_2$-SS-DTT.
16. Add 50 µL polyethleneimine. The polyethleneimine will interfere with the electrostatic interaction between anionic materials such as nucleic acids and the TAPS-modified proteins and thus decrease precipitation.
17. Dialyze the TAPS-modified solution against 10% acetic acid for 12 h at 4°C to precipitate most of the bacterial proteins, which are anionic under acidic conditions. Because the TAPS-modified RNase fusion proteins are cationic at low pH due to the net charge of the RNase (very basic proteins with pIs in excess of 9.0), these proteins will remain in solution. Continue the dialysis for an additional day but now dialyze against H$_2$O, changing the H$_2$O frequently (approx 100 vol). Centrifuge at 16,000 rpm (30,000g) for 20 min. The

TAPS-modified fusion protein is usually >90% pure at this step and because the soluble fraction does not contain nucleic acids, the amount of protein recovered can be estimated by UV absorption. Determine protein concentration assuming $E_{1\%} = 10.0$.

18. Add an equal volume of 6 M guanidine-HCl, 0.1 M Tris-HCl, pH 8.0. Add 2-mercaptoethanol to a final concentration of 30 mM. Incubate for 15 min at 37°C. Follow **steps 15–18** in **Subheading 3.3.2.** For this method protein concentration was determined by absorbance (*see* **step 17**).

19. Apply the centrifuged refolded protein to a CM-Sephadex C-50 column (4 mL resin per 160 mg protein determined in **step 15** in **Subheading 3.3.1.** or 3 mL resin for protein folded using the methods described in **Subheadings 3.3.2.** or **3.3.3.** Whenever possible CM-Sephadex C-50 should be the first column of choice as the majority of bacterial contaminating proteins will not adhere to the strongly cationic exchanger resin. RNases such as angiogenin, pancreatic RNase A and amphibian RNases are basic proteins and thus adhere to this resin. For the human eosinophil RNase, EDN, heparin-Sepharose is the appropriate first column. Perform this step at 4°C.

20. Wash the column with 2 column volumes of chromatography buffer A.

21. Strip elute the column with 2–4 column volumes of chromatography buffer B followed by 1 column volume of chromatogaphy buffer C. The majority of RNase fusion protein will be contained in the buffer B eluate. If the fusion protein contains a histidine tag, proceed to **step 22**. If there is no tag proceed to **step 25**.

22. If the protein contains a histidine tag, add imidizole and Triton X-100 to a final concentration of 0.8 mM and 1%, respectively. Add 0.6 mL Ni^{2+}-NTA agarose (for 320 mg of refolded protein determined in **step 15**, **Subheading 3.3.1.** or 0.2 mL resin for protein folded according to **Subheading 3.3.2.** or **3.3.3.** The low level of imidazole and the Triton X-100 reduce the binding of impurities to the resin. Keep the amount of resin used as low as possible to reduce the nonspecific binding of other proteins to the column and to maximize the final concentration of fusion protein (*see* **Note 11**).

23. Rotate the slurry (Ni^{2+}-NTA agarose and sample) end over end for several hours or overnight at 4°C before collecting it as a column.

24. Wash the column with 10 mL 20 mM Tris-HCl, pH 7.5, containing 10% glycerol and 0.8 mM imidazole. Step elute the column with 1 column volume each of the same buffer made 40, 50, 60 ,100, 200, 300, 400, and 500 mM imidazole (*see* **Note 12**). Proceed to **step 27**.

25. If no histidine tag is present, dialyze the sample against chromatography buffer A.

26. Apply the centrifuged sample (10 min at 3000 rpm) to either a Mono S HR 5/5 column or Mono Q HR 5/5 column equilibrated with chromatography buffer A. Elute the sample with a 30-min gradient between 0 and 80% chromatography buffer C with a final 10-min hold on 80% chromatography buffer C. This step should be performed on an analytical scale first to determine which column (Mono S or Mono Q HR 5/5) and elution conditions are most suitable for the final purification of the fusion protein. The conditions described here work for many different RNase fusion proteins. If contaminants are present after chromatography, dialyze the sample as described in **step 25** and reapply to the same column adjusting the chromatograpy conditions so that the gradient is more shallow in the area in which the protein elutes. Often there are different isomers of the same protein due to the refolding process. These can be visualized and separated by FPLC or HPLC.

27. Analyze the fractions by SDS-polyacrylamide gel electrophoresis and pool the appropriate fractions.

28. Store the purified pooled RNase fusion protein at 4°C. Avoid freezing to prevent aggregation of the sample. Samples should be stored in the presence of 10% glycerol and 0.1 M NaCl or imidazole to prevent precipitation. Samples can be filter sterilized without loss of protein with a Millipore Millex-HV filter. Other filters such as Millex-GV low protein binding filters have been tried and have resulted in large losses of protein concentration.

3.4. Characterization of the Binding of the RNase-sFv

1. For binding to adherent cells, the cells are plated 1 d prior to the assay into a 24-well plate. The cells should be approx 80% confluent on the day of assay. Wash the cells twice with ice cold PBS to remove dead cells or nonadherent cells that might interfere with the assay. Add 500 μL 1% BSA/PBS to each well. For binding to nonadherent cells, centrifuge the cells, wash twice with ice-cold PBS, resuspend in 1% BSA/PBS to a concentration of 8×10^5 cells/mL. Add 250 μL of the cell suspension to 1.5 mL Eppendorf tubes. Keep the cells cold to prevent or slow down the rate of internalization of cell surface receptors.
2. Apply 10 μL of varying concentrations of intact IgG antibody, the RNase-sFv, or buffer (control to determine the maximum amount of binding of labeled antibody) to the appropriate wells or tubes. A preincubation of 15–30 min may be incorporated to help a weaker binding monovalent sFv bind to the receptor before the addition of the intact bivalent-labeled antibody. Bivalent antibodies or antibody fragments usually bind with higher affinities than monovalent Fab or sFv fragments (37).
3. Apply 10 μL [^{125}I] labeled antibody to the cells (5000–10,000 cpm per reaction) and incubate the plate or tubes for 2 h on ice.
4. Wash the cells three times with ice cold 1% BSA/PBS using an aspirator to carefully remove the washes without disturbing the cells.
5. Add 0.1 N NaOH to the cells and incubate 30 min at 37°C. Determine the radioactivity of the lysed cells using a gamma counter.
6. Determine the % maximal binding as follows:

$$\frac{\text{cpm of reaction containing cold antibody or fusion protein}}{\text{cpm of reaction containing labeled antibody alone}} \times 100$$

Plot the % maximal binding on the Y-axis vs the concentration of cold antibody or fusion protein on the X-axis and calculate the EC_{50}, the amount of RNase fusion protein or unlabeled intact IgG antibody required to displace 50% of the [^{125}I] labeled antibody from the cells.

3.5. Characterization of Ribonuclease Activity of the RNase Fusion Protein

1. Determine the pH at which ribonuclease activity is optimal as follows (note that gloves must be worn to avoid contamination of the assay with RNases found on hands): Add 100 μL of each of the following solutions to numbered sterile disposable 1.5 mL screw cap tubes contained on ice: tRNA (stock concentration, 1.0 mg/mL), HSA (stock concentration 0.5 mg/mL), buffer at pH 6.0, 7.5, or 8.0 (*see* **Subheading 2.5.**, **step 5**).
2. Add 10 μL dilution buffer, RNase, or RNase fusion protein to the appropriate tubes (*see* **Note 13**).
3. Initiate the reaction by placing all tubes at 37°C and incubating for the appropriate length of time. The incubation time varies with the RNase. Some example incubation times for

nonfused RNases are: EDN and pancreatic RNase, 15 min; angiogenin, 18 h; onconase, 2 h. The incubation time of the fused RNases may need to be adjusted due to a decrease in ribonuclease activity.

4. Terminate the assay by placing the tubes on ice, adding 700 µL 3.4% ice-cold perchloric acid and incubating for 10 min.

5. Centrifuge the tubes for 10 min in an Eppendorf centrifuge (or equivalent centrifuge) at full speed. Read the absorbance of the supernatant at 260 nm. Average the replicate tubes, subtract the blank (those tubes containing dilution buffer only), and choose the pH at which the enzymatic activity was the highest for further characterization of the RNase fusion protein.

6. Determine the K_m (the substrate concentration at which the reaction velocity is half maximal) and the catalytic constants as follows (*see* **Note 14**): Add 100 µL of each solution to the appropriately labeled reaction tubes: tRNA (stock concentration to be varied from 0.25–10 mg/mL), HSA (stock concentration 0.5 mg/mL), buffer at which the enzymatic activity was optimal (*see* **step 5** above).

7. Follow **steps 2–5** described above.

8. Plot the data in a Lineweaver-Burk graph as follows: plot the reciprocal of the substrate, 1/s, on the *x*-axis; plot the reciprocal of the enzymatic activity, $1/v_o$ (the absorbance at 260 nm for each substrate concentration with the appropriate blank value subtracted), on the *Y*-axis. The intercept of the line on the *Y*-axis is 1/Vmax. The intercept of the line on the *X*-axis is $-1/K_m$. Convert K_m from mg/mL to a molar value using the M_r for tRNA of 28,100 *(38)* and V_{max} from absorbance to a molar value by dividing the absorbance at 260 nm by 7×10^5. Use the equation $K_{cat} (E_o) = V_{max}/t$ where E_o is the molar concentration of the enzyme used and t is the incubation time in seconds to calculate the K_{cat} (catalytic constant or turnover number). The final units are s^{-1}. The efficiency of the enzyme is K_{cat}/K_m, (an indicator of catalytic efficiency). The units are $M^{-1}s^{-1}$.

3.6. Characterization of In Vitro Activity of the RNase Fusion Protein

1. Using the media in which the cells are normally grown, plate 2500 (adherent) or 10,000 (nonadherent) cells in a final volume of 0.1 mL per well of a 96-well microtiter plate one day before treatment.

2. On the day of treatment, prepare sterile (*see* **Subheading 3.3.**, **step 28**) dilution curves of the nonfused RNase and RNase fusion protein in sterile dilution buffer (*see* **Note 13**). Include the buffer in which the RNase is stored as some cells are sensitive to glycerol and imidazole. Apply 10 µL to the appropriate well (test each sample at least in triplicate).

3. Incubate the plates for 3 d in a humidified CO_2 incubator.

4. To determine cell viability, use WST-1 and follow the manufacturer's instructions. To determine protein synthesis inhibition, replace the serum-containing media with serum- and leucine-free RPMI, add 10 µL $[^{14}C]$ leucine (0.1 mCi), and incubate for an additional 2–4 h at 37°C. Harvest the cells onto glass fiber filters using a PHD cell harvester, wash with H_2O, dry with ethanol, and count the filters in a scintillation counter.

5. Average the triplicate determinations and express the results as % of buffer-treated cells calculated as follows:

$$\frac{\text{cpm (or absorbance for WST-1) of sample-treated cells}}{\text{cpm (or absorbance for WST-1) of buffer-treated cells}} \times 100$$

Plot % of control (protein synthesis or cell viability) on the *Y*-axis vs sample concentration on the *X*-axis. Determine the IC_{50}, the concentration of sample that inhibits protein synthesis or cell viability by 50% from the plot.

3.7. Characterization of Toxicity of the RNase Fusion Protein In Vivo

1. Inject mice i.p. or i.v. with multiple concentrations (in 0.2 mL volume for i.v. injection and 0.4 mL for i.p. injection) of sterile RNase fusion protein, the RNase alone, or the buffer control. Use DPBS as the diluent. Inject the RNase fusion protein at the highest concentration achievable. Continue the injections for a total of five consecutive days.
2. Monitor the weight of the animals daily, and look for signs of toxicity, such as coat ruffling, and changes in gait. Death is the final endpoint. Continue monitoring the animals until the animals regain any weight loss that occurred during the injection period.
3. If no toxicity is observed, increase the number of injections per day (*see* **Note 15**).
4. Report the data as LD_{50} (mg test substance/kg body weight of animal or mg test substance administered/day) that caused death in 50% of the animals.

3.8. Characterization of the In Vivo Activity of the RNase Fusion Protein

3.8.1. Model 1: Survival

1. Two days before the injection of cells, inject (i.v.) 0.2 mL ASGM-1.
2. The next day, irradiate the animals with 200 rads for 0.9 s. Immunosuppression promotes survival of many types of human tumor cells in the nude mouse *(39)*.
3. The following day, prepare the cells as follows (for the best results the cells should be in log phase of growth):
   a. Remove the media from ten flasks and rinse each flask twice with DPBS.
   b. Apply 1X trypsin-EDTA solution (7 mL per 150 cm^2 flask) taking care to coat the flask evenly. Remove 5 mL.
   c. Allow the flask to sit 30 s before tapping the flask to dislodge the cells.
   d. Add 10 mL media to the first flask, resuspend the cells, add this solution to the next flask, resuspend the cells and continue until the cells of 10 flasks are resuspended in the same solution. Repeat this procedure for each set of 10 flasks.
   e. Adjust the volume with media to 50 mL for each set of 10 flasks.
   f. After centrifuging the cells for 5 min at 2300 rpm, resuspend all the cells in a final volume of 40 mL DPBS.
   g. Repeat **step f**.
   h. Centrifuge as described in **step f** and resuspend the cells in a final volume of 10 mL DPBS.
   i. Pour the cells through a cell strainer and count viable cells using the trypan blue exclusion assay following the manufacturer's instructions.
   j. Adjust the cell number with DPBS for a 0.2 mL injection volume.
4. Begin treatment 3–10 d after the injection of cells. Inject (i.v.) the RNase fusion protein, antibody alone, RNase alone, the combination of antibody and RNase, and the vehicle in a volume of 0.2 mL (*see* **Note 16**).
5. Treat the animals twice weekly for 3 wk (*see* **Note 17**).
6. Either death or the number of tumor foci in a target organ can be the final endpoint. To determine tumor foci, terminate the experiment at a designated time, fix the tissue of interest in 10% formalin or Bouin's fixative, and count the number of tumor nodules present in the tissue.

3.8.2. Model 2: Flank Model

1. Follow **step 3** in **Subheading 3.8.1.** for cell preparation.
2. Inject the cells subcutaneously into the flank of the mouse.
3. Begin treatment when the tumor diameter reaches 0.5–1.0 cm. The best route of injection is intravenous.
4. Monitor tumor growth using in situ caliper measurements to determine tumor volume, using the following equation $TV = 1/2LW^2$ where TV = tumor volume, L = length, and W = perpendicular diameter.

4. Notes
4.1. Construction of the RNase Fusion Gene

1. The pET vector system was specifically designed for the expression of toxic proteins *(25)*. There are a variety of pET vectors available containing different peptide tags for affinity purification and for use in detection of the fusion protein by Western analysis. If desired these tags can be removed after purification with proteases following the manufacturer's instructions.
2. The last three amino acid residues of the C-terminal region of the human serum RNase, angiogenin, are involved in an active center subsite *(40)*. Attachment of an sFv to the C-terminus of angiogenin resulted in loss of enzymatic activity *(19,22)*. Conversely, the N-terminal pyroglutamic acid folds back into the active site center of the amphibian RNase, onconase *(41)*. Expression of onconase with a methionine as the first residue resulted in a severe loss of RNase and cytotoxic activity *(42,43)*.
3. If a spacer is not required to separate the RNase from the cell targeting agent such as has been observed for RNase-growth factor fusion proteins *(17,18,21,* and unpublished observations), the primer described in (b) should contain the last 21 bp of the RNase gene and the first 21 bp of the cell targeting agent and be in the antisense direction for (b) and the sense direction for (c).
4. For those fusion proteins lacking a spacer, each half of the fusion protein now contains 21 bp of complementary sequence of the other half of the fusion protein and thus the technique of splicing by overlap extension can be used as described in **Subheading 3.1., step 6**.
5. Splicing by overlap extension is a simple method of fusing two genes together that eliminates the need for compatible restriction enzyme sites. It also eliminates one ligation reaction. The most common reason for PCR 3 not to work is a mistake in the primer sequence or in the design of the primers. If there is no product in the PCR 3 reaction and the design of the primers are found to be correct, check the yield of DNA to determine if losses occurred during the DNA purification procedure. If the yield of product from the PCR 3 reaction is low, try adding 5–10 µL of DMSO to the PCR reaction as DMSO oftentimes can increase the yield of the PCR product.
6. The procedure for dephosphorylating the restricted vector is as follows: after restricting overnight, 2 µL calf intestinal phosphatase (Roche, 1 U/µL) is added and incubation is continued for 15 min at 37°C. The phosphatase is inactivated by a 10 min incubation at 65°C. The restricted and dephosphorylated vector is then purified as described in **Subheading 3.1., step 5**.
7. Any host lacking the T7 RNA polymerase gene (for example; XL1-Blue, JM109, HB101) is suitable for the generation of plasmid DNA. Note that the amount of bacteria used in the transformation can be scaled down to 10 µL per reaction with the proper adjustment of the other components of the reaction. If no colonies result, the amount of DNA should

be adjusted before deciding that the ligation did not work. Lack of colonies can result from too much as well as too little DNA.

8. The presence of a positive clone can also be determined by PCR as follows: pick a colony with a sterile tip, touch the tip to a fresh LB/ampicillin plate to have a record of the plasmid, rinse the tip containing the colony in 50 μL sterile water, vortex, and boil the water containing the colony for 5 min. After centrifuging the boiled sample for 5 min in an eppifuge, perform the PCR reaction as described in **Subheading 3.1., step 3**, with the following modifcations; decrease the final reaction volume to 50 μL, use 10 μL of the boiled colony mixture as the DNA source, and increase the cycle number to 35. Analyze 10 μL of the PCR reaction on a 1% agarose gel.

4.2. Analysis of Protein Expression

9. Before beginning large scale production of the RNase-sFv protein, it is necessary to do a pilot protein expression because not all plasmids with an insert of the correct size will express a protein of the appropriate molecular weight. PCR error can result in a mutation encoding a termination signal or the insertion or deletion of a bp, resulting in a truncated or nonsense protein product.

10. Rifampicin inhibits protein expression in some bacteria by forming a stable complex with bacterial RNA polymerases *(44)* thus allowing the expressed protein to be visualized with reduced interference from bacterial proteins. Studies by Studier et al. *(25)* demonstrate that BL21 bacteria are sensitive to rifampicin.

4.3. Purification of the Recombinant RNase Fusion Protein from E. coli Bacteria

11. Some RNase fusion proteins - not all - can be concentrated by using a very small DEAE or CM-Sephadex C-50 column (0.2 mL) and strip eluting with multiple one column volume aliquots of chromatography buffer B. This involves dialysis or dilution before application to the column, which usually leads to loss of sample due to precipitation. Other methods such as Centricon cartridges, Diaflo ultrafiltration (Amicon) with a YM3 membrane or simply packing the sample in a dialysis bag and surrounding it with dry G100 resin have been tried and proven unsuccessful.

12. For some RNase-sFv fusion proteins, a protein of appropriate molecular weight elutes in the 40–60 m*M* imidazole range. This species is discarded because of the other impurities present.

4.4. Characterization of Ribonuclease Activity of the RNase Fusion Protein

13. The dilution buffer (0.5 mg/mL HSA) is a good diluent for RNases and RNase fusion proteins. RNases diluted with this buffer maintain full enzymatic activity at very low concentrations and low blank values are obtained in the presence of HSA. Keep the enzyme in the linear range of the assay and do not limit the substrate (50–100 times the enzyme concentration). All buffer components should be included in the standards to control for buffer effects.

14. A preliminary assay should be performed to determine an approximate K_m. Perform the assay using a wide range of substrate concentrations. Choose five different substrate concentrations spanning 0.5–5.0 times the approximate K_m. Prepare buffer blanks (dilution buffer and no enzyme) for each substrate concentration as the blank values will be different for each substrate concentration.

4.5. Characterization of Toxicity of the RNase Fusion Protein In Vivo

15. Mice can tolerate 300–500 mg/kg anti-CD22 antibody RNase conjugates without serious toxicity (*23* and unpublished observations). To achieve these concentrations, the anti-CD22 antibody RNase conjugates were administered as 300–500 μg injections in 0.4 mL i.p. injections, four times per day for five consecutive days. Weight loss occurred during the injection period, but was reversed upon cessation of treatment.

4.6. Characterization of the In Vivo Activity of the RNase Fusion Protein

16. The antibody is included as a control because of possible anti-tumor effects due to the antibody alone (*45–47*) while the combination of antibody and RNase is included to demonstrate that the activity observed is due to the covalent coupling between the RNase and antibody and not to an additive or synergistic effect between the two proteins.
17. Different dosing schedules should be tried. For the first evaluation, the RNase fusion protein can be administered 24 h after the injection of cells. If activity is observed, treatment can be tried at later times after tumor cell injection (3, 5, or 7 d later). In some experiments treatment is daily for five consecutive days.

Acknowledgments

This project has been funded in whole or in part with federal funds from the National Cancer Institute, National Institutes of Health, under Contract No. NO1-CO-56000. The content of this publication does not necessarily reflect the views or policies of the Department of Health and Human Services, nor does mention of trade names, commercial products, or organizations imply endorsement by the US government. The publisher or recipient acknowledges right of the US government to retain a nonexclusive, royalty-free license in and to any copyright covering the article.

References

1. Vitetta, E. S., Thorpe, P. E., and Uhr, J. W. (1993) Immunotoxins: magic bullets or misguided missiles. *TiPS* **14,** 148–154.
2. Pastan, I. (1997) Targeted therapy of cancer with recombinant immunotoxins. *Biochim. Biophys. Acta* **1333,** C1–C6.
3. Sawler, D. L., Bartholomew, R. M., Smith, L. M., and Dillman, R. (1985) Human immune response to multiple injections of murine monoclonal IgG. *J. Immunol.* **135,** 1530–1535.
4. Schroff, R. W., Foon, K. A., Beatty, S. M., Oldham, R., and Morgan, A. (1985) Human anti-murine immunoglobulin response in patients receiving monoclonal antibody therapy. *Cancer Res.* **45,** 879–885.
5. Harkonen, S., Stoudemire, J., Mischak, R., Spitler, L., Lopez, H., and Scannon, P. (1987) Toxicity and immunogenicity of monoclonal antimelanoma antibody-ricin A chain immunotoxins in rats. *Cancer Res.* **47,** 1377–1385.
6. Rybak, S. M. and Youle, R. J. (1991) Clinical use of immunotoxins: monoclonal antibodies conjugated to protein toxins. *Immunol. Allergy Clin. N. Am.* **11,** 359–380.
7. Soler-Rodriguez, A. M., Ghetie, M.-A., Oppenheimer-Marks, N., Uhr, J. W., and Vitetta, E. S. (1993) Ricin A-chain and ricin A-chain immunotoxins rapidly damage human endothelial cells: Implications for vascular leak syndrome. *Exp. Cell Res.* **206,** 227–234.
8. Thrush, G. R., Lark, L. R., Clinchy, B. C., and Vitetta, E. S. (1996) Immunotoxins: An Update. *Ann. Rev. Immunol.* **14,** 49–71.

9. Khazaeli, M. B., Conry, R. M., and LoBuglio, A. F. (1994) Human immune response to monoclonal antibodies. *J. Immunother.* **15,** 42–52.

10. Stephens, S., Emtage, S., Vetterlein, O., Chaplin, L., Bebbington, C., Nesbitt, A., et al. (1995) Comprehensive pharmacokinetics of a humanized antibody and analysis of residual anti-idiotypic responses. *Immunology* **85,** 668–674.

11. Rybak, S. M. and Newton, D. L. (1999) Immunoenzymes, in *Antibody Fusion Proteins* (Chamow, S. M. and Ashkenazi, A., eds.), John Wiley & Sons, New York, NY, pp. 53–110.

12. Rybak, S. M., Saxena, S. K., Ackerman, E. J., and Youle, R. J. (1991) Cytotoxic potential of ribonuclease and ribonuclease hybrid proteins. *J. Biol. Chem.* **266,** 21,202–21,207.

13. Newton, D. L., Ilercil, O., Laske, D. W., Oldfield, E., Rybak, S. M., and Youle, R. J. (1992) Cytotoxic ribonuclease chimeras: Targeted tumoricidal activity *in vitro* and *in vivo*. *J. Biol. Chem.* **267,** 19,572–19,578.

14. Jinno, H., Ueda, M., Ozawa, S., Kikuchi, K., Ikeda, T., Enomoto, K., and Kitajima, M. (1996) Epidermal growth factor receptor-dependent cytotoxic effect by an EGF-ribonuclease conjugate on human cancer cell lines: a trial for less immunogenic chimeric toxin. *Can. Chemother. Pharmacol.* **38,** 303–308.

15. Newton, D. L., Nicholls, P. J., Rybak, S. M., and Youle, R. J. (1994) Expression and characterization of recombinant human eosinophil-derived neurotoxin and eosinophil-derived neurotoxin-anti-transferrin receptor sFv. *J. Biol. Chem.* **269,** 26,739–26,745.

16. Zewe, M., Rybak, S. M., Dubel, S., Coy, J. F., Welschof, M., Newton, D. L., and Little, M. (1997) Cloning and cytotoxicity of a human pancreatic RNase immunofusion. *Immunotechnology* **3,** 127–136.

17. Psarras, K., Ueda, M., Yamamura, T., Ozawa, S., Kitajima, M., Aiso, S., et al. (1998) Human pancreatic RNase1-human epidermal growth factor fusion: an entirely human immunotoxin analog with cytotoxic properties against squamous cell carcinomas. *Prot. Eng.* **11,** 1285–1292.

18. Yoon, J. M., Han, S. H., Kown, O. B., Kim, S. H., Park, M. H., and Kim, B. K. (1999) Cloning and cytotoxicity of fusion proteins of EGF and angiogenin. *Life Sci.* **64,** 1435–1445.

19. Newton, D. L., Xue, Y., Olson, K. A., Fett, J. W., and Rybak, S. M. (1996) Angiogenin single-chain immunofusions: Influence of peptide linkers and spacers between fusion protein domains. *Biochemistry* **35,** 545–553.

20. Rybak, S. M., Hoogenboom, H. R., Meade, H. M., Raus, J. C., Schwartz, D., and Youle, R. J. (1992) Humanization of immuntoxins. *Proc. Natl. Acad. Sci. USA* **89,** 3165–3169.

21. Futami, J., Seno, M., Ueda, M., Tada, H., and Yamada, H. (1999) Inhibition of cell growth by a fused protein of human ribonuclease 1 and human basic fibroblast growth factor. *Prot. Eng.* **12,** 1013–1019.

22. Newton, D. L., Pollock, D., DiTullio, P., Echelard, Y., Harvey, M., Wilburn, B., et al. (2000) Functional properties of human ribonuclease fusion proteins expressed in *Escherichia coli* or transgenic mice. *J. Int. Soc. Tumor Targ.* **1,** 70–81.

23. Newton, D. L., Hansen, H. J., Mikulski, S. M., Goldenberg, D. M., and Rybak, S. M. (2001) Potent and specific antitumor effects of an anti-CD22 targeted cytotoxic ribonuclease: potential for the treatment of non-Hodgkin's lymphoma. *Blood* **97,** 528–535.

24. Horton, R. M., Cai, Z. L., Ho, S. N., and Pease, L. R. (1990) Gene splicing by overlap exension: tailor made genes using the polymerase chain reaction. *BioTechniques* **8,** 528–535.

25. Studier, F. W., Rosenberg, A. H., Dunn, J. J., and Dubendorff, J. W. (1990) Use of T RNA polymerase to direct expression of cloned genes. *Methods Enzymol.* **185**, 60–89.

26. Futami, J., Tsushima, Y., Tada, H., Seno, M., and Yamada, H. (2000) Convenient and efficient *in vitro* folding of disulfide-containing globular protein from crude bacterial inclusion bodies. *J. Biochem (Tokyo)* **127**, 435–441.

27. Seno, M., DeSantis, M., Kannan, S., Bianco, C., Tada, H., Kim, N., et al. (1998) Purification and characterization of a recombinant human cripto-1 protein. *Growth Factors* **15**, 215–229.

28. Inoue, M., Akimaru, J., Nishikawa, T., Seki, N., and Yamada, H. (1998) A new derivatizing agent, trimethylammoniopropyl methanethiosulphonate, is efficient for preparation of recombinant brain-derived neurotrophic factor from inclusion bodies. *Biotechnol. Appl. Biochem.* **28**, 207–213.

29. Terzyan, S. S., Peracaula, R., de Llorens, R., Tsushima, Y., Yamada, H., Seno, M., et al. (1999) The three-dimensional structure of human RNase 4, unliganded and complexed with d(Up), reveals the basis for its uridine selectivity. *J. Mol. Biol.* **285**, 205–214.

30. Mallorqui-Fernandez, G., Pous, J., Peracaula, R., Aymami, J., Maeda, T., Tada, H., et al. (2000) Three-dimensional crystal structure of human eosinophil cationic protein (RNase 3) at 1.75 A resolution. *J. Mol. Biol.* **300**, 1297–1307.

31. Sambrook, J., Fritsch E. F., and Maniatis, T. (1989) *Molecular Cloning: A Laboratory Manual.* Cold Spring Harbor Laboratory Press, Cold Spring Harbor, NY.

32. Harlow, E. and Lane, D. (1988) *Antibodies: A Laboratory Manual.* Cold Spring Harbor Laboratory Press, Cold Spring Harbor, NY.

33. Bond, M. D. (1988) An in vitro binding assay for angiogenin using placental ribonuclease inhibitor. *Anal. Biochem.* **173**, 166–173.

34. Gart, J., Krewski, D., Lee, P., Tarone, R., and Wahrendorf, J. (1986) *Statistical Methods in Cancer Research.* International Agency for Research on Cancer, NY.

35. Tai, M. S., Mudgett-Hunter, M., Levinson, D., Wu, G.-M., Haber, E., Oppermann H., and Huston, J. S. (1990) A bifunctional fusion protein containing Fc-binding fragment B of staphylococcal protein A amino terminal to antidigoxin single-chain Fv. *Biochemistry* **29**, 8024–8030.

36. Buchner, J., Pastan, I., and Brinkmann, U. (1992) A method for increasing the yield of properly folded recombinant fusion proteins: Single-chain immunotoxins from renaturation of bacterial inclusion bodies. *Anal. Biochem.* **205**, 263–270.

37. Crothers, D. M. and Metzger, H. (1972) The influence of polyvalency on the binding properties of antibodies. *Immunochem.* **9**, 341–357.

38. Rosenberg, H. F. and Dyer, K. D. (1995) Eosinophil cationic protein and eosinophil-derived neurotoxin. Evolution of novel function in a primate ribonuclease gene family. *J. Biol. Chem.* **270**, 21,539–21,544.

39. Giovanella, B. C., Stehlin, J. S., Shepard, R. C., and Williams, L. J. (1979) Hyperthermic treatment of human tumors heterotransplanted in nude mice. *Cancer Res.* **39**, 2236–2241.

40. Russo, N., Nobile, V., DiDonato, A., Riordan, J. F., and Valee, B. L. (1996) The C-terminal region of human angiogenin has a dual role in enzymatic activity. *Proc. Natl. Acad. Sci. USA* **93**, 3243–3247.

41. Mosimann, S. C., Ardelt, W., and James, M. N. G. (1994) Refined 1.7 A X-ray crystallographic structure of P-30 protein, an amphibian ribonuclease with anti-tumor activity. *J. Mol. Biol.* **236**, 1141–1153.

42. Boix, E., Wu, Y., Vasandani, V. M., Saxena, S. K., Ardelt, W., Ladner, J., and Youle, R. J. (1996) Role of the N terminus in RNase A homologues: Differences in catalytic activity, ribonuclease inhibitor interaction and cytotoxicity. *J. Mol. Biol.* **257,** 992–1007.

43. Newton, D. L., Xue, Y., Boque, L., Wlodawer, A., Kung, H. F., and Rybak, S. M. (1997) Expression and characterization of a cytotoxic human-frog chimeric ribonuclease: Potential for cancer therapy. *Protein Eng.* **10,** 463–470.

44. Wehrli, W., Knusel, F., Schmid, K., and Staehelin, M. (1968) Interaction of rifamycin with bacterial RNA polymerase. *Proc. Natl. Acad. Sci. USA* **61,** 667–673.

45. Goldenberg, D. M., Horowitz, J. A., Sharkey, R. M., Hall, T. C., Murthy, S., Goldenberg, H., et al. (1991) Targeting, dosimetry, and radioimmunotherapy of B-cell lymphomas with iodine-131-labeled LL2 monoclonal antibody. *J. Clin. Oncol.* **9,** 548–564.

46. Ghetie, M. A. J., Richardson, J., Tucker, T., Jones, D., Uhr, J. W., and Vitetta, E. S. (1991) Antitumor activity of Fab' and IgG-anti-CD22 immunotoxins in disseminated human B lymphoma grown in mice with severe combined immunodeficiency disease effect on tumor cells in extranodal sites. *Cancer Res.* **51,** 5876–5880.

47. Kreitman, R. J., Hansen, H. J., Jones, A. L., FitzGerald, D. J. P., Goldenberg, D. M., and Pastan, I. (1993) Pseudomonas Exotoxin-based immunotoxins containing the antibody LL2 or LL2-Fab' induce regression of subcutaneous human B-cell lymphoma in mice. *Cancer Res.* **53,** 819–825.

18

Bispecific Diabodies for Cancer Therapy

Michaela Arndt and Jürgen Krauss

1. Introduction

Natural killer (NK) cells represent a potent subset of lymphocytes for targeting and lysing tumor cells. In contrast to T lymphocytes, they do not need to be preactivated in vitro because they constitutively express cytolytic functions against a number of different targets (*1,2*). Their inherent cytolytic activity can be stimulated via the FcγIIIA receptor (CD16), which is expressed on the surface of NK cells, macrophages, and activated monocytes (*3,4*). Bispecific antibodies binding to both CD16 and a tumor-associated antigen are therefore of great interest as potential reagents for cancer immunotherapy.

To target NK cells against Hodgkin's disease (HD), a mouse hybrid hybridoma bispecific monoclonal antibody (MAb) was constructed with specificities for CD16 and CD30 (*5*). CD30 is expressed on virtually all Hodgkin and Reed-Sternberg cells and on only a small proportion of activated lymphocytes in normal tissue (*6*). The antibody was able to induce the specific lysis of CD30+ tumor cells in vitro. Administration of the bispecific antibody in a severe combined immunodeficiency (SCID) mouse model resulted in the complete remission of subcutaneously established tumors after one single injection (*5*). More recently, the bispecific monoclonal antibody (biMAb) was used to treat patients with refractory HD in Phase I/II clinical trials with promising results (*7–9*). However, human anti-mouse Ig antibodies were found in most patients and some patients developed an allergic reaction after attempted retreatment.

In addition to the problem of immunogenicity, hybrid hybridoma biMAbs are extremely difficult to isolate as a homogenous molecule from the large number of molecules generated by the random associations of the various light and heavy chains. We therefore constructed an anti-CD30/anti-CD16 bispecific diabody comprising only the variable domains of the hybrid hybridoma. A diabody consists of two fusion proteins comprising the V_H domain of one antibody connected by a short linker to the V_L domain of another antibody. Both fusion proteins associate noncovalently in the periplasm of the bacteria to a bispecific diabody (*10–13*) (*see*

From: *Methods in Molecular Biology, vol. 207: Recombinant Antibodies for Cancer Therapy: Methods and Protocols*
Edited by: M. Welschof and J. Krauss © Humana Press Inc., Totowa, NJ

Fig. 1B). Their relatively small size is expected to enable a better penetration of tumor tissue compared to the murine monoclonal equivalent. Crystallographic studies have shown that the two antigen-binding domains of diabodies are located on opposite sides of the complex, thus capable of binding two cells *(14)*.

In this chapter we describe the construction and production of a bispecific diabody followed by its characterization in vitro and in vivo. The protocol will describe: (1) the generation of a bispecific diabody from hybridoma cell lines by polymerase chain reaction (PCR), (2) the purification of the expressed soluble protein in the periplasm of *E. coli*, (3) its in vitro characterization by flow cytometry and its capability to mediate the specific killing of tumor cells using the JAM-test assay *(15)*, (4) its in vivo administration in SCID mice bearing xenografted tumors.

2. Materials

2.1. Cloning Procedures

1. Total RNA isolation: RNeasy Midi Kit (Qiagen, Valencia, CA).
2. Poly A+ mRNA isolation from total RNA: Oligotex mRNA Kit (Qiagen).
3. First-strand cDNA synthesis: Reverse Transcriptases Omniscript™ or Sensiscript™ (Qiagen).
4. Thermal Cycler PTC 150-16 (MJ Research Inc., Waltham, MA).
5. Primer for amplification of the light chain and the heavy chain, respectively (*see* **Table 1**).
6. Vectors used for the cloning and expression of scFvs and diabody (*see* **Fig. 1A,B**).
7. *Vent* DNA polymerase (New England Biolabs Inc., Beverly, MA) or *Expand™ High Fidelity* DNA polymerase (Roche Diagnostics Corp., Indianapolis, IN).
8. 10X Thermopol buffer (New England Biolabs) for *Vent* polymerase or 10X Expand HiFi buffer (Roche) for *Expand™ High Fidelity* polymerase.
9. 100 mM dNTPs (New England Biolabs).
10. Sterile deonized water.
11. Molecular weight marker: 100 bp DNA ladder, Lambda DNA-BstEII Digest (New England Biolabs).
12. QIAquick Gel Extraction Kit (Qiagen).
13. QIAquick-spin PCR purification kit (Qiagen).
14. Restriction endonucleases with 10X restriction enzyme buffers: *Nco*I, *Hin*dIII, *Eco*RV, *Not*I, *Bam*HI, *Bgl*II, *Xba*I (New England Biolabs).
15. Calf Intestinal Phosphatase (CIP) (Roche).
16. T4 DNA Ligase with 10X ligation buffer (includes ATP) (Roche).
17. 3 M Sodium acetate, pH 5.3.
18. Ethanol absolute.
19. Glycogen MB grade (20 mg/mL) (Roche).
20. 80% (v/v) Ethanol.
21. SOC medium (Life Technologies, Rockville, MD).
22. Table-top microcentrifuge.
23. Forward sequencing primer: Dp1-5'ATTAAAGAGGAGAAATTAACCA3'; backward sequencing primer: Dp2-5'TATTGATGCCTCAAGCTAGC3' (*see* **Note 1**).

Table 1
Oligonucleotides for the Amplification of Immunoglobulin Variable Regions of Mouse and Rat[a]

Primer Name	Sequence	Restriction sites	Reference
κ chain variable domain			
Bi6	5'- GGTG<u>ATATC</u>GTGAT(A/G)AC(C/A)CA(G/A)GATGAACTCTC	EcoRV	Duebel et al. 1994
Bi7	5'- GGTG<u>ATATC</u>(A/T)TG(A/C)TGACCCAA(A/T)CTCCACTCTC	EcoRV	Duebel et al. 1994
Bi8	5'- GGTG<u>ATATC</u>GT(G/T)CTCAC(C/T)CA(G/A)TCTCCAGCAAT	EcoRV	Duebel et al. 1994
κ chain constant domain			
Bi5	5'- GGGAAGATG<u>GGATCC</u>AGTTTGGTGCAGCATCAGC	BamHI	Duebel et al. 1994
λ chain variable domain			
Kr1	5' AGAGA<u>CGCGT</u>ACAGGCTGTTGTGACTCAGG	MluI	Arndt et al. 1999
λ chain constant domain			
Kr2	5'GACTG<u>CGGCCGC</u>AGACTTGGGCTGGCC	NotI	Arndt et al. 1999
Heavy chain variable domain			
Bi3	5'- GAGGTGAAGC<u>TGCAG</u>GAGTCAGGACCTAGCCTGGTG	PstI	Duebel et al 1994
Bi3b	5'- AGGT(C/G)(A/C)AA<u>CTGCAG</u>(C/G)AGTC(A/T)GG	PstI	Duebel et al. 1994
Bi3c	5'- AGGT(C/G)(A/C)AG<u>CTGCAG</u>(C/G)AGTC(A/T)GG	PstI	Duebel et al. 1994
Bi3f	5'- CAGCCGGC<u>CATGG</u>CGCAGGT(C/G)<u>CAGCTGCAG</u>(C/G)AG	NcoI, PvuII, PstI	Unpublished
γ chain constant domain			
Bi4	5'- CCAGGGGCCAGTGGATAGACA<u>AGCTT</u>GGGTGTCGTTTT	HindIII	Duebel et al. 1994

[a]Restriction sites are underlined.

A

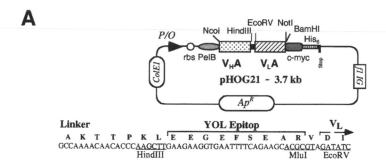

Linker | YOL Epitop | V_L
A K T T P K L E E G E F S E A R V D I
GCCAAAACAACACCC**AAGCTT**GAAGAAGGTGAATTTTCAGAAGC**ACGCGT**AG**ATATC**
.................................HindIII..MluI.......EcoRV

B

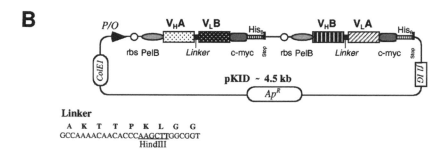

Linker
A K T T P K L G G
GCCAAAACAACACCC**AAGCTT**GGCGGT
.................................HindIII

C

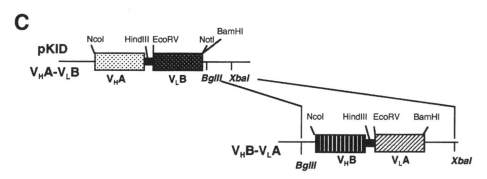

Fig. 1. Schematic representation of the scFv encoding plasmid pHOG21 (**A**), the bispecific diabody encoding plasmid pKID (**B**) and the assembly of the diabody expression plasmid (**C**). Restriction sites used for the cloning of variable domains are indicated. Ap^R denotes the ampicillin resistance gene; rbs, the sequence of ribosome-binding site; pelB the leader peptide sequence of bacterial pectate lyase from *Erwinia carotovora*; c-myc, a sequence encoding an epitope recognized by the MAb 9E10; His₆, a sequence encoding for hexahistidine residues and Stop the stop codons. Nucleotide sequences of linkers connecting variable domains are shown.

2.2. Bacterial Large Scale Production of Diabody (see Note 2)

1. *E. coli* XL1-Blue electrocompetent cells (Stratagene, La Jolla, CA).
2. Incubator Shaker (Infors GmbH, Eisenbach, Germany).
3. Sorvall centrifuge RC-5C PLUS with a set of fixed-angle rotors (SS-34, SLA-1500, SLA-3000) (Kendro Laboratory Products, Newtown, CT) or comparable centrifuge.
4. 2YT medium: 270 mM NaCl, 1% Yeast Extract, 0.5% Tryptone, pH 7.0 (*see* **Note 3**).
5. Stock solution of 2 M glucose.
6. 2YT$_{GA}$: 2YT medium containing 100 mg/L ampicillin and 100 mM glucose.
7. Sucrose powder.
8. 2YT$_{SA}$: Dissolve 274 g sucrose powder in 2 L 2YT containing 100 mg/L ampicillin to obtain a final concentration of sucrose of 0.4 M.
9. Isopropyl-β-D-thiogalactopyranoside (IPTG): 1 M stock solution stored at –20°C.

2.3. Isolation and Purification of Diabody
from Bacterial Periplasma and Culture Supernatant

1. Magnetic stirrer.
2. PPP-Solution: 50 mM Tris-HCl, 20% Sucrose, 1 mM EDTA, pH 8.0 (*see* **Note 4**).
3. 5 M Stock solution of Imidazole, filtered, store at 4°C.
4. Ammonium sulfate powder.
5. Buffers (*see* **Note 5**):
   P1: 1 M NaCl, 50 mM Tris-HCl, pH 7.0; 4°C
   P2: 1 M NaCl, 50 mM Tris-HCl, 50 mM Imidazole, pH 7.0; 4°C
   P3: 1 M NaCl, 50 mM Tris-HCl, 250 mM Imidazole, pH 7.0; 4°C.
6. SPECTRA/POR Dialysis Membrane No.4, MWCO 12,000 to 14,000 Dalton (Spectrum Laboratories Inc., Rancho Dominguez, CA) (*see* **Note 6**).
7. C16/20 column (Amersham Pharmacia Biotech Inc., Piscataway, NJ).
8. Fraction collector (Amersham Pharmacia Biotech).
9. Chelating Sepharose, Fast flow (Amersham Pharmacia Biotech).
10. 1 M Stock solution of CuSO$_4$.
11. Phosphate-buffered saline (PBS), pH 7.4.
12. PBSI: PBS containing 50 mM Imidazole, pH 7.4. Filter and store at 4°C.
13. Biomax-10 Ultrafree-15 Centrifugal Filter Device (Millipore, San Jose, CA).
14. Bio-Rad Protein Assay Kit (Bio-Rad, Life Science Research, Hercules, CA).

2.4. In Vitro Assays for Diabody Characterization

2.4.1. Isolation of Granulocytes from Whole Blood of a Human Donor

1. Polysucrose solution with density of 1.077, e.g., Histopaque® 1077 (Sigma-Aldrich Corp., St. Louis, MO).
2. Polysucrose solution with density of 1.119, e.g., Histopaque® 1119 (Sigma-Aldrich).
3. PBS.
4. Centrifuge with swinging bucket rotor.
5. 50 mL Centrifuge tubes.
6. Serologic pipets 10 mL and 25 mL (Sarstedt Inc., Newton, NC).
7. Microscope.
8. EDTA- or Heparin-coated syringes.
9. Human whole blood from donor.

2.4.2. Flow Cytometry

1. Flow Cytometer FACScan (Becton-Dickinson, Mountain View, CA).
2. FACS buffer: PBS, 2% fetal bovine serum (FBS), 0.1% sodium azide.
3. 96-Well tissue culture dish, round or V bottomed (Nalgene Nunc International, Rochester, NY).
4. Anti-c-myc antibody 9E10 (Abcam Ltd, Cambridge, UK).
5. Goat anti-mouse IgG FITC-labeled (Life Technologies).
6. Propidium iodide (Sigma-Aldrich).

2.4.3. Cytotoxicity Assay

1. $CD30^+$ tumor cells: L540CY *(16)*.
2. RPMI-1640 Medium (Sigma-Aldrich).
3. Penicillin-Streptomycin solution (Life Technologies).
4. L-Glutamine 200 mM (Life Technologies).
5. Fetal bovine serum (FBS), heat inactivated.
6. RPMI complete medium (RPMI-CM): RPMI, 10% FBS, 2 mM glutamine, 100 U penicillin, 100 µg/mL streptomycin.
7. Peripheral blood lymphocytes (PBL).
8. Ficoll/Hypaque (Amersham Pharmacia Biotech).
9. PBS-F: PBS containing 5% FBS.
10. Tissue culture flasks, 75 cm² (Nalgene Nunc International).
11. 96-Well tissue culture dish, round bottomed (Nalgene Nunc International).
12. Cell Harvester, Betaplate (Amersham Pharmacia Biotech).
13. Liquid Scintillation Beta Counter (LKB-Wallac, Turku, Finland).
14. Glassfiber filtermats (Perkin-Elmer Wallac GmbH, Freiburg, Germany).
15. HiSafe liquid scintillation cocktail (Perkin-Elmer Wallac GmbH).

2.5. In Vivo Analysis of Diabody

2.5.1. Enzyme-Linked Immunosorbent Assay (ELISA)
for Testing SCID Mice of Functional Lymphocyte Deficiency

1. 96-Well flat-bottom ELISA microplates (Nalgene Nunc International).
2. Rabbit anti-mouse immunglobulins (Jackson Immuno Research Laboratories Inc., West Grove, PA).
3. PBS-T: PBS, 0.05% Tween-20.
4. PBA-B: PBS, 1% BSA.
5. PBS-TB: PBS, 0.05% Tween-20/1% BSA.
6. 5–10 µL Serum from BALB/c mouse.
7. 5–10 µL Serum from SCID mice.
8. Purified mouse IgG (ICN Pharmaceutics, Frankfurt/Main, Germany).
9. Alkaline phosphatase-goat anti-mouse IgG+A+M(H+L) (ZYMED Laboratories, San Francisco, CA).
10. Diethanolamine buffer: 96.5 mL of 1 M diethanolamine solution, 47 mg $MgCl_2$, 0.1 g sodium azide, adjust pH to 9.8 with 1 N HCl (*see* **Note 7**).
11. PNPP, Paranitrophenylphosphat (Sigma-Aldrich).
12. Substrate solution for one 96-well ELISA plate (*see* **Note 8**): resolve 10 mg PNPP/100 mL diethanolamine buffer.
13. 3 N NaOH.

2.5.2. Xenotransplantation of Tumor Cells to SCID Mice

1. Pathogen-free female mice with severe combined immunodeficiency (SCID C.B-17) (Charles River Laboratories, San Diego, CA).
2. Anti-Asialo-GM1 antibody solution (Wako Chemicals USA, Inc., Richmond, VA).
3. L540CY cells.
4. Syringes (1 mL).
5. 26-Gauge needle.
6. PBS.
7. Caliper rule.

3. Methods
3.1. Construction of Antibody Fragments
3.1.1. Cloning of ScFv's from Mouse Hybridomas

1. Grow hybridoma cells up to 1×10^7 and collect cells in the logarithmic growth phase to obtain the maximum amount of mRNA. Perform the isolation of total RNA followed by preparation of Poly A^+ mRNA according to the manufacturer's protocol.
2. For first strand cDNA synthesis use the Reverse Transcriptases Omniscript™ kit and follow the manufacturer's instruction.
3. Amplify cDNA of the heavy and light chain variable gene segments by PCR using the set of primer combinations described in **Table 1**. Carry out PCR in a total volume of 50 µL, containing 2 µL of cDNA, 0.5 µ*M* of each primer, 200 µ*M* dNTPs, 5 µL 10X PCR reaction buffer and 1 U of DNA polymerase (*see* **Note 9**). Run PCR with the following program: One cycle 5 min at 94°C denaturation, followed by 25–30 cycles 80 s at 94°C, 80 s at 58–52°C (*see* **Note 10**), 2 min at 72°C, and final extension at 72°C for 5 min.
4. Analyze 5 µL of the PCR product by gel electrophoresis using a 1.5% agarose gel. If DNA of correct fragment length can be visualized run a preparative gel to recover DNA. Cut out the specific amplified DNA fragments. Extract the DNA from the gel using a QIAquick gel extraction kit.
5. Digest 5 µg of vector pHOG21 (*see* **Fig. 1A**) with 20–30 U of appropriate restriction endonucleases for 4 h at 37°C. Dephosphorylate the vector by adding 0.5 U calf intestine phosphatase (CIP) to the reaction mixture. After 2 h add another 0.5 U CIP to the restriction digest. Inactivate CIP by adding EDTA, pH 8.0, to a final concentration of 5 m*M* and incubate the sample at 65°C for 20 min. Purify and recover the linearized vector by agarose gel electrophoresis followed by gel extraction.
6. For cloning of the heavy chain and light chain of the variable domains into the bacterial expression vector, digest 250 ng of PCR product from **step 4** with 20 U each of the appropriate restriction endonucleases and incubate for 4 h at 37°C. Purify the digested PCR products using the QIAquick-spin PCR purification kit.
7. Ligate the inserts successively into expression vector using a molar ratio of insert: vector = 3:1. Perform ligation overnight at 16°C in a volume of 10 µL, using 1 U T4 ligase, 1 µL 10X ligation buffer, 50 ng vector DNA, and appropriate amount of insert DNA.
8. Precipitate the ligation reaction mix by adding 2.5 vol ethanol absolute, 1/10 vol 3 *M* sodium acetate and 20 µg glycogen. Incubate for at least 3 h at –20°C and centrifuge the precipitated DNA for 30 min at 10,000*g* and 4°C, wash the pellet three times with 500 µL 80% EtOH, followed by centrifugation for 5 min at 10,000*g* and 4°C. Discard ethanol and let pellet air-dry for 10 min. Dissolve the pellet in 10 µL H_2O.

9. For transformation, pipet 5 μL of the ligation product, 4 μL of electrocompetent *E. coli* cells to a fresh 1.5 mL tube and add H_2O to a final volume of 50 μL. Mix gently on ice. Transfer the suspension into a precooled cuvet and perform electroporation at 1700 V, 200 Ω, 25 μF. Add 1 mL SOC medium as quick as possible and transfer suspension into a 15 mL polypropylene tube. Shake suspension for 1 h at 280 rpm at 37°C. Spread 20–50 μL onto 2YT agar plates containing 100 mg/L ampicillin and 2% (w/v) glucose (*see* **Note 11**) and incubate at 37°C overnight.

10. Sequence at least five clones of the scFv. Perform an alignment of the sequences for the light chain and heavy chain, respectively. As a reference, align these sequences to the most homologous entries in the KABAT database (*see* **Note 12**).

3.1.2. Cloning of a Bispecific Diabody Derived from ScFv's

The construction of the vector pKID (**Fig. 1B**), containing a dicistronic operon for cosecretion of soluble fusionproteins V_HA-V_LB and V_HB-V_LA has been described in detail *(17)*. A schematic representation of the cloning steps for the diabody anti-CD16/CD30 is shown in **Fig. 1C**. The diabody gene can be sequenced using Dp1 as forward primer and Dp2 as backward primer. Prepare glycerol stocks and plasmid DNA stocks.

3.2. Expression and Purification of Diabodies

3.2.1. Growth and Induction of Bacteria Culture

1. Inoculate 50 mL of 2YTGA with 10 μL bacteria containing the diabody-expression-plasmid from a glycerol stock and incubate at 37°C overnight (*see* **Note 13**).
2. Prepare 2 L of YT_{GA} and add the over night culture. Divide the 2 L into two 3-L Erlenmeyer flasks and shake (180–220 rpm) at 37°C until $OD_{600} = 0.7$–0.8 (*see* **Note 14**).
3. Harvest bacteria culture by centrifugation at 1500g for 15 min and 20°C (Sorvall rotor SLA-3000).
4. Discard supernatant and resuspend the pellet in 2 L YT_{SA} medium. Add IPTG to a final concentration of 1 mM (*see* **Note 15**) and incubate bacterial culture by shaking at 21°C (*see* **Note 16**) for 15–21 h (*see* **Note 17**).

3.2.2. Isolation of Recombinant Protein from Bacterial Periplasm and Preparation of Supernatant for Ammonium Sulfate Precipitation

1. Harvest induced bacteria culture by centrifugation at 6200g for 15 min and 4°C (Sorvall rotor SLA-3000).
2. Transfer supernatant in fresh centrifuge tubes and centrifuge for 1 h at 30,000g and 4°C (Sorvall rotor SLA-3000). Store the supernatant at 4°C in a 5-L jar for ammonium sulfate precipitation.
3. Resupend (*see* **Note 18**) bacteria pellet in 100 mL ice-cold PPP-solution (1/20 of the original culture volume) and incubate for 1 h on ice by gentle agitation.
4. Centrifuge the cell suspension for 1 h at 4°C at 30,000g (30 mL tubes, Sorvall rotor SS34) and recover supernatant with the soluble periplasmic protein carefully. Pool the soluble periplasmic extract and the supernatant from **step 2**.

3.2.3. Ammonium Sulfate Precipitation

1. For ammonium sulfate precipitation place the 5-L jar, containing the combined periplasmic extract and the supernatant on a magnetic stirrer at 4°C. Add ammonium sulfate powder gradually (!) to a final concentration of 70% of saturation (472 g/L). Stir for 2–3 h (*see* **Note 19**).

2. Collect the protein precipitate by centrifugation for 1 h at 30,000g and 4°C (500 mL tubes, Sorvall rotor SLA-3000).
3. Decant supernatant carefully (*see* **Note 20**) and resuspend (*see* **Note 21**) the protein pellet in 200 mL buffer P1 (1/10 of the initial volume).
4. Dialyze the resuspended protein using previously washed Spectra/Por 4 tubular membrane in a 1 L cylinder. Cut two one meter pieces from the tubular membrane and split the 250 mL protein sample by filling into the two Spectrapor tubes. Dialyze antibody preparation at 4°C for 24 h against buffer P1. Change buffer two times (2× 2 L).

3.2.4. Binding of the His-Tagged Protein to Cu²⁺-Sepharose (see *Note 22*)

1. For Immobilized Metal Affinity Chromatography (IMAC), prepare a Cu^{2+}-sepharose column (*see* **Note 23**): Load column with 1–2 mL of Sepharose per 1 L of bacteria culture. Wash out residual EtOH from the sepharose (*see* **Note 24**) with five bed volumes of distilled water. Charge the sepharose with Cu^{2+} by applying 0.7 bed volume of 0.1 M $CuSO_4$-solution onto the column. Remove unbound Cu^{2+} by washing the Sepharose-column with ten bed volumes of distilled water. Equilibrate the Cu^{2+} charged column with five column volumes of equilibration buffer P1 (4°C) (*see* **Note 25**).
2. Centrifuge the dialyzed protein-sample from **Subheading 3.2.3., step 4** for 1 h at 30,000g and 4°C (250 mL tubes, Sorvall rotor SLA-1500).
3. All following chromatography steps should be carried out at 4°C. Pass the soluble protein over the equilibrated Cu^{2+}-Sepharose column by gravity flow (*see* **Note 26**).
4. Connect the column to an UV unit and read absorbance at 280 nm. Wash column with 100 mL of buffer P1. To remove unspecific bound, host-related proteins from the Cu^{2+}-Sepharose, continuously wash with buffer P2 until the absorbance of the effluent is minimal (about 400 mL).
5. Elute the desired protein with buffer P3 and collect about 20 1.0 mL fractions (*see* **Note 27**).
6. Analyze the eluted protein by SDS-PAGE.
7. If the IMAC preparation of the recombinant protein does not contain major impurities, pool diabody containing fractions and dialyse against PBS, 50 mM Imidazole, pH 7.0–7.4. If not, *see* purification protocol for bispecific antibody fragments in **Subheading 3.4.** in Chapter 19 of this volume.
8. Determine the protein concentration with the Bio-Rad Protein Assay Kit according to the Bradford method (*18*). Concentrate the purified antibody preparations to 1.0–2.0 mg/mL using Ultrafree-15 centrifugal filter units.
9. The purified protein samples can be stored at −80°C after adding bovine serum albumin (BSA) to a final concentration of 10 mg/mL.

3.3. In Vitro Analysis of Antibody Fragments

3.3.1. Preparation of Granulocytes from Blood by Gradient Density Centrifugation (19)

Since there is no FcγRIII (CD16) positive cell line commercially available, we isolated granulocytes from whole blood of healthy donors as a source for CD16 antigen.

1. Dilute 12 mL of whole blood 1:2 with PBS (*see* **Note 28**).
2. Form a double gradient in a 50 mL centrifuge tube (*see* **Note 29**) by careful layering an equal volume (12 mL) of Histopaque® 1077 over Histopaque® 1119 (*see* **Note 30**).
3. Load diluted blood (24 mL) carefully onto the gradient.

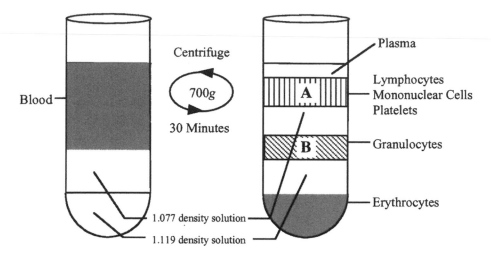

Fig. 2. Separation of granulocytes from venous blood by double gradient density centrifugation.

4. Centrifuge at 700*g* for 30 min at room temperature. Run centrifuge without brake to maintain gradient!
5. Carefully remove tubes from centrifuge. Two distinct opaque layers should be visible (*see* **Fig. 2**). Granulocytes are found in the 1077/1119 interphase, whereas lymphocytes, other mononuclear cells and platlets are located in the plasma/1077 interphase.
6. Collect granulocytes by carefully aspirating the 1077/1119 interphase with a 10 mL serological pipet and transfer to a fresh tube (*see* **Note 31**).
7. Wash the cells with 25 mL cold PBS and centrifuge at 200*g* for 10 min at 4°C.
8. Resuspend the cells with 25 mL cold PBS and repeat washing for two more times.
9. Count the cells and resuspend the cells in an appropriate volume of PBS.

3.3.2. Determination of Binding Activities of Recombinant Antibody Fragments by Flow Cytometry (FACS)

1. A convenient way of preparing multiple FACS stains is to perform the staining in a 96-well microplate. Use $2–5 \times 10^5$ cells per staining. Wash cells with 200 µL of FACS buffer and centrifuge at 200*g* for 2 min at 4°C.
2. For flowcytometric analysis of crude periplasmic preperations of scFv or diabody (*see* **Note 13**) take 100 µL of the dialyzed antibody solution. Purified protein from a large-scale production can be used at a concentration of 1–50 µg/mL. Resuspend cells with 100 µL of antibody solution and incubate for 45 min on ice.
3. Wash the cells twice with 200 µL FACS buffer and centrifuge at 200*g* for 2 min at 4°C.
4. Incubate the cells with 100 µL of 10 µg/mL anti-c-myc antibody for 45 min on ice.
5. Repeat **step 3**.
6. Incubate cells with 100 µL of FITC-labeled goat anti-mouse IgG (1:100) in the dark, for 45 min on ice.
7. Repeat **step 3**.
8. Resuspend the cells in 200 µL FACS buffer containing 1 µg/mL propidium iodide solution to exclude dead cells from the measurement.

9. Perform flow cytometry.

3.3.3. Determination of Cytotoxicity Mediated by Bispecific Diabody

The ability of the bispecific diabody to mediate tumor cell lysis by redirecting NK cells was tested by using the JAM-test method *(15)*. The assay is based on the measurement of DNA fragmentation of apoptotic cells.

1. Grow L540CY cells in 75 cm^2 plastic tissue culture flasks using RPMI-CM under standard conditions. Subculture growing cells the day before labeling at about 5×10^6/mL.
2. To label target cells, add [^{3}H]thymidine to a final concentration of 2.5–5 µCi/mL and let them grow for 4–6 h (*see* **Note 32**). Pellet the cells carefully and wash them once shortly before the assay. Resuspend the target cells in RPMI-CM to a concentration of 1×10^5 cells /mL.
3. Isolate PBL from 50 mL of whole blood of a healthy donor by density gradient centrifugation. Dilute blood 1:2 with PBS at room temperature and layer 25 mL of diluted blood carefully onto 25 mL Ficoll/Hypaque at room temperature in a 50 mL tube. Centrifuge at 200g for 30 min at room temperature without brake! Remove the PBL interphase and wash two times with PBS-F. Centrifuge the cells between washing steps at 200g for 10 min at 4°C.
4. To deplete mononuclear cells from the PBL suspension, resuspend the cells after the final washing step with 50 mL RPMI-CM and incubate for 1 h in two 75 cm^2 plastic tissue culture flasks at 37°C and 5% CO_2. Monocytes will adhere to the plastic flask and PBL can be recovered easily. Centrifuge the monocyte-depleted PBL and resuspend to 2×10^7 cells/mL in RPMI-CM (*see* **Note 33**).
5. To investigate the cytotoxicity mediated by the diabody at different effector:target ratios, dilute PBL suspension serially. Plate 100 µL of PBL (2×10^7 cells /mL) in triplicates into 96-well round-bottomed microwell plates and dilute 50 µL from each of these wells into fresh wells containing 50 µL RPMI-CM medium. Set up a titration from 1×10^6 PBL to 7.8×10^3 PBL.
6. Add 50 µL of diabody solution in various dilutions (*see* **Note 34**), control antibodies or medium as negative control to triplicates.
7. After adding 100 µL of target cells (1×10^5 cells /mL) incubate the plates at 37°C and 5% CO_2 for 3–4 h.
8. Harvest the cells by aspiration onto glassfibre filtermats using a cell harvester.
9. After washing and drying the filters, place them in sample bags, add 10 mL of liquid scintillation cocktail, and seal the bag. Place sample bag with filtermat into a filter cassette and count radioactivity on filters by using a Betaplate liquid scintillation counter.
10. For calculating % specific killing, the standard equation for the JAM test is: % specific killing = (S-E)/S × 100, with E = experimentally retained DNA in the presence of effector cells (in cpm) and S = retained DNA in the absence of effector cells (spontaneous) (*see* **Note 35**).

3.4. In Vivo Application of the Diabody in a SCID Mouse Model

To determine the in vivo efficiency, mice with SCID-bearing xenotransplanted tumors were treated with the bispecific diabody. As a control, we used the parental bispecific MAb.

3.4.1. Testing SCID Mice for Functional Lymphocyte Deficiency by ELISA

SCID mice possess a genetic autosomal recessive mutation, which impairs the differentiation of both T and B lymphocytes. However, approx 15% of SCID mice show spontaneously rearranged TCRγ- and TCRβ-alleles *(20)* or express immunoglobulins in the serum *(21)*. The following ELISA-method is to test the animals for "leakiness."

1. Coat 96-well ELISA flat bottom plate, except wells A1-D1(blank), with 100 µL/well of a 1:500 diluted rabbit anti-mouse antibody solution in PBS at 4°C overnight (*see* **Fig. 3**).
2. Wash plate five times with 200 µL/well PBS-T.
3. Incubate wells with 200 µL/well PBS-B at 37°C for 1 h, wash three times with 200 µL/well PBS-T.
4. For standard curve, dilute mouse IgG 1:30,000 in PBS-TB and dilute 100 µL serially from wells A2-4 to H2-4 to set up a titration of twofold dilutions (*see* **Fig. 3**).
5. As a positive control, dilute serum from a BALB/c mouse 1:40,000 in PBS-TB, and add 100 µL to wells A5-7 (*see* **Fig. 3**).
6. Dilute serum from SCID mice 1:100, and add 100 µL/well in triplicates. Serum of 20 SCID mice can be tested per ELISA plate (*see* **Fig. 3**).
7. Incubate ELISA plate at 37°C for 90 min.
8. Wash plate five times with 200 µL/well PBS-T.
9. Dilute alkaline phosphatase conjugated antibody 1:1500 in PBS-TB and add 100 µL/well, except blank wells.
10. Incubate ELISA plate at 37°C for 90 min.
11. Wash four times with 200 µL/well PBS-T.
12. For detection, add 100 µL/well substrate solution (*see* **Note 7**) and incubate in the dark for 30 min at room temperature.
13. To stop reaction, add 50 µL/well 3 *N* NaOH.
14. Read absorbance at 405 nm using an ELISA Reader.
15. Exclude mice from experiment with immunoglobulin titers exceeding 0.05 µg/mL.

3.4.2. Eradication of Natural Killer (NK) Cells in SCID Mice

To eradicate residual murine NK cells, administer 100 µL of anti-asialo-GM1 antibody solution intraperitoneally, starting 3 d before tumor cell grafting and every fifth subsequent day, until d 17 after tumor cell injection.

3.4.3. Xenotransplantation of Hodgkin Tumor in SCID Mice and Treatment with Antibodies

1. Harvest exponentially growing L540CY cells and wash two times with PBS. Inject 1×10^7 tumor cells (*see* **Note 36**) per mouse in a volume of 200 µL PBS subcutaneously into the right flank with a 26-gauge needle (*see* **Note 37**).
2. Divide tumor-bearing animals with established tumors of 4–6 mm in diameter randomly into different groups.
3. Isolate human peripheral blood lymphocytes by density gradient centrifugation and deplete mononuclear cells according to description in **Subheading 3.3.3.** To obtain sufficient amounts of PBL, use a buffy coat from a blood donor.
4. Inject treatment groups 1×10^7 monocyte-depleted PBL together with 100 µg antibody in 200 µL PBS intravenously through the tail vein (*see* **Note 38**). Control groups receive

	1	2	3	4	5	6	7	8	9	10	11	12
		Standard Curve Titration			Positive Control Serum BALB/c Mouse							
A	Blank	c	c	c	sample 1 →	→	→	sample 8 →	→	→	sample 16	sample 16
B	Blank	c/2	c/2	c/2	sample 2 →	→	→	sample 9 →	→	→	sample 16	sample 17
C	Blank	c/4	c/4	c/4	sample 3 →	→	→	sample 10 →	→	→	sample 17	sample 17
D	Blank	c/8	c/8	c/8	sample 4 →	→	→	sample 11 →	→	→	sample 18	sample 18
E	BC	c/16	c/16	c/16	sample 5 →	→	→	sample 12 →	→	→	sample 18	sample 19
F	BC	c/32	c/32	c/32	sample 6 →	→	→	sample 13 →	→	→	sample 19	sample 19
G	BC	c/64	c/64	c/64	sample 7 →	→	→	sample 14 →	→	→	sample 20	sample 20
H	BC	c/128	c/128	c/128				sample 15 →	→	→	sample 20	

Fig. 3. Pipetting scheme for SCID mouse "Leaky-Test" using a 96-well microplate. Row 1 controls: A1–D1 (Blank) = no rabbit anti-mouse immunglobulins (Ig); E1–H1 (background control, BC) = rabbit anti-mouse Ig + AP conjugated goat anti-mouse Ig + substrate. Rows 2–4: titration for standard curve, serial dilutions of mouse Ig with a starting concentration (c) of about 400 ng/mL (A2-4). Positive control well A5-A7 = serum from BALB/c mouse (1:40,000).

1×10^7 PBL in 200 µL PBS or 200 µL PBS only.

5. Measure tumor development with caliper rule every second day. The tumor volume can be calculated as follows: Volume $= d^2 \times D \times \pi/6$, with d as the smaller and D as the larger diameter.

6. Sacrifice mice when the tumor size exceeds 1.5 cm in diameter, corresponding to a tumor volume of approx 0.4–0.6 cm^3.

7. Data on tumor volumes and survival times should be evaluated by statistical methods to ascertain statistical significance.

4. Notes

1. Both primers can be used for sequencing of scFvs and diabodies in their respective expression vectors.

2. Data are given for protein-purification from a 2 L bacteria culture.

3. Prepare 5 L 2XYT for protein purification from a 2 L culture.

4. Prepare 500 mL and filter (0.2 µm). Solution should be ice-cold before usage.

5. In order to purify protein from 2 L bacteria culture, prepare
   P1: 5 L and filter 1L (0.2 µm) for chromatography steps,
   P2: 1 L and filter (0.2 µm) for chromatography steps,
   P3: 500 mL and filter (0.2 µm) for chromatography steps.

6. Remove glycerol and small impurities by washing with distilled water. Dialysis membranes can be stored at 4°C in distilled water containing 0.1% sodium azide.

7. Diethanolamine buffer can be stored up to one month in the dark.

8. Prepare substrate solution shortly before usage.

9. Perform a "hot start" PCR, add the DNA polymerase after 3 min of denaturation to minimize loss of DNA polymerase activity and the degradation of the primers due to the 3'→5' exonuclease activity of the *Vent* or *Expand™ High Fidelity* DNA polymerase .

10. Initially, the annealing temperature should be 58°C; if no specific band ($\approx$400 bp for γ; $\approx$350 bp for κ/λ) appears, gradually decrease temperature.

11. Addition of glucose is necessary to repress the expression of the recombinant protein.

12. If sequences of all clones differ from the KABAT database reference clone at a particular position, it is very likely that this is not a PCR introduced mutation but the original sequence of the particular antibody. Because the 5' sequence is dictated by the 5' primer, it is important to do a proper alignment with the reference clone from the KABAT database, especially within this region. If the sequence differs within this region from the KABAT reference clone due to the used 5' primer, it could necessitate mutagenesis according to the sequence of the reference clone to restore binding activity of the expressed fragments.

13. To verify the binding activity of the recombinant antibody fragments, prepare crude periplasmic extracts from 5 mL small-scale cultures *(22)*, which usually yield sufficient recombinant protein to test the activity by flow cytometry.

14. It takes approx 3–5 h to reach $OD_{600} = 0.7$–0.8.

15. It is recommended to optimize the IPTG concentration for induction for every diabody within a range of 0.1 m*M*–2 *M* in small-scale experiments.

16. Induction temperatures considerably higher than 21°C lead to a decrease in recombinant protein production in the periplasm.

17. Significant amounts of antibody protein can be found in the culture supernatant of XL1-Blue cells in a time-dependent manner. However, a lengthy induction results in a decrease of protein in the bacterial periplasm. Thus the optimal induction length should be determined for every diabody.

18. For easy resuspension use an Ultra-Turrax dispenser at the lowest speed (T 50 basic ULTRA-TURRAX®, IKA Works Inc. Wilmington, NC).

19. The protein precipitates and appears as foam on the surface.

20. The protein is not completely pelleted after centrifugation. Use a plastic pipet for aspiration of the supernatant to prevent loss of protein not being pelleted.

21. Distribute buffer P1 to each tube and put the tubes on ice. The protein starts to resolve on its own, shake the tubes from time to time by cyclical movement.

22. The sequence of the histidine-containing tag itself, as well as the amino acid sequence surrounding the tag, can influence the selectivity and affinity for an immobilized metal ion *(23)*. The prime candidate for an IMAC tag for recombinant antibody fragments is a hexahistidine sequence (His$_6$), generally fused to the C-terminus of the antibody fragment.

23. The Cu^{2+}-Sepharose column can be prepared 1–2 d in advance. Keep Cu^{2+}-Sepharose-columns at 4°C.

24. 20% (v/v) Ethanol is used as a preservative for the sepharose.

25. Do not let the sepharose column run dry; the sepharose should always be covered with at least 1 mL of buffer.

26. To save time, it is possible to incubate Cu^{2+}-Sepharose and His-tagged protein in a 400 mL tumbler for 2–3 h at 4°C by gentle stirring.

27. To regenerate the used IMAC column, wash with five column volumes of: (a) 50 mM EDTA, (b) 0.5 M NaOH, (c) ddH$_2$O. Wash the column in a final step with 20% (v/v) EtOH if not used frequently.

28. All solutions for the preparation should have room temperature.

29. Do not use high-binding plastics such as polystyrene to avoid cell-binding to centrifuge tube.

30. In our experience it is easier to pipet the solution with lesser density (Histopaque® 1077) first, followed by under-layering with the solution of higher density (Histopaque® 1119). Prepare with caution to avoid mixing up the two phases. Prepare gradient shortly before use.

31. If lymphocytes or mononuclear cells are recovered at the same time, aspirate layer A prior to granulocytes containing layer B. While aspirating granulocytes, try to avoid aspiration of erythrocytes.

32. The labeling procedure depends on the growth rate of the cells. Slow growing cells can be labeled overnight. The optimal labeling conditions should be tested for each new cell line.

33. The remaining PBL contain approx 7–12% NK cells, which are the effector cells and do not need to be preactivated in vitro to obtain their cytolytic activity.

34. Concentrations of the diabody should range between 10 μg/mL and 0.01 μg/mL.

35. The total incorporated counts *(T)* should be measured in the presence of a detergent each time.

36. Prior to the experiment, the amount of tumor cells needed to obtain an established tumor of 4–6 mm in diameter within a period of 2 wk, should be tested for each cell line.

37. Determine number of animals for treatment and control groups according to standard statistical procedures.
38. To ease the injection, let the animals sit for a while under infrared light. The cells should be injected continuously and very slowly.

References

1. Gudelj, L., Deniz, G., Rukavina, D., Johnson, P. M., and Christmas, S. E. (1996) Expression of functional molecules by human CD3-decidual granular leucocyte clones. *Immunology* **87,** 609–615.
2. Herberman, R. B. and Ortaldo, J. R. (1981) Natural killer cells: the role in defense against disease. *Science* **214,** 24–30.
3. Fanger, M. W., Morganelli, P. M., and Guyre, P. M. (1993) Use of bispecific antibodies in the therapy of tumors. *Cancer Treat. Res.* **68,** 181–194.
4. Moretta, A., Tambussi, G., Ciccone, E., Pende, D., Melioli, G., and Moretta, L. (1989) CD16 surface molecules regulate ths cytolytic function of CD3-CD16⁺ human natural killer cells. *Int. J. Cancer* **44,** 727–730.
5. Hombach, A., Jung, W., Renner, C., Sahin, U., Schmits, R., Wolf, J., et al. (1993) A CD16/CD30 bispecific monoclonal antibody induces lysis of Hodgkin's cells by unstimulated natural killer cells *in vitro* and *in vivo. Int. J. Cancer* **55,** 830–836.
6. Stein, H., Mason, D. Y., Gerdes, J., O'Connor, N., Wainscoat, J., Pallesen, G., et al. (1985) The expression of the Hodgkin's disease associated antigen Ki-1 in reactive and neoplastic lymphoid tissue: evidence that Reed-Sternberg cells and histiocytic malignancies are derived from activated lymphoid cells. *Blood* **66,** 848–858.
7. Hartmann, F., Renner, C., Jung, W., Deisting, C., Juwana, M., Eichentopf, B., et al. (1997) Treatment of refractory Hodgkin´s disease with an anti-CD16/CD30 bispecific antibody. *Blood* **89,** 2042–2047.
8. Hartmann, F., Renner, C., Jung, W., and Pfreundschuh, M. (1998) Anti-CD16/CD30 bispecific antibodies as possible treatment for refractory Hodgkin's disease. *Leuk. Lymphoma* **31,** 385–392.
9. Renner, C., Hartmann, F., Jung, W., Deisting, C., Juwana, M., and Pfreundschuh, M. (2000) Initiation of humoral and cellular immune responses in patients with refractory Hodgkin's disease by treatment with an anti-CD16/CD30 bispecific antibody. *Cancer Immunol. Immunother.* **49,** 173–180.
10. Atwell, J. L., Pearce, L. A., Lah, M., Gruen, L. C., Kortt, A., and Hudson, P. (1996) Design and expression of a stable bispecific scFv dimer with affinity for both glycophorin and N9 neurominidase. *Mol. Immunol.* **33,** 1301–1312.
11. Holliger, P., Prospero, T., and Winter, G. (1993) "Diabodies": Small bivalent and bispecific antibody fragments. *Proc. Natl. Acad. Sci. USA* **90,** 6444–6448.
12. Holliger, P., Brissinck, J., Williams, R. L., Thielmans, K., and Winter, G. (1996) Specific killing of lymphoma cells by cytotoxic T-cells mediated by a bispecific diabody. *Prot. Eng.* **9,** 299–305.
13. Zhu, Z., Zapata, G., Shalaby, R., Snedecor, B., Chen, H., and Carter, P. (1996) High-Level secretion of a humanized bispecific diabody from *Escherichia coli. Biotechnology* **14,** 192–196.
14. Perisic, O., Webb, P. A., Holliger, P., Winter, G., and Williams, R. L. (1994) Crystal structure of a diabody, a bivalent antibody fragment. *Structure* **2,** 1217–1226.

15. Matzinger, P. (1991) The JAM test. A simple assay for DNA fragmentation and cell death. *J. Immunol. Methods* **145,** 185–192.

16. von Kalle, C., Wolf, J., Becker, A., Sckaer, A., Munck, M., Engert, A., et al. (1992) Growth of Hodgkin cell lines in severely combined immunodeficient mice. *Int. J. Cancer* **52,** 887–891.

17. Kipriyanov, S. M., Moldenhauer, G., Srauss, G., and Little, M. (1998) Bispecific CD3 × CD19 diabody for T cell-mediated lysis of malignant human B cells. *Int. J. Cancer* **77,** 763–772.

18. Bradford, M. M. (1976) A rapid and sensitive method for the quantitation of microgram quantities of protein utilizing the principle of protein-dye binding. *Anal. Biochem.* **72,** 248–254.

19. English, D. and Andersen, B. R. (1974) Single-step separation of red blood cells. Granulocytes and mononuclear leukocytes on discontinuous density gradients of Ficoll-Hypaque. *J. Immunol. Methods* **5,** 249–252.

20. Bosma, G. C., Custer, R. P., and Bosma, M. J. (1983) A severe combined immunodeficiency mutation in the mouse. *Nature* **301,** 527–530.

21. Schuler, W., Weiler, I. J., Schuler, A., Phillips, R. A., Rosenberg, N., Mak, T. W., et al. (1986) Rearrangement of antigen receptor genes defective in mice with severe combined immune deficiency. *Cell* **46,** 963–972.

22. Kipriyanov, S. M., Moldenhauer, G., and Little, M. (1997) High level production of soluble single chain antibodies in small-scale *Escherichia coli* cultures. *J Immunol. Methods* **200,** 69–77.

23. Sharma, S. K., Evans, D. B., Vosters, A. F., Chattopadhyay, D., Hoogerheide, J. G., and Campbell, C. M. (1992) Immobilized metal affinity chromatography of bacterially expressed proteins engineered to contain an alternating-histidine domain, in *Methods: A Companion to Methods in Enzymology* (Arnold, F., ed.) Academic Press, NY, pp. 57–67.

24. Duebel, S., Dübel, S., Breitling, F., et al. (1994) Isolation of IgG antibody Fv-DNA from various mouse and rat hybridoma cell lines using the polymerase chain reaction with a simple set of primers. *J. Mol. Methods* **175,** 89–95.

25. Arndt, M., Krauss, J., Kipriyanov, S. M., et al. (1999) A bispecific diabody that mediates natural killer cell cytotoxicity against xenotransplantated human Hodgkin's tumors. *Blood* **94,** 2562–2568.

19

Generation and Characterization of Bispecific Tandem Diabodies for Tumor Therapy

Sergey M. Kipriyanov

1. Introduction

Bispecific antibodies (BsAb) provide an effective means of retargeting cytotoxic effector cells against tumor cells *(1)*. They have mainly been produced using murine hybrid hybridomas *(2)* or by chemical crosslinking *(3,4)*. However, the immunogenicity of BsAb derived from rodent monoclonal antibodies (MAbs) is a major drawback for clinical use *(5)*. They are also difficult to produce and purify in large quantities. Recent advances in recombinant antibody technology have provided several alternative methods for constructing and producing BsAb molecules *(6)* (**Fig. 1**). For example, single chain Fv (scFv) fragments have been genetically fused with adhesive polypeptides *(7)* or protein domains *(8)* to facilitate the formation of heterodimers (**Fig. 1A**). The genetic engineering of scFv-scFv tandems linked with a third polypeptide linker has also been carried out in several laboratories *(9,10)* (**Fig. 1B**). A bispecific diabody was obtained by the non-covalent association of two single chain fusion products consisting of the V_H domain from one antibody connected by a short linker to the V_L domain of another antibody *(11,12)* (*see* Chapter 18 of Arndt and Krauss in this issue) (**Fig. 1C**). The two antigen binding domains have been shown by crystallographic analysis to be on opposite sides of the diabody such that they are able to crosslink two cells *(13)*. However, the co-secretion of two hybrid scFv fragments can give rise to two types of dimer: active heterodimers and inactive homodimers. A second problem is that the two chains of diabodies are held together by noncovalent associations of the V_H and V_L domains and can diffuse away from one another. Moreover, to ensure the assembly of a functional diabody, both hybrid scFv fragments must be expressed in the same cell in similar amounts. This latter requirement is difficult to uphold in eukaryotic expression systems such as yeast, which are often preferred because high yields of enriched product can be obtained *(14,15)*. Finally, the small size of bispecific diabodies (50–60 kDa) leads to their rapid clearance from the bloodstream through the kidneys,

From: *Methods in Molecular Biology, vol. 207: Recombinant Antibodies for Cancer Therapy: Methods and Protocols*
Edited by: M. Welschof and J. Krauss © Humana Press Inc., Totowa, NJ

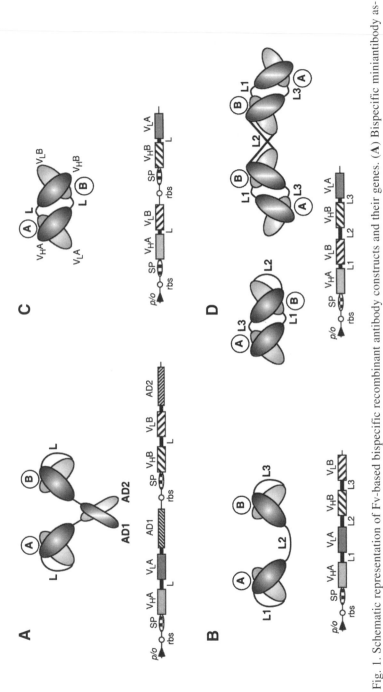

Fig. 1. Schematic representation of Fv-based bispecific recombinant antibody constructs and their genes. (**A**) Bispecific miniantibody assembled from dimerization cassettes based either on leucine zippers (Jun and Fos) (**7**) or on the antibody first constant domains (C_H1 and CL) (**8**). In this case, two scFv antibody fragments of different specificities (A and B) are fused to adhesive self-associating peptide or protein domains (AD). (**B**) Bispecific scFv-scFv tandem [(scFv)$_2$] and four-domain gene construct for its production. (**C**) Bispecific diabody formed by non-covalent association of two hybrid scFv fragments consisting of V_H and V_L domains of different specificities. (**D**) Single chain four-domain gene construct for production of dimeric or tetrameric bispecific molecules. Depending on the linker length, either single-chain diabody (left), or tetravalent tandem diabody (right) can be formed. Antibody variable domains (V_H, V_L), peptide linkers (L) and antigen-binding sites (A or B) of Fv modules are indicated. The locations of promoter/operator (*p/o*), ribosome binding sites (rbs), and signal peptides for secretion in bacteria (SP) are also shown.

thus requiring the application of relatively high doses for therapy. In contrast to native antibodies, all of the aforementioned bispecific molecules have only one binding domain for each specificity. However, bivalent binding is an important means of increasing the functional affinity and possibly the selectivity for particular cell types carrying densely clustered antigens.

To circumvent the drawbacks of diabodies and to increase the valence, stability, and therapeutic potential of recombinant bispecific antibodies, we have recently constructed single-chain molecules comprising four antibody variable domains (V_H and V_L) of two different specificities in an orientation preventing Fv formation *(16)*. They can either form bivalent bispecific antibodies by diabody-like folding ("sc-diabodies") or dimerize with the formation of tetravalent BsAbs with M_r 115,000 kDa ("tandem diabodies") (**Fig. 1D**). The efficacy of tandem diabody (Tandab) formation is dependent on the length of the linker between two halves of the molecule. The Tandabs are both bispecific and have higher avidity resulting from the bivalency for each specificity. For example, the constructed CD3 × CD19 Tandabs were more potent than the diabody for inducing human T cell proliferation in the presence of irradiated CD19+ B cells. In cytotoxic assays, Tandabs were able to retarget human T lymphocytes to malignant B cells. The efficacy of Tandab mediated cell lysis also compared favorably to that obtained with a diabody of the same dual specificity *(16)*. In vivo studies demonstrated that tetravalent Tandabs were both more stable and retained longer in the blood of normal mice compared to scFv and diabodies. Treatment of severe combined immunodeficient (SCID) mice bearing established Burkitt's lymphoma (5 mm in diameter) with human peripheral blood lymphocytes (PBL), Tandab and anti-CD28 MAb resulted in the complete elimination of tumors in all animals within 10 d. In contrast, mice receiving human PBL in combination with either the diabody alone or diabody plus anti-CD28 MAb showed only partial tumor regression *(17)*. This bispecific antibody format could therefore prove to be particularly advantageous for cancer immunotherapy.

In this chapter, generation of genetic constructs coding for bispecific Tandab as well as the protocols for bacterial expression and purification of active bispecific molecules will be described. Generation of plasmids for high-level expression of bispecific Tandab in *Escherichia coli* includes the following steps:

1. Construction of genes encoding hybrid scFv fragments consisting of the V_H domain from one antibody (V_HA) connected by a 5–10 amino acid linker to the V_L domain of another antibody (V_LB).
2. Joining the two dimerizing parts, V_HA-V_LB and V_HB-V_LA, with a peptide linker of 10–20 amino acids in length.

As an example, the primers used for the generation of genetic constructs coding for CD3 × CD19 Tandab *(16)* are listed in **Table 1**.

2. Materials
2.1. Gene Construction

1. Thermocycler PTC 150-16 (MJ Research, Watertown, MA).
2. *Vent* DNA polymerase (New England Biolabs, Beverly, MA).

Table 1
Oligonucleotides for PCR Amplification of DNA Fragments Used in Assembly
of Bispecific CD3 × CD19 Tandem Diabody Gene

(A) Construction of Hybrid V_H3-V_L19 and V_H19-V_L3 scFv genes
V_H Domains
DP1 ($n = 42$)
5' TCA CAC A<u>GA ATT C</u>TT <u>AGA TCT</u> ATT AAA GAG GAG AAA TTA ACC
          *Eco*RI   *Bgl*II
DP2 ($n = 40$)
5' AGC ACA C<u>GA TAT C</u>AC CGC C<u>AA GCT T</u>GG GTG TTG TTT TGG C
          *Eco*RV   *Hin*dIII
V_L Domains
DP3 ($n = 43$)
5' AGC ACA C<u>AA GCT T</u>GG CGG T<u>GA TAT C</u>TT GCT CAC CCA AAC TCC A
          *Hin*dIII   *Eco*RV
DP4 ($n = 57$)
5' AGC ACA C<u>TC TAG A</u>GA CAC AC<u>A GAT C</u>TT TAG TGA TGG TGA TGG TGA TGT
         *Xba*I   *Bgl*II   GAG TTT AGG

(B) Construction of a Gene Encoding Four Domain Fusion Protein V_H3-V_L19-Linker-V_H19-V_L3
V_H3-V_L19-Linker
Bi3sk ($n = 33$)
5' CAG CCG G<u>CC ATG G</u>CG CAG GTG CAA CTG CAG CAG
         *Nco*I
Li-2 ($n = 57$)
5' TAT ATA CTG <u>CAG CTG</u> CAC CTG CGA CCC TGG GCC ACC AGC GGC CGC AGC
         *Pvu*II   ATC AGC CCG

3. 10X *Vent* buffer (New England Biolabs).
4. Sterile deionized water.
5. 100 m*M* dNTPs (New England Biolabs).
6. Bovine serum albumin (BSA), nonacetylated (10 mg/mL) (New England Biolabs).
7. Lambda *Bst*EII DNA molecular weight marker (New England Biolabs).
8. Agarose (FMC BioProducts, Rockland, ME).
9. 50X TAE buffer: Dissolve 242 g Trizma base (Sigma-Aldrich Chemie GmbH, Steinheim, Germany) in distilled water. Add 57.1 mL glacial acetic acid, 100 mL 0.5 *M* EDTA, and water to a total volume of 1 L.
10. 1X Tris-acetate electrophoresis buffer (1X TAE buffer): Prepare a stock solution of 50X TAE and dilute it 1:50 with water before use.
11. 0.5 *M* EDTA.
12. Ethidium bromide (10 mg/mL) (Merck, Darmstadt, Germany).
13. Table-top microcentrifuge.
14. QIAquick Gel Extraction Kit (Qiagen, Hilden, Germany).
15. QIAquick-spin PCR Purification Kit (Qiagen).
16. *Afl*II, *Bgl*II, *Eco*RI, *Eco*RV, *Hin*dIII, *Nco*I, *Nde*I, *Pvu*II and *Xba*I restriction endonucleases (New England Biolabs).

17. 10X Restriction enzyme buffers (New England Biolabs).
18. Calf intestine alkaline phosphatase (CIP, New England Biolabs).
19. T4 DNA-ligase (Stratagene).
20. 10X T4 DNA-ligase buffer (Stratagene).
21. 3 *M* Sodium acetate, pH 4.8.
22. Glycogen from mussels, molecular biology grade (20 µg/mL) (Boehringer GmbH).
23. Absolute ethanol.
24. 80% (v/v) Ethanol.

2.2. Preparation of Bacterial Culture

1. 85 mm-Petri dishes (Greiner, Frickenhausen, Germany).
2. Sterile glass Erlenmeyer flasks, 100, 1000, and 5000 mL.
3. Thermostatic Shaker (Infors GmbH, Einsbach, Germany).
4. Sorvall centrifuge with a set of fixed-angle rotors (Kendro Laboratory Products GmbH, Hanau, Germany).
5. Either *E. coli* K12 XL1-Blue (Stratagene, La Jolla, CA) or RV308 (Δ*lac*ψ74*gal*ISII:: OP308strA) *(18)* competent cells (*see* **Note 1**).
6. 2YT medium: 1 L contains 16 g bacto-tryptone, 10 g bacto-yeast extract, 5 g NaCl, pH 7.5 (*see* **Note 2**).
7. 2YT$_{GA}$: 2YT medium containing 0.1 g/L ampicillin and 2% (w/v) glucose.
8. 2YT$_{GA}$ agar plates. Media and agar plates are prepared according to standard protocols as described *(19)*.
9. 2YT$_{SA}$: 2YT medium containing 0.1 g/L ampicillin and 0.4 *M* sucrose (*see* **Note 3**).
10. YTBS: 2YT medium containing 0.1 g/L ampicillin, 1 *M* sorbitol, and 2.5 m*M* glycine betaine.
11. 100 m*M* Solution of isopropyl-β-D-thiogalactopyranoside (IPTG). Store at –20°C.

2.3. Isolation of Recombinant Product
from Soluble Periplasmic Fraction and Culture Medium

1. Ammonium sulfate powder.
2. Magnetic stirrer.
3. Molecularporous dialysis tubes with a 12–14 kDa cut-off (Spectrum Laboratories Inc., Rancho Dominguez, CA).
4. Buffer A: 50 m*M* Tris-HCl, 20% sucrose, 1 m*M* EDTA, pH 8.0.
5. Buffer B: 50 m*M* Tris-HCl, 1 *M* NaCl, pH 7.0.
6. Buffer C: 50 m*M* Tris-HCl, 1 *M* NaCl, 50 m*M* imidazole, pH 7.0.
7. Buffer D: 50 m*M* Tris-HCl, 1 *M* NaCl, 250 m*M* imidazole, pH 7.0.
8. C16/20 column (Amersham Pharmacia Biotech, Freiburg, Germany).
9. Chelating Sepharose Fast Flow (Amersham Pharmacia Biotech).
10. 0.1 *M* CuSO$_4$.

2.4. Protein Purification and Analysis of Molecular Forms

1. Mono S HR5/5 column (Amersham Pharmacia Biotech).
2. Mono Q HR5/5 column (Amersham Pharmacia Biotech).
3. Superdex 200 HR10/30 column (Amersham Pharmacia Biotech).
4. 50 m*M* Imidazole-HCl, pH 6.4. Filter (0.2 µm) and store at 4°C.
5. 50 m*M* Imidazole-HCl, 1 *M* NaCl, pH 6.4. Filter (0.2 µm) and store at 4°C.
6. 20 m*M* Tris-HCl, pH 8.0. Filter (0.2 µm) and store at 4°C.

7. 20 m*M* Tris-HCl, 1 *M* NaCl, pH 8.0. Filter (0.2 μm) and store at 4°C.
8. Phosphate-buffered saline (PBS): 15 m*M* sodium phosphate, 0.15 *M* NaCl, pH 7.4. Filter (0.2 μm) and store at 4°C.
9. PBSI: PBS containing 50 m*M* imidazole, pH 7.4. Filter (0.2 μm) and store at 4°C.
10. Biomax-10 Ultrafree-15 Centrifugal Filter Device (Millipore GmbH, Eschborn, Germany).
11. PD-10 prepacked disposable columns containing Sephadex G-25 (Amersham Pharmacia Biotech).
12. High and Low Molecular Weight Gel Filtration Calibration Kits (Amersham Pharmacia Biotech).
13. Bio-Rad Protein Assay Kit (Bio-Rad Laboratories GmbH, Munich, Germany).
14. 20% Human Serum Albumin (Immuno GmbH, Heidelberg, Germany).

2.5. Analysis of Antigen-Binding Activities by Enzyme-Linked Immunosorbent Assay (ELISA)

1. 96-Well Titertek polyvinylchloride ELISA microplates (Flow Laboratories).
2. 50 m*M* Sodium carbonate/bicarbonate buffer, pH 9.6. Store at 4°C.
3. PBS/Tween-20: 0.05% (v/v) Tween-20 in PBS. Store at room temperature.
4. 2% (w/v) Skimmed milk in PBS (milk/PBS). Store frozen at –20°C.
5. Mouse monoclonal antibody (MAb) 9E10 specific for the *c-myc* oncoprotein (Cambridge Research Biochemicals, Cambridge, UK).
6. Goat anti-mouse IgG conjugated to hoarse radish peroxidase (HRP) (Jackson Immuno Research Laboratories, Inc.).
7. 3,3',5,5'-Tetramethylbenzidine (TMB) peroxidase substrate (Kirkegaard & Perry Laboratories Inc.).

3. Methods

3.1. Generation of Plasmids for Expression of Four Domain Molecule

3.1.1. PCR Amplification

1. Perform the PCR amplification of DNA fragments in a total volume of 50 μL containing 50 ng of plasmid DNA, 25 pmol of each primer, 300 μ*M* dNTPs, 5 μL of 10X PCR buffer, 5 μg BSA, and 1 U *Vent* DNA polymerase.
2. Run 15–20 PCR cycles on a thermocycler. The thermal cycle is 95°C for 1 min (denaturation), 57°C for 2 min (annealing) and 75°C for 2 min (extension). At the beginning of the first cycle incubate for 3 min at 95°C and at the end of the last cycle incubate for 5 min at 75°C.
3. Analyze the amplified DNA fragments by electrophoresis on a 1.5% agarose gel prestained with ethidium bromide.

3.1.2. Cloning into Expression Vector (see **Note 4**)

1. Digest 10 μg of appropriate vector with suitable restriction endonucleases in presence of alkaline phosphatase (CIP). Incubate at least 2 h at temperature recommended by the supplier.
2. Purify the PCR fragments and linearized vector by agarose gel electrophoresis followed by extraction using a QIAquick gel extraction kit.
3. Digest isolated PCR fragments with restriction endonucleases suitable for cloning into the vector of choice.
4. Remove stuffer fragments and purify the digested PCR products using the QIAquick-spin PCR purification kit.

5. Ligate the vector and insert using a molar ratio between 1:1 and 1:3. The reaction mixture consists of 50 ng DNA, 1 U of T4 ligase, ligation buffer and H_2O to a final volume of 10–20 μL. Incubate overnight at 16°C.

6. Precipitate the DNA by adding 1/10 vol of 3 M sodium acetate, 20 μg glycogen, and 2.5X vol absolute ethanol. Incubate for at least 3 h at –20°C. Sediment the precipitate by centrifugation for 15 min at 10,000g, 4°C (minifuge). Wash the pellet four times with 500 μL 80% ethanol followed by centrifugation for 10 min at 10,000g, 4°C. Allow the pellet to dry at room temperature. Dissolve the dry pellet in 5 μL H_2O.

7. Use the products of one ligation reaction for the electroporation of 40 μL electrocompetent *E. coli* cells according to the supplier's protocol. Plate the bacteria on 2YT agar plates containing 0.1 g/L ampicillin and 2% (w/v) glucose. Incubate overnight at 37°C.

8. Test individual colonies for the presence of the desired insert by plasmid minipreps (*see* **Note 5**).

3.2. Preparation and Cultivation of Bacterial Culture

1. Inoculate a few milliliters of 2YTGA with an individual bacterial colony and let it grow overnight at 37°C when using *E. coli* XL1-Blue or at 26°C when using RV308.

2. Dilute an overnight bacterial culture 40 times with fresh $2YT_{GA}$ and incubate at 37°C (XL1-Blue) or at 26°C (RV308) with vigorous shaking (180–220 rpm) until $OD_{600} = 0.8$–0.9.

3. Harvest bacteria by centrifugation at 1500g for 10 min and 20°C.

4. Resuspend the pelleted bacteria in the same volume of either fresh $2YT_{SA}$ or YTBS medium (*see* **Note 6**). Add IPTG to a final concentration of 0.2 mM (*see* **Note 7**) and incubate the bacterial culture for 14–16 h with shaking at room temperature (22–24°C).

5. Collect the cells by centrifugation at 6200g for 20 min and either discard the culture supernatant (RV308) or retain it and keep on ice (XL1-Blue) (*see* **Note 8**).

3.3. Isolation of Soluble Secreted Recombinant Product

1. Resuspend the pelleted bacteria in 5% of the initial volume of ice-cold Buffer A and incubate on ice for 1 h with occasional stirring.

2. Centrifuge the cell suspension at 30,000g for 40 min at 4°C, carefully collect the supernatant (soluble periplasmic extract). In case of using RV308, go to **step 5**. In case of using XL1-Blue, combine the culture supernatant and the soluble periplasmic extract.

3. Concentrate the bispecific recombinant product by ammonium sulfate precipitation. Place the beaker with the culture supernatant and the soluble periplasmic extract on a magnetic stirrer. Slowly add ammonium sulfate powder to a final concentration 70% of saturation (472 g per 1 L of solution). Continue stirring for at least another 2 h at 4°C.

4. Collect the protein precipitate by centrifugation (30,000g, 4°C, 30 min) and dissolve it in 1/10 of the initial volume of Buffer B.

5. Thoroughly dialyze the concentrated protein against Buffer B at 4°C. Clarify the dialyzed material by centrifugation (30,000g, 4°C, 60 min).

6. For IMAC, prepare a column of Chelating Sepharose (1–2 mL of resin per 1 L of flask culture), wash with 5 bed volumes of water. Charge the column with Cu^{2+} by loading 0.7 bed volume of 0.1 M $CuSO_4$ (*see* **Note 9**), wash the excess of ions with 10 bed volumes of water, equilibrate with 3 volumes of Buffer B (*see* **Note 10**).

7. Pass the soluble periplasmic proteins over a Chelating Sepharose column either by gravity flow or using a peristaltic pump. Wash the column with 10 bed volumes of start Buffer B followed by Buffer C containing 50 mM imidazole (*see* **Note 11**) until the absorbance (280 nm) of the effluent is minimal (20–30 column volumes). Perform all chromatography steps at 4°C.

8. Elute bound antibody fragments with a Buffer D containing 250 mM imidazole (*see* **Note 12**).
9. Analyze the purity of eluted material by SDS-PAGE *(20)*.

3.4. Final Purification of Bispecific Antibody Fragments and Analysis of Molecular Forms

1. If the IMAC yields in homogeneous preparation of recombinant protein according to reducing SDS-PAGE, go to **step 6** (*see* **Note 13**). Otherwise, calculate the isoelectric point (pI) of your bispecific product on the basis of amino acid composition of antibody fragment (*see* **Note 14**).
2. Subject the protein material eluted from the IMAC column to buffer exchange either for 50 mM imidazole-HCl, pH 6.0–7.0, or 20 mM Tris-HCl, pH 8.0–8.5, using prepacked PD-10 columns (*see* **Note 15**). Remove the turbidity of protein solution by centrifugation (30,000g, 4°C, 30 min).
3. Load the protein solution either on a Mono Q or Mono S column equilibrated either with 20 mM Tris-HCl (pH 8.0–8.5) or 50 mM Imidazole-HCl (pH 6.0–7.0), respectively. Wash the column with a least 10 vol of the start buffer.
4. Elute the bound material using a linear 0–1 M NaCl gradient in the start buffer, collect 1 mL fractions.
5. Perform the SDS-PAGE analysis of eluted fractions.
6. Pool the fractions containing pure recombinant antibodies. Determine the protein concentration (*see* **Note 16**).
7. Perform a buffer exchange for PBSI, pH 7.0–7.4 (*see* **Note 17**), and concentrate the purified antibody preparations up to 1.0–2.0 mg/mL using Ultrafree-15 centrifugal filter units.
8. Equilibrate a Superdex 200 column with PBSI buffer, calibrate the column using High and Low Molecular Weight Gel Filtration Calibration Kits.
9. For analytical size-exclusion chromatography, apply 50 µL of the concentrated preparation of bispecific product to a Superdex HR10/30 column. Perform gel-filtration at 4°C, monitor the UV-absorption of effluent at 280 nm and, if necessary, collect 0.5 mL fractions.
10. For long term storage, stabilize purified antibody fragments by adding Human Serum Albumin (HSA) to a final concentration of 10 mg/mL. Store the sample at –80°C (*see* **Note 18**).

3.5. Analysis of Binding Properties of Bispecific Tandab in ELISA

1. Coat 96-well ELISA microplates with 100 µL/well of a 10 µg/mL solution of antigen in 50 mM sodium carbonate/bicarbonate buffer, pH 9.6, overnight at 4°C.
2. Wash the wells five times with PBS/Tween-20 and incubate with 200 µL of milk/PBS at room temperature for 2 h.
3. Load 100 mL of purified Tandab at various dilutions in milk/PBS into the wells and incubate for another 2 h at room temperature.
4. Wash the wells ten times with PBS/Tween-20, add 100 µL of 1/4000 dilution of MAb 9E10 in milk/PBS, incubate the plates for 1 h at room temperature (*see* **Note 19**).
5. Wash the wells ten times with PBS/Tween-20, add 100 µL of 1/4000 dilution of goat anti-mouse IgG-peroxidase conjugate in milk/PBS, incubate the plates for 1 h.
6. Wash the wells ten times with PBS/Tween-20, add 100 µL of a TMB peroxidase substrate, incubate at room temperature for 20–40 min. Read the absorbance of the colored product at 655 nm on a Microplate Reader.

4. Notes

1. Both XL1-Blue and RV308 are suitable hosts for expression of BsAb fragments in shake-flask bacterial cultures. XL1-Blue has the following advantages: electro-competent bacterial cells are commercially available (Stratagene) and standard DNA isolation protocols yield in pure DNA preparations for restriction digests and sequencing. However, RV308 is a more robust, fast-growing strain suitable for high-cell density fermentation *(21)*. Moreover, unlike XL1-Blue no leakage of antibody fragments into the culture medium was observed for RV308.

2. LB (Luria Bertani) broth can also be used. However, we observed that the simple substitution of LB for somewhat richer 2YT medium gave an essential increase in the yield of soluble bispecific molecules.

3. 2YT$_{SA}$ medium is prepared directly before use by dissolving 137 g of sucrose powder in 1 L of sterile 2YT medium containing 0.1 g/L ampicillin.

4. The protocols were established for vectors pHOG21 *(22)* and pSKK *(16)* designed for periplasmic expression of single recombinant product.

5. All DNA manipulations and transformation experiments are performed according to standard cloning protocols *(19)*.

6. The change of medium and induction of protein synthesis in bacteria under osmotic stress significantly increases the yield of dimers, such as Tandab, since these conditions favor domain-swapping and promote the formation of dimers *(16)*.

7. This concentration of IPTG was found to be optimal for vectors containing scFv gene under the control of wt *lac* promoter/operator such as pHOG21 *(22)* or pSKK *(16)*. Nevertheless, performing small-scale experiments to optimize the induction conditions is recommended for each vector.

8. For XL1-Blue either due to the leakiness of the outer membrane or due to the partial cell lysis, a significant fraction of antibody fragments is found in the culture medium. Therefore, supernatant should also be used as a starting material for isolation of recombinant protein.

9. IMAC can be also performed on Ni^{2+}-charged Chelating Sepharose or Ni-NTA-Superflow resin (Qiagen). However, the use of Cu^{2+} instead of Ni^{2+} is recommended for isolation of antibody fragments for clinical applications *(23)*.

10. Tris-HCl buffer is usually not recommended for IMAC because of the presence of amines interacting with immobilized metal ions. However, we have found that such conditions do not influence the absorption of strong binders containing six histidines, while preventing nonspecific interactions of some *E. coli* proteins with the Chelating Sepharose.

11. Unlike Chelating Sepharose, the Ni-NTA columns should not be washed with buffers containing imidazole at concentrations higher than 20 mM.

12. To avoid the unnecessary dilution of eluted scFv, collect 0.5–1.0 mL fractions and monitor the UV absorbance at 280.

13. The purity of the antibody fragments eluted from the IMAC column depends on the expression level of particular recombinant protein.

14. Isoelectric point of the protein can be calculated using a number of computer programs, e.g., DNAid+1.8 Sequence Editor for Macintosh (F. Dardel and P. Bensoussan, Laboratoire de Biochimie, Ecole Polytechnique, Palaiseau, France). The calculated pI value gives you hint what ion exchange matrix and buffer system should be used.

15. For bispecific molecules with pI values below 7.0, we recommend using the anion exchanger such as a Mono Q with linear 0–1 M NaCl gradient in 20 mM Tris-HCl, pH 8.0. For

proteins with p*I* values higher than 7.0, the cation exchange chromatography on a Mono S column with linear 0–1 *M* NaCl gradient in 50 m*M* imidazole-HCl buffer (pH 6.0–7.0) can be recommended. Moreover, we found that by exchanging the buffer after IMAC for 50 m*M* imidazole-HCl, pH 6.4–6.7, most of the contaminating bacterial proteins precipitate while the recombinant antibody fragments remain soluble *(16)*.

16. For determination of protein concentrations, we recommend using a Bradford dye-binding assay because it is easy to use, sensitive, and fast *(24)*.

17. We recommend using PBSI buffer because, in our experience, PBS alone appeared to be unfavorable for the stability of some antibody fragments. The presence of imidazole stabilizes the antibody fragments. It was determined empirically that PBS with 50 m*M* imidazole, pH 7.0–7.5, is a suitable buffer for various antibody fragments kept at relatively high concentrations (2–3 mg/mL). Moreover, this buffer does not interfere with antigen binding and does not show any toxic effects after incubation with cultured cells or after injection into mice (intravenous injection of 200 μL) *(16)*.

18. Alternatively recombinant protein can be stabilized by adding bovine serum albumin (BSA) or fetal calf serum (FCS). HSA is recommended for antibody fragments developed for clinical applications. The recombinant antibodies stabilized by albumin can be stored at −80°C for years without loss of activity. These preparations may be used for a number of biological assays such as ELISA, FACS analysis, analyses of anti-tumor activity both in vitro and in vivo.

19. If different epitopes are used for immunodetection (non *c-myc*), the corresponding antibodies should be used.

References

1. Fanger, M. W., Morganelli, P. M., and Guyre, P. M. (1992) Bispecific antibodies. *Crit. Rev. Immunol.* **12**, 101–124.

2. Bohlen, H., Hopff, T., Manzke, O., Engert, A., Kube, D., Wickramanayake, P. D., et al. (1993) Lysis of malignant B cells from patients with B-chronic lymphocytic leukemia by autologous T cells activated with CD3 × CD19 bispecific antibodies in combination with bivalent CD28 antibodies. *Blood* **82**, 1803–1812.

3. Brennan, M., Davidson, P. F., and Paulus, H. (1985) Preparation of bispecific antibodies by chemical recombination of monoclonal immunoglobulin G1 fragments. *Science* **229**, 81–83.

4. Glennie, M. J., McBride, H. M., Worth, A. T., and Stevenson, G. T. (1987) Preparation and performance of bispecific F(ab'γ)₂ antibody containing thioether-linked Fab'γ fragments. *J. Immunol.* **139**, 2367–2375.

5. Khazaeli, M. B., Conry, R. M., and LoBuglio, A. F. (1994) Human immune response to monoclonal antibodies. *J. Immunother.* **15**, 42–52.

6. Plückthun, A. and Pack, P. (1997) New protein engineering approaches to multivalent and bispecific antibody fragments. *Immunotechnology* **3**, 83–105.

7. de Kruif, J. and Logtenberg, T. (1996) Leucine zipper dimerized bivalent and bispecific scFv antibodies from a semi-synthetic antibody phage display library. *J. Biol. Chem.* **271**, 7630–7634.

8. Müller, K. M., Arndt, K. M., Strittmatter, W., and Plückthun, A. (1998) The first constant domain (CH1 and CL) of an antibody used as heterodimerization domain for bispecific miniantibodies. *FEBS Lett.* **422**, 259–264.

9. Gruber, M., Schodin, B. A., Wilson, E. R., and Kranz, D. M. (1994) Efficient tumor cell lysis mediated by a bispecific single chain antibody expressed in *Escherichia coli*. *J. Immunol.* **152,** 5368–5374.

10. Kurucz, I., Titus, J. A., Jost, C. R., Jacobus, C. M., and Segal, D. M. (1995) Retargeting of CTL by an efficiently refolded bispecific single-chain Fv dimer produced in bacteria. *J. Immunol.* **154,** 4576–4582.

11. Holliger, P., Prospero, T., and Winter, G. (1993) "Diabodies": small bivalent and bispecific antibody fragments. *Proc. Natl. Acad. Sci. USA* **90,** 6444–6448.

12. Holliger, P., Brissinck, J., Williams, R. L., Thielemans, K., and Winter, G. (1996) Specific killing of lymphoma cells by cytotoxic T-cells mediated by a bispecific diabody. *Protein Eng.* **9,** 299–305.

13. Perisic, O., Webb, P. A., Holliger, P., Winter, G., and Williams, R. L. (1994) Crystal structure of a diabody, a bivalent antibody fragment. *Structure* **2,** 1217–1226.

14. Ridder, R., Schmitz, R., Legay, F., and Gram, H. (1995) Generation of rabbit monoclonal antibody fragments from a combinatorial phage display library and their production in the yeast *Pichia pastoris*. *Biotechnology* **13,** 255–260.

15. Shusta, E. V., Raines, R. T., Plückthun, A., and Wittrup, K. D. (1998) Increasing the secretory capacity of *Saccharomyces cerevisiae* for production of single-chain antibody fragments. *Nat. Biotechnol.* **16,** 773–777.

16. Kipriyanov, S. M., Moldenhauer, G., Schuhmacher, J., Cochlovius, B., Von der Lieth, C. W., Matys, E. R., and Little, M. (1999) Bispecific tandem diabody for tumor therapy with improved antigen binding and pharmacokinetics. *J. Mol. Biol.* **293,** 41–56.

17. Cochlovius, B., Kipriyanov, S. M., Stassar, M. J., Schuhmacher, J., Benner, A., Moldenhauer, G., and Little, M. (2000) Cure of Burkitt's lymphoma in severe combined immunodeficiency mice by T cells, tetravalent CD3 × CD19 tandem diabody, and CD28 costimulation. *Cancer Res.* **60,** 4336–4341.

18. Maurer, R., Meyer, B., and Ptashne, M. (1980) Gene regulation at the right operator (O_R) bacteriophage λ. I. O_R3 and autogenous negative control by repressor. *J. Mol. Biol.* **139,** 147–161.

19. Sambrook, J., Fritsch, E. F., and Maniatis, T. (1989) *Molecular Cloning: A Laboratory Manual*, Cold Spring Harbor Laboratory Press, Cold Spring Harbor, NY.

20. Laemmli, U. K. (1970) Cleavage of structural proteins during the assembly of the head of bacteriophage T4. *Nature* **227,** 680–685.

21. Horn, U., Strittmatter, W., Krebber, A., Knupfer, U., Kujau, M., Wenderoth, R., et al. (1996) High volumetric yields of functional dimeric miniantibodies in *Escherichia coli*, using an optimized expression vector and high-cell-density fermentation under non-limited growth conditions. *Appl. Microbiol. Biotechnol.* **46,** 524–532.

22. Kipriyanov, S. M., Moldenhauer, G., and Little, M. (1997) High level production of soluble single chain antibodies in small-scale Escherichia coli cultures. *J. Immunol. Methods* **200,** 69–77.

23. Casey, J. L., Keep, P. A., Chester, K. A., Robson, L., Hawkins, R. E., and Begent, R. H. (1995) Purification of bacterially expressed single chain Fv antibodies for clinical applications using metal chelate chromatography. *J. Immunol. Methods* **179,** 105–116.

24. Bradford, M. M. (1976) A rapid and sensitive method for the quantitation of microgram quantities of protein utilizing the principle of protein-dye binding. *Anal. Biochem.* **72,** 248–254.

20

Generation of Recombinant Multimeric Antibody Fragments for Tumor Diagnosis and Therapy

Barbara E. Power, Alexander A. Kortt, and Peter J. Hudson

1. Introduction

Single chain recombinant antibody fragments can multimerise to provide high binding avidity and unique specificity for target antigens and can be used to replace the parent antibody or Fab derivatives *(1)*. A unique advantage in using bacterial expression systems is the high yield and low cost, especially when the V_H and V_L domains are tethered by a single-chain linker (scFv). This chapter describes expression systems for production of new types of scFv molecules with size, flexibility, and valency suited to in vivo cell-targeting, tumor imaging, and therapy. Further, we review the design of expression cassettes that create multi-specific scFv dimers suited to crosslinking target antigens for T-cell recruitment, viral delivery, and immunodiagnostics. Choice of the linker length that joins V_H and V_L domains dictates precisely whether the (scFv) product is a soluble monomer or a high-avidity multimer (dimer, trimer, etc.). Based on the Kabat numbering system *(2)* and X-ray structures of Fv domains *(3,4)*, we define the C-terminal end of the V_H domain as $Ser^{H\,112}$ or Arg^{L107} of V_L. In either V_H-V_L or V_L-V_H orientation, single chain Fv fragments (scFvs, $\approx$30 kDa) are predominantly monomeric when the Fv domains are joined by polypeptide linkers of at least 12 residues *(5)*. An scFv molecule with a linker of 3–12 residues cannot fold into a functional Fv domain and instead associates with a second scFv molecule to form a bivalent dimer (diabody, $\approx$60 kDa) *(5,6)*. Reducing the linker length below three residues can force scFv association into trimers (triabodies, $\approx$90 kDa) or tetramers ($\approx$120 kDa) depending on linker length, composition, and Fv domain orientation *(7–10)*. The increased binding valency in these scFv multimers results in high avidity (long off-rates). A particular advantage for tumor targeting is that molecules of $\approx$60–100 kDa have increased tumor penetration and fast clearance rates compared to the parent Ig (150 kDa) *(1,11–14)*. A number of cancer-targeting scFv multimers have recently undergone preclinical evaluation for in vivo stability and efficacy *(11–14)*. Bi- and tri-specific multimers

From: *Methods in Molecular Biology, vol. 207: Recombinant Antibodies for Cancer Therapy: Methods and Protocols*
Edited by: M. Welschof and J. Krauss © Humana Press Inc., Totowa, NJ

can be formed by association of different scFv molecules and, in the first examples, have been designed as crosslinking reagents for T-cell recruitment into tumors (immunotherapy) and as red blood cell agglutination reagents (immunodiagnostics) *(1,15,16)*.

Bacterial synthesis of scFv molecules was originally performed in expression vectors using leaky promoters (*lac*, *trp* and *tac*), all of which are not effectively repressed. For example, *lac* promoters are controlled inefficiently by the *lac* repressor and are induced by the addition of isopropyl-β-galactosidase (ITPG). Although these expression systems can be improved *(17,18)* the levels of protein recovered are usually low (below 1 mg/L from shake flasks). A far more effective strategy is to use strong promoters (*tet*, *pho*A, *ara*BAD, and lambda), initially with tight repression to ensure efficient cell/vector growth, followed by short burst of induction *(19–23)*. In these systems, the recombinant protein can be over 50% of the total bacterial proteins and can be recovered in yields greater than 10 mg/L and sometimes up to 1 g/L. Antibody fragments fold efficiently only in the oxidizing extracellular environment, so should be targeted to the periplasm using secretion signals (most commonly *pel*B and *omp*A). This chapter describes our preferred vector, pPOW *(19,23)*, and protocols for high-level scFv synthesis into the bacterial periplasm, ulitizing procedures for recovery by either osmotic shock or by denaturation and refolding. Purification is achieved by affinity chromatography using a tag tail such as the octa-peptide (FLAG) fused to the C-terminus of the antibody construct *(23)*.

2. Materials

2.1. Bacterial Expression Vector

The pPOW3 expression vector is shown in **Fig. 1** and comprises the following features (the vector is available from the authors on request *(23)*. The vector encodes the F1 origin for designed point mutations (via phage production and site-directed mutagenesis using single-strand DNA). Expression of the inserted scFv gene is controlled by the lambda left and right promoters in tandem. The promoters are controlled by the temperature-sensitive repressor gene *cI*857. Protein synthesis is induced by heat-shock, which inactivates the repressor (*see* **Note 1**). Constitutive expression of the repressor gene from the plasmid allows a wide range of host cells to be used for expression (*see* **Note 2**). The 5' cloning sites for antibody scFv genes are *Sfi*I, *Nco*I and *Msc*I, in the *pel*B gene that encodes the signal sequence, (the N-terminal PelB signal sequence is removed by signal sequence peptidases immediately following secretion of the PelB-scFv fusion protein). The 3' cloning sites for antibody scFv genes are *Bam*HI, *Eco*RI, or *Sal*I sites, retaining the termination codons (one in each reading frame) in the *Eco*RI or *Sal*I sites (**Fig. 2**). There is no in-frame peptide tag-tail in the vector to aid in the protein purification so if desired this should be encoded within the reverse polymerase chain reaction (PCR) primer before the termination codon.

2.2. Primers

General pPOW3 oligonucleotides for sequencing or insert size analysis by PCR as listed.

N2175   5' TGT GTG ATA CGA AAC GA 3' (17-mer).

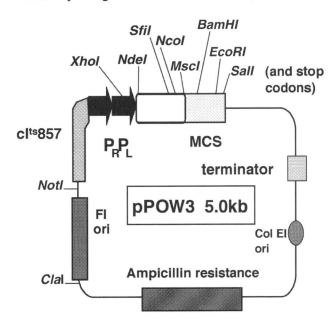

Fig. 1. pPOW3 vector diagram, showing PelB secretion signal, MCS (multiple cloning site) containing *Sfi*I and *Nco*I sites, translational stop codons, and an FI origin of replication.

The forward sequencing primer binds 50 bp upstream of the *pel*B sequence, before the *Xho*I site.

N2357   5' GCG CGT CGG GCT CTA GA 3' (17-mer).

The reverse sequencing primer binds 8 bp downstream of the multiple cloning site. It is a reverse primer and it can be used to sequence any DNA that has been cloned into the multiple cloning site.

2.3. Media Recipes

Purified water should be used for all solutions. All chemicals are analytical reagent grade unless otherwise indicated.

1. 2X YT + Amp Bacterial Cell Growth Media and YT + A Agar Plates: Prepare as 8.0 g Tryptone (Difco- Bacto), 5.0 g Yeast Extract (Difco), 5.0 g NaCl, (for YT + A agar plates add 15 g Difco-Bacto agar) in 1 L of water. Autoclave and cool then add Ampicillin to 100 µg/mL. Alternative bacterial cell growth SB (superbroth) media can be used (*see* **Note 3**).

2. Ampicillin:Prepare stock at 100 mg/mL by weighing out 100 mg of ampicillin powder (Sigma), and dissolve in 1 mL of water. Filter through 0.22 µm filter to sterilize. Store at –20°C. Use at 100 µg/mL.

3. Antifoam: PPG-antifoam, (ALDRICH chemicals) 2 µL is added to 300 mL of culture media, before the induction of protein synthesis to prevent foaming and denaturation of proteins.

*Xho*I
ggggtgtgtgatacgaaacgaagcattggcgc*ctcgag*taatttaccaacactactacgttttaactgaaacaa

RBS   *Nde*I
actggagact*cat* **ATG AAA TAC CTA TTG CCT ACG GCA GCC GCT**
            M   **K**   **Y**   **L**   **L**   **P**   **T**   **A**   **A**   **A**

                         *Sfi*I   *Nco*I *Msc*I
GGA TTG TTA TTA CTC GCG GCC CAG CCG GCC ATG GCC
 G   **L**   **L**   **L**   **L**   **A**   **A**   **Q**   **P**   **A**   **M**   **A**

*Bam*HI   *Eco*RI   *Sal*I
aa*ggatcc*taagtaagta*gaattc*tgagtaggtaa*gtcgac*aatcgcgtctagagccccgacgcgctggg
    *   *   *   *   *   *

Fig. 2. Nucleotide sequence over the promoter/RBS region and multiple cloning sites in the pPOW3 vector. Restriction sites for cloning are 5'; *Sfi*I (GGCCCAGC/CGGCC), *Nco*I (C/CATGG) or *Msc*I (TGG/CCA) and 3' *Bam*HI (G/GATCC), *Eco*RI (G/AATTC) and *Sal*I (G/TCGAC). The codons for the PelB secretion signal are in bold, and the corresponding amino acids underneath. The translational stop codons are indicated with an asterisk.

4. Competent (host) cells: Competent cell strains such as TOP™ 10 (Invitrogen), TOPP™ 6 (Stratagene) may be purchased or prepared as electrocompetent cells by the method of Dower *(24)* (*see* **Notes 2** and **4**). Store at –70°C for up to 6 mo. The competent cells are thawed on ice then transformed with plasmid DNA, using the Bio-Rad Gene Pulser apparatus following the instructions of the manufacturer (12.5 kV/cm, 25 μF, 200 ohms).

5. Lysozyme extraction buffer: Lysozyme (Sigma) at 0.2 mg/mL, is dissolved in 20 m*M* Tris-HCl, pH 8.0, 0.1% Tween-20 (Sigma–polyoxyethylene sorbitan monolaurate) for the extraction buffer. Prepare on the day of use and store at 4°C. The pH of this buffer may need to be altered depending on the pI of the expressed protein.

6. 10X TBS (Tris-buffered saline): Prepared at 80.0 g NaCl, 2.0 g KCl, 30.0 g Tris base in 800 mL water. Adjust the pH to 8.0 with 1 *M* HCl and the volume to 1 L. Sterilize by autoclaving. Store at room temperature. Dilute 1:10 for 1X TBS.

7. 3 m*M* ATP in 1X TBS: Dilute 100 mL of 10X TBS to 1 L with deionized water. Weigh out 1.8 g of ATP (adenosine 5'-triphosphate) (Amersham Pharmacia Biotech) and dissolve in the 1X TBS buffer. Make up fresh reagent on the day of use.

8. 4 *M* Urea/1X TBS: Dissolve 240 g urea in a small volume of 1X TBS, then adjust volume to 1 L with 1X TBS. Store at room temperature.

9. GEB (Gentle Elution Buffer) from (Pierce) or use Affinity elution buffer (AEB): prepared at 3 *M* MgCl$_2$, 20 m*M* MES buffer, pH 7.0, 0.25% ethylene glycol. Store at 4°C.

10. Anti-FLAG affinity resin: Couple the anti-FLAG antibody (FLYTAG™ Silenus, Australia) to the affinity resin (Mini Leak™ Low Resin Kem-En-Tec, Denmark) according to manufacturer instructions.

3. Methods

This section describes the cloning of a gene encoding an antibody scFv into the pPOW3 temperature induced bacterial expression vector, transforming a suitable host cell, preferred conditions for protein synthesis, and isolation by affinity chromatography followed by a brief description of product stability and analysis of binding affinity to the target antigen.

3.1. Cloning of an Antibody scFv Gene into pPOW3

The gene to be inserted into pPOW3 preferably encodes only the mature scFv protein. No leader or presequence is required as the pPOW3 vector provides the PelB secretion signal leader (**Figs. 1** and **2**). The preferred 5' cloning sites for antibody scFv genes in pPOW3 are *Sfi*I, *Nco*I, or *Msc*I, all in the *pel*B gene that encodes the signal sequence. Insertion is most efficient using the sticky-end *Sfi*I or *Nco*I sites in preference to the blunt ended *Msc*I site. The preferred 3' cloning sites for the antibody gene are sticky-end ligation into either *Bam*HI or *Eco*RI sites, which both provide stop codons immediately downstream in all three reading frames. The alternative 3' ligation into the *Sal*I site requires addition of an in-frame stop codon. There is no in-frame peptide tag-tail in the vector to aid in the protein purification so the desired tag should be provided (encoded) within the reverse PCR primer before the termination codon.

3.1.1. PCR Primers for Cloning
into the Sfi*I or* NcoI *Sites Within the* pelB *Gene*

PCR primers should be an exact complement to their target sequence for 50% of their length.

1. The forward V_H PCR primer must create an additional sequence 5' to the scFv gene that encodes *pel*B so that insertion into *Sfi*I (GGCCCAGCCGGCC) or *Nco*I sites (underlined), that partially overlaps with the *Msc*I site (TGGCCA), within the *pel*B gene creates the exact *Pel*B-scFv fusion protein.

   ```
                  SfiI              NcoI MscI
   TTA TTA CTC GCG GCC CAG CCG GCC ATG GCC
    L   L   L   A   A   Q   P   A   M   A //scFv
   ```

2. When cloning into the *Nco*I site, the forward V_H domain PCR primer must encode the *Nco*I site (C/CATGG, 4 base 5' overhang, shown underlined) and also provide the additional nucleotides encoding (MA) positioned immediately 5' to the first codon of the scFv gene. The insertion recreates the correct PelB signal sequence and directs correct signal processing between PelB and scFv. For example, if the mature protein of the scFv begins with N-terminal Glutamine (CAG) and there are no *Nco*I sites in the gene, then the forward PCR primer would be designed as follows:

   V_H forward primer 5'→3' (30-mer)

   ```
              NcoI
   5'   CAG CCG GCC ATG GCC CAG GTA CAG GTA CAG 3'
         Q   P   A   M   A   Q   V   Q   LQ
                  pelB //V_H gene
   ```

3. When a PCR product made with this primer is cut with NcoI, the 5' end of the gene will now be in-frame for expression. Extra nucleotides are added at the 5' end of all of the PCR primers to help the restriction enzyme recognize its cleavage sequence. If the antibody gene contains an internal *Sfi*I or *Nco*I site then cloning into these sites within the *pel*B leader is unsuitable. In this case, blunt-end ligation into the *Msc*I site is required (*see* **Note 5**).

3.1.2. Primers for Addition of Gly₄Ser Linker Residues to Synthesize Diabodies

Short linkers of 3–10 residues joining the V_H and V_L domain direct the formation of diabodies *(7)*.

1. Our preferred linker is the 5 residue linker residues GlyGlyGlyGlySer (6), added to the 3' end of the V_H domain Ser_{112} so that the last two GlySer residues of the linker incorporated a *Bam*HI site. The V_H domain can then be cloned into pPOW3 as *Nco*I-*Bam*HI fragment.

   V_H reverse 5 residue primer 5'→3' (38-mer) *Bam*HI site underlined

   TG GAT GTC <u>GGA TCC</u> GCC TCC TCC TGA GAC GGT GAC CGG
                   S   G   G   G   G   S   V   T   V   P

2. The "overlap" PCR primer for amplifying the V_L domain therefore also encodes a *Bam*HI site positioned for in-frame fusion in the Gly₄Ser linker region. The V_L domain is cloned as a *Bam*HI-*Eco*RI fragment, completing the linker region.

   V_L forward 5 residue primer 5'→3' (39-mer) *Bam*HI site underlined

   GGA GGC <u>GGA TCC</u> GAC ATC CAG ATG ACC CAG AGC CCA AGC
     G   G   G   S   D   I   Q   M   T   Q   S   P   S

3. When the 3' end of the V_L domain gene sequence encodes C-terminal Arginine:

   ...   CTG GAA ATC AAA CGT 3'
          Leu Glu Ile   Lys Arg

   a restriction enzyme site (*Eco*RI) needs to be added and an optional tag tail. The reverse primer to insert a V_L gene into the *Eco*RI site of pPOW3 with a C-terminal FLAG tail would be:

   V_L reverse primer 5'→3' with FLAG peptide tail, *Eco*RI site and stop codon (80-mer)

   AA CGA <u>GAA TTC</u> TTA CTT GTC ATC GTC GTC CTT GTA ATC CCG
           *Eco*RI   K   D   D   D   D   K   Y   D   R
   TTT GAT TTG CAG CTT GGT CCC TTG GCC GAA CGT GAA GGG
     K   I   Q   L   K   T   G   Q   G   F   T   F   P

3.1.3. C-Terminal Peptide Tags

A short polypeptide tail is usually added to the C-terminus to help with expressed product identification, affinity purification, or subsequent radiolabeling. Our preferred tag is the octapeptide FLAG sequence DYKDDDDK, which is encoded by additional nucleotide sequence between the C-terminal (Arg) codon and the *Eco*RI site in the example above (*see* **Note 6**).

3.1.4. Direct Linkage of V-Domains to Synthesize Triabodies

An easy way of converting a diabody into a triabody is to remove the 5' residue linker and instead directly link the C-terminus of V_H (Ser_{112}) to the N-terminus of V_L (Asp_1). This can be most easily achieved by restriction endonuclease excision of the linker followed by PCR-assisted reconstruction of the V_H-V_L junction. For example, some antibodies contain a *Bst*EII site near the C-terminus of V_H ($VTVS_{112}$), so restriction digestion with *Bst*EII and *Eco*RI will remove the linker and V_L domain followed by insertion of a new V_L domain (*Bst*EII-*Eco*RI fragment) created using a forward PCR primer as below:

V_L forward PCR primer 5'→3' for a triabody (scFv 0-mer); *Bst*EII underlined.

GGG ACC CC<u>G GTC ACC</u> GTC TCC GAC ATC CAG ATG ACC CAG
 G   T   P   V   T   V   S   D   I   Q   M   T   Q

3.1.5. PCR Amplification

Typical PCR cycle times for *pfu* polymerase were: (94°C for 2 min) 1 cycle, (94°C for 30 s, 55°C for 30 s, 72°C for 30 s) 35 cycles, (72°C for 2 min) 1 cycle, then store at 4°C. The PCR product is phenol extracted (to inactivate the polymerase), ethanol precipitated and resuspended in water. For subcloning, the DNA is then digested with the appropriate restriction enzymes (*Nco*I + *Eco*RI), isolated from a gel (either agarose or acrylamide depending on the fragment size).

3.1.6. Ligation of the scFv Gene, Transformation, and Colony Selection

1. The gel-purified PCR scFv fragment is ligated into *Nco*I + *Eco*RI digested pPOW3 vector and transformed into electro-competent *E. coli* host cells using our published methods *(23)*.
2. Electrocompetent cells are thawed on ice then transformed with plasmid DNA, using the Bio-Rad Gene Pulser apparatus following the instructions of the manufacturer (12.5 kV/cm, 25 µF, 200 ohms). Calcium-competent cells should not be used since the heat-shock step inactivates the lambda repressor in pPOW3, activates expression, and interferes with cell growth. Our preferred host cell strains are XL10-GOLD™ (Stratagene) for DNA preps and TOP™ 10 (Invitrogen), TOPP™ 6 (Stratagene) for protein synthesis, purchased from scientific suppliers or prepared as electrocompetent cells *(24)*.
3. The vector contains the Ampicillin resistance gene so YT + A plates (30°C, *see* **Note 1**) are used to select after transformation with suitable competent host cells.
4. Positive transformants are identified by colony screens using PCR with N2175 and N2357 primers, checking for a correct-size band by either acrylamide or agarose gel chromatography. If the vector contains no insert, a PCR product of 215 bp will be amplified. This size represents the distance between the *Xho*I site, the *pel*B signal and the 3' cloning site. If the transformant contains an insert, a PCR band of (the insert size) + 215 bp will be amplified.
5. With the selected clone, prepare a 100 mL cell culture in 1X YT + Amp media (30°C) and isolate plasmid DNA (*see* **Note 1**). The scFv gene insert can be sequenced using double-stranded DNA sequencing and the N2175 (forward) and N2357 (reverse) primers.
6. The plasmid DNA is stored frozen as the most stable stock of the expression vector. Before each protein synthesis experiment, use this stable plasmid DNA to transform com-

petent host cells and select fresh colonies from YT + A plates for each protein synthesis experiment described below (to ensure maximal plasmid copy number) (*see* **Note 7**).

3.2. Protein Expression

3.2.1. Small Scale Expression Screen to Determine Optimum Induction Time

For maximum expression yield two times are important. The time required for repressor inactivation and the subsequent time for protein synthesis. For pPOW3, we find that optimal product synthesis occurs by continual repressor inactivation and concomitant protein synthesis using a constant temperature over 37°C (preferably 42°C). Ideally, the bacterial cells should be in exponential growth phase and induction completed before the bacterial cells reach stationary phase. The following protocol is to determine the optimal total induction time (*see* **Notes 1, 2, 4, 7**, and **8**).

1. Pick a colony from a YT + A plate (grown specifically for this experiment at 30°C as described earlier). Inoculate 1 mL of culture medium using a 10 mL tube. Incubate for a maximum of 16 h at 30°C.
2. On the following day, use 500 µL of the starter culture to inoculate 5 mL of 2X YT + Amp media in a 50 mL tube so that the A_{600} is between 0.5–0.8.
3. Incubate the cells for 4 h at 30°C in the orbital shaker at 150–200 rpm (assume that it will take four hours to reach an A_{600} of 4.0–5.0).
4. Take a zero time sample as a preinduction control (500 µL).
5. Induce the culture by increasing the temperature to 42°C and hold at this temperature. Take 500 µL samples at the 1 h, 2 h, 3 h, 4 h, and overnight time points (*see* **Notes 8** and **9**). Store samples on ice or at 4°C.
6. Determine protein expression by SDS-PAGE. Vortex time-point samples; take 30 µL and add 30 µL of SDS sample dye, boil, and load 15 µL onto duplicate 12.5% SDS-PAGE gels. Run one gel for Coomassie Blue stain and another for Western-Blot analysis with scFv-specific probing.
7. An induced Coomassie-stained band should be seen accumulating over time compared to the uninduced sample (0 time control) (*see* **Fig. 3**).
8. The earliest time point with highest levels of expression is the optimal induction time.

3.2.2. Shake Flask Expression (1 L) and Cell Fractionation

1. Pick a colony from a YT + A plate and prepare a cell suspension using 1 mL of culture medium and inoculate 100 mL of 2X YT + Amp media in a 1-L flask. Incubate for a maximum of 16 h at 30°C.
2. Use 25 mL of the overnight starter culture to inoculate 225 mL of fresh 2X YT + Amp media in each of four 1-L flasks previously autoclaved and cooled. (A_{600} should be 0.5–0.8.) Set the orbital shaker speed to 150–200 rpm and temperature to 30°C.
3. Monitor A_{600} at hourly intervals until it reaches mid to late exponential phase before induction. It usually takes about four hours to reach an A_{600} of 4.0 (This is assuming a max. OD of 7.0.)
4. Take a 1-mL sample as a zero-time preinduction control. Before inducing the sample add 2 µL of anti-foam (*see* **Subheading 2.3.**) to each flask, then induce the culture by increasing the temperature to 42°C and incubate for the optimal time determined from the small scale experiment earlier (usually 1 h, *see* **Notes 8** and **9**).

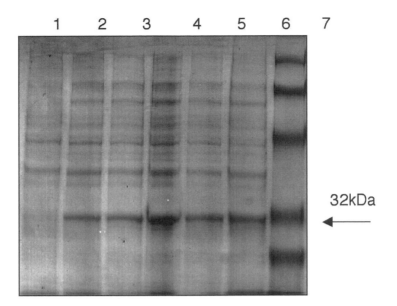

Fig. 3. 12.5% SDS-PAGE gel of time course induction, stained with Coomassie Blue R-250. Each time point sample was thoroughly mixed to resuspend the cells in the culture medium. Then 15 μL of each time point sample was mixed with sample loading buffer, boiled, then loaded onto the gel. Arrow indicated protein band (~32 kDa) accumulating over time. Lane 1, preinduced; lane 2, 1 h postinduction; lane 3, 2 h postinduction; lane 4, 3 h postinduction; lane 5, 4 h postinduction; lane 6, 20 h postinduction; lane 7, low-range molecular-weight markers; 107, 74, 49.3, 36.4, 28.5 kDa. Western-blot analysis of a duplicate gel showed that the 32 kDa bands contain the peptide tag as they react with anti-FLAG antibody (data not shown).

3.2.3. Expressed Protein Location and Isolation

For 1 L of shake flask culture use the following conditions:

1. Spin down the samples in a refrigerated centrifuge at 4°C for 5 min × 6000 rpm. Remove the supernatant and discard, as it is unlikely to contain any of the expressed protein (*see* **Note 10**).
2. Resuspend the cell pellet in 100 mL of lysozyme extraction buffer (*see* **Subheading 2.3.**).
3. Leave cell pellet on ice for 1 h.
4. Cells will become thick and viscous. Homogenize with ultra turrex for 30 s to break up DNA.
5. Spin for 10 min × 12,000 rpm at 4°C. Retain the aqueous phase (lysozyme wash, fraction A). Freeze if affinity chromatography step of this fraction is not done on the same day.
6. Resuspend the cell pellet in 100 mL of ice-cold sterile water. Leave on ice for 30 min. This osmotic shock step releases soluble product from the periplasmic space.
7. Spin for 5 min × 12,000 rpm at 4°C. Collect the aqueous phase which contains soluble proteins released by osmotic shock (fraction B), add 1/10 vol of 10X TBS. Freeze if affinity chromatography step is not done on the same day.

8. Freeze the cell pellet and thaw, ensuring the temperature remains always below 10°C during thawing. Add 100 mL of ice-cold sterile water. Leave on ice for 30 min.

9. Spin for 5 min × 12,000 rpm at 4°C. Collect the aqueous phase (fraction C), add 1/10 vol 10X TBS. Freeze if affinity chromatography step is not done on the same day.

10. The fractions A, B, and C should be analyzed by SDS-PAGE to determine which fraction contains the greatest amount of expressed protein product (*see* **Note 11**). If there is significant protein expressed in all three fractions, they can be combined as the total soluble fraction and affinity purified in one batch.

11. The bacterial cell pellet may contain a significant quantity of expressed product. This protein can be recovered from the pellet by solubilization with denaturants such as urea or guanidine.

12. Resuspend the cell pellet in 50 mL of 4 M urea in TBS, pH 8.0. Leave on ice for 1 h (*see* **Note 12**).

13. Spin for 5 min × 12,000 rpm at 4°C. Load the sample into dialysis tubing (3000 MW cutoff) and dialyze against 1X TBS buffer. Initially use volume of buffer equal to the volume of the protein sample, allow to equilibrate then dilute the dialysate 1:1 with 1X TBS buffer, and allow to equilibrate overnight. Slowly increase the volume in a 1:1 ratio stepwise. After this initial slow dialysis of ≈4 changes subsequent buffer changes can be done using the larger volumes of buffer to remove the residual urea. This procedure minimizes the amount of expressed protein precipitating compared with "rapid" removal of denaturant.

14. Recover the solution from the dialysis tubing including a white precipitate that may have formed during dialysis. Spin the dialyzed sample 5 min × 12,000 rpm. The aqueous phase contains the solubilized refolded proteins. The precipitate contains the insoluble material including misfolded scFv aggregates. Analyze the solubilized fraction by sodium dodecyl sulfate polyacrylamide gel electrophoresis (SDS-PAGE) to assess the amount of solubilized expressed protein recovered.

15. Load the samples on 12% SDS-PAGE gels. Typical volumes are as follows; Culture supernatant 20 μL, Periplasm (osmotic shock) 10 μL, Cell pellet 2 μL (*see* **Notes 13–16**).

3.3. Affinity Chromatography

The soluble expressed protein product is recovered with an affinity resin specific to the C-terminal tag used. We have generally used the FLAG peptide as an affinity tag. The preferred procedure is to use the affinity resin in a batch method. This minimizes proteolytic degradation and aggregation of the protein often observed when extracts are concentrated prior to affinity column purification.

1. Determine the total protein concentration of the soluble protein fractions (usually ≈3 mg/mL).

2. Dilute the pooled periplasmic fraction (300 mL) to just less than ≈1 mg/mL, using 1X TBS buffer.

3. Place the sample into a 2-L flask. Add 2 mL of affinity resin (*see* **Subheading 2.3.**) and gently swirl on a bench top shaker at 4°C for 1 h (*see* **Note 17**).

4. Filter the mixture through a scintered-glass filter under vacuum.

5. Release the vacuum and wash the resin (while still on the filter) with 10 mL of 1X TBS containing 3 mM ATP (*see* **Subheading 2.3.**) (to dissociate interaction of GroEL with expressed scFv in the soluble osmotic shock fraction; *see* **Fig. 4**).

6. Apply the vacuum and rinse with 10 mL of 1X TBS.

7. Release the vacuum and wash the resin into a 5 mL column. Allow the resin to settle and pack.

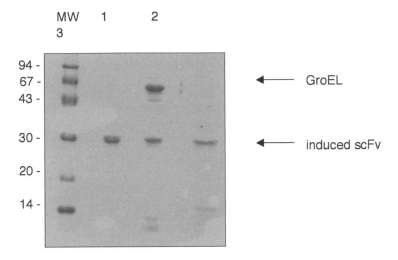

Fig. 4. Effect 3 m*M* of ATP wash on the affinity purification of soluble extracts eluted from the anti-FLAG column using GEB buffer. Coomassie blue G-250 stained SDS gel of anti-FLAG purified scFv trimer. Lanes 2 and 3 are before and after 3 m*M* ATP treatment (respectively), showing the loss of a GroEL protein band. The GroEL in complex with scFv binds to the anti-FLAG affinity resin but is not detected during Western blotting and probing with anti-FLAG antibody. Samples from left are: Molecular mass markers 94, 67, 43, 30, 20, 14 kDa. Affinity purified scFv, lane 1, urea refolded scFv; lane 2, soluble scFv from soluble periplasmic fraction; lane 3, soluble scFv from periplasmic fraction after washing with ATP.

8. Connect the 5-mL column into a FPLC system (e.g., Bio-Rad Econo system) and wash the column with 1X TBS (*see* **Subheading 2.3.**)
9. Elute the bound protein with GEB buffer or AEB (*see* **Subheading 2.3.**). Monitor the A_{280} absorbance and collect the peak.
10. The urea solubilized fraction is processed in the same way but the wash with ATP is not required.
11. Run a sample of the eluted protein on size exclusion columns (e.g., Superose 12) to determine oligomeric composition and size *(5–10)*. More precise measurement of molecular mass can be determined by analytical ultracentrifugation *(5,8)*.

3.4. Stability and Binding Affinity

1. Expression yields can be enhanced by point mutations or by codon usage (*see* **Notes 15** and **16**) and by choice of fermenter conditions *(21)*.
2. ScFv with linkers of 12 or more residues preferentially form monomers (≈30 kDa), but have a propensity to dimerise into diabodies (≈60 kDa). ScFv with 3–12 residues preferentially form diabodies and with less than 3 residues form triabodies (≈90 kDa) or higher aggregates. In some cases the trimers are not homomgeneous forms, but remain in equilibrium *(10)*.
3. Preferred storage is frozen at –20°C or –80°C, providing that cycles of freeze/thaw does not cause unwanted aggregation or unfolding. Although, when an scFv trimer is present as an equilibrium mixture, cycles of freeze/thaw at –20°C can drive the equilibrium to the trimeric form. Alternatively, store in 0.02% azide at 4°C.

4. Protein samples should be checked for stability to concentration (greater than 1 mg/mL can cause aggregation *(25)*.

5. Check size by size-exclusion chromatography, comparing elution times with standards.

6. Check binding affinity to (immobilized) target antigen by ELISA or with BIAcore/IAsys biosensors. It is difficult to quantitate accurate kinetic constants from binding data measured for multivalent binding interactions *(26)*.

7. The gain in functional affinity for scFv dia/triabodies compared to scFv monomers is significant and is seen primarily in reduced biosensor off-rates *(8,27)*.

8. Functional valency and Fv orientation can also be assessed by electron microscopy analysis of antigen complexes *(28)*.

9. Recombinant scFv monomers and multimers can be radiolabelled according to protocols described in other chapters in this book.

The significant gain in avidity (functional affinity) through multivalent binding makes multimeric scFvs attractive for in vivo tumor imaging and offers a significant improvement over monovalent scFv and Fab fragments *(11–14)*.

4. Notes

1. All liquid and plated cell cultures prior to protein synthesis must be done below 33°C, preferably 30°C. pPOW is a heat-inducible vector and to ensure good cell growth rates the repressor must be active and functional.

2. We have found that for protein synthesis it is best to choose a bacterial host cell strain that does not produce an *E. coli* protein at the same size as the expected synthesized protein. Use the following strains as a guide:

protein size	14 kDa use cell strain	LE392 or SURE or TGI
27 kDa		LE392 or SURE or NM514
32 kDa		LE392 or SURE or NM514

These cell strains produce slightly different *E. coli* banding patterns upon heat induction, when used for protein synthesis in conjunction with a cloned insert in the pPOW vector. Some cells are more susceptible to releasing the soluble proteins from the osmotic shock fraction. Try TOP™ 10 (Invitrogen), BL21, TOPP™ 6 (Stratagene) for greater cell permeability.

3. SB (Superbroth) media, alternative bacterial cell growth media for antibody scFv protein synthesis: 20 g Tryptone, 10 g Yeast Extract, 5 g NaCl, 2.5 g K_2HPO_4, 1 g $MgSO_4\cdot7H_2O$. Make to 1 L with water. Autoclave, cool, then add filtered stocks; 1 mL 0.1 mg/mL biotin, 1 mL 1 mg/mL thiamine, 3 mL trace element solution, 1 mL 100 mg/mL ampicillin. Trace element solution (100 mL) 1.6 g $FeCl_3$, 0.2 g $ZnCl_2\cdot4H_2O$, 0.2 g $CoCl_2\cdot6H_2O$, 0.2 g $Na_2MoO_4\cdot2H_2O$, 0.1 g $CaCl_2\cdot2H_2O$, 0.1 g $CuCl_2$, 0.5 g H_3BO_3, 10 mL conc. HCl. Stir until dissolved. Adjust volume to 100 mL. Store frozen –20°C. When this supplement is added to the medium, the medium will become slightly hazy. This does not affect the performance of the medium.

4. Use electrocompetent cells for transformations but do not heat shock if using calcium competent cells.

5. Cloning into the blunt-end *Msc*I site to regenerate the final alanine of the PelB signal sequence. The forward PCR primer must contain two extra nucleotides (CX) added to the blunt-ended scFv, positioned immediately 5' to the DNA encoding the first amino acid of the scFv gene (refer to **Fig. 2**). *Msc*I cleaves TGG/CCA, in the last codon of the *pel*B gene

at the sequence G/CC so, to keep the translation in-frame for expression, the last amino acid codon (Alanine = GCX) needs to be reformed. The nucleotides to be added to scFv are CX with X being any of the four nucleotides (*see* **Table 1** for a list of restriction enzymes that cleave DNA leaving CX after cleavage) and can be easily incorporated in the PCR oligonucleotide primer used to assemble the gene fragment for subsequent cloning. For example, if the mature protein of the gene to be expressed begins with N-terminal Lysine (AAG) and there are no *Msc*I sites in the gene, then the forward PCR primer would be designed as follows:

    *Msc*I
5' G*ATGGCC* AAG CCA CAG GCA CCC 3' (22-mer)
    Lys
encoding GCC AAG CCA CAG GCA CCC
        Ala Lys
   *pel*B foreign gene

*Msc*I cleaves TGG\CCA. When a PCR product made with this primer is cut with *Msc*I, the 5' end of the gene will now be in-frame for expression. Extra nucleotides are added at the 5' end of all of the PCR primers to help the restriction enzyme recognise its cleavage sequence.

6. Other frequently used tag-tails for purification are hexa-his (*18*) and strep-tag (*29*).
7. It is preferabe to use freshly transformed cells to ensure maximal plasmid copy number, and it is important to use cells or colonies that are only 2–3 d old at most.
8. Cell division (OD levels) and product synthesis continues for about 4 h postinduction. It is unlikely that more than 4 h cultures are needed postinduction because no additional accumulation of the synthesized product has been observed after an overnight culture. Pay close attention to the bacterial cell A_{280} OD units as induction of protein synthesis should be done when the cells are rapidly dividing in the exponential growth phase.
9. It may take 45 min or more for the culture temperature to increase to 42°C required for induction (measure fluid temperature with a thermometer). If optimal induction is at 42°C for 1 h, reduce the temperature to 20°C for a further 1 h maximum. The reason for this is that the bacterial cells will still be in a rapidly dividing state during protein synthesis and we have found that a further 1 h incubation at 20°C allows sufficient time for the last generation of bacterial cells to produce protein which greatly increases the overall protein yield. This method is unlikely to allow secretion of the protein into the supernatant.
10. When using long overnight induction times, protein may be recovered from the supernatant, but the levels of protein synthesis are lower than periplasm recovery. Small amounts of protein can be recovered by affinity chromatography directly from the culture supernatant. This is likely to be owing to cell rupture or lysis and is not detected in the early time points of the rapidly growing bacterial cell population. Therefore, long induction times can lead to cell death (the culture will be in stationary phase) and increase the amount of protein recoverable from the culture supernatant.
11. Sonication may be used to release more soluble proteins from the cells.
12. 4 *M* Urea solubilizations give better quality product with little or no aggregate after affinity chromatography, whereas the 8 *M* urea solubilizations often result in 50% aggregate formation.
13. The secretion signal PelB is efficiently excised after export through the inner membrane into the periplasm. By SDS-PAGE, there should be a predominant product in total cell extracts. A minor product ~ 2kDa larger can be due to unprocessed precursor containing

Table 1
Blunt End Restriction Enzymes that Can Be Used
at the 5' End to PCR a New Gene into the pPOW Vector

*Alu*I	AG/CT
*Hae*III	GG/CC
*Msc*I	TGG/CCA
*Nru*I	TGG/CGA
*Nsp*BII	CCG/CGG
*Pvu*II	CAG/CTG
*Stu*I	AGG/CCT
*Tha*I	CG/CG

the PelB leader, but this contaminant is usually lost during purification since the hydrophobic PelB leader causes aggregation.

14. Periplasmic product may be retained in the periplasmic or secreted through the outer membrane into the culture supernatant. Relative levels in each compartment can be assessed by SDS-PAGE after fractionation. The periplasmic aggregates can be further separated into soluble components that are released by osmotic shock, and insoluble aggregates that require denaturation, purification, and refolding. The optimum conditions for protein synthesis into each of these fractions can be controlled by the culture medium, the age of the bacterial population at time of induction, and length of induction. At the highest level of protein synthesized (50% of the total cell protein), one antibody V_H domain was predominantly in insoluble aggregates and could be recovered by a simple denaturation and dialysis refolding process to 30 mg/L in shake flasks *(19)*.

15. Some scFv antibodies can be synthesized at higher yields due to their intrinsic solubility. Several key residues have been identified as being important for increasing the levels of soluble expression, particularly V_H residue 6 should be Glu, V_H position 84 Asp and other positions *(1,30)*.

16. Gene expression can be effected by codon usage and replacement of codons favoring those of *E. coli* preferred should be considered *(31)*. The main two are Proline CCG and Leucine CUG.

17. Purify the protein samples by pre-adsorbing to an affinity matrix in a batch method rather than by using columns. The batch method is a lot faster and results in better protein product of the correct size. Keep the samples cold (4°C) at all times. The protein sample should be diluted with 1X TBS to just under ≈1 mg/mL before binding to the resin. Gently swirl the affinity resin during the binding phase, do not use magnetic stirrers, as these tend to be too vigorous in their action causing protein denaturation.

Acknowledgments

We thank all our colleagues in the antibody engineering program at CSIRO Health Sciences and Nutrition for their helpful advice on the design and expression of scFv molecules. We also thank the fermentation group for their hints on microbial physiology and fermenter conditions.

References

1. Hudson, P. J. (1999) Recombinant antibody fragments in cancer therapy. *Curr. Opin. Immunol.* **11,** 548–557
2. Kabat, E. A., Wu, T. T., Perry, H. M., Gottensman, K. S., and Foeller, C. (1991) *Sequences of Proteins of Immunological Interest.* U.S. Department of Health and Human Service, U.S. Public Health Service, NIH, Bethesda, MD.
3. Malby, R., Caldwell, J., Gruen, L., Harley,V., Ivancic, N., Kortt, A., et al. (1993) Recombinant anti-neuraminidase single chain antibody: expression, characterization and crystallisation in complex with antigen *Proteins Struct. Funct. Genet.* **16,** 57–63.
4. Malby, R. L., McCoy, A. J., Kortt, A. A., Hudson, P. J., and Colman, P. M. (1998) Single-chain Fv/neuraminidase complexes: different stoichiometry in solution and crystals. *J. Mol. Biol.* **279,** 901–910.
5. Kortt, A., Malby, R., Caldwell, J., Gruen, L., Ivancic, N., et al. (1994) Recombinant antineuraminidase single chain Fv antibody: characterization, formation of dimer and higher molecular mass multimers and the solution of the crystal structure of the scFv-neuraminidase complex. *Eur. J. Biochem.* **221,** 151–157.
6. Holliger, P., Prospero, T., and Winter, G. (1993) "Diabodies": small bivalent and bispecific antibody fragments. *Proc. Natl. Acad. Sci. USA* **90,** 6444–6448.
7. Atwell, J. L., Breheney, K. A., Lawrence, L. J., McCoy, A. J., Kortt, A. A., and Hudson, P. J. (1999) scFv Multimers of the anti-neuraminidase antibody NC10: length of the linker between V$_H$ and V$_L$ domains dictates precisely the transition between diabodies and triabodies. *Protein Eng.* **12,** 101–108.
8. Kortt, A. A., Lah, M., Oddie, G. W.,Gruen, L. C., Burns, J. E., Pearce, L. A., et al. (1997) Single Chain Fv Fragments of anti-neuraminidase antibody NC10 containing five and ten residue linkers form dimers and with zero residue linker a trimer. *Protein Eng.* **10,** 423–433.
9. Iliades, P., Kortt, A. A., and Hudson, P. J. (1997) Triabodies: Single Chain Fv Fragments without a linker form trivalent trimers. *FEBS Lett.* **409,** 437–441.
10. Dolezal, O., Pearce, L. A., Lawrence, L. J., McCoy, A. J., Hudson, P. J., and Kortt, A. A. (2000) ScFv Multimers of the anti-neuraminidase antibody NC10: shortening of the linker in single-chain Fv fragment assembled in V$_L$ to V$_H$ orientation drives the formation of dimers, trimers, tetramers and higher-molecular-mass multimers. *Protein Eng.* **13,** 56–574.
11. Adams, G. P., Schier, R., McCall, A. M., Crawford, R. S., Wolf, E. J., Weiner, L. M., and Marks, J. D. (1998) Prolonged *in vivo* tumor retention of a human diabody targeting the extracellular domain of human HERk2/*neu Br. J. Cancer* **77,** 1405–1412.
12. Wu, A. M., Williams, L. E., Zieran, L., Padma, A., Sherman, M., Bebb, G. G., et al. (1999) Anti-carcinoembryonic antigen (CEA) diabody for rapid tumor targeting and imaging. *Tumor Target.* **4,** 47–58.
13. Viti, F., Tarli, L., Giovannoni, L., Zardi, L., and Neri, D. (1999) Increased binding affinity and valence of recombinant antibody fragments lead to improved targeting of tumoral angiogenesis. *Cancer Res.* **59,** 347–352.
14. Adams, G. P., Shaller, C. C., Chappell, L. L., Wu, C., Horak, E. M., Simmons, H. H., et al. (2000) Delivery of the alpha-emitting radioisotope bismuth-213 to solid tumors via single-chain Fv and diabody molecules. *Nucl. Med. Biol.* **27,** 339–346

15. Atwell, J. L., Pearce, L. A., Lah, M., Gruen, L. C., Kortt, A. A., and Hudson, P. J. (1996) Design and expression of a stable bispecific scFv dimer with affinity for both glycophorin and N9 neuraminidase. *Mol. Immunol.* **33**, 1301–1312.

16. Holliger, P., Brissinck, J., Williams, R. L., Thielemans, K., and Winter, G. (1996) Specific killing of lymphoma cells by cytotoxic T-cells mediated by a bispecific diabody. *Protein Eng.* **9**, 299–305.

17. Coia G., Hudson, P. J., and Lilley G. G. (1996) Construction of recombinant extended single-chain antibody peptide conjugates for use in the diagnosis of HIV1 and HIV2. *J. Immunol. Methods.* **192**, 13–23.

18. Kipriyanov, S. M., Moldenhauer, G and Little, M. (1997) High level production of soluble single chain antibodies in small-scale *Escherichia coli* cultures. *J. Immunol. Methods* **200**, 69–77.

19. Power, B. E., Ivancic, N., Harley, V. R., Webster, R. G., Kortt, A. A., Irving, R. A., and Hudson, P. J. (1992) High-level temperature-induced synthesis of an antibody V_H –domain in *Escherichia coli* using the PelB secretion signal. *Gene* **113**, 95–99.

20. Skerra, A. (1994) Use of the tetracycline promoter for the tightly regulated production of a murine antibody fragment in *Escherichia coli*. *Gene* **151**, 131–135.

21. Kortt, A. A., Guthrie, R. E., Hinds, M. G., Power, B. E., Ivancic, N., Caldwell, J. B., et al. (1995) Solution properties of *E. coli* expressed V_H domain of anti-neuraminidase antibody NC41. *J. Protein Chemistry* **14**, 167–178.

22. Zhu, Z., Zapata, G., Shalaby, R., Snedecor, B., Chen, H., and Carter, P. (1996) High level secretion of a humanised bispecific diabody from *E. coli*. *Nature Biotechnol,* **14**, 192–196.

23. Power, B. E. and Hudson, P. J. (2000) Synthesis of high avidity antibody fragments (scFv multimers) for cancer imaging. *J. Immunol. Methods* **242**, 193–204.

24. Dower, W. J. (1990) Electroporation of bacteria: a general approach to genetic transformation. *Genet. Eng. (NY)* **12**, 275–295.

25. Arndt, K. M., Muller, K., M., and Plückthun, A. (1998) Factors influencing the dimer to monomer transition of an antibody single-chain Fv fragment. *Biochemistry* **37**, 12,918–12,926.

26. Muller, K. M., Arndt, K. M., and Plückthun, A. (1998) Model and simulation of multivalent binding to fixed ligands. *Anal. Biochem.* **261**, 149–158.

27. Plückthun, A. and Pack, P. (1997) New protein engineering approaches to multivalent and bispecific antibody fragments. *Immunotechnology* **3**, 83–106.

28. Lawrence, L. J., Kortt, A. A., Iliades, P., Tulloch, P. A., and Hudson, P. J. (1998) Orientation of antigen binding sites in dimeric and trimeric single chain Fv antibody fragments. *FEBS Lett.* **425**, 479–484.

29. Schmidt, T. G. and Skerra, A. (1994) One-step affinity purification of bacterially produced proteins by means of the "Strep tag" and immobilised recombinant core streptavidin. *J. Chromatogr. A.* **676**, 337–345.

30. Nieba, L., Honegger, A., Krebber, C., and Plückthun, A. (1997) Disrupting the hydrophobic patches at the antibody variable/constant domain interphase: improved *in vivo* folding and physical characterisation of an engineered scFv fragment. *Protein Eng.* **10**, 435–444.

31. Ernst, J. F. (1988) Codon usage and gene expression. *TIBTECH* **6**, 196–199.

21

Construction and Characterization of Minibodies for Imaging and Therapy of Colorectal Carcinomas

Paul J. Yazaki and Anna M. Wu

1. Introduction

1.1. Optimization of Antibody Characteristics for In Vivo Imaging and Therapy

Engineering of antibodies specific for tumor-associated antigens provides great flexibility in improving their properties for eventual use in the clinic, for the detection of cancer, or as a therapeutic. In some instances, murine monoclonal antibodies (MAbs) have been identified with innate biological anti-tumor activity. Production of chimeric or humanized (CDR-grafted) antibodies lowers the immunogenicity of murine MAbs, a necessary modification if repeat administration is desired (1,2). Chimerization or humanization can also increase the ability of murine MAbs to interact with the human immune system. The anti-lymphoma and anti-breast cancer antibodies Rituxan™ (Rituximab) and Herceptin™ (Trastuzumab) are robust examples of this path to a clinically useful reagent (3,4). Production of chimeric or humanized antibodies with Fc regions of a suitable subclass allows engagement of human host immune responses (complement activation, antibody-dependent cellular cytotoxity). Many anti-tumor MAbs, however, must be further "armed" in some fashion in order to be useful as therapeutics. Alternate approaches, described in detail elsewhere in this volume, include fusion of antibodies to toxins or cytotoxic proteins such as ribonuclease, production of bispecific antibodies for recruitment of effector T cells, or direct activation of T cells through chimeric T-cell receptors.

One of the classic approaches toward arming antibodies has been radiolabeling. Antibodies can be tagged with radionuclides such as ^{99m}Tc, ^{111}In, ^{123}I, or many other isotopes that emit gamma rays, and be used for imaging purposes. The approach can be extended to radiolabeling with positron-producing radionuclides such as ^{18}F, ^{64}Cu, ^{124}I, and so on, for positron emission tomography (PET), affording higher resolution and better quantitation than single-photon approaches. By switching to radionuclides

From: *Methods in Molecular Biology, vol. 207: Recombinant Antibodies for Cancer Therapy: Methods and Protocols*
Edited by: M. Welschof and J. Krauss © Humana Press Inc., Totowa, NJ

that emit alpha or beta particles on decay, a therapeutic effect can be delivered specifically to tumor deposits.

Recombinant approaches can be utilized to optimize several characteristics of antibodies that will be radiolabeled for clinical use. As mentioned earlier, chimerization or humanization are essential first steps to reduce patient immune responses and allow multiple or long-term administration. Alternately, fully human antibodies can be isolated from transgenic animals or by phage-display technology. Protein engineering can be used to produced antibodies of improved affinity or modified specificity. Recombinant antibody fragments can be tailored with regard to molecular weight, valency, domain composition, flexibility, and orientation of binding sites. Furthermore, modifications can be introduced into engineered antibodies to facilitate radiolabeling, such as addition of a peptide sequence capable of chelating a radiometal. These characteristics are readily modified by genetic engineering and can have a large impact on the in vivo targeting properties and potential utility of radiolabeled antibodies.

1.2. Pharmacokinetic Properties of Antibodies and Engineered Fragments

A critical characteristic of antibodies under development for in vivo use is their pharmacokinetic properties. For example, for most therapeutic applications, a longer half-life in the circulation is often desirable in order to allow ample time for exposure of the target tissue to the therapeutic agent. However, when antibodies are radiolabeled, the issue of background activity in blood and normal tissues becomes a major factor. Intact antibodies typically have circulating half-lives of several days. As a result, when radiolabeled intact antibodies are used for in vivo imaging, typically 2–7 d must elapse following administration in order for background activity to clear and allow optimal visualization of target tumors. An analogous problem arises when therapeutic radionuclides are coupled to antibodies for radioimmunotherapy. Prolonged persistence in the circulation results in substantial delivery of radioactivity to normal tissues, with bone marrow toxicity frequently becoming the limiting factor in the doses that can be administered. Enzymatic digestion of antibodies with papain or pepsin yields Fab or F(ab')$_2$ fragments with improved properties, especially for imaging. Fragments lacking the Fc region exhibit much more rapid disappearance from the circulation, as they no longer interact with the Fc receptors on the surface of immune cells or the FcRB (Brambell receptor, also known as FcRn or FcRp) responsible for maintaining plasma persistence of antibodies (5).

The use of genetically engineered antibody fragments provides an approach for modifying the targeting and clearance properties of antitumor antibodies. A useful first step is conversion of native antibody combining sites into the single-chain Fv format (scFv) (6). This provides the antigen recognition function in a single polypeptide, encoded by a single gene, and greatly facilitates expression in heterologous systems. Many groups have developed scFv from antibodies specific for a variety of tumor-associated antigens, using conventional cloning and reformatting, or through phage display. Several have been evaluated in radiolabeled form in preclinical models of human cancer, specifically, using human tumor xenografts in immunodeficient mice. Rapid, specific targeting has been observed, but the absolute levels of radioactivity delivered to xenografts have been consistently low *(7)*. Of note, two clinical studies of scFv targeting in patients have been completed with analogous results *(8,9)*. Thus, the potential of anti-tumor scFv for radioimmunoimaging or radioimmunotherapy appears limited.

Larger engineered fragments, based on scFvs as building blocks, have been generated. Diabodies, noncovalent dimers of scFvs, are readily produced by the use of constructs with short interdomain linkers *(10)*. When the linker is too short to allow the variable regions of an scFv to associate with each other, (generally under about 12 aa residues) the protein can readily associate with a second scFv polypeptide through domain exchange. Several groups have reported that diabodies exhibit superior xenograft targeting in mouse models, compared to the corresponding scFv *(11–14)*. This is likely due to the increased valency and molecular weight of the diabody format. Bispecific diabodies open further possibilities for targeting of therapeutic moieties to tumors. The concept has been further extended into larger multivalent molecules such as triabodies and tetrabodies.

Alternately, larger fragments have been built by fusion of antibody variable regions to a broad range of protein domains. Fusion to human immunoglobulin domains such as IgG1 C_H3 can be used to add mass and promote dimerization *(15)*; fusion to human Ig hinge-Fc regions can add also add effector functions. Multimerization can be promoted by fusion to heterologous protein domains from multimeric proteins. For example, fusion of scFv to short amphipathic helices have been used to produce miniantibodies *(16)*. Domains from proteins that form heterodimers (such as fos/jun) can be used to produce bispecific molecules *(17)*; alternately homodimerization domains can be engineered to form heterodimers by engineering strategies such as "knobs into holes" *(18)*. Finally, fusion protein partners can be selected that provide both multimerization as well as an additional function, e.g., streptavidin *(19)*. As fusion proteins are designed and developed for use in vivo, attention must be paid to characteristics such as molecular weight (whether the final product will be above or below the threshhold for first-pass renal clearance), overall pI, potential immunogenicity of the fusion partner, and other factors.

1.3. Carcinoembryonic Antigen and Colorectal Carcinoma as a Model System

Carcinoembryonic antigen (CEA), which is overexpressed in human colorectal carcinomas, has been extensively studied as a tumor-associated marker *(20)*. The CEA gene family is a subset of the immunoglobulin gene superfamily. CEA is a GPI-linked cell-surface glycoprotein, with a molecular weight of 180,000 Dalton. CEA was originally described as a classic oncofetal antigen, appearing early during human development in the fetal gut, but not widely expressed in the normal adult. Development of colorectal carcinoma is accompanied by reexpression of CEA in the tumor, as well as shedding of antigen into the serum. More recently, a close look reveals that CEA is expressed in a limited number of adult tissues, primarily on the apical surface of the columnar epithelium in the colon, but also in limited cells in the stomach, tongue, esophagus, cervix, sweat glands, and prostate *(21)*. In human tumors, CEA is widely expressed in colorectal, gastric, pancreatic, gallbladder, urinary bladder, and ovarian carcinomas; lung adenocarcinoma, small cell lung carcinoma, and to a lesser extent in breast carcinoma *(21)*.

Antibody-directed targeting of CEA-positive tumors has been progressively developed and refined as the understanding of the CEA gene family, including commonly expressed, closely related antigens has matured. Concomitantly, many laboratories have developed antibodies with high affinity and high specificity for CEA that lack cross-reactivity with cross-reacting family members such as BGP and NCA. Goldenberg and co-workers were the first to propose labeling anti-CEA antibodies for radioimmunodetection and radioimmunotherapy *(22,23)*. Subsequent studies demonstrated the potential advantages of antibody fragments for clinical imaging *(24,25)*, and ultimately CEA-Scan™ (Arcitumomab), a ^{99m}Tc-labeled murine Fab' fragment, received approval for marketing as an imaging agent for colorectal carcinoma. Work in many laboratories continues, directed toward imaging products with reduced immunogenicity and improved targeting properties. Furthermore, the therapeutic potential of intact chimeric or humanized anti-CEA antibodies, radiolabeled with ^{131}I or ^{90}Y, is being investigated.

1.4. Construction and Characterization of scFv-C$_H$3 Minibodies

The tumor targeting and pharmacokinetic properties of a series of anti-CEA antibody fragments, including scFv, diabody, scFv-C$_H$3 (minibody), F(ab')$_2$, and intact forms, have been evaluated in xenografted athymic mice, using the CEA-positive human colorectal carcinoma cell line, LS174T, as the target. Results indicate that the minibody format exhibits a combination of properties that may be optimal for imaging, including rapid, high-level uptake into tumors, and concomitant rapid blood clearance *(15,26)*. The combination of high activity deposited in the tumor and low background activity allows visualization of antigen-positive tumors within a few hours of injection in murine models, and the kinetics of minibody targeting are well-suited to labeling with radionuclides of intermediate half-life such as [123]I (13.2 h) or [64]Cu (12.7 h) *(15,27)*. An additional advantage of an ^{123}I minibody is that liver and kidney activities are low, presumably due to the activity of dehalogenases present in these tissues. In contrast, radiometal labeled minibodies, and/or their radiolabeled metabolites, demonstrate localization and persistence in the liver.

Further development and evaluation of scFv-C$_H$3 minibodies is warranted in several areas. An important next step is evaluation of the tumor targeting, normal tissue distribution, and blood clearance of radioiodinated minibodies in humans. While murine models are helpful to select candidates for further development, reliable extrapolation of results to the clinical setting is impossible. A key question will be determining the pharmacokinetics of minibodies in humans. A second open issue is the potential of the minibody format for radioimmunotherapy of colorectal and other cancers. The clearance properties in humans will have a significant impact on the blood and bone marrow doses. Another concern is the observed high liver activity of radiometal-labeled minibodies in the mouse studies. The issue should be explored first by imaging in humans using radiometals such as ^{111}In or ^{64}Cu. Targeting and dosimetry studies will reveal whether an scFv-C$_H$3 minibody can deliver sufficient dose to tumors without excessive toxicity to bone marrow and other normal tissues. Improvements might be made in the chemistry of the chelate and conjugation methods, with the goal of obtaining an agent whose radiolabeled metabolites clear from the liver. Finally, it is important to extend studies to additional antibodies and antigen systems and derive general principles for production of engineered antibody fragments specifically for in vivo targeting and therapeutic purposes.

An engineered antibody fragment optimized for targeting cancer in vivo should have the following properties: high specificity and affinity for target antigen; bivalency or multivalency; low immunogenicity; single-chain format to facilitate expression. In addition, the recombinant fragment must demonstrate favorable kinetics in vivo, including rapid, high-level targeting of tumors. The blood clearance kinetics must be compatible concurrently with adequate time of exposure to the tumor as well as rapid clearance to minimize unwanted activity in normal organs.

The scFv-C$_H$3 minibody format has demonstrated favorable xenograft targeting properties in murine models and is a promising candidate for further development. Several variables can be considered in minibody design. It is helpful to begin with a well-characterized scFv, in which issues such as order of the variable regions, and length and sequence of the intervariable domain linker have been addressed, and retention of high affinity and specificity has been demonstrated. Fusion to the C$_H$3 domain can be direct, through a short peptide spacer, or via an immunoglobulin hinge region. The latter allows formation of disulfide-linked covalent dimers, and evidence indicates improved performance in vivo. Choice of expression system will dictate the nature of the ribosome binding site and signal peptide (for secretion) that must be fused to the N-terminus of the gene construct. Both bacterial (*E. coli*) and mammalian (Sp2/0, NS0, COS cells) expression systems have been employed; however, susceptibility to proteolysis at the hinge region limited the recovery of the scFv-hinge-C$_H$3 minibody from bacteria *(15)*. Eukaryotic systems, including mammalian cells, may be preferable for production of larger, multi-subunit antibody fragments.

Protocols are described below for the assembly of genes encoding a minibody by the PCR-splice overlap extension method. Methods for stable mammalian expression are given. Expansion of high-expressing transfectomas into hollow-fiber bioreactors can provide sufficient material for pilot clinical trials such as radioimmunoimaging or radioimmunotherapy, where relatively small quantities of protein are required (low milligram doses) *(28)*. A general purification method that utilizes mild chromatography and elution conditions, that has proved successful for a variety of diabodies and minibodies, is described. These protocols are assembled as an example of a successful path for production of minibodies for evaluation of in vivo targeting, but alternate expression vectors, systems, and purification approaches should also be considered.

2. Materials

2.1. Construction of the Minibody Gene

1. Murine hybridoma cells secreting antibody of interest.
2. TRIzol (Life Technologies, Rockville, MD).
3. Gene-Amp kit (Perkin-Elmer Cetus, Foster City, CA).
4. AMV reverse transcriptase (Promega, Madison, WI).
5. Synthetic oligonucleotide primers (various commercial sources).
6. Thermal cycler (Perkin-Elmer Cetus or other supplier).
7. Agarose gel electrophoresis apparatus (various suppliers).
8. SeaKem LE agarose (FMC, Chicago, IL).
9. Restriction enzymes (various commercial sources).
10. Manual DNA sequence analysis reagents/equipment or automated DNA sequencing facility.
11. QIAquick spin columns (QIAgen, Valencia, CA).

2.2. Stable Transfection of Minibody in NS0 Cells

2.2.1. Transfection

1. Murine myeloma NS0 cells (Lonza Biologics, Slough, UK).
2. Disposable sterile cultureware (Falcon, Franklin Lakes, NJ).
3. Nonselective media: 2 mM glutamine enriched DME media (JRH Biosciences, Lenexa, KS, cat. no. 51435) supplemented to 10% with heat-inactivated fetal bovine serum (FBS) (HyClone, Logan, UT).
4. L-Glutamine (Irvine Scientific, Irvine, CA, cat. no. 9317).
5. Phosphate buffered saline (PBS) sterile (Irvine Scientific, cat. no. 9240).

2.2.2. Cell Culture

1. Trypan blue T8154 (Sigma Chemical, St. Louis, MO).
2. Hemocytometer (VWR-Scientific Products, cat. no. 15170-172).
3. Micropure-EZ Enzyme Remover (Millipore, Bedford, MA, cat. no. 42529).
4. Gene Pulser II electroporation unit and cuvets (Bio-Rad Laboratories, Hercules, CA).
5. Multiporator electroporation unit and cuvets (Eppendorf, Hamburg, Germany).
6. Hypo-osmotic buffer (Eppendorf, cat. no. 4308070.501).
7. Selective media: glutamine-free enriched DME media high modified (JRH Biosciences, cat. no. 51435) supplemented to 10% with heat inactivated dialyzed fetal bovine serum (HyClone) and GS supplement (JRH Biosciences, cat. no. 58672).
8. Flat-bottomed 96-well sterile plates (Costar Inc., Corning, NY, cat. no. 3585).
9. Bottom viewing mirror (Dynatech, Chantilly, VA).
10. Freeze media: 20% FBS (Hyclone), 10% dimethyl sulfphoxide hybri-max (DMSO) (Sigma, cat. no. D2650), DME media (JRH Biosciences).

2.2.3. ELISA

1. Coating buffer: 0.2 M sodium bicarbonate buffer, pH 9.6, 0.02% sodium azide (Sigma).
2. PBST: PBS + 0.05% Tween 20 (Bio-Rad Laboratories).
3. Blocking solution: 5% bovine serum albumin (BSA) (Sigma, cat. no. A9647) in PBST.
4. Conjugated antibody: Goat anti-human IgG Fc alkaline phosphatase antibody (Jackson ImmunoResearch, West Grove, PS, cat. no. 109-055-098).
5. Sigma 104 Phosphatase substrate 104-40 (Sigma).
6. Bio-Rad 450 plate reader (Bio-Rad Laboratories).

2.3. Hollow Fiber Bioreactor Production

1. Cell Pharm 100 bioreactor (Unisyn Technologies, Hopkinton, MA).
2. Hollow fiber Flowpath 10,000 kDa exclusion (Unisyn Technologies, cat. no. 22010663).
3. Autoharvester and Flowpath (Unisyn Technologies, cat. no. 12340637).

2.4. Purification of Minibodies

1. All solutions are made with nanopurified water or water for injection.
2. Diethylaminoethyl cellulose (DE 52) (Whatman, Maidstone, UK).
3. 0.2 μm PES vacuum 1L filter (Corning, Corning, NY, cat. no. 431098).
4. AG1-X8, 100-200 mesh (Bio-Rad Laboratories).
5. 50 mM 2-[N-Morpholino]ethanesulfonic acid sodium salt, (MES) pH 6.5 (Sigma, cat. no. M2933).
6. Macro-Prep ceramic hydroxyapatite (HA), Type I, (Bio-Rad Laboratories).
7. Advanced Purification (AP) column bodies (Waters, Milford, MA, cat. no. WAT021901; WAT027501).
8. 0.04 M $KH_2PO_4 \cdot 3H_2O$ (Mallinkrodt Baker, Phillipsberg, NJ), 50 mM MES, pH 6.5.
9. 50 mm N-[2-hydroxyethyl]piperazine-N'-[2-ethanesulfonic acid] (HEPES) pH 7.4 #54457 (Fluka Chemical Milwaukee, WI, cat. no. 54457).
10. Source 15Q (Amersham Pharmacia Biotech, Piscataway, NJ).
11. 0.2 M NaCl (Fluka), 50 mM HEPES, pH 7.4.
12. 20 mM Sodium phosphate, pH 7.4 (Fluka).
13. Centriprep 30 (Millipore, cat. no. 4306).
14. 4 mm Syringe filter 0.2 μm (Whatman, cat. no. 6780-0402).

2.5. Characterization of Expressed Minibodies

1. Ready-Gels, 10% polyacrylamide (Bio-Rad Laboratories, cat. no. 161-1305).
2. 10X Tris, Glycine, SDS buffer (Bio-Rad Laboratories, cat. no. 161-0732).
3. Kaleidoscope Prestained standards (Bio-Rad Laboratories, cat. no. 74815).
4. Bio-Safe Coomassie (Bio-Rad Laboratories, cat. no. 161-0786).
5. Mini Trans-blot electrophoretic transfer cell (Bio-Rad Laboratories).
6. 10X Tris/Glycine buffer (Bio-Rad Laboratories, cat. no. 161-0734).
7. Nitrocellulose membrane (Bio-Rad Laboratories, cat. no. 162-0115).
8. Superdex 75 HR 10/30 (Amersham Pharmacia Biotech).
9. Alkaline phosphatase buffer: 0.1 M Tris, 0.1 M NaCl, 5 mM MgCl, pH 9.6.
10. Development buffer: 33 μL of 5-bromo-4-chloro-3-indoyl phosphate (BCIP) and 66 μL of nitro blue tetrazolium (NBT) (Promega, Madison, WI, cat. no. S3771) in 10 mL of alkaline phosphatase buffer.
11. Bio-Rad Protein Assay kit I (Bio-Rad Laboratories, cat. no. 500-0001).
12. rProtein L-agarose (Actigen, Cambridge, UK, cat. no. 201-2).
13. 100 mM Tri-sodium citrate, not pH-adjusted (Fluka, cat. no. 71404).
14. 20 mM Sodium citrate, 20 mM sodium phosphate pH 7.4/ 0.5 M NaCl.
15. 100 mM Citric acid anhydrous, not pH-adjusted (Fluka, cat. no. 27487).
16. EZ-Link Sulfo-NHS-LC-Biotinylation kit (Pierce Chemical, Rockford, IL, cat. no. 21430ZZ).
17. BIAcore 1000, biosensor SA chips, reagents and BIAevaluation 3.0 software (BIAcore Inc., Piscataway, NJ).

3. Methods

3.1. Construction of Minibody Gene

3.1.1. Amplification of Variable Region Genes from Hybridoma Cell Lines

1. Prepare total RNA from 2×10^7 or more hybridoma cells expressing the monoclonal antibody of interest, using a standard method such as guanidine thiocyanate/cesium chloride ultracentrifugation *(29)* or using a product such as TRIzol (Life Technologies).
2. Set up separate RT-PCR reactions, one for the heavy chain and one for the light chain variable region. Each RT-PCR reaction should contain 5 µg total RNA, 20 pmol of upstream (V-region consensus) and downstream (constant region) primers, 2.5 m*M* dNTPs, 10X PCR buffer, and 0.1 m*M* DTT in a 50 µL reaction. Commercially available kits such as Gene-Amp (Perkin-Elmer Cetus) provide a convenient source of reagents (*see* **Note 1**).
3. Denature the reaction at 70°C for 10 min.
4. Add 10 U of AMV reverse transcriptase and allow cDNA synthesis to proceed at 37°C for 15 min.
5. Add 2 U of *Taq* polymerase (AmpliTaq, Perkin-Elmer Cetus, or equivalent) polymerase and amplify in a thermal cycler programmed for 30 cycles at 1 min, 94°C, 1 min, 58°C, 2 min, 72°C.
6. Gel purify the PCR products, clone into the plasmid of interest, and confirm that the appropriate variable regions have been isolated by DNA sequence analysis.

3.1.2. Gene Assembly by Splice Overlap Extension PCR (SOE-PCR)

1. Fusion primers should be designed to extend across the planned junction of the two starting gene segments, with a six amino acid (18 nucleotide) overlap on each side. Each gene segment is then amplified separately using a flanking (outside) primer and the appropriate overlap primer using standard PCR conditions, 25–30 cycles, to create modified gene segments that now include a short overlap.
2. Purify PCR products by agarose gel electrophoresis, and include a DNA standard of known concentration for quantitation. Following ethidium bromide staining, estimate the amount of PCR product.
3. Recover the PCR fragment from the agarose using the QIAquick (QIAgen) protocol or similar method, according to the manufacturer's instructions.
4. Set up the overlap extension to include: 100 ng of each overlap fragment; 2 µL of 250 µM dNTP mix; 5 µL 10X PCR buffer, 0.5 U *Taq* polymerase and H$_2$O to a final volume of 50 µL.
5. Perform overlap extension in a thermal cycler programmed to run six cycles of 1 min, 94°C, 2 min, 37°C, 4 min, 72°C.
6. Transfer 10 µL of the above reaction to a fresh tube and add: 1 µL 250 µM dNTP mix; 4 µL 10X PCR buffer, 20 pmol each flanking (outside) forward and backward primers; 0.5 U *Taq* polymerase and H$_2$O to a final volume of 50 µL. Amplify 25–30 cycles using standard PCR program.
7. Gel-purify fused PCR gene product and insert into a plasmid to be grown up for DNA sequence analysis and confirmation that the correct fusion has been produced. Transfer the engineered antibody gene to an expression vector. The following example is based on use of the vector pEE12, which contains the cytomegalovirus immediate early region with promotor and intron, a multi-cloning site, and polyadenylation signal for expression of the gene of interest. A selectable marker is provided by a glutamine synthetase mini-gene *(30,31)*.

3.2. Stable Transfection of Minibody in NS0 Cells

3.2.1. Transfection

1. Grow host NS0 cells in nonselective media and expand in a T-150 flask. Harvest cells in log phase by centrifugation, wash in PBS and count viable cells by trypan blue exclusion using a hemocytometer.
2. Linearize 100 µg each of pEE12 minibody plasmid and a pEE12 control, using restriction enzyme *Sal*I. Spin-filter using a Micropure-EZ Enzyme Remover (Millipore) to remove BSA and restriction enzyme from sample. Ethanol precipitate, resuspend the DNA in sterile water, and quantify by gel electrophoresis.
3. Electroporate a 0.4 cm electrode gap cuvet containing 800 µL of PBS, 40 µg of DNA and 10^7 NS0 cells using two pulses at 1500 V, 3 µF using a Gene Pulser II™.
4. Alternately, electroporate a cuvet containing 400 µL hypo-osmotic buffer, 10 µg DNA and 2×10^6 cells using 1 pulse at 200 V, 100 µs using a Multiporator™, according to the manufacturer's instructions (*see* **Note 2**).
5. Place on ice for 5 min, then carefully pipet cells into a T-75 flask containing 10 mL of pre-warmed nonselective media, and place into a humidified 37°C, 10% CO_2 incubator.

3.2.2. Cell Culture

1. After 72 h, count the viable cells by trypan blue exclusion using a hemocytometer.
2. Dilute the transfected cells from each cuvet to a density of 5×10^4 cell/mL with selective media (glutamine-deficient), and pipet 10^3–10^4 cells in a volume of 200 µL into each well of ten 96-well plates (*see* **Note 3**).
3. Return plates to the incubator and leave undisturbed for 3 wk.
4. Using a bottom viewing mirror, mark wells containing single colonies.
5. When lightly confluent, determine antibody expression by removal of 100 µL of supernatant for an ELISA (*see* **Subheading 3.2.3.**) and refeed the clones. Score as either positive or negative.
6. When confluent, expand 96 of the positive wells into 24-well plates. A day prior to transfer, add 100 µL of fresh selective media, and the next day transfer to 24-well plates (2 mL). Refeed the 96-well plates as a backup.
7. When the 24-well plates are confluent, assay by ELISA for antibody quantitation.
8. Transfer the 24 highest producing clones to 6-well plates (in 3 mL selective media), and repeat quantitation assay.
9. Expand the 6–12 best stable producers into T-25 flasks (10 mL) and repeat quantitation assay.
10. At first available opportunity, freeze a limited number of cell-culture stocks in 20% FBS/ 10% DMSO at −80°C.
11. Select three clones, subclone by limiting dilution, adapt to 2% FBS or if possible serum-free conditions, and freeze stocks in liquid nitrogen.

3.2.3. ELISA

1. Coat 96-well plates with antigen, e.g., 100 µL of a 2 µg/mL N-A3 recombinant CEA fragment *(32)* in ELISA coating buffer overnight at 4°C.
2. Wash plates three times for 5 min with PBST, tap dry and block with 5% BSA/PBST for 1 h at room temperature.
3. Serially dilute culture supernatant and add 0.1 mL of each dilution to each well. Incubate at 37°C for 1 h, and wash three times with PBST.

4. Detect using secondary antibody conjugated to alkaline phosphatase (AP). The human C_H3 domain can be detected using anti-human Fc-AP at a 1:20,000 dilution. Wash plates three times in PBST, tap dry. Develop color by the addition of phosphatase substrate, wait 15–30 min and read absorbance using a ELISA plate reader. Serial dilutions of a standard (e.g., parental chimeric antibody) should be assayed at the same time.

3.3. Hollow Fiber Bioreactor Production

1. Set-up Cell Pharm 100 (CP100) bioreactor equipped with a single 1.5 sq. ft. hollow fiber Flowpath (mw exclusion 10 kDa). Use selective media supplemented with 2% FBS on the intracapillary space (ICS) and the extracapillary space (ECS). Monitor pH, glucose, lactate, and ammonia levels every other day. Make adjustments to the incoming O_2 and CO_2 levels to maintain the pH between 7–7.2. The ICS feed rate should be approx 2 L/wk and the recirculation rate should be 130 mL/min.
2. Inoculate 10^8 cells into the ECS.
3. Connect an Autoharvester to the ECS and initially collect two harvests/day for a total of 5 mL/d and gradually increase to 12 harvests/day for a total of 20 mL/d (*see* **Note 4**).

3.4. Purification of Minibodies

3.4.1. Processing of Bioreactor Harvest

1. Add to the bioreactor harvest a 50% slurry of DE 52/PBS to a final concentration of 5% (v/v).
2. Slowly rotate overnight at 4°C. Pour mixture into a 0.2 μm PES vacuum filter unit, allow the DE52 to settle, and apply the vacuum.
3. Repeat procedure using the anion exchanger, AG1-X8 for complete removal of phenol red.
4. Store material at 4°C until purification (*see* **Notes 5** and **6**).

3.4.2. Ceramic Hydroxyapatite (HA) Chromatography

1. Dialyze the supernatant against 10 vol of 50 m*M* MES, pH 6.5, three changes, overnight at 4°C.
2. Prepare HA column (2 cm id × 10 cm) by pre-equilibration with 50 m*M* MES, pH 6.5.
3. Apply the supernatant (2 mL/min), and wash until the absorbance at 280 nm returns to baseline.
4. Elute using a linear gradient from 0–0.04 *M* potassium phosphate, 50 m*M* MES, pH 6.5, over 20 column volumes (CV) at 5 mL/min collecting 10 mL fractions.
5. Analyze fractions by Coomassie blue-stained SDS-PAGE under nonreducing conditions. Pool minibody fractions and dilute with 4 vol of 50 m*M* HEPES, pH 7.4.

3.4.3. Anion Exchange Chromatography

1. Prepare a Source 15Q (1 cm id × 10 cm) by pre-equilibration with 50 m*M* HEPES, pH 7.4.
2. Apply the HA peak at 2.5 mL/min and wash with 50 m*M* HEPES, pH 7.4.
3. Elute by a linear gradient from 0–0.2 *M* NaCl, 50 m*M* HEPES, pH 7.4 over 20 CV.
4. Analyze fractions by SDS-PAGE, pool purified minibody, and dialyze against 20 m*M* sodium phosphate, pH 7.4, or PBS overnight at 4°C.
5. Concentrate the purified minibody to 8–20 mg/mL using a Centriprep-30.
6. Under aseptic conditions, filter the sample using an 0.2 μm filter.

3.5. Characterization of Expressed Minibody

3.5.1. SDS-PAGE

1. Electrophorese aliquots of sample along with molecular weight standards on precast SDS-PAGE gels under nonreducing conditions *(33)*.
2. Detect proteins by staining with Coomassie Blue.

3.5.2. Western-Blot Analysis

1. Electrotransfer a duplicate SDS-PAGE gel to nitrocellulose using established techniques *(34)*.
2. Use anti-human Fc AP antibody in 1:10,000 dilution as reporting antibody.
3. Develop blot in dark in development buffer.

3.5.3. Size-Exclusion Chromatography

1. Preequilibrate and standardize elution on a Superdex 75 column in PBS (0.5 mL/min).
2. Following chromatography under isocratic conditions, analyze aliquots of fractions.

3.5.4. Protein Determination

1. Determine initial protein concentrations by Bradford assay using bovine gamma globulin as a standard.
2. Determine final protein concentration by amino acid composition analysis.

3.5.5. Protein L Antibody Quantitation

1. Preequilibrate Protein L column (1 cm id × 2.5 cm h) in 50 mM sodium citrate, pH 7.4 (1 mL/min).
2. Inject 100 μL of sample, wash with 20 mM sodium citrate, 20 mM sodium phosphate, pH 7.4, 0.5 M NaCl (10 CV).
3. Elute with linear gradient from 100 mM sodium citrate to 100 mM citric acid (15 CV). Monitor absorbance at 280 nm and calculate the area of the minibody peak. A previously purified lot of protein (concentration determined by amino acid analysis) should be used as a standard.

3.5.6. Affinity Analysis by BIAcore

1. Biotinylate antigen using a kit such as the EZ-Link Sulfo-NHS-LC-Biotin kit (Pierce).
2. Immobilize to SA biosensor chip that result in a R_{max} of 250 response units.
3. Perform kinetic analysis on concentration of minibody (6.25–500 nM), regenerating the antigen surface between runs.
4. Calculate affinity using bivalent model of BIAevaluation 3.0 software.

4. Notes

1. When cloning antibody variable regions by RT-PCR, it is important to bear in mind that mutations can arise in any PCR reaction. A error occuring early in the amplification cycles can be propagated to many of the final clones. Thus, the DNA sequence must be determined from clones that have been generated in at least two independent RT-PCR reactions. Sequences should be checked to determine that endogenous kappa chain transcripts have not been cloned. Comparison with databases such as Kabat (immuno.bme.nwu.edu) will provide a useful indication as to whether the sequences cloned represent *bona fide* variable region genes.

2. Electroporation is the most common method for introduction of foreign genes into myeloma cells, and the majority of our work involving the expression of anti-CEA minibodies employed the Bio-Rad Gene Pulser II™. Subsequently the Eppendorf Multiporator™ was tested as an alternative, using buffers and conditions recommended by the manufacturer. While both instruments provided acceptable results, the Multiporator™ required 10-fold fewer cells, less DNA, and the hypo-osmotic buffer called for in the protocol allowed use of gentler electroporation conditions.

3. As the process of selecting a stable high-producing clone is time consuming, it is important to initially expand a sufficient number of independent clones to ensure that a stable producer is obtained. Typical production levels obtained in T-flasks were 20–50 µg/mL.

4. Production in the small hollow-fiber bioreactor (Unisyn CP100) usually resulted in a fivefold higher level of activity compared to T-flasks. Pilot runs produced between 100 and 300 mg of minibody in the harvested supernatant over a period of 2–4 mo. Scale-up production in a larger hollow-fiber bioreactor (Unisyn CP2000) resulted in gram quantities of crude minibody, ample for purification for pilot clinical trials.

5. An excellent general source of information on antibody purification can be found in *Purification Tools for Monoclonal Antibodies* by Pete Gagnon *(35)*.

6. The clarification steps (DE52 and AG1-X8) greatly enhanced the protein purification process. Reduction of cellular debris, DNA, and removal of the pH indicator dye, phenol red, have contributed to higher resolution and improved reproducibility of the chromatography steps. Chromatography conditions have been optimized for the anti-CEA minibody (p*I*, approx 5), and conditions may need to be modified depending on the p*I* and chromatographic properties of the protein of interest.

Acknowledgments

We are grateful to Chia-wei Cheung, Louise Shively, Cheryl Clark, and Giselle Tan for their expert technical assistance in developing the protocols outlined here. We also thank the many participants in the City of Hope Radioimmunotherapy Program for ongoing support and contributions. Funding was provided by National Institutes of Health grants CA 43904 and CA 33572.

References

1. Morrison, S. L., Johnson, J. M., Herzenberg, L. A., and Oi, V. T. (1984) Chimeric antibody molecules: Mouse antigen-binding domains with human constant region domains. *Proc. Natl. Acad. Sci. USA* **81,** 6851–6855.

2. Jones, P. T., Dear, P. H., Foote, J., Neuberger, M. S., and Winter, G. (1986) Replacing the complementarity-determining regions in a human antibody with those from a mouse. *Nature* **321,** 522–525.

3. Grillo-Lopez, A. J., White, C. A., Varns, C., Shen, D., Wei, A., Mcclure, A., and Dallaire, B. K. (1999) Overview of the clinical developent of rituximab: First monoclonal antibody approved for the treatment of lymphoma. *Seminars in Oncol.* **26,** 66–73.

4. Baselga, J., Tripathy, D., Mendelsohn, J., Baughman, S., Benz, C. C., Dantis, L., et al. (1996) Phase II study of weekly intravenous recombinant humanized Anti-p185[HER2] monoclonal antibody in patients with HER2/neu-overexpressing metastatic breast. *J. Clin. Oncol.* **14,** 737–744.

5. Junghans, R. P. (1997) Finally! The Brambell receptor (FcRB). Mediator of transmission of immunity and protection from catabolism for IgG. *Immunol. Res.* **16,** 29–57.

6. Bird, R. E., Hardman, K. D., Jacobson, J. W., Johnson, S., Kaufman, B. M., Lee, S. M., et al. (1988) Single-chain antigen-binding proteins. *Science* **242,** 423–426.

7. Huston, J. S., George, A. J. T., Adams, G. P., Stafford, W. F., Jamar, F., Tsai, M.-S., et al. (1996) Single-chain Fv radioimmunotargeting. *Q. J. Nuc. Med.* **40,** 320–323.

8. Begent, R. H. J., Verhaar, M. J., Chester, K. A., Casey, J. L., Green, A. J., Napier, M. P, et al. (1996) Clinical evidence of efficient tumor targeting based on single-chain Fv antibody selected from a combinatorial library. *Nature Med.* **2,** 979–984.

9. Larson, S. M., El-Shirbiny, A. M., Divgi, C. R., Sgouros, G., Finn, R. D., Tschmelitsch, J., et al. (1997) Single chain antigen binding protein (sFv CC49). First human studies in colorectal carcinoma metastatic to liver. *Cancer* **80,** 2458–2468.

10. Holliger, P., Prospero. T., and Winter, G. (1993) "Diabodies": Small bivalent and bispecific antibody fragments. *Proc. Natl. Acad. Sci. USA* **90,** 6444–6448.

11. Wu, A. M., Chen, W., Raubitschek, A. A., Williams, L. E., Fischer, R., Hu, S., et al. (1996) Tumor localization of anti-CEA single chain Fvs: Improved targeting by non-covalent dimers. *Immunotechnology* **2,** 21–36.

12. Adams, G. P., Schier, R., McCall, A. M., Crawford, R. S., Wolf, E. J., Weiner, L. M., and Marks, J. D. (1998) Prolonged *in vivo* tumour retention of a human diabody targeting the extracellular domain of human HER2/*neu*. *Br. J. Cancer* **77,** 1405–1412.

13. Pavlinkova, G., Beresford, G. W., Booth, B. J. M., Batra, S. K., and Colcher, D. (1999) Pharmacokinetics and biodistribution of engineered single-chain antibody constructs of MAb CC49 in colon carcinoma xenografts. *J. Nucl. Med.* **40,** 1536–1546.

14. Viti, F., Tarli, L., Giovannoni, L., Zardi, L., and Neri, D. (1999) Increased binding affinity and valence of recombinant antibody fragments lead to improved targeting of tumoral angiogenesis. *Cancer Res.* **59,** 347–352.

15. Hu, S., Shively, L., Raubitschek, A. A., Sherman, M., Williams, L. E., Wong, J. Y. C., et al. (1996) Minibody: A novel engineered anti-CEA antibody fragment (single-chain Fv-CH3) which exhibits rapid, high-level targeting of xenografts. *Cancer Res.* **56,** 3055–3061.

16. Pack, P. and Pluckthun, A. (1992) Miniantibodies: Use of amphipathic helices to produce functional, flexibly linked dimeric Fv fragments with avidity in *Escherichia coli*. *Biochemistry* **31,** 1579–1584.

17. Kostelny, S. A., Cole, M. S., and Tso, J. Y. (1992) Formation of a bispecific antibody by the use of leucine zippers. *J. Immunol.* **148,** 1547–1553.

18. Ridgway, J. B., Presta, L. G., and Carter, P. (1996) "Knobs-into-holes" engineering of antibody C_H3 domains for heavy chain heterodimerization. *Protein Eng.* **9,** 617–621.

19. Dübel, S., Breitling, F., Kontermann, R., Schmidt, T., Skerra, A., and Little, M. (1995) Bifunctional and multimeric complexes of streptavidin fused to single chain antibodies (scFv). *J. Immunol. Methods* **178,** 201–209.

20. Shively, J. E. and Beatty, J. D. (1985) CEA-related antigens: molecular biology and clinical significance. *Crit. Rev. Oncol. Hematol.* **2,** 355–399.

21. Hammarström, S. (1999) The carcinoembryonic antigen (CEA) family: structures, suggested functions and expression in normal and malignant tissues. *Semin. in Cancer Biol.* **9,** 67–81.

22. Goldenberg, D. M. and Larson, S. M. (1992) Radioimmunodetection in cancer identification. *J. Nucl. Med.* **33,** 803–814.

23. Goldenberg, D. M. (1993) Monoclonal antibodies in cancer detection and therapy. *Am. J. Med.* **94,** 297–312.

24. Buchegger, F., Haskell, C. M., Schreyer, M., Scazziga, B. R., Randin, S., Carrel, S., and Mach, J. P. (1983) Radiolabeled fragments of monoclonal antibodies against carcino-embryonic antigen for localization of human colon carcinoma grafted into nude mice. *J. Exp. Med.* **158,** 413–427.

25. Moffat, F. L. Jr., Pinsky, C. M., Hammershaimb, L., Petrelli, N. J., Patt, Y. Z., Whaley, F. S., and Goldenberg, D. M. (1996) Clinical utility of external immunoscintigraphy with the IMMU-4 technetium-99m Fab' antibody fragment in patients undergoing surgery for carcinoma of the colon and rectum: results of a pivotal, phase III trial. *J. Clin. Oncol.* **14,** 2295–2305.

26. Wu, A. M. and Yazaki, P. J.. (2000) Designer genes: recombinant antibody fragments for biological imaging. *Q. J. Nucl. Med.* **44,** 268–283.

27. Wu, A. M., Yazaki, P. J., Tsai, S., Nguyen, K., Anderson, A.-L., McCarthy, D. W., et al. (2000) High-resolution microPET imaging of carcinoembryonic antigen-positive xenografts using a copper-64 labeled engineered antibody fragment. *Proc. Natl. Acad. Sci. USA* **97,** 8495–8500.

28. Yazaki, P. J., Shively, L., Clark, C., Cheung, C.-W., Le, W., Szpikowska, B., et al. (2001) Mammalian expression and hollow fiber bioreactor production of recombinant anti-CEA diabody and minibody for clinical applications. *J. Immunol. Methods* **253,** 195–208.

29. Chirgwin, J. M., Przybyla, A. E., MacDonald, R. J., and Rutter, W. J.. (1979) Isolation of biologically active ribonucleic acid from sources enriched in ribonuclease. *Biochemistry* **18,** 5294.

30. Bebbington, C. R. 1991. Expression of antibody genes in nonlymphoid mammalian cells. *Methods Companion Methods Enzymol.* **2,** 136–145.

31. Bebbington, C. R., Renner, G., Thomson, S., King, D., Abrams, D., and Yarranton, G. T. (1992) High-level expresion of a recombinant antibody from myeloma cells using a glutamine synthetase gene as an amplifiable selectable marker. *Bio/Technology* **10,** 169–175.

32. You, Y. H., Hefta, L. J., Yazaki, P. J., Wu, A. M., and Shively, J. E. (1998) Expression, purification, and characterization of a two domain carcinoembryonic antigen minigene (N-A3) in *Pichia Pastoris*. The essential role of the N-domain. *Anticancer Res.* **18,** 3193–3202.

33. Laemmli, U. K. (1970) Cleavage of structural proteins during assembly of the head of bacteriophage T4. *Nature* **227,** 680–685.

34. Towbin, H., Staehlin, T., and Gordon, J. (1979) Electrophoretic transfer of proteins from polyacrylamide gels to nitrocellulose sheets: procedure and some applications. *Proc. Natl. Acad. Sci. USA* **76,** 4350–4354.

35. Gagnon, P. *Purification Tools for Monoclonal Antibodies*, Validated Biosystems, Inc., Tuscon, AZ, 1996.

22

Generation, Expression, and Monitoring of Recombinant Immune Receptors for Use in Cellular Immunotherapy

Andreas Hombach, Claudia Heuser, and Hinrich Abken

1. Introduction

Cellular immunotherapy has attracted increasing interest in genetic modification of immunologically competent cells in order to activate the effector cell after binding to predefined antigen. The chimeric immune-receptor strategy utilizes recombinant receptor molecules that are grafted on the surface of effector cells and comprise an extracellular antigen-binding domain and an intracellular signaling domain. The antigen-binding domain is a scFv (single-chain fragment of variable regions) derived from an antibody and is fused to a transmembrane moiety and an intracellular signaling domain that mediates cellular activation upon receptor crosslinking by binding of the scFv domain to antigen. This design of a chimeric receptor molecule combines the specific binding to predefined ligands with the initiation of intracellular signaling pathways for cellular activation (1).

We have generated a panel of chimeric receptor molecules that contain a scFv domain with specificity for a tumor-associated antigen and an intracellular signaling domain derived from the γ-chain of the high-affinity IgE receptor (FcεRIγ) or, alternatively, the CD3-ζ signaling chain of the T-cell receptor (TCR) complex (for review, see refs. 2,3). The antigen binding domain is fused directly or, alternatively, via a human IgG1-derived Fc domain to the transmembrane moiety. Expression of the recombinant receptor in T cells results in predetermined specificity of the grafted cell bypassing the major histocompatibility complex (MHC) restriction of target cell recognition.

Clinical application of the recombinant immune-receptor strategy requires highly efficient gene transfer into host cells and stable expression of the receptor in sufficient amounts on the cell surface. Retroviral gene transfer is currently the most efficient procedure to express heterologous molecules in primary lymphocytes. Because current retroviral gene transfer protocols result in high transduction rates, the majority of

From: *Methods in Molecular Biology, vol. 207: Recombinant Antibodies for Cancer Therapy: Methods and Protocols*
Edited by: M. Welschof and J. Krauss © Humana Press Inc., Totowa, NJ

recently developed retroviral vectors of the second generation lack selectable marker genes in order to reduce immunogenicity of transduced cells. In order to produce infectious retroviruses, producer cells are transfected with a MuLV-derived retroviral vector together with plasmid DNAs encoding retroviral helper functions. High titers of replication-deficient recombinant retroviruses are obtained from the supernatant of both stably and transiently transfected producer cells *(4)*. Transient production of recombinant retroviruses circumvents time-consuming generation of stable producer lines and dramatically reduces the probability of recombination events that increases significantly with prolonged cultivation periods and results in generation of replication competent retroviruses.

We here present step-by-step protocols for the generation of modular composed immune receptors, the retroviral transduction and expression of these receptors in peripheral blood T cells. The recombinant receptor molecules were primarily cloned into and expressed by the eukaryotic expression vector pRSVneo *(1)*. As shown in **Fig. 1**, the expression casssette contains the DNA sequences encoding an IgG kappa light chain leader peptid, a single chain antibody (scFv) with specificity for TNP (tri-nitro-phenyl), and the transmembrane and intracytoplasmatic part of the human IgE Fc receptor γ-chain or the TCR/CD3 ζ-chain, respectively. We substituted the anti-TNP-scFv domain by a number of scFv domains with specificity for tumor-associated antigens, e.g., CEA, CA19-9, CA72-4, CD30, melanoma-associated antigens (for review, *see* **ref. *3***). Some of the receptor molecules were additionally modified by insertion of a DNA sequence coding for the constant immunoglobulin CH2CH3 domain derived from the human IgG1 *(5–7)*. The expression cassettes for the recombinant immune receptors were inserted into the LXSN derived retroviral expression vector pBULLET. The 5' LTR U3 region in pBULLET was replaced by the CMV IE promotor *(4)*. To produce infectious retroviruses, DNA of the retroviral expression vector was cotransfected with DNA of the retroviral packaging plasmids pHIT60 and pCOLT *(4,7)* coding for the MuLV gag-, pol-, and the GALV env genes, respectively, into 293 cells. Infectious retroviruses produced after transient transfection of 293 cells were found to be suitable to transduce efficiently primary lymphocytes and to stably engraft T cells with chimeric receptor molecules for use in adoptive cellular immunotherapy.

2. Materials

1. DNA encoding a scFv antibody fragment of desired specificity. The scFv can be generated by phage-display techniques, e.g., utilizing the "Recombinant Phage Antibody System" (Amersham Pharmacia Biotech, Uppsala, Sweden).
2. dNTP-mix: 20 *mM* each of dATP, dCTP, dGTP and dTTP in ddH$_2$O (Roche Diagnostics, Mannheim, Germany). Store in aliquots at –20°C.
3. *Taq* polymerase and 10X PCR buffer (Roche Diagnostics).
4. Nucleic acid molecular size and quantitation standards (Life Technologies Ltd., Paisley, UK).
5. *Xba*I, *Bam*HI, *Bgl*II, *Nco*I restriction enzymes (Roche Diagnostics).
6. T4 DNA ligase and 10X ligase buffer (Roche Diagnostics).
7. Competent *E. coli* DH5a (Life Technologies Ltd.).
8. Cell lines: MD45 cells (murine T lymphocyte hybridoma cell line *[1]*); 293 cells (human embryonal kidney cell line, ATCC CRL 1573, American Type Culture Collection

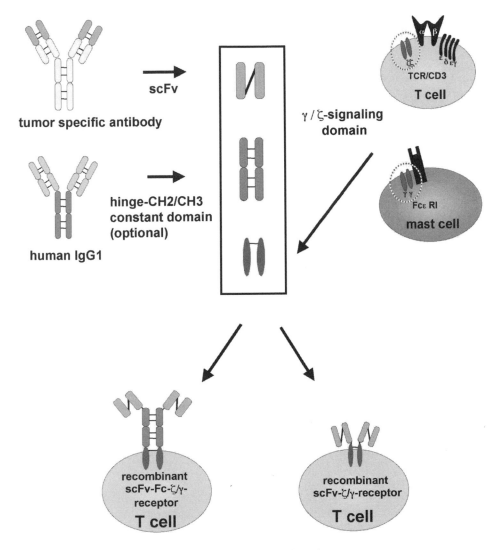

Fig. 1. Modular composition of recombinant immune receptors.

[ATCC], Rockville, MD); Jurkat cells (human T leukemia cell line, ATCC TIB 153, ATCC, Rockville, MD).

9. Culture medium and supplements: RPMI 1640 medium, DMEM, fetal calf serum (FCS), antibiotics (Life Technologies Ltd.)
10. Electroporation cuvets (Bio-Rad, Hercules, CA).
11. G418-stock solution: 50 mg/mL G418 (Sigma, St. Louis, MO) in PBS. Sterilize by passing through a 0.22-micron filter. Store in aliquots at 4°C.
12. Phosphate-buffered saline (PBS), pH 7.4: 8 g/L NaCl, 0.2 g/L KCl, 1.44 g/L Na_2HPO_4, 0.24 g/L KH_2PO_4. Adjust pH to 7.4 with NaOH and autoclave.

13. Calcium phosphate transfection reagents:
    Calcium Solution: 2 M CaCl$_2$. Dissolve 10.8 g of CaCl$_2$·6H$_2$O in 20 mL of distilled H$_2$O. Sterilize by passing through a 0.22-micron filter. Store in aliquots at –20°C. 2X HEPES-buffered saline (HBS): 280 mM NaCl, 1.5 mM Na$_2$HPO$_4$, 50 mM HEPES, pH 7.12 (!). To prepare 100 mL of solution dissolve 1.6 g NaCl, 0.027 g Na$_2$HPO$_4$·2H$_2$O, and 1 g of HEPES in 90 mL H$_2$O. Carefully adjust pH to 7.12 with 1 N NaOH and adjust volume to 100 mL with H$_2$O. Sterilize the solution by filtration through a 0.22-micron filter (*see* **Note 1**).

14. Plasticware (Nunc, Roskilde, Denmark).

15. Mitogenic anti-human CD3 MAb (OKT3 MAb derived from OKT3 hybridoma cells (ATCC CRL 8001, ATCC, Rockville, MD).

16. IL-2 (Roche Diagnostics).

17. Primary and secondary antibodies and detection reagents: Phycoerythin (PE)-conjugated anti-CD3 antibody (Dako, Hamburg, Germany), goat anti-human IgG1 Fc antibody, goat-anti-mouse IgG1 antibody, FITC-conjugated F(ab)'$_2$-goat-anti-human IgG1 Fc antibody (Southern Biotechnology, Malvern, PA), peroxidase-labeled streptavidin (Roche Diagnostics).

18. ELISA plates, e.g., PolySorb™ and MaxiSorb™ (both Nunc, Roskilde, Denmark).

19. Coating buffer for plastic-immobilization of antibodies: Mix 0.8 mL of 0.2 M NaHCO$_3$ solution (stock A) with 1.7 mL of 0.2 M Na$_2$CO$_3$ solution (stock B) and add ddH$_2$O to a final volume of 10 mL, pH 9.8. If required, scale up to a higher volume.

20. Washing buffer for use in ELISA: PBS + 1% (v/v) Tween-20 (Merck, Darmstadt, Germany).

21. Blocking buffer for use in ELISA: 3% (w/v) bovine serum albumin (BSA) in PBS + 1% (v/v) Tween-20.

22. Human IFN-γ ELISA reagents: e.g., anti-human IFN-γ capture MAb, biotinylated anti-human IFN-γ MAb, recombinant IFN-γ standard (all Endogen, Woburn, MA).

23. Peroxidase substrate solution: 1 mg/mL ABTS® in ABTS-substrate buffer (Roche Diagnostics).

24. Staining buffer for immunofluorescence: PBS containing 0.1% (v/v) NaN3 (optional plus 1% [w/v] BSA).

25. Propidium iodide: stock solution 1 mg/mL in ddH$_2$O.

26. Special laboratory equipment: cytofluorometer (FACScan™ cytofluorometer equipped with the Cellquest™ analysis software, Becton Dickinson, Mountain View, CA); thermocycler (OmniGene Thermocycler, MWG Biotech GmbH, Ebersberg, Germany); centrifuge with cooling and operation at >10,000g (Labofuge 5804 (R), Eppendorf, Hamburg, Germany); electroporation device (Gene Pulser II System, Bio-Rad, Hercules, CA); ELISA reader (MWG Biotech GmbH).

3. Methods

3.1. Generation of Expression Cassettes for Recombinant Receptors

Owing to the modular composition of receptor molecules, the antigen-binding and signaling domains can be replaced to generate a receptor with desired specificity and function (*see* **Fig. 1**). To generate the expression cassette coding for the recombinant receptor, we amplified the DNA coding for the scFv-, spacer-, and signaling domains, respectively, by polymerase chain reaction (PCR) techniques utilizing primer oligonucleotides (*see* **Tables 1–3**) that introduce restriction sites suitable for the subsequent cloning steps (*see* **Note 2**). The expression cassettes for the recombinant receptors are shown in **Fig. 2**.

3.1.1. PCR Amplification and Modification of the scFv DNA and pRSV-scFv-γ/ζ DNA

Isolation of mRNA from mouse spleen cells or hybridoma cells, respectively, was performed utilizing the Oligotex™ mRNA-purification system (Qiagen, Hilden, Germany). Synthesis of the cDNA, PCR amplification, and assembly of the immunoglobulin V_H- and V_L-regions and isolation of antigen-specific scFv was done by means of the "Recombinant Phage Antibody System" (Pharmacia) according to the manufacturer's recommendations. To amplify scFv generated by other systems the primer oligonucleotides described below (*see* **Table 1**) must be modified accordingly.

1. In a 0.5-mL PCR tube mix 10 ng of template DNA, 50 pmol of both the 5' and 3' primer oligonucleotides (*see* **Table 1**), 20 mM of each deoxynucleotide triphospate (dNTP-mix), 10 µL of 10X PCR buffer (Roche Diagnostics) and 1 U of *Taq* DNA polymerase (Roche Diagnostics) in a total volume of 100 µL.
2. Run PCR in an automatic thermocycler with an initial denaturation step for 2 min at 95°C followed by 30 cycles of 1 min denaturation at 94°C, 2 min annealing at 54°C, 2 min extension at 72°C. Finally, run 1 min denaturation at 94°C, 2 min annealing at 54°C, 4 min extension at 72°C.
3. Analyze 5 µL of the PCR reaction mixture by electrophoresis in a 1% agarose gel and visualize DNA to verify amplification. A DNA band of ~750 bp in size should be present indicating the desired scFv DNA.
4. Remove unincorporated primer oligonucleotides by gel filtration (e.g., utilizing S400 HR™-Columns, Pharmacia Amersham).
5. Digest 500–1000 ng of the scFv DNA and the pRSV-γ/ζ vector DNA (*see* **Note 3**), respectively, with 10 U of the restriction enzymes *Xba*I and *Bam*HI, respectively, and isolate the cleaved DNA fragments by preparative gel electrophoresis (*see* **Note 4**).

3.1.2. Ligation of scFv into the Mammalian Expression Vectors pRSV-γ/ζ

1. Estimate the amount of cleaved scFv DNA and pRSV-γ/ζ vector-DNA by agarose gel electrophoresis along with a standard of known DNA concentration (DNA Quantification standard, Life Technologies Ltd.).
2. Set up the ligation reaction by mixing vector DNA (50–200 ng DNA) and scFv DNA (we recommend a 1:1–1:3 molar ratio of vector:insert), 1 U of T4 DNA ligase (Roche Diagnostics) and 1 µL of 10X ligase buffer (Roche Diagnostics). Add ddH_2O to a final volume of 10 µL.
3. Incubate the ligation reaction for 16 h (overnight) at 12°C.
4. Transform the ligated DNA into competent *E. coli* DH5α cells according to Hanahan (*8*) (*see* **Note 5**).

3.1.3. Amplification, Modification, and Insertion of the DNA Encoding the Human IgG Fc Domain into the Expression Cassette of the Recombinant Receptor

Recombinant γ-chain receptors of the minimal design (scFv-trans-membrane domain-γ-signaling domain) are expressed and functionally active in peripheral blood T cells. In contrast to γ-chain receptors, recombinant ζ-chain receptors were found to

Table 1
Nucleotide Sequences of Primer Oligonucleotides Used for PCR Amplification of scFv DNA that is Clonedin the Phagemid Vector pCANTAB 5E[a]

Name	Sequence	T_m
V_H5'-$XbaI$	5'-[GCGGCCCAGT<u>CTAGA</u>ATGGCCCAG]-3' *XbaI*	60°C
E tag/V_L3'-$BamHI$1	5'-[GGTTCCAGC<u>GGATCC</u>GGATACGGC]-3' *BamHI*	64°C
HRS3-scFv/V_L3'-$BamHI$[b,c]	5'-[ACCT<u>GGATCC</u>GCCCGTTTGATTTCCAGC]-3' *BamHI*	56°C

[a]The scFv DNA is modified by introducing 5' the *XbaI* restriction site and 3' the *BamHI* site suitable for insertion into the mammalian expression vector pRSV-γ/ζ.

[b]ScFv that are amplified from pCANTAB5E by means of the E tag/V_L3'-*BamHI* oligonucleotide contain coding sequences for 9 amino acids of the E tag peptide (the complete sequence for the E-tag peptide is: *GCGGCCGCA GGTGCGCCGGTGCCGTATCCGGATCCGCTGGAACCGCGT*; the underlined sequence is incorporated into the sequence for the scFv-γ/ζ receptor; *italics* indicate a *NotI* and *BamHI* restriction site, respectively). This peptide is suitable as a minimal spacer domain of immune receptors of the scFv-γ type. For generation of scFv-Fc-γ/ζ receptors this peptide sequence may be deleted utilizing modified primer oligonucleotides.

[c]This oligonucleotide was used for cloning of the anti-CD30 HRS3-scFv into the scFv-Fc-γ/ζ receptor without the E-tag sequences (*7*). The *NotI* site of the E-tag sequence was mutated to *BamHI*.

Table 2

Nucleotide Sequences of Primer Oligonucleotides Used for PCR Amplification of the Human IgG1 Constant Hinge-Fc-Domain[a]

Name	Sequence	T_m
hIgG-5'*BamHI*	5'-[CTGAAGGATCCCGCCGAGCCCAAATCTCCTGACAAAACT]-3' BamHI	62°C
hIgG-3'*BglII*	5'-[CCCACCCAGATCTTTTTTACCCGGAGACAGGGAGAGGCTCTTCTG]-3' BglII	65°C

[a]The DNA coding for the human IgG hinge-Fc region is modified by adding restriction sites suitable for insertion of the DNA between the scFv DNA and signaling domain DNA.

Table 3

Primer Oligonucleotides for PCR Amplification of the DNA Encoding the Recombinant scFv-Fc-γ/ζ Receptors

Name	Sequence	T_m
Lκ-5'	5'-[CTACGTACCATGGATTTTCAGGTGCAGATTTTC]-3' NcoI	59°C
γ-3'	5'-[AAGATCTGATATCTGATCACTAGTCTAAAGCTACTGTGGTGGTTTCTCATG]-3' BglII EcoRV BclI SpeI	54°C
ζ-3'	5'-[GGCAGATCTGTCGACCTGTTAGCGAGGGGGCAGGG]-3' BglII SalI	59°C

[a]The expression cassettes for the recombinant receptors are modified by introducing restriction sites suitable for subcloning into the retroviral expression vector pBULLET.

A: Expression cassette of recombinant receptors in pRSV

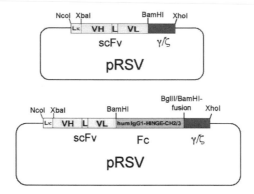

B: Expression cassette of recombinant receptors in pBULLET

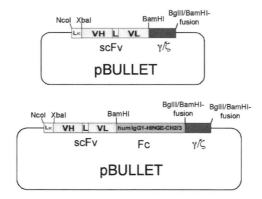

Fig. 2. Expression cassettes coding for recombinant immune receptors inserted into the mammalian expression vector pRSV (**A**) and in the MuLV-derived retroviral expression vector pBULLET (**B**).

require an additional spacer domain inserted between the scFv domain and the transmembrane domain for stable and functional expression *(3,9)*. We generated recombinant receptor molecules that are composed of the antigen-binding scFv-domain, the ζ- or γ-chain signaling domain and the human IgG1 hinge-Fc (CH2/3) constant domain inserted between the scFv and transmembrane domain. This type of receptor is functionally expressed in T cells. The extracellular constant IgG domain, moreover, can be used staining with an anti-human IgG Fc specific antibody to monitor recombinant receptor expression on the surface of T cells. This is a useful procedure for the detection of recombinant receptors when scFv-specific reagents, e.g., anti-idiotypic antibodies, are not available.

1. In a 0.5-mL-PCR tube mix 10 ng template DNA (*see* **Note 6**), 50 pmol of both the 5' and 3' primer oligonucleotides (*see* **Table 2**), 20 m*M* of each desoxynucleotide triphospate (dNTP-mix), 10 µL of 10X PCR buffer (Roche Diagnostics) and 1 U of *Taq* polymerase (Roche Diagnostics) in a total volume of 100 µL.
2. Run PCR in an automatic thermocycler and analyze the PCR product by agarose gel electrophoresis as described above (DNA encoding the IgG-hinge-Fc domain is about 800 bp in size).
3. Remove unincorporated primers by gel filtration (by utilizing MicroSpin™ Columns, Pharmacia).
4. Digest 500–1000 ng of the IgG hinge-Fc DNA with the restriction enzymes *Bam*HI and *Bgl*II (about 10 U each) and about 1000 ng of the pRSV-scFv-γ/ζ vector DNA with 10 U *Bam*HI (*see* **Note 7**). Isolate the cleaved DNA fragments by preparative gel electrophoresis (*see* **Note 4**).
5. Estimate the amount of cleaved scFv- and pRSV-γ/ζ vector DNA by agarose gel electrophoresis and set up the ligation reaction by mixing *Bam*HI digested vector-DNA and *Bam*HI/BglII digested IgG-hinge-Fc insert DNA (about 50–200 ng total DNA) as described in **Subheading 3.1.2.**
6. Transform the ligated DNA into competent cells (e.g., *E. coli* DH5α) as described in **Subheading 3.1.2.**

3.1.4. Generation of the Retroviral Expression Cassette Encoding the Recombinant Receptor

Retroviral gene transfer is the method of choice to express proteins in human lymphocytes. In order to express chimeric receptors in peripheral blood lymphocytes (PBL), the expression cassette encoding the scFv-(Fc)-γ chain or -ζ chain receptor can be transferred *in toto* into the retroviral expression vector pBULLET *(4)*. The DNA encoding the recombinant receptor (*see* **Fig. 2**) is amplified by PCR techniques utilizing modifying oligonucleotide primers that introduce a *Nco*I (5') and a *Bgl*II (3') restriction site (*see* **Table 3**). The amplified DNA is inserted into the *Nco*I/*Bam*HI sites of pBULLET DNA.

1. Set up PCR with oligonucleotide primers (*see* **Table 3**) as described in **Subheading 3.1.3.** The scFv-γ receptor is about 1 kb in size, the scFv-Fc-γ DNA is about 2 kb, the scFv-Fc-ζ DNA is about 2.2 kb in size)
2. Purify amplified DNA, digest DNA (about 500–1000 ng) with *Nco*I and *Bgl*II (about 10 U each). Digest the retroviral vector DNA pBULLET (about 500–1000 ng) with *Nco*I and *Bam*HI (10 U each). Purify digested DNAs as described in **Subheading 3.1.1.**
3. Ligate the *Nco*I/*Bgl*II digested DNA encoding the recombinant receptor into the *Nco*I/*Bam*HI cleaved pBULLET vector DNA as described in **Subheading 3.1.2.** Herewith, a *Bgl*II/*Bam*HI fusion site is created (*see* also **Note 7**).
4. Transform competent *E. coli* bacteria (e.g., DH5α) as described in **Subheading 3.1.2.**

3.2. Expression of Recombinant Receptors

3.2.1. Stable Expression of Recombinant Receptors in T-Cell Lines

After DNA transfection, we stably expressed recombinant receptors on the surface of murine MD45 T cells *(1)*. The protocol described in the following steps, however, may also be suitable for a transfection of a number of human T-cell lines including Jurkat.

1. Wash MD45 cells once in RPMI 1640 medium containing 10% (v/v) FCS (referred here as complete medium).
2. Resuspend 5×10^7 cells/mL complete medium.
3. Transfer 0.8 mL of cell suspension into an electroporation cuvet with 0.4 cm gap (0.4 cm cuvets, Bio-Rad) and keep on ice.
4. Add pRSV-scFv-(Fc)-γ/ζ DNA (50–100 µg), mix, and keep on ice for 20 min.
5. Place the cuvet into the electroporation chamber and treat the cells with one pulse at 250 V and 2400 µF (*see* **Note 8**).
6. Transfer the cells immediately to a culture flask containing 10 mL of complete medium. Allow the cells to stand at room temperature for 10 min and incubate for 48 h at 37°C in a humidified atmosphere with 5% CO_2.
7. Add an equal volume of selective medium containing the neomycin analogue G418 (final concentration 2 mg/mL).
8. Plate the cells onto 96-well TC-plates (200 µL/well) (Nunc), incubate at 37°C in a humidified atmosphere with 5% CO_2. Isolate individual colonies that stably express the chimeric receptor.

3.2.2. Transient Expression of the Recombinant Receptor in 293 Cells

Expression of successfully assembled recombinant receptor molecules can be rapidly tested after transient transfection of 293 cells.

1. Plate 2×10^6 293 cells in 10 mL DMEM supplemented with 10% (v/v) FCS (referred to as complete medium) 24 h prior to transfection into 100-mm-culture dishes and culture overnight at 37°C in a humidified atmosphere with 10% CO_2.
2. Feed cells 3 h before transfection with fresh complete medium.
3. For each 100-mm-culture dish prepare 0.5 mL of calcium chloride-DNA suspension as follows: Dissolve the plasmid DNA coding for the recombinant receptor (20 µg DNA of pBULLET or pRSV; *see* **Note 9**) in 440 µL (final volume) sterile H_2O. Add 60 µL of calcium chloride solution and mix gently (*see* **Note 1**).
4. Place 0.5 mL of 2X HBS, sufficient for one 100-mm-culture dish, into a sterile 1.5-mL tube. Bubble the 2X HBS solution using a mechanical pipettor attached to a 1 mL plastic pipet and add the calcium chloride/DNA suspension dropwise. A fine precipitate should become visible. Allow the solution to stand for 20 min at room temperature, finally vortex (*see* **Note 10**).
5. Add the precipitate to the culture dish and gently mix the culture medium by agitating the plate several times.
6. Incubate the cells overnight at 37°C in humidified atmosphere with 10% CO_2.
7. Replace 10 mL of medium by fresh complete medium and incubate for additional 2 d.
8. Harvest the cells and analyze for recombinant receptor expression.

3.3. Co-Transfection of 293 Cells with Retroviral Vector DNA and Plasmid DNA Encoding Helper Functions for Transient Generation of Amphotropic Retrovirus

3.3.1. Isolation and Activation of T Cells

1. Dilute heparinisized peripheral blood or alternatively the content of a buffy coat 1:1 with PBS.
2. Overlay 15 mL of Ficoll-Paque solution containing 5.7 % (w/v) Ficoll 400 and 9% (w/v) sodium diatrizoate (Ficoll-Paque PLUS, Amersham Pharmacia Biotech, Upsala, Sweden) with 30 mL diluted blood in a 50 mL conical tube.

3. Spin the density gradient at 400g for 30 min at room temperature (switch off the brake!). The mononuclear cells will focus in the interface between plasma and Ficoll-solution.
4. Remove most of the plasma and collect the mononuclear cells carefully from the interface and wash the cells three times in PBS (*see* **Note 11**).
5. Resuspend the cells at a density of 1–2 × 10^6 cells/mL in RPMI 1640 medium supplemented with 10% (v/v) FCS [alternatively human serum (HS)], 200 U/mL IL-2, and 100 ng/mL anti-CD3 antibody (OKT3).
6. Culture the cells for 2 d at 37°C in a humidified atmosphere with 5% CO_2.
7. Collect the cells, wash twice with complete medium and resuspend in RPMI 1640 medium supplemented with 10% FCS (alternatively HS) and 200 U/mL IL-2.
8. Start co-culture with co-transfected producer cells as described below, alternatively co-culture with retrovirus-containing cell-free supernatant for several days (*see* **Note 12**).

3.3.2. Co-Transfection of 293 Cells with Retroviral Vector DNA and Helper Plasmid DNA

This protocol is used for transient generation of GALV-pseudotyped amphotropic retroviruses that are secreted into the culture supernatant upon co-transfection of the retroviral vector DNA and helper plasmid DNAs encoding the MuLV *gag-*, *pol-*, and GALV-*env* genes *(4)* (*see* **Fig. 3**) (*see* **Note 13**).

1. Plate 1–2 × 10^6 293 cells in 10 mL DMEM containing 10% (v/v) FCS into 100-mm-culture dishes 24 h prior to co-transfection. Culture cells overnight at 37°C in a humidified atmosphere with 10% CO_2.
2. Feed cells 3 h before co-transfection with fresh DMEM medium, 10% (v/v) FCS.
3. For each 100-mm-dish prepare 0.5 mL of calcium phosphate-DNA precipitate as follows: Dissolve 7 µg DNA of the pBULLET vector coding for the recombinant receptor and 7 µg DNA each of the helper plasmids pCOLT and pHIT60 *(4)* coding for MuLV *gag-*, *pol*, and GALV *env* helper functions (*see* **Note 14**) in 440 µL (final volume) sterile H_2O. Add 60 µL of calcium chloride solution and mix gently. Scale up accordingly for transfection of more than one 100-mm-dish with the same construct.
4. Place 0.5 mL of 2X HBS into a sterile 1.5-mL tube. Use a mechanical pipettor attached to a 1-mL plastic pipet and bubble the 2X HBS solution, meanwhile add the calcium chloride/DNA suspension dropwise. A fine precipitate should become visible. Scale up accordingly for transfection of more than one 100-mm-dish. Incubate the solution for 20 min at room temperature and subsequently vortex.
5. Add the precipitate to the culture medium and gently mix by agitating the plate several times (*see* **Note 1**).
6. Incubate the cells overnight at 37°C in a humidified atmosphere with 10% CO_2.
7. Replace the medium and add 3 × 10^6 preactivated T cells in 10 mL of fresh RPMI 1640 medium supplemented with 10% FCS (alternatively human serum) and 100 U/mL IL-2.
8. Co-culture for 36 h as described above, recover T cells by careful aspiration of the medium. Analyze the cells for receptor expression by immunofluorescence.

3.4. Monitoring of Recombinant Receptor Expression and Function

3.4.1. Flow Cytometric Analysis of Cells Expressing the Recombinant Receptor

1. Pipet transfected 293 cells or transduced T cells (approx 2 × 10^5 cells) into a 4-mL polypropylen test tube.

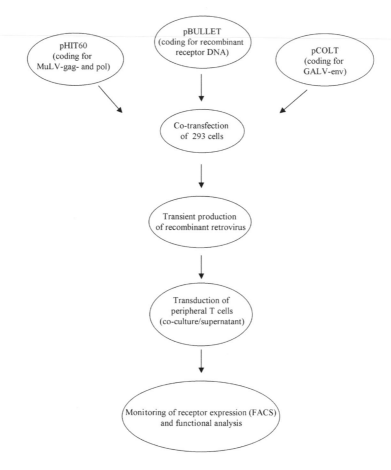

Fig. 3. Flow chart illustrating the strategy of expression and monitoring of chimeric receptors in peripheral blood T cells for use in adoptive immunotherapy.

2. Centrifuge the cell suspension for 3 min at 400g, discard supernatant by inversion of the tube, and wash the cells once in ice-cold PBS.
3. Discard the washing solution and resuspend the cells in 100 μL of staining buffer containing an appropriate dilution of a fluorochrome-conjugated anti-human IgG1 Fc antibody (e.g., F(ab)$_2$ goat-anti-human IgG1-FITC, 1:100 diluted in PBS; Southern Biotechnology, Malvern, PA). Vortex test tubes prior to incubation!
4. Incubate 30 min on ice.
5. Wash the cells twice with ice-cold PBS.
6. Discard the washing solution, resuspend the cells in 100 μL of staining buffer containing 1 μg/mL propidium iodide (1:1000 dilution of a 1 mg/mL stock solution in ddH$_2$O, Sigma). Analyze cells by flow cytometry. To exclude dead cells, set appropriate life gates prior to analysis (*see* **Note 15**).

3.4.2. Functional Analysis of Recombinant Receptor Grafted T Cells

Receptor-grafted T cells are activated in a MHC-independent fashion upon antigen-specific receptor crosslinking resulting in T cell proliferation, secretion of certain cytokines, and efficient target cell lysis. Here we give a protocol to monitor receptor-mediated cellular activation based on secretion of IFN-γ into the culture supernatant by activated T cells.

3.4.2.1. IFN-γ SECRETION OF scFv-Fc-γ/ζ RECEPTOR GRAFTED T CELLS UPON CROSSLINKING BY A PLASTIC IMMOBILIZED ANTI-HUMAN IgG1 Fc ANTIBODY

1. Prepare a solution of 10 μg/mL of an anti-human IgG1 Fc antibody and, for control, of an anti-mouse IgG1 antibody (Southern Biotechnology) in coating buffer and pass through a 0.2-μm filter.
2. Coat the wells of an ELISA plate (PolySorp™, Nunc) with the diluted antibody (50 μL/well) and incubate overnight at 4°C.
3. Aspirate the antibody solution and wash the plate three times with 200 μL/well sterile PBS.
4. Wash transduced T cells three times with RPMI 1640 medium to remove residual IL-2 and resuspend $0.5–1 \times 10^6$ cells per mL in RPMI 1640 medium, 10% FCS.
5. Add $1–2 \times 10^5$ lymphocytes in 200 μL/well to the coated microtiter plate and incubate for 48 h at 37°C.
6. Analyze 100 μL of cell free supernatant per well for IFN-γ as described below.

3.4.2.2. IFN-γ SECRETION OF RECOMBINANT RECEPTOR GRAFTED T CELLS UPON CO-CULTURE WITH ANTIGEN EXPRESSING TARGET CELLS

Specific, MHC-independent signaling of receptor grafted T cells upon binding to antigen can be monitored by coculture of grafted T cells with allogenic or autologeous tumor cells that express the antigen recognized by the scFv domain of the receptor.

1. Wash transduced T cells and, for control, non-transduced T cells three times with RPMI 1640 medium to remove residual IL-2 and resuspend 2×10^6 cells per mL RPMI 1640 medium, 10% FCS.
2. Suspend target cells, that express the antigen recognized by the receptor, in RPMI 1640 medium, 10% FCS (5×10^5 cells/mL).
3. Prepare serial dilutions of the effector T cells in 96-well round-bottom microtest plates starting from 2×10^5 cells in 100 μL medium/well.
4. Add a 100-μL-suspension of target cells (i.e., 5×10^4 cells/well) to effector cells and incubate for 48 h at 37°C.
5. Remove 100 μL/well of the supernatant and analyze for IFN-γ as described below.

3.4.2.3. HUMAN IFN-γ ELISA

1. Prepare a dilution of an anti-human IFN-γ antibody (e.g., 1 μg/mL mouse anti-human IFN-γ antibody, Endogen, Woburn, MA) in coating buffer.
2. Coat the wells of an ELISA plate (MaxiSorp™, Nunc) with the anti-human IFN-γ antibody (capture antibody) (100 μL/well) and incubate overnight at 4°C.
3. Discard the antibody coating solution, wash plate three times with washing buffer (3 × 200 μL/well) and incubate for at least 2 h at room temperature with blocking buffer (200 μL/well).

4. Wash once with washing buffer (200 µL/well).
5. Prepare a standard of IFN-γ concentration (e.g., recombinant human IFN-γ, Endogen) with serial dilutions of 20 ng IFN-γ /mL in RPMI 1640 medium, 10% FCS. Add 100 µL of cell culture supernatant and of standard dilution, respectively, per well. Optional apply dilutions of the cell-culture supernatant in RPMI 1640 medium, 10% FCS. Incubate for 2 h at room temperature.
6. Discard the supernatants and wash five times with washing buffer (200 µL/well).
7. Add 100 µL of a biotin-conjugated anti-human IFN-γ detection antibody (biotinylated mouse anti-human IFN-γ antibody, Endogen) (0.5 µg/mL) and incubate for 1 h at room temperature.
8. Repeat **step 6**.
9. Add 100 µL of peroxidase labeled streptavidin (e.g., 1:10,000 dilution in PBS, Roche Diagnostics) and incubate for 30 min at room temperature.
10. Repeat **step 6**.
11. Prepare the peroxidase substrate solution (ABTS®, Roche Diagnostics) according to the manufacturer's recommendation and add 100 µL peroxidase substrate solution per well to the test plate. Incubate for at least 30 min. Record OD photometrically at 405 nm utilizing an ELISA reader. A positive reaction is indicated by green color.

4. Notes

1. We routinely use the calcium phosphate transfection kit (Life Science, Life Technologies) for transfection of 293 cells. Alternatively, transfections can be performed utilizing nonliposomal reagents (e.g., FuGENE®, Roche Diagnostics) according to the manufacturer's recommendations. We found that the FuGENE® protocol also works for transient receptor expression as well as transient production of retroviruses by 293 cells.
2. DNA coding for the spacer and signaling domains can also be directly amplified by RT-PCR from mRNA of appropriate cells, for example, Jurkat cells (human T leukemia cell line, ATCC TIB 153, ATCC), can be used to amplify the CD3 ζ-chain, TPH-1 cells (ATCC TIB202, ATCC), to amplify the FcεRI γ-chain and B cells from peripheral blood to amplify the IgG hinge-Fc domains. The mRNA can be prepared as described in **Subheading 3.1.1.**, cDNA can be generated from mRNA of these cells utilizing random oligonucleotide primers according to the manufacturer's recommendations (e.g., TimeSaver™ cDNA synthesis kit, Amersham Pharmacia Biotech, Uppsala, Sweden), and the cDNA encoding the spacer and signaling domains can specifically be amplified utilizing the primer oligonucleotides listed below (*see* **Tables 3** and **4**). Alternatively, specific DNA can be directly amplified from the mRNA via a RT-PCR-system (e.g., Titan One Tube RT-PCR System, Roche Diagnostics) according to the manufacturer's recommendation.
3. To create recombinant scFv-γ/ζ receptors, the cleaved scFv DNA fragments are inserted into pRSV-γ/ζ DNA. The pRSV-(anti-TNP)scFv-γ/ζ expression vector (*1*) contains a murine IgG kappa light-chain leader and an anti-TNP scFv that are fused to DNA coding for the transmembrane and intracellular part of the γ-chain signaling subunit of the human high-affinity IgE receptor (FcεRIγ) or the ζ-chain signaling subunit of CD3ζ, respectively. The DNA coding for the anti-TNP scFv can be removed by *Xba*I and *Bam*HI digestion. Owing to the neomycin-resistance gene, transfected cells that express the recombinant receptor can be selected.
4. Isolation of DNA restriction fragments from the agarose gels can be done using commercially available purification systems (e.g., QIAquick™ Gel Extraction Kit, Qiagen GmbH).

Table 4
Primer Oligonucleotides for PCR Amplification of the DNA Encoding the Human CD3 ζ- and FcRI γ-Chain[a]

Name	Sequence	T_m
Lκ-scFv-5[b]	5'-[GTA<u>CCATGG</u>ATTTTCAGGTGCAGATTTTCAGCTTCCTGCTAA *Nco*I	
	TCAGTGCCTCAGTCATAGCGGGCCCAGT<u>CTAGA</u>ATGGCCCAGG]-3' *Xba*I	60°C
γ-5'2[c]	5'-[AGCG<u>GGATCC</u>TCAGCTCTGCTATATCCTGGATGCCATCC]-3' *Bam*HI	60°C
ζ-5'2[c]	5'-[GCT<u>GGATCCC</u>AAACTCTGCTACCTGCTGGATGGA]-3' *Bam*HI	57°C

[a]The primers can be used for RT-PCR amplification and for amplification from a cDNA pool that was generated by reverse transcription utilizing random oligonucleotides. We additionally list the sequence for an oligonucleotide (Lκ-scFv-5') that 5' includes a DNA sequence coding for the Ig κ light-chain leader peptide suitable for scFv expression in mammalian cells.
[b]The Lκ-scFv-5' primer can be combined with the E tag/V$_L$3'-*Bam*HI oligonucleotide as listed in **Table 1**.
[c]These primer oligonucleotides can be combined with the γ-3'- and ζ-3' oligonucleotides listed in **Table 3**.

5. A detailed protocol for the generation of competent *E. coli* DH5α and transformation of plasmid DNA is described by Sambrook et al. *(8)*.

6. The cDNA sequence encoding the human IgG1 CH2CH3 constant region is amplified by PCR techniques utilizing the plasmid SCADCLCH1 *(9)* as template and primer oligonucleotides that introduce 5' a *Bam*HI and 3' a *Bgl*II restriction site (*see* **Table 2**).

7. DNA restriction with *Bam*HI and *Bgl*II generates compatible 3' DNA extensions that can be ligated to the *Bam*HI site of pRSV-scFv-γ/ζ DNA. Because ligation of a *Bgl*II restriction site into a *Bam*HI site destroys the *Bam*HI restriction site, the orientation of the inserted IgG-hinge-Fc DNA can easily be tested by appropriate restriction analysis.

8. These electroporation conditions work well with MD45 T cells and may also work with Jurkat cells. However, optimal voltage and capacity of the pulse must be determined individually for each cell line.

9. We routinely use the retroviral vector pBULLET to express the chimeric receptor. However, we found that this protocol works with similar efficiency utilizing the mammalian expression vector pRSV *(1)* that expresses the coding DNA under control of the RSV LTR.

10. Scale up accordingly for transfection of more than one 100-mm dish with the same construct.

11. We routinely depleted the number of monocytes by plastic adherence as follows: Ficoll-isolated mononuclear cells were resuspended in RPMI 1640 medium without serum (about 5×10^6 cells/mL) and incubated in 150 mm tissue culture plates for 1 h at 37°C. Nonadherent cells were collected, counted, and activated as described in **Subheading 3.3.1.**

12. Transduction with cell free supernatant generally results in lower transduction efficiencies than transduction by co-culture with virus-producing cells. To improve transduction rates, we recommend to culture activated T cells for 3 d in virus-containing supernatant replacing the medium every day by virus-containing medium, which is freshly generated and diluted 1:1 in RPMI 1640 medium, 10% FCS or HS, or in AIM V medium (Life Technologies).

13. Production and handling of recombinant amphotropic retrovirus fall within the NIH-Biosafety Level 2 criteria or corresponding national guidelines. Please inform yourself about the appropriate safety guidelines before starting to work. Most potential hazards can be avoided by good tissue-culture techniques.

14. According to the protocol described in **Subheading 3.3.2.**, infectious retrovirus can also be generated by utilizing any MuLV-derived retroviral expression vector (Stratagene, LaJolla, CA) and the commercially available helper plasmids pVPack-GP and pVPack-10A1 (both Stratagene).

15. We identified transduced T cells by double immunofluorescence by simultaneous incubation with an phycoerytin (PE)-conjugated anti-CD3 antibody (Dako) and a FITC-conjugated anti-human IgG Fc antibody (Southern Biotechnology). Recombinant receptors without an extracellular spacer domain must be detected by reagents with specificity for the scFv antigen-binding domain, e.g., an anti-idiotypic antibody. We identified transduced T cells that harbor this type of recombinant receptor by simultaneous staining with 10 μg/mL of a scFv-specific anti-idiotypic MAb (IgG1) and 5 μg/mL of the anti-CD3 MAb OKT3 (IgG2a). Bound antibodies were detected by a FITC-conjugated F(ab)'$_2$ goat-anti-mouse IgG1 and a PE-conjugated F(ab)'$_2$ goat-anti-mouse IgG2a antibody, respectively (each diluted 1:1,000, Southern Biotechnology).

References

1. Eshhar, Z., Waks, T., Gross, G., and Schindler, D. G. (1993) Specific activation and targeting of cytotoxic lymphocytes through chimeric single chains consisting of antibody-binding domains and the or subunits of the immunoglobulin and T-cell receptors. *Proc. Natl. Acad. Sci. USA* **90,** 720–724.
2. Abken, H., Hombach, A., Reinhold, U., and Ferrone, S. (1998) Can combined T cell- and antibody-based immunotherapy outsmart tumor cells? *Immunol. Today* **19,** 2–5.
3. Hombach, A., Pohl, C., Reinhold, U., and Abken, H. (1999) Grafted T cells with tumor specificity: the chimeric receptor strategy for use in immunotherapy of malignant disease. *Hybridoma* **18,** 57–61.
4. Weijtens, M. E., Willemsen, R. A., Hart, E. H., and Bolhuis, R. L. (1998) A retroviral vector system 'STITCH' in combination with an optimized single chain antibody chimeric receptor gene structure allows efficient gene transduction and expression in human T lymphocytes. *Gene Ther.* **5,** 1195–1203.
5. Hombach, A., Sircar, R., Heuser, C., Tillmann, T., Diehl, V., Kruis, W., et al. (1998) Chimeric anti-TAG72 receptors with immunoglobulin constant Fc domains and gamma or zeta signaling chains. *Int. J. Mol. Med.* **2,** 99–103.
6. Hombach, A., Koch, D., Sircar, R., Heuser, C., Diehl, V., Kruis, W., et al. (1999) A chimeric receptor that selectively targets membrane-bound carcinoembryonic antigen (mCEA) in the presence of soluble CEA. *Gene Ther.* **6,** 300–304.
7. Hombach A., Heuser C., Gerken M., Fischer B., Lewalter K., Diehl V., et al. (2000) T cell activation by recombinant FcepsilonRI gamma-chain immune receptors: an extracellular spacer domain impairs antigen-dependent T cell activation but not antigen recognition. *Gene Ther.* **7,** 1067–1075.
8. Sambrook, J., Fritsch, E. F., and Maniatis, T. (1989) *Molecular Cloning: A Laboratory Manual*, 2nd ed, Cold Spring Harbor Laboratory, Cold Spring Harbor Press, NY.
9. Moritz D. and Groner B. (1995) A spacer region between the single chain antibody- and the CD3 zeta-chain domain of chimeric T cell receptor components is required for efficient ligand binding and signaling activity. *Gene Ther.* **2,** 539–546.

23

Tailoring Natural Effector Functions

Antibody Engineering Beyond Humanization

Ole H. Brekke and John E. Thommesen

1. Introduction

A large number of new biological drugs in clinical development from the biotechnology industry are based on recombinant antibodies. The Food and Drug Administration (FDA) has recently approved several of these drugs including reagents against cancer *(1,2)*, transplant rejection *(3)*, rheumatoid arthritis, and Crohn's diseases *(4,5)* as well as antiviral prophylaxis *(6)*. At present 30% of all biological proteins in application for FDA approvals are recombinant antibodies. Some are based on fusions of murine variable regions with human constant region, called chimeric antibodies. Others are more sophisticated being "humanized" from their mouse monoclonal parent molecule, whereas more recently full human antibodies from phage antibody libraries have been generated *(7)*.

Therapeutic antibodies are used in a variety of ways such as blocking reagent, crosslinkers for intracellular signaling or as direct targeting agents for the subsequent elimination of the target cell. Targeting antibodies should either carry effector moieties such as toxins and radionuclides, or they can possess optimized natural effector functions. A series of publications have revealed binding sites and structural requirements for binding and activation of the complement system as well as the interaction with cellular Fc-receptors *(8–14)*. This information gives us the opportunity to design novel human IgG molecules with predetermined effector functions, e.g., one can envisage the design of antibodies with only Fc-receptor (i.e., antibody-dependent cell-mediated cytotoxicity [ADCC], and phagocytosis) binding capacities, rendering the complement activation impossible. On the contrary, even cytolytic antibodies with strong complement activation potential can be generated *(15,16)*.

Antibody-dependent complement mediated lysis (ADCML) is initiated by the binding of two or more IgGs to the surface of target cells, followed by a multivalent inter-

From: *Methods in Molecular Biology, vol. 207: Recombinant Antibodies for Cancer Therapy: Methods and Protocols*
Edited by: M. Welschof and J. Krauss © Humana Press Inc., Totowa, NJ

action between the IgGs and C1q *(17)*. C1q is part of C1, the first component of the complement cascade. Although it is generally accepted that recognition of IgG by C1q occurs via a site in the C_H2 domain *(18–22)*, the precise location of the amino acids constituting the site is still a matter of debate. However, a few main requirements can be listed: the two heavy chains must be disulfide bound *(16,23)*, the C_H2 domains must be glycosylated *(24)*, and they must have paired C_H3 domains because their removal reduces complement activation by 50% below optimum *(25)*. Thus, only intact glycosylated IgG molecules can activate complement.

The systematic mutagenesis of accessible charged residues in the C_H2 domain of mouse IgG2b and a peptide mimic assay have revealed that three residues, Glu-318, Lys-320, and Lys-322 (EU numbering), constitute an essential binding motif *(8)*. The residues are conserved in all human IgGs and most of all mouse, rat, rabbit, and guinea pig IgGs. No obvious correlation exists between primary structure and complement fixing ability. For example, the "inactive" isotypes, human IgG4 and mouse IgG1 contain the motif, yet they bind C1q very weakly and are also poor complement activators. An earlier view that the hinge region might be modulating effector functions has been strongly disputed *(13)*, and it now appears that for human IgG4 individual amino acids in the C_H2 domain is responsible for the lack of activity *(10)*.

The following protocols should be read as examples only for the engineering of human effector functions, implying that your own oligonucleotides, polymerase chain reaction (PCR) conditions, and so on, should be applied for your experiments. The protocols are optimized in our lab for the purpose of altering the constant heavy-chain genes of human IgG1, IgG3, and IgG4 for the detection of structural parts that are involved in complement activation. The engineered antibodies are expressed in the mouse myeloma cell line J558L. All the antibodies show specificity to the hapten NIP. All alterations being made are addressed to the human Fc part of the IgG molecules and thus serve as model antibodies for the study of human IgG effector functions.

2. Materials

2.1. PCR-Mutagenesis

1. 1 *M* NaOH, 0.1 *M* HCL.
2. 1.5 mL Tubes and 0.2 mL PCR tubes (Eppendorf).
3. *Vent* DNA polymerase (New England Biolabs).
4. Streptavidin coated magnetic beads M280 (Dynal, Oslo, Norway).
5. Oligonucleotides were synthesized at Eurogentec.

Frw-CH2-biotin	5'bio-GAC AGG TGC CCT AGA GTG GC
Rev-CH2-biotin	5'bio-CAC TCC ACG GCG ATG TCG TC
K322A, forward primer	5'GAG TAC AGG TGC **gc**G GTC TCC AAC
K322A, reverse primer	5'GGT GGA GAC **Cgc G**CA CTT GTA CTC

Mismatches are shown in lower case letters, restriction sites are bold.

2.2. Purification of Digested PCR Products

1. 96% EtOH, 70% EtOH.
2. *Sac*II (New England Biolabs).

3. Centriflex™ Protein cartridges (Advanced Genetic Technologies Corp.).
4. Streptavidin (Boehringer Mannheim).

2.3. Cloning into the Mammalian Expression Vector pLNOH₂

1. *Bst*UI and Phosphatase (New England Biolabs).
2. Ampicillin (Sigma).

2.4. Antibody Expression in J558L Cells

1. Maxisorp 96-well plates (NUNC, Roskilde, Denmark).
2. 10- and 75-mL screw-cap incubator flasks, 24- and 96-well cell-culturing plates, 10- and 25-mL pipets (Greiner).
3. BTX sterile 4 mm electroporation cuvets. (BTX, Genetronics Inc.).
4. RPMI 1640 medium, fetal calf serum (FCS), streptomycin, penicillin, and Geneticine™ (Neomycine, G418-sulphate) (Gibco).
5. Sepharose 4B (Pharmacia).

3. Methods
3.1. PCR-Mutagenesis (see Fig. 1)

1. The first two sets of PCR reactions (**Fig. 1B**) are set up with 10 ng template IgG3 (*see* **Note 1**), 200 µ*M* dNTPs, with 2 U *Vent* DNA polymerase in 1X Thermopol buffer and 20 pmol of each primer sets (*see* **Notes 2** and **3**) Frw-CH2-biotin/ K322A, forward primer and Rev-CH2-biotin/ K322A, reverse primer. The reactions are mixed to a final volume of 50 µL and run for 20 cycles at 95°C, 30 s, 52°C, 30 s, and 72°C 30 s.
2. The two PCR products are denatured by adding 0.15 *M* NaOH.
3. The biotinylated strands are removed by streptavidin coated magnetic beads (M280, Dynal, Oslo, Norway).
4. Nonbiotinylated mutant DNA strands are neutralized with 20 m*M* HCl.
5. The two mutant strands are pooled and hybridized by heating to 65°C and then placed on ice (**Fig. 1C**).
6. The second PCR is run for 25 cycles at 95°C, 30 s, 50°C, 30 s, and 72°C, 30 s with the hybridized strands as template and 20 pmol each of the biotinylated primers Frw-CH2-biotin Rev-CH2-biotin with 2 U *Vent* polymerase in 1X thermopol buffer.

3.2. Purification of Digested PCR Products (see Note 4 and Fig. 2)

1. The PCR products are digested with *Sac*II 2 h at 37°C in a total volume of 100 µL 1X enzyme buffer.
2. Add 50 µg Streptavidin to the 100 µL digestion reaction.
3. Incubate for 30 min at room temperature (RT).
4. Apply on a Centriflex™ column and spin at 13000 rpm.
5. Isolated fragment can be used directly or concentrated by EtOH precipitation as described in **ref.** *(27)*.

3.3. Cloning into the Mammalian Expression Cector pLNOH₂ (see Note 5 and Fig. 3)

The cloning and transformation procedures are as described in **ref.** *27*.

1. The purified mutant DNA fragment is subcloned into a *Sac*II-digested and dephosphorylated intact heavy chain constant region gene of human IG3 in pUC19 *(28)*.

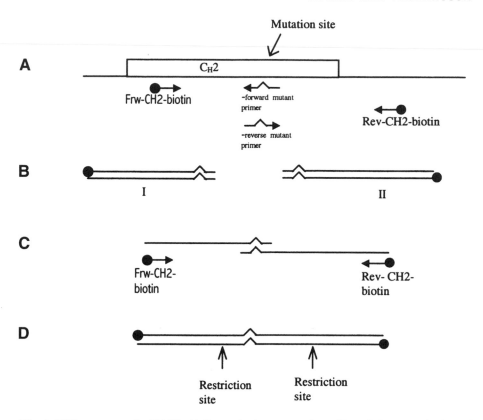

Fig. 1. PCR mutagenesis. (**A**) The C_H2 exon is shown as enlarged box. Primers are indicated as arrows. Two sets of primers are used. First set: Frw-C_H2-biotin and forward mutant primer, second: Rev-C_H2-biotin and reverse mutant primer. The mutations are incorporated in the reverse and forward primers. (**B**) Frw-C_H2-biotin and forward primer amplifies PCR product I, Rev-C_H2-biotin and reverse primer amplifies PCR product II. (**C**) Products I and II are hybridized and amplified by using the Frw-C_H2-biotin and Rev-C_H2-biotin. (**D**) The final biotinylated PCR product is cut with restriction enzymes.

2. The correct sequence of the insert is verified (*see* **Note 6**) by digestion with *Bst*UI followed by sequencing.
3. The intact mutant IgG3 constant region gene is cloned into the mammalian antibody expression vector pLNOH$_2$ (*29*) on *Hind*III and *Bam*HI sites (*see* **Fig. 3**).

3.4. Antibody Expression in J558L Cells

1. The murine myeloma cells J558L are maintained in RPMI 1640 medium supplemented with 10% FCS and penicillin100 U/mL and streptomycin 100 µg/mL (PS) in 25-mL or 75-mL sterile filter screw-caps flasks and grown at 37°C with 5% CO_2.
2. 1×10^7 cells are collected by centrifugation at 1200 rpm and washed twice in RPMI 1640 medium at RT. The pelleted cells are resuspended in 400 µL RPMI 1640 medium (RT) and transferred to a 4 mm electroporation cuvet (BTX inc). Add 20 µg plasmid DNA.

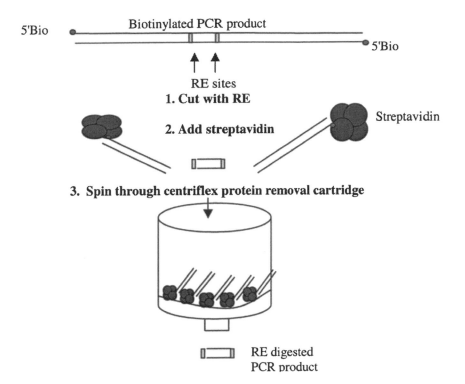

5'Bio Biotinylated PCR product

5'Bio

RE sites
1. Cut with RE

2. Add streptavidin Streptavidin

3. Spin through centriflex protein removal cartridge

RE digested
PCR product

Fig. 2. Outline of the PCR product purification process.

3. The cells are electroporated with a pulse of 175 V with a capacitance of 1300 µF. The cells are immediately diluted into 10 mL prewarmed (37°C) RPMI-PS-FCS medium and plated in a 96-well plate. The transfected cells are grown overnight.

4. After 24 h add selection medium containing G418-sulphate to a final concentration of 800 µg/mL.

5. Supernatant from individual clones are harvested after approx 2 wk and checked for the presence of antibody by ELISA with BSA-NIP (1 µg/mL). Detected with HRP-conjugated α-human Fc antibodies, developed with ABTS and read at 405 nm after 10 min.

6. The best producing clones are expanded in 75 mL flasks. Supernatant is collected from outgrown cell culture.

7. The mutant antibodies are affinity purified with the hapten NIP-sepharose.

3.5. Measuring IgG Effector Functions

The in vitro assays to evaluate the effector functions of the mutant antibodies are beyond the scope of this chapter. However, the methods are previously published in **ref. 30**.

3.6. Concluding Remarks

The methods described above resulted in a mouse/human chimeric anti-NIP IgG3 antibody with a single mutation in the position 322 in the C_H2 domain. This amino

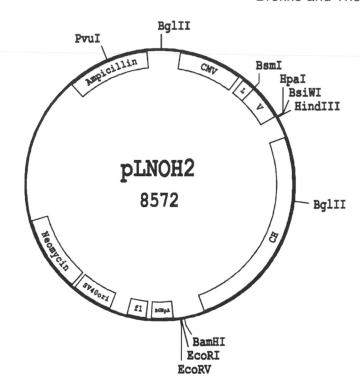

Fig. 3. The antibody expression vector pLNOH$_2$. L, Murine κ leader region; V, variable domain exon; C$_H$, constant heavy chain region gene; CMV, Cytomegalovirus promoter.

acid substitution from a Lysine to an Alanine altered the antibody ability to activate complement significantly *(31)*. The original "Magic Bullet" concept is still alive and recombinant antibodies are the preferred targeting agents. Antibody fragments derived from human antibody libraries can be regenerated as intact fully human antibodies. These antibodies can be subjected to further manipulation for the optimization of their effector functions. By exchanging the variable genes in such antibody expression vectors as described in this chapter, we can design any kind of specificity to any engineered human effector function. The described vector system also contains light chain vectors for the expression on any correct light chain in myeloma cells such as Ns0 cells *(28)*. We have earlier generated mutant human IgG3 molecules with cytolytic activity 50 times higher than natural occurring IgG3 *(15,16)*. Such molecules may be important taking into consideration the in vivo administration of therapeutic antibodies.

4. Notes

1. We have introduced specific restriction enzyme-cleavage sites (RE) flanking the mutation site(s) (some by silent mutations if located within the coding region) in the constant region genes of the human IgG subclasses for the easy substitution of mutant PCR-gener-

ated DNA fragments. The human IgG3 heavy-chain constant region gene is used as template for PCR mutagenesis as described in **Fig. 1**.

2. Two invariant primers are designed such that they flank the area of mutations. These primers should be designed such that they can be used for any kind of mutations within the same exon, i.e., they can reside in the introns or in the exon not being subjected to mutagenesis. These primers are biotinylated for isolation and purification purposes (*see* **Note 4**).

3. Mutagenic primers are made antiparallel to the forward and reverse biotinylated invariant primers. These primers should in addition introduce a novel RE site (silent) for the easy detection of positive mutations. The mutagenic primers introduce a *Bst*UI site for the Lys322Ala substitution for the easy verification of inserted mutation.

4. The protocol is derived from **ref. 26**. It is based on the isolation of completely digested PCR products by the retention of partially digested biotinylated PCR products on a protein-binding membrane. The method gives digested PCR products of very high purity and avoids gel purification with the unwanted use of ethidium bromide and UV-light visualization.

5. pLNOH$_2$ contains the exon encoding a variable heavy-chain domain with specificity for the hapten 5-iodo-4-hydroxy-3-nitro-phenacetyl (NIP), and the constant- and variable-region genes together encode complete immunoglobulin heavy chains The expression of these heavy chains can pair with the λ_1 light chain produced endogenously by the murine myeloma cell line J558L. The products are MAbs with specificity for NIP.

6. If several inserts have been ligated as concatamers due to common RE sites at each end of the insert, it can be revealed by performing a PCR reaction with the two invariant primers.

Acknowledgments

We would like to thank Geir Åge Løset, Affitech AS, and Vigdis Lauvrak, University of Oslo for helpful comments.

References

1. Cragg, M. S., French, R. R., and Glennie, M. J. (1999). Signalling antibodies in cancer therapy. *Curr. Opin. Immunol.* **11**, 541–547.

2. Farah, R. A., Clinchy, B., Herrera, L., and Vitetta, E. S. (1998) The development of monoclonal antibodies for the therapy of cancer. *Crot. Rev. Eukaryot. Gene Exp.* **8**, 321–356.

3. Berard, J. L. (1999) A review of interleukin–2 receptor antagonists in solid organ transplantations. *Pharmacotherapy* **19**, 1127–1137.

4. Maini, R., St. Clair, E. W., Breedveld, F., et al. (1999) Infliximab (chimeric anti-tumour necrosis factor alpha monoclonal antibody) versus placebo in rheumatoid arthritis patients receiving conconiminant methotrexate: a randomised phase III trial. *Lancet* **254**, 1932–1939.

5. Sandborn, W. J. and Hanauer, S. B. (1999) Antitumor necrosis factor therapy for inflammatory bowel disease: a review of agents, pharmacology, clinical results and safety. *Inflamm. Bowel Dis.* **5**, 119–133.

6. Saez-Llorens, X., Castano, E., Null, D., et al. (1998) Safety and pharmacokinetics of an intramuscular humanised antibody monoclonal antibody to respiratory syncitial virus in premature infants with brochopulmonary dysplasia. *Pediatr. Infect. Dis.* **17**, 787–791.

7. Huls, G. A., Heijnen, I. A., Cuomo, M. E., et al. (1999) A recombinant, fully human

monoclonal antibody with antitumor activity constructed from phage-displayed antibody fragments. *Nature Biotechnol.* **17**, 276–280.

8. Duncan, A. R. and Winter (1988) The binding site for C1q on IgG. *Nature* **322**, 738–740.
9. Tao, M. H., Canfield, S. M., and Morrison, S. L. (1991) The differential ability of human IgG1 and IgG4 to activate complement is determined by the COOH-terminal sequence of the C_H2 domain. *J. Exp. Med.* **173**, 1025–1028.
10. Brekke, O. H., Michaelsen, T. E., Aase, A., et al. (1994) Human IgG isotype-specific amino acid residues affecting complement-mediated cell lysis and phagocytosis. *Eur. J. Immunol.* **24**, 2542–2547.
11. Xu, Y., Oomen, R., and Klein, M. H. (1994) Residue position 331 in the IgG1 and IgG4 C_H2 domains contribute to their differential ability to bind and activate complement. *J. Biol. Chem.* **269**, 3469–3474.
12. Morgan, A., Jones, N. D., Nesbitt, A. M., et al. (1995) the N-terminal end of the C_H2 domain of chimeric human IgG1 anti HLA-DR is necessary for C1q, FcgRI and FcgRII binding. *Immunology* **86**, 319–324.
13. Brekke, O. H., Michaelsen, T. E., and Sandlie, I. (1995) The structural requirements for complement activation by IgG: does it hinge on the hinge? *Immunol. Today* **16**, 85–90.
14. Idusogie, E. E., Presta, L. G., Gazzano-Santora, H., et al. (2000) Mapping the C1q binding site on Rituxan, a chimeric antibody with a human IgG1 Fc. *J. Immunol.* **164**, 4178–4184.
15. Sandlie, I., Aase, A., Westby, C., et al. (1989) C1q binding to chimeric monoclonal IgG antibodies consisting of mouse variable regions and human constant regions with shortened hinge containing 15 to 47 amino acids. *Eur. J. Immunol.* **19**, 1593–1603.
16. Brekke, O. H., Michaelsen, T. E., Sandin, R., and Sandlie, I. (1993) Activation of complement by an IgG molecule without a genetic hinge. *Nature* **363**, 628–630.
17. Burton, D. R., Boyd, J., Bramton, A. D., et al. (1980) The C1q receptor site on immunoglobulin G. *Nature* **288**, 338.
18. Connell, G. E. and Porter, R. R. (1971) A new enzymic fragment (Facb) of rabbit immunoglobulin G. *Biochem. J.* **124**, 53.
19. Colomb, M. and Porter, R. R. (1975) Characterization of a plasmin-digest fragment of rabbit immunoglobulin gamma that binds antigen and complement. *Biochem. J.* **145**, 177–183.
20. Yasmeen, D., Ellerson, J. R., Dorrington, K. J., and Painter, R. H. (1976) The structure and function of immunoglobulin domains. IV. The distribution of some effector functions among the Cgamma2 and Cgamma3 homology regions of human immunoglobulin G1. *J. Immunol.* **116**, 518–526.
21. Painter, R. H., Foster, D. B., Gardner, B., and Hughes-Jones, N. C. (1982) Functional affinity constants of subfragments of immunoglobulin G for C1q. *Mol. Immunol.* **19**, 127–131.
22. Tao, M. H., Canfield, S. M., and Morrison, S. L. (1991) The differential ability of human IgG1 and IgG4 to activate complement is determined by the COOH-terminal sequence of the C_H2 domain. *J. Exp. Med.* **173**, 1025–1028.
23. Michaelsen, T. E., Brekke, O. H., Aase, A., et al. (1994) One disulfide bond in front of the second heavy chain constant region is necessary and sufficient for effector functions of human IgG3 without a genetic hinge. *Proc. Natl. Acad. Sci. USA* **91**, 9243–9247.
24. Jefferis, R., Lund, J., and Pound, J. D. (1998) IgG-Fc-mediated effector functions: molecular definition of interaction sites for effector ligands and the role of glycosylation. *Immunol. Rev.* **163**, 59–76.
25. Utsumi, S. M., et al. (1985) Preparation and biologic characterization of fragments containing dimeric and monomeric C gamma 2 domain of rabbit IgG. *Mol. Immunol.* **22**, 811–819.

26. Ihle, O. and Michaelsen, T. E. (2000) Efficient purification of DNA fragments using a protein binding membrane. *Nucleic Acid Res.* **28,** E76.

27. Sambrook, J., Fritsch, E. F., and Maniatis, T. (1989) *Molecular Cloning: A Laboratory Manual*, 2nd ed. Cold Spring Harbor Laboratory Press, Cold Spring Harbor, NY.

28. Brekke, O. H., Bremnes, B., Sandin, R., et al. (1993) Human IgG3 can adopt the disulfide bond pattern characteristic for IgG1 without resembling it in complement mediated cell lysis. *Mol. Immunol.* **30,** 1419–1425.

29. Norderhaug, L., Olafsen, T., Michaelsen, T. E., et al. (1997) Versatile vectors for transient and stable expression of recombinant antibody molecules. *J. Immunol. Methods* **204,** 77–87.

30. Sandlie, I. and Michaelsen, T. E. (1996) Choosing and manipulating effector functions, in *Antibody Engineering: A Practical Approach* (McCafferty, Hoogenboom, and Chiswell, eds.) IRL Press, Oxford Press, pp. 187–202.

31. Thommesen, J. E., Michaelsen, T. E., Loset, G. A., et al. (2001) Lysine 322 in the human IgG3 CH2 domain is crucial for antibody dependent complement activation. *Mol. Immunol.* **37,** 995–1004.

24

Single-Chain Fv-Based Affinity Purification of the Cellular Stress Protein gp96 for Vaccine Development

Christian Kleist, Danièle Arnold-Schild, Martin Welschof, Martina Finger, Gerhard Opelz, Hans-Georg Rammensee, Hansjörg Schild, and Peter Terness

1. Introduction

Cellular stress proteins like the classical heat-shock proteins (HSPs) hsp70 (*1–3*), hsp90 (*3*) and hsp110 (*4*); the glucose-regulated proteins gp96/GRP94 (*3,5*) and grp170 (*4*); as well as the endoplasmic chaperone calreticulin (*6,7*) have been shown to induce cytotoxic T-cell responses and protective immunity when isolated from tumor or infected cells and used to vaccinate animals (*8–10*; reviewed in **refs.** *11–17*). The specificity of the immune responses is owing to antigenic peptides associated with the HSPs (*18–26*). The HSP-peptide complexes are taken up by professional antigen-presenting cells (APCs) for effective presentation of the peptides to T cells (*19,27–33*). The extensively studied endoplasmic reticulum-resident chaperone gp96 is most efficient and promising in this regard (*34–39*); encouraging clinical studies with human cancer patients (*40*).

Application in immunization protocols requires the rapid and efficient isolation of HSP molecules from tumors and infected tissues. Monoclonal antibodies (MAbs) would be an ideal tool for the specific purification of HSP molecules via antibody-based affinity chromatography, even from limited amounts of cancerous material. Furthermore, it would be of great importance to obtain the HSP in its native form in order to isolate HSP-peptide complexes, still carrying the immunogenic peptides.

The perfect source for antibodies with these properties are recombinant antibody phage-display libraries. The complexity of these libraries provides a pool of antigen binding proteins with specificities against any antigenic entity, potentially exceeding that of the natural B-cell repertoire (*41–54*). This is partly based on the in vitro joining of heavy and light chains, which results in newly formed combinations. Furthermore, very promising are semi- or fully synthetic libraries, which theoretically have the poten-

From: *Methods in Molecular Biology, vol. 207: Recombinant Antibodies for Cancer Therapy: Methods and Protocols*
Edited by: M. Welschof and J. Krauss © Humana Press Inc., Totowa, NJ

tial to carry antigen binding proteins to all possible antigenic epitopes including the so-called "self-antigens," which are removed in vivo during B-cell maturation via the negative selection process *(55–58)*. Antibody fragments such as F(ab) or single-chain Fv (scFv) *(59)* can be selected for conformational epitopes that specifically recognize the native, correctly folded antigen. An additional advantage of antibody libraries is the circumvention of the usage of experimental animals in order to create antibodies of desired specificities.

Since HSPs belong to the self-antigen group and have been highly conserved throughout vertebrate phylogeny *(60,61)*, we chose a semi-synthetic scFv antibody phage-display library *(58)* in order to increase the likelihood of selecting antibody specificities directed against the gp96 protein. After the enrichment of a polyclonal pool of anti-gp96 scFv-expressing phage particles, during four screening rounds with native gp96, distinct monoclonal phagemids were isolated and characterized. In order to generate soluble scFv proteins in *Escherichia coli* *(62)*, the gene cassettes, encoding the variable domains of the heavy and light chains, were recloned into an appropriate bacterial-expression vector *(63)*. Subsequently, the soluble scFv antibody fragments were expressed on a small scale for specification of the properties of the scFv antibodies in immunoassays such as ELISA, dot blot, and immunoprecipitation. Large-scale expression of the binding clones resulted in high amounts of scFv proteins to produce affinity chromatography columns for rapid one-step purification of native gp96-peptide complexes from various tumor cell lines *(64,65)*.

2. Materials

Labware and equipment that are routinely available in a research laboratory such as disposable tubes and standard centrifuges are not specifically mentioned in the Materials section, though they may appear in the Methods section when this information might help the researcher with experimental performance. Reagents, labware, and equipment suggested are related to our experiences and availability. Therefore, equivalent materials can be obtained from other sources provided that quality and application are comparable to those described herein. Additionally, companies for standard reagents such as Tris-HCl base or sodium chloride are not listed in some cases because major suppliers for these chemical products are well-known. Additional information on general materials and methods can be found in the laboratory manual by Sambrook et al. *(66)*, as well as in the references provided with the specific procedures.

2.1. Selection of gp96-Specific scFv Ab-Expressing Phages from a Semi-Synthetic Phage-Display Antibody Library

2.1.1. Screening of a Phage-Display Antibody Library to Rescue Specific scFv-Antibody Fragments

The materials and methods for the screening of the phage display scFv antibody library are according to the protocols in Chapter 6, **Subheadings 2.4.–2.5.** and **3.5.–3.9.** provided by Welschof et al. Changes to the materials used in our current protocol are as follows:

1. Human semi-synthetic scFv antibody library in the phage display vector pHEN1 *(46)*, officially called "Synthetic scFv Library (#1)" *(58)* (Medical Research Council [MRC], Cambridge, UK).
2. Antigen: purified native murine protein gp96 (1 mg/mL) in 1 m*M* phosphate buffer containing 200 m*M* sodium chloride (NaCl) (IMMATICS Biotechnologies, Tübingen, Germany). Stored at –70°C (*see* **Note 1**).

See also **Subheading 3.1.1.** for further information on the antibody library used.

2.1.2. Isolation of Monoclonal scFv-Expressing Phagemid Particles

1. *E. coli* K12 TG1 infected with the phagemid pHEN1 coding for the selected scFv antibodies (MRC).
2. LB (Luria Bertani) broth: Dissolve 10 g bacto-tryptone, 5 g yeast extract (both from Becton Dickinson Microbiology Systems, Sparks, MD), and 10 g NaCl in 950 mL distilled H₂O, adjust the pH to 7.0 with 1 M NaOH, add distilled H₂O to a total volume of 1 L, and autoclave.
3. LB-GA medium: LB broth supplemented with 100 m*M* glucose and 50 µg/mL ampicillin.
4. 2 *M* Glucose, sterile-filtered.
5. Ampicillin (5 mg/mL) (Roche Diagnostics, Mannheim, Germany) in H₂O, sterile-filtered and stored in aliquots at –20°C.
6. H₂O ad inj. (Braun, Melsungen, Germany).
7. 0.5 *M* EDTA: Dissolve 186.1 g of disodium ethylenediamine-tetraaceticacetate in distilled H₂O. Adjust pH to 8.0 and add H₂O to a final volume of 1 L. Autoclave to sterilize.
8. 50X Tris-acetate electrophoresis buffer (50X TAE buffer stock): Dissolve 242 g Tris-HCl base in distilled H₂O. Add 57.1 mL glacial acetic acid, 100 mL of 0.5 *M* EDTA, pH 8.0, and H₂O to a final volume of 1 L.
9. 1X TAE buffer: Dilute the 50X TAE stock 1:50 in H₂O before use.
10. 6X DNA sample buffer: 0.25% (w/v) bromophenol blue, 0.25% (w/v) xylene cyanol and 15% ficoll type 400 (Amersham Biosciences Europe, Freiburg, Germany).
11. Mineral oil (Sigma-Aldrich Chemie, Taufkirchen, Germany).
12. Ethidium bromide (EtBr) stock solution (10 mg/mL in H₂O) (Sigma) (*see* **Note 2**).
13. Restriction enzymes: *Alu*I (8000 U/mL), *Bst*NI (10,000 U/mL), *Nco*I (10,000 U/mL), *Not*I (10,000 U/mL), *Rsa*I (10,000 U/mL), the appropriate buffers (NEBuffer 1-4), and 100X BSA (10 mg/mL) (New England Biolabs, Beverly, MA).
14. DNA molecular-weight markers: 100 bp ladder (Amersham) and λ DNA *Bst*EII digest (New England Biolabs).
15. Plasmid isolation mini and midi kits (QIAGEN, Hilden, Germany or Sigma-Aldrich).
16. Agarose (Hybaid, Heidelberg, Germany).

2.2. Production of Soluble scFv Antibody Fragments

2.2.2. Cloning of scFv Fragments into the Bacterial Expression Vector pHOG21

1. Shaking incubator (Infors, Einsbach, Germany).
2. Gene pulser transfection apparatus for bacterial cell electroporation (Bio-Rad Laboratories, Munich, Germany).
3. Gene pulser cuvets for *E. coli* electroporation (0.1 cm electrode gap) (Bio-Rad).
4. Single clones of *E. coli* K12 XL1-blue or TG1 infected with the phagemid pHEN1, which codes for the selected scFv antibodies.

5. *E. coli* K12 XL1-blue transformed with the pHOG21 plasmid, which carries any scFv fragment (for isolation of vector pHOG21).
6. Electroporation-competent *E. coli* K12 XL1-blue (Stratagene Cloning Systems, La Jolla, CA).
7. LB-GA medium.
8. SOB-GA medium agar plates: Add 920 mL of distilled H_2O to 15 g bacto agar, 20 g bacto tryptone, 5 g bacto yeast extract, and 0.5 g NaCl, and autoclave. After the medium has cooled to 55°C, add 10 mL of sterile $MgCl_2$, 50 mL of 2 *M* glucose, and 20 mL of sterile-filtered ampicillin (5 mg/mL), and pour quickly into Petri dishes (85 m*M* in diameter).
9. SOB medium (*see* **step 8** without bacto agar and ampicillin).
10. SOC medium: SOB medium supplemented with 20 m*M* glucose.
11. 2 *M* Glucose, sterile-filtered.
12. Ampicillin (5 mg/mL) in H_2O, sterile-filtered and stored in aliquots at –20°C.
13. H_2O ad inj. (Braun).
14. Ethanol pA, absolute (EtOH) and ethanol p.A. 80%.
15. 1X TAE buffer.
16. Ethidiume bromide (EtBr) stock solution (10 mg/mL in H_2O).
17. 3 *M* sodium acetate, pH 4.6.
18. Glycogen from mussels, molecular biology grade (20 µg/µL) (Roche).
19. Restriction enzymes: *Nco*I (10,000 U/mL), *Not*I (10,000 U/mL), NEBuffer 3, and 100X BSA (10 mg/mL) (New England Biolabs).
20. Calf intestine phosphatase (CIP), alkaline (Roche).
21. DNA molecular weight markers: 100 bp ladder (Amersham) and λ DNA *Bst*EII digest (500 µg/mL) (New England Biolabs).
22. Plasmid isolation mini and midi kits (QIAGEN).
23. QIAquick gel extraction kit (QIAGEN).
24. Rapid DNA ligation kit (Roche).
25. Agarose (Hybaid).

2.2.3. Small-Scale Expression of scFv Antibody Fragments

1. Shaking incubator (Infors).
2. UV/Visible spectrophotometer (Amersham).
3. Erlenmeyer flasks, 100 mL, sterilized.
4. Disposable sample concentrating devices: Vivaspin 15 mL with molecular-weight cut-off of 10,000 (Sartorius Vivascience, Göttingen, Germany).
5. Disposable cuvets (Müller ratiolab, Dreieich, Germany).
6. Disposable 50 mL syringes (Becton Dickinson, Heidelberg, Germany).
7. Sterile, low protein binding syringe driven filter units with 0.22 µm and 5.0 µm pore sizes (Millipore).
8. *E. coli* K12 XL1-blue transformed with the expression vector pHOG21, which carries the anti-gp96 scFv DNA fragments.
9. LB-GA medium containing 100 m*M* glucose and 50 µg/mL ampicillin.
10. 2X YT medium: Dissolve 16 g bacto-tryptone, 10 g yeast extract, and 5 g NaCl in 950 mL distilled H_2O, adjust the pH to 7.0, add distilled H_2O to a final volume of 1 L and autoclave.
11. 2X YT-GA medium: 2X YT medium supplemented with 100 m*M* glucose and 75 µg/mL ampicillin.
12. 2X YT-SA medium: 2X YT medium containing 400 m*M* sucrose and 75 µg/mL ampicillin.
13. 2 *M* Glucose, sterile-filtered.

14. 2 *M* Sucrose, sterile-filtered.
15. Ampicillin (5 mg/mL) in H$_2$O, sterile filtered and stored in aliquots at –20°C.
16. 100 m*M* isopropyl-b-galactopyranoside (IPTG) (Hybaid) in H$_2$O. Stored in aliquots at –20°C.
17. Shock solution for the preparation of the bacterial periplasmic fraction: 50 m*M* Tris-HCl, pH 8.0, 20% (w/v) sucrose, 1 m*M* EDTA in H$_2$O. Store at 4°C.
18. 100 m*M* Pefabloc (Merck, Darmstadt, Germany) in H$_2$O. Aliquot in volumes of 1–2 mL and store at –20°C.
19. Protease inhibitor cocktail tablets complete, EDTA-free (mini and regular size) (Roche).
20. 1 *M* Dithiothreitol (DTT) in H$_2$O. Store at –20°C.
21. Sodium azide (Merck) (*see* **Note 3**).
22. 2X SDS protein sample buffer: 100 m*M* Tris-HCl, pH 6.8, 4% (w/v) sodium dodecyl sulphate (SDS), 0.02% (w/v) bromophenol blue (Amersham), and 20% (v/v) glycerol. Add dithiothreitol (DTT) to a final concentration of 200 m*M* prior to use. When storage is required after the addition of DTT, displace the remaining air in the tube with nitrogen gas, to prevent oxidization of DTT, and maintain tightly closed at room temperature.
23. Dialysis buffer: 50 m*M* Tris-HCl and 1 *M* NaCl, pH 7.0. Sterilize through filtration and store at 4°C.
24. Dulbecco's phosphate-buffered saline (PBS) (Invitrogen, Karlsruhe, Germany): 8.1 m*M* Na$_2$HPO$_4$, 1.5 m*M* KH$_2$PO$_4$, 0.142 *M* NaCl, and 2.7 m*M* KCl. Adjust pH to 8.0, sterilize by filtration, and store at 4°C.
25. Cellulose tubular dialysis membrane (Carl Roth, Karlsruhe, Germany) with a 12,000–14,000 molecular-weight cut-off. Treat the membrane as specified by the supplier prior to use for dialysis and store the pretreated membrane at 4°C in 20% (v/v) ethanol until needed.

2.2.4. Purification of the Isolated Soluble scFv Antibodies Using Immobilized Metal Ion Affinity Chromatography (IMAC)

1. Automated chromatography system/Fast Performance Liquid Chromatography (FPLC) system (Amersham).
2. UV/Visible spectrophotometer (Amersham).
3. Empty chromatography columns (e.g., Amersham; Bio-Rad; Kronlab, Sinsheim, Germany).
4. Dialysis buffer: 50 m*M* Tris-HCl and 1 M NaCl, pH 7.0. Sterilize through filtration and store at 4°C.
5. Washing buffer: dialysis buffer containing 50 m*M* imidazole, pH 7.0.
6. Elution buffer: dialysis buffer containing 300 m*M* imidazole, pH 7.0.
7. Dialysed solution containing the soluble anti-gp96 scFv antibody fragments.
8. Bovine serum albumin (BSA); 50 mg/mL (Sigma-Aldrich) and/or glycerol.
9. 100 m*M* Pefabloc in H$_2$O.
10. Bio-Rad protein assay kit containing a bovine gamma globulin standard (Bio-Rad).
11. Chelating Sepharose Fast Flow (Amersham).

2.3. Detection and Characterization of Soluble scFv Fragment Expression

2.3.1. Detection of scFv Expression Using SDS-PAGE and Western Blotting

1. Mini electrophoresis cell (Bio-Rad).
2. Mini electrophoretic transfer cell (Bio-Rad)
3. Electrophoresis power supply (Amersham).
4. Gel dryer (Owl Scientific Plastics, Cambridge, MA).

5. Automatic film processor with required reagents (Agfa, Cologne, Germany).
6. Autoradiography cassettes with intensifying screens (Amersham).
7. Precast polyacrylamide gels (12%) containing 10 and/or 15 wells or reagents and equipment for casting of gels (Bio-Rad).
8. Samples from the scFv antibody expression and purification process (*see* **Subheadings 3.2.3.**, **3.4.1.**, and **3.4.2.**).
9. 2X SDS protein sample buffer.
10. Electrophoresis running buffer: 25 mM Tris-HCl, pH 8.3, 192 mM glycine, and 0.1% (w/v) SDS.
11. Transfer buffer: 25 mM Tris-HCl, pH 8.3, 192 mM glycine without SDS(!).
12. Coomassie R 350 staining solution. Use Ph astGel Blue R tablets (Amersham) to prepare a 0.2% stock and 0.02% final staining solution as described by the supplier.
13. Destaining solution for polyacrylamide gels: 30% (v/v) methanol, 10% (v/v) acetic acid in distilled H$_2$O.
14. Solutions for gel drying procedure:
    a. 5% (v/v) glycerol in dionized H$_2$O; and
    b. 40% (v/v) methanol, 10% (v/v) glycerol, 7.5% (v/v) acetic acid.
15. Ponceau S protein staining solution: 0.1% (w/v) in 5% (v/v) acetic acid (Sigma-Aldrich).
16. Washing buffer: TBS (10 mM Tris-HCl, 150 mM NaCl, pH 7.5) and TNT (10 mM Tris-HCl, 150 mM NaCl, 0.05 % (v/v) Tween-20, pH 7.5).
18. Blocking buffer: 5% (w/v) skimmed milk powder in TBS, 0.1% (v/v) Tween-20.
19. Mouse anti-human-c-myc monoclonal antibody (MAb) (IgG1, Clone 9E10, Santa Cruz Biotechnology, Santa Cruz, CA). Dilute 1:4000 in 2% (w/v) skimmed milk powder in PBS.
20. Peroxidase-conjugated rabbit anti-mouse immunoglobulins (DAKO, Glostrup, Denmark). Dilute 1:5000 in 2% (w/v) skimmed milk powder in PBS.
21. ECL Western blotting analysis system (Amersham) for chemiluminescent detection including ECL protein molecular weight markers.
22. Protein molecular weight marker: SDS-7 (Sigma-Aldrich).
23. Gel drying film (Promega, Madison, WI).
24. Nitrocellulose membrane, Protran BA 83, 0.2 μm (Schleicher & Schuell, Dassel, Germany).
25. Whatman 3MM chromatography paper (Whatman International, Maidstone, UK).
26. High performance chemiluminescence film (Hyperfilm ECL) (Amersham).
27. Clear plastic sheets.

2.3.2. Enzyme-Linked Immunosorbent Assay (ELISA)

1. Absorbance microplate reader (Tecan, Crailsheim, Germany).
2. Microtier immuno-plates, Maxisorp surface, 96 wells (Nunc, Roskilde, Denmark).
3. Rotating shaker (neoLab Migge, Laborbedarf, Heidelberg, Germany).
4. Washing buffers:
   a. PBS, pH 7.4, sterilized by filtration.
   b. PBS/Tween (PBST): 0.05% (v/v) Tween 20 in PBS. Store at room temperature.
5. Blocking buffer: 2% (w/v) skimmed milk powder in PBS (MPBS).
6. Dilution buffer for the gp96 antigen: 10 mM sodium phosphate, 0.38 M NaCl, pH 7.0.
7. 3,3',5,5'-Tetramethylbenzidine (TMB) peroxidase substrate system (Kirkegaard & Perry Laboratories, Gaithersburg, MD).
8. Purified native heat shock protein gp96 (IMMATICS).

9. Anti-gp96 scFv antibodies (from **step 14** in **Subheading 3.2.3.**; IMAC-purified samples from **Subheadings 3.2.4.** or **3.4.2.**). Make up a dilution series in MPBS.
10. Rat anti-Grp94 MAb, IgG2a, Clone 9G10 (StressGen Biotechnologies, Victoria, B.C., Canada), 1:1000 dilution in MPBS.
11. Mouse anti-human-c-myc MAb (IgG1, Clone 9E10, Santa Cruz), 1:4000 dilution in MPBS.
12. Peroxidase-conjugated rabbit anti-mouse immunoglobulins (DAKO), 1:5000 dilution in MPBS.
13. Peroxidase-conjugated rabbit anti-rat immunoglobulins (DAKO), 1:5000 dilution in MPBS.

2.3.3. Dot-Blot Analysis

1. Multi-axle rotating mixer or rotating shaker (neoLab-Migge).
2. End-over-end rotator or multi-axle rotating mixer (neoLab-Migge).
3. Protein sample buffers:
   a. Dilution buffer for native gp96: 10 mM sodium phosphate, 0.38 M NaCl, pH 7.0.
   b. 2X Sample buffer (denaturing): 125 mM Tris-HCl, pH 7.5, 4% SDS, 10% glycerol.
   c. 2X Sample buffer (denaturing and reducing): 125 mM Tris-HCl, pH 7.5, 4% SDS, 10% glycerol, 10% 2-mercaptoethanol, or 10% DTT.
4. Blocking buffer: 2% (w/v) skimmed milk powder in PBS (MPBS).
5. Washing buffers (for Western blot membranes): TBS (10 mM Tris-HCl, 150 mM NaCl, pH 7.5) and TNT (10 mM Tris-HCl, 150 mM NaCl, 0.05 % [v/v] Tween-20, pH 7.5).
6. Stock solutions for chromogenic detection by horseradish peroxidase conjugates:
   a. Cobalt chloride (1% w/v): dissolve 100 mg $CoCl_2$ (Merck) in 10 mL 1X TBS, dispense in aliquots of 250 µL, and store at –20°C until use.
   b. Diaminobenzidine (DAB) (25 mg/mL): dissolve 250 mg 3-3'-diaminobenzidine tetrahydrochloride (Sigma-Aldrich) in 10 mL PBS, dispense in aliquots of 250 µL, and store at –20°C.
   c. Perhydrol 30% H_2O_2 (Merck) (*see* **Note 4**).
7. Horseradish peroxidase substrate solution: add 200 µL of $CoCl_2$ stock to 9.8 mL of 1X TBS. Mix well by inversion or vortexing. Add 200 µL of DAB stock and 1 µL 30% of H_2O_2 and mix well (*see* **Note 5**).
8. Purified native heat shock protein gp96 (IMMATICS).
9. Anti-gp96 scFv antibody fragments.
10. Rat anti-Grp94 MAb, IgG2a, Clone 9G10 (StressGen).
11. ScFv or other antibody nonreactive to gp96.
12. Mouse anti-human-c-myc MAb, IgG1, Clone 9E10 (Santa Cruz).
13. Peroxidase-conjugated rabbit anti-mouse immunoglobulins (DAKO).
14. Peroxidase-conjugated rabbit anti-rat immunoglobulins (DAKO).
15. Nitrocellulose membrane, Protran BA 83, 0.2 µm (Schleicher & Schuell).
16. Whatman 3MM chromatography paper (Whatman).

2.3.4. Immunoprecipitation of Native gp96

1. Materials for SDS-PAGE (*see* **Subheading 2.3.1.**).
2. Gel dryer (Bio-Rad).
3. Phosphoimager, e.g., FujiFilm BAS1500 (Fuji Photo Film, Düsseldorf, Germany).
4. Image plate, e.g., FujiFilm BAS-MS (Fuji Photo Film).

5. 250 mL Tissue culture flask (Greiner, Frickenhausen, Germany).
6. Glass douncer (2 mL, small gap) (Braun).
7. Methionine-free RPMI 40 medium (Invitrogen).
8. 35S-methionine (NEN Life Science Products, Zaventem, Belgium).
9. Dialyzed and sterilized fetal calf serum (FCS) (Invitrogen).
10. Detergent lysis buffer: PBS, 0.5% (v/v) Nonidet P-40 (NP-40) (Sigma-Aldrich), 1 μ*M* leupeptin and 1 μ*M* pepstatin (Roche), 20 μ*M* phenylmethylsulfonyl fluoride (PMSF) (Sigma-Aldrich).
11. Hyptonic lysis buffer: 30 m*M* NaHCO$_3$, pH 7.1, 1 μ*M* leupeptin, 1 μ*M* pepstatin, 20 μ*M* PMSF, iodoacetamide (0.95 mg/mL) (Sigma-Aldrich).
12. Beads washing buffer: 1 m*M* HCl.
13. 0.2 *M* Glycine, pH 8.0–8.5.
14. Coupling buffer: 0.1 *M* NaHCO$_3$, 0.5 *M* NaCl, pH 8.3.
15. Washing buffers:
    a. 0.1 *M* Sodium acetate, 0.5 *M* NaCl, pH 4.0; and
    b. 0.1 *M* Tris-HCl, 0.5 *M* NaCl, pH 8.0.
16. Blocking buffer: 0.1 *M* Tris-HCl, pH 8.0.
17. Gel fixation solution: 10% (v/v) glacial acetic acid, 20% (v/v) methanol in H$_2$O.
18. Cell culture in exponential growth phase (murine and/or human).
19. Purified anti-gp96 scFv antibodies.
20. CNBr-activated Sepharose 4B (Amersham).
21. Whatman 3MM chromatography paper (Whatman).
22. Saran Wrap.

2.4. Large Scale Expression and Purification of Soluble scFv Antibodies

The large scale expression of 5 L of bacterial culture is a direct upscaling of the method described in **Subheading 2.2.3.** Note that this scale is much more time-consuming and the procedure must be well-planned in advance.

In the following subheadings, only changes are mentioned that are strictly due to the scale.

2.4.1. Induction of Soluble scFv Fragments

1. Erlenmeyer flasks: 500 mL, 2 L, and 5 L, sterilized.
2. 2X YT-GA and 2X YT-SA media: at least 5 L of each.

2.4.2. Purification of the scFv Antibodies by Immobilized Metal Ion Affinity Chromatography (IMAC)

1. Speed adjustable peristaltic pump (Millipore, Eschborn, Germany).
2. Magnetic stirrer and stir bar.
3. Spiral-wound membrane cartridge S3Y10 with a membrane cut-off of 10,000 molecular weight and a membrane area of 1 ft^2 (Amicon, Beverley, MA).
4. Spiral-cap filter capsule (0.8/0.2 μm) (PALL Gelman Laboratory, Dreieich, Germany).
5. Erlenmeyer flasks, 5 L, sterilized.
6. Three-neck round-bottom flask, sterilized.
7. Tubing, glass parts (air-leak tubes and cones with gound joints) and clamps for pump-cartridge-flask connections (*see* **Fig. 1**).
8. Dialysis buffer: 50 m*M* Tris-HCl and 1 M NaCl, pH 7.0, approx 15 L.

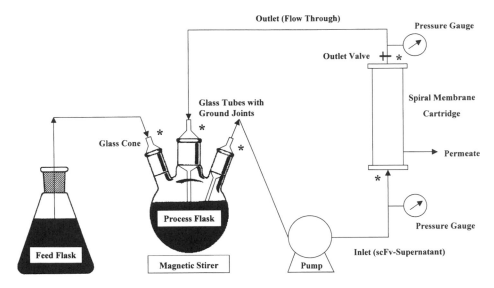

Fig. 1. Schematic representation of the configuration of the equipment for the concentration and diafiltration of the scFv-containing supernatant in large scale expression. Ensure that the tubings are tightly connected to the cartridge, the process, and feed flasks at the indicated sites (*) in order to create a closed system.

2.4.3. Determination of Expressed scFv Fragments and Verification of the Binding Characteristics

The materials used are the same as in **Subheading 2.3.**

2.5. Purification of gp96 Using scFv Antibody Fragments Coupled to Sepharose Beads

2.5.1. Production of gp96-Specific Affinity Columns

1. Multi-axle rotating mixer or rotating shaker (neoLab-Migge).
2. UV/Visible spectrophotometer (Amersham Pharmacia).
3. Empty chromatography columns in different sizes (2.5 mL, 5 mL, 10 mL) with lids, filters, and stop-cocks (MoBiTec, Göttingen, Germany).
4. 0.2 M Glycine, pH 8.0–8.5.
5. Coupling buffer: 0.1 M NaHCO$_3$, 0.5 M NaCl, pH 8.3.
6. Washing buffers:
   a. 0.1 M Sodium acetate, 0.5 M NaCl, pH 4.0; and
   b. 0.1 M Tris-HCl, 0.5 M NaCl, pH 8.0.
7. Blocking buffer: 0.1 M Tris-HCl, pH 8.0.
8. Column storage solution: 20% (v/v) ethanol in H$_2$O or PBS containing 0.02% (w/v) sodium azide (*see* **Note 3**).
9. Purified anti-gp96 scFv antibodies.
10. Bovine serum albumin (BSA) or human serum albumin (HSA) (Sigma-Aldrich).
11. Disposable PD-10 desalting columns (Amersham).
12. CNBr-activated Sepharose Fast Flow or 4B (Amersham).

2.5.2. One-Step Affinity Purification of gp96

1. Ultracentrifuge (Beckman, Fullerton, CA)
2. Polyallomer ultracentrifuge tubes (Herolab, Wiesloch, Germany).
3. Disposable sample concentrating devices: Vivaspin 5 mL with molecular weight cut-off of 30,000 (Sartorius Vivascience).
4. Chromatography columns based on CNBr-activated sepharose coupled with anti-gp96 scFv antibodies.
5. Glass douncer (Braun).
6. Cell pellet washed three times with cold PBS (freshly prepared or stored at –70°C).
7. Protease inhibitor stocks: 100 mM Pefabloc SC in H$_2$O (Merck), 2 mg/mL pepstatin in dimethyl sulfoxide (DMSO), 2 mg/mL leupeptin in DMSO, and protease inhibitor cocktail tablets complete (mini and regular size) (all from Roche). Make aliquots of inhibitor solutions and store at –20°C.
8. Hypotonic lysis buffer: 30 mM NaHCO3, pH 7.1. Directly before use add protease inhibitors: Pefabloc (1:500), leupeptin, and pepstatin (each 1:1000) and one cocktail tablet (mini to 10 mL and regular to 50 mL lysis buffer).
9. Washing buffers:
   a. PBS, pH7.4; and
   b. PBS containing 0.5 M NaCl.
10. Elution buffer: PBS, pH 7.4, containing 1.3 M NaCl.
11. Column regeneration buffer: PBS, pH 7.4, containing 2 M NaCl.
12. Column storage solution:
    a. 20% (v/v) ethanol in H$_2$O; or
    b. PBS containing 0.02% (w/v) sodium azide.
13. 0.2 M glycine, pH 8.0.
14. Dilution buffer for the antigen gp96: 10 mM sodium phosphate, 0.38 M NaCl, pH 7.0.

3. Methods

3.1. Selection of gp96-Specific scFv Ab-Expressing Phages from a Semi-Synthetic Phage-Display Antibody Library

3.1.1. Screening of a Phage-Display Antibody Library to Rescue Specific scFv-Antibody Fragments

As mentioned briefly in **Subheading 2.1.1.**, materials and methods for the screening of the phage display scFv antibody library are according to the protocols in Chapter 6, **Subheadings 2.4.–2.5.** and **3.5.–3.9.** Please note, however, that instead of the natural modular human antibody library cloned into the phagemid pSEX81 *(45,52)*, our protocol is based on the selection of specific anti-gp96 scFv antibody fragments from a semi-synthetic scFv antibody library *(58)*, which uses the phagemid vector pHEN1 *(46)*. Using pHEN1, scFv antibody fragments are also displayed on the tip of filamentous phage particles, where they are anchored in the phage surface as fusion proteins to the minor phage coat protein pIII *(44)*. The restriction sites of the *Nco*I and *Not*I endonucleases flanking the scFv encoding cassette are compatible with the cloning sites in the phagemid vector pSEX81 and the bacterial expression vector pHOG21 *(63)*. The latter is used to express soluble scFv fragments in *E. coli* after the scFv antibody cassette, comprising the coding sequences for the variable heavy chain, linker, and variable light chain, has been cloned into the corresponding site. The expressed scFv fragments carry a human-c-myc-tag and a 6-his-tag that allow specific detection via anti-c-myc-antibodies and the purification through immobilized metal ion affinity chromatography, respectively *(67,68)*.

3.1.2. Isolation of Distinct Monoclonal scFv-Expressing Phagemid Particles

After the generation of single phagemid clones from the polyclonal pool of the last screening round, each expressing one distinct scFv antibody fragment, one should check the diversity of these clones in order to determine distinct scFv antibody clones for the subsequent expression of soluble scFv fragments. For preselection, a so-called "fingerprinting" analysis of the scFv clones is performed *(55)*. Restriction endonucleases such as *Alu*I, *Bst*NI, and *Rsa*I, which recognize DNA sequences frequently encoded by human DNA, preferentially cut the different human scFv fragments. A distinct digestion pattern for each antibody clone can be generated if the clones encode different immunoglobulin sequences and possess restriction sites at different positions. After the fingerprinting analysis and grouping of clones with similar digestion patterns, these inserts can then be cloned into the expression vector. In order to distinguish exactly the monoclonal scFv fragments from each other, the composition of the DNA encoding the scFv fragments must be determined by nucleotide sequencing *(69)*.

3.1.2.1. DNA FINGERPRINTING OF THE SCFV CLONES

1. Inoculate 5 mL LB-GA medium with *E. coli* transfected with scFv-carrying pHEN1 phagemids that have been proved to be positive for binding to the antigen gp96 in a single clone phage-ELISA (*see* Chapter 6, **Subheading 3.9.**). Incubate at 37°C and 280 rpm overnight.
2. Harvest the bacterial cells by spinning the cultures for 15 min at 2800g and 4°C.
3. Follow the instructions of the supplier of the mini plasmid preparation kit for the isolation of the phagemid DNA. When using the kit from QIAGEN, dissolve the washed and precipitated DNA pellet well (but carefully) in 40 µL H_2O. Use 80–100 µL H_2O to elute the DNA from the column with the Sigma kit. Dissolved DNA can be stored at –20°C.
4. Check for successful plasmid DNA isolation by running 10 µL of each phagemid DNA sample (4 µL phagemid DNA, 5 µL H_2O, 2 µL DNA sample buffer) and 5 µL of the l BstEII molecular-weight marker on a 0.8% (w/v) agarose gel (1X TAE and 0.5 µg/mL EtBr) at 5–7 V/cm gel for approx 1–2 h. Check the gel on a UV transilluminator and photograph for documentation. Repeat the plasmid preparation procedure for the samples that did not show any DNA in the gel.
5. Digest 4 µL of plasmid DNA with 10 U of *Nco*I, 10 U of *Not*I, and 1 µL of NEBuffer 3 in a final volume of 10 µL at 37°C for 90 min. Add 2 µL of DNA sample buffer to each digest and run on a 0.8–1.5 % (w/v) agarose gel along with 10 µL of the 100 base pair marker. Bands with a molecular weight near 800 bp indicate clones that most likely carry an scFv antibody insert.
6. Digest 4 µL of the scFv encoding clones for 90 min with:
   a. 10 U of *Alu*I at 37°C,
   b. 10 U of *Bst*NI at 60°C, and
   c. 10 U of *Rsa*I at 37°C in a total volume of 10 µL containing the appropriate buffer and 10 µg of RNase (*see* **Note 6**).

7. After the addition of 2 µL of DNA sample buffer, run digested samples along with the 100 bp marker on a 3% TAE-agarose gel at approx 6 V/cm for 2–3 h. Document as in **step 4** and group the scFv clones according to similar digestion banding patterns (*see* **Note 7**).

3.1.2.2. DNA SEQUENCING OF THE PRESELECTED SCFV CLONES

Because the preselection of monoclonal scFv clones based on the DNA fingerprinting cannot be exact due to missing restriction sites, minimal molecular-weight differences in the resulting fragments, and interpretation difficulties of slightly nonlinear gel running conditions, DNA sequencing *(69)* should be performed on at least two clones of each preselected group (*see* **Note 8**).

Sequencing services are available from different companies such as Sequence Laboratories (Göttingen, Germany) and MediGenomix (Planegg-Martinsried, Germany) with the latter offering very good customer service and sequencing packages (*see* **Note 9**).

3.2. Production of Soluble scFv Antibody Fragments

3.2.2. Cloning of the scFv Fragments into the Bacterial Expression Vector pHOG21

1. Prepare o/n cultures in 50 mL LB-GA of the different *E. coli* clones that carry monoclonal scFv antibody fragments and isolate the scFv-pHEN1 phagemid DNA according to the protocol for medium size procedure of the supplier of the preparation kit. Also include a clone transformed with the expression vector pHOG21 alone or pHOG21 encoding any scFv fragment.

2. Check the isolated phagemid DNA as described in **steps 4** and **5** in **Subheading 3.1.2.1.**

3. Measure the OD of the phagemid DNA at 280 nm and 260 nm in a spectrophotometer. Calculate the concentration of the DNA by using an OD_{260} of 1 corresponding to approx 50 µg plasmid DNA/mL. The purity of the DNA preparation can be checked by dividing the value of the OD measurement at 260 nm by that at 280 nm and should lie between 1.8 and 2.0 *(66)*.

4. Set up a preparative DNA digest by using 5 µg of plasmid DNA, 25 U of each of the restriction endonucleases *Nco*I and *Not*I, 5 µL of the NEBuffer 4, and 5 µg of RNase A in a total volume of 50 µL. Incubate at 37°C for 2 h. After the digest add 0.5 U of CIP to the sample containing the vector pHOG21 and incubate for an additional 2 h at 37°C. CIP will remove the 5'-phosphate of the vector DNA and therefore prevent the religation of pHOG21 to itself.

5. Add sample buffer and run the digested samples on a 1% TAE-agarose gel for approx 2.5 h at 5–6 V/cm. Split each sample into two equal aliquots and run them in adjacent lanes, leaving one lane without sample between different clones in order to prevent cross-contamination.

6. Check the gel on a long-wave UV transilluminator and excise the gel bands containing the *Nco*I/*Not*I-scFv inserts and the pHOG21 vector, respectively.

7. Extract the DNA from the gel blocks using the QIAquick gel extraction kit.

8. Run 1/50 of each sample along with increasing amounts of the λ *Bst*EII digestion marker (0.125 µg, 0.25 µg, 0.5 µg and 1 µg) on a 1.5% TAE-agarose gel. Determine the concentration of the extracted DNA (*see* **Note 10**).

9. Ligate the vector and insert using a molar ratio of between 1:1 and 1:3 according to the protocol provided with the ligation kit (*see* **Note 11**).

10. Precipitate the ligated DNA with 1/10 vol of 3 M sodium acetate, pH 7.5, 20 µg of glycogen and 2.5X volume absolute EtOH at –20°C for at least 1 h. Sediment the precipitated DNA by centrifugation for 30 min at 20,000g (14,000 rpm in Universal 16R centrifuge, Hettich). Wash the pellet three times with 500 µL 80% EtOH. Allow the pellet to dry at room temperature and subsequently resuspend in 5 µL H_2O.

11. Use the products of one ligation reaction for the transformation of a 40 µL aliquot of electrocompetent *E. coli* XL1-blue with the gene pulser electroporating device according to the supplier's protocol.

12. Plate out the bacteria on SOB-GA agar plates in dilutions of 1:1, 1:10, 1:100 and 1:1000, and incubate overnight at 37°C.

13. Pick several colonies per clone and check for pHOG21 containing scFv inserts as described in **Subheading 3.1.2.1.** and generate 20% (v/v) glycerol stocks from overnight cultures containing the scFv inserts. Store them at –80°C.

3.2.3. Small Scale Expression of scFv Antibody Fragments (63)

1. Inoculate 5 mL LB-GA medium with *E. coli* that had been transformed with anti-gp96 scFv antibody fragment carrying pHOG21. Incubate overnight at 37°C and 280 rpm.

2. Transfer 2.5 mL to 50 mL 2X YT-GA in a 100 mL Erlenmeyer flask and grow the culture to an OD_{600} of approx 0.6–0.8.

3. Transfer 2 mL of the culture to a new tube. This will be the "negative control" that will not be induced to produce soluble scFv antibody fragments.

4. Spin all cultures for 10 min at 1500g at room temperature (3000 rpm in Heraeus Megafuge, Kendro) and discard the supernatant (*see* **Note 12**).

5. Gently resuspend the bacterial pellet of the "negative control" in 2 mL 2X YT-GA, but use the original volume of 50 mL 2X YT-SA (no glucose!) for the remaining majority of pelleted *E. coli* cells. Just before the incubation add IPTG to a final concentration of 0.1 mM and shake all cultures overnight at room temperature at 280 rpm (*see* **Note 13**).

6. Measure the OD_{600} of the cultures. Take 100 µL of the induced and uninduced cultures, and centrifuge at 17,000g for 5 min at room temperature (14,000 rpm in Heraeus Biofuge). Discard the supernatant and resuspend the pellets, according to the measured OD_{600}, in SDS sample buffer (OD_{600} / 10 = volume of sample buffer in µL to be used).

7. Spin the remaining cultures for 15 min at 2800g and 4°C (4000 rpm in Heraeus Megafuge, Kendro). Save the supernatant (SN-1) and store on ice.

8. Resuspend the cell pellets in 5% of the original culture volume (=2.5 mL) of ice-cold shock solution and incubate on ice for approx 1 h. Shake gently from time to time (*see* **Note 14**).

9. Transfer to 1.5 mL tubes and centrifuge at 20,000g (14,000 rpm in Universal 16R centrifuge, Hettich) and 4°C for 45 min. The resulting supernatant contains the soluble periplasmic scFv antibody fraction. Take 50 µL and add to 50 µL 2X SDS sample buffer. Combine the remaining periplasmic supernatant with the corresponding sample of **step 10**.

10. Spin SN-1 (**step 7**) for 1 h at 6200g and 4°C (6000 rpm in Heraeus Megafuge, Kendro). Take 50 µL and add to 50 µL 2X SDS sample buffer. Combine the supernatant with the appropriate periplasmic fraction of **step 9**.

11. Sterile filter the samples using low protein binding syringe driven units of 0.22 µm preceded by a 5.0-µm filtration step.

12. Transfer into tubular dialysis membranes and thoroughly dialyze against one of the following buffers including three buffer changes every several hours at 4°C (*see* **Note 15**):

    a. Dialysis buffer (if the sample will be purified by IMAC), or

    b. PBS (if the sample will be stored for subsequent assays).

13. Fill into concentrating cups and spin at 4°C and approx 800*g* (2,200 rpm in Heraeus Megafuge, Kendro) to yield 1/10 of the original culture volume.

14. Make an additional SDS sample by adding 50 µL of the concentrated soluble scFv solutions to 50 µL of 2X SDS sample buffer. Add Pefabloc to the remaining solution at a final concentration of 200 µ*M* and 0.02% (w/v) sodium azide, then dispense into aliquots and store at –20°C or preferably at –80°C. Keep a sample at 4°C to be used in characterization assays such as SDS-PAGE, Western Blot, and ELISA (*see* **Note 16**).

15. Heat all SDS samples for 5 min at 95°C with vigorous shaking. Cool down immediately for a short time on ice. Spin the samples from the bacterial pellets for 5 min at 18,000*g* (14,300 rpm in Heraeus Biofuge, Kendro). Transfer the supernatant to a new tube and store all samples at –20°C.

3.2.4. Chromatographic Purification of Isolated Soluble scFv Antibodies (67,68)

1. Equilibrate a column containing chelating sepharose with approx 5 column volumes of dialysis buffer at a linear flow rate of 1–3 mL/min. Set the baseline on the recorder of the FPLC apparatus (*see* **Note 17**).

2. Load the dialysed scFv containing sample several times (at least twice) onto the column (*see* **Note 18**).

3. Wash the column with at least 10 column volumes wash buffer until the baseline is reached.

4. Wash the column with at least 10 column volumes wash buffer containing 50 m*M* imidazole (*see* **Note 19**).

5. Elute the scFv fragments with 5–10 column volumes wash buffer containing 250–300 m*M* imidazole. Collect the eluate in fractions (*see* **Note 20**).

6. Prepare SDS samples according to the elution profile (especially the peaks) recorded during the elution step and run an SDS-polyacrylamide gel and check the fractions for scFv and purity as described in **Subheading 3.3.1.**

7. Pool the scFv antibody fragment containing fractions and estimate the protein concentration by measuring the absorbance at 260 nm and 280 nm and applying the Warburg Christian equation (*70*) (*see* **Note 21**).

8. Transfer into tubular dialysis membranes and extensively dialyze against dialysis buffer at 4°C. Ensure that the buffer will be changed at least three times every few hours.

9. Concentrate the sample to a value of approx 0.5–1 mg protein/mL with concentrating devices and determine the concentration using a protein quantification assay, e.g., Bradford (Bio-Rad) (*71,72*).

10. Add Pefabloc at a final concentration of 200 µ*M* and 0.02% (w/v) sodium azide, prepare aliquots, and store at –80°C (*see* **Note 22**).

11. Check the binding activity of the purified scFv antibody fragments with the methods described in **Subheading 3.3.**

3.3. Detection and Characterization of Expressed Soluble scFv Fragments

3.3.1. Detection of the Expressed scFv Using SDS-PAGE and Western Blot

3.3.1.1. SDS-Polyacrylamide Gel Electrophoresis (SDS-PAGE) *(73)*

1. Thaw the SDS protein samples from the scFv expression and purification procedure. Allow the samples to equilibrate at room temperature to dissolve the SDS completely.
2. Assemble the electrophoresis apparatus, fill with running buffer, and load up to 15 μL (15-well comb) or 30 μL (10-well comb) of the protein samples into the wells of the pre-cast 12% polyacrylamide gel (*see* **Note 23**). Do not forget to also load approx 8–10 μL of the SDS-7 protein marker onto the gel for Coomassie staining. Use 10 μL of ECL protein marker (1 μg sample ECL marker in 9 μL of 2X SDS sample buffer) for the gel to be blotted (*see* **Note 24**).
3. Run the gel with at least 60 V (4–6 V/cm) and approx 3–4 W (measured at start) for about 1–1.5 h or until the blue dye front reaches the lower end of the gel (*see* **Note 25**).
4. Disassemble the gel chamber. Use one gel for Coomassie staining and the other for Western blotting.
5. Coomassie staining: place the gel into a tray containing 0.02% Coomassie staining solution so that it is well-covered. Incubate gently on a rocking shaker for at least 1 h or overnight.
6. Incubate the gel at room temperature by shaking in destaining solution with several changes of the solution until the background is completely removed and only the protein bands are visible.
7. Dry the gel overnight between two transparent gel drying sheets on a gel dryer according to the supplier's instructions. The dried gels are perfectly suited for documentation.

3.3.1.2. Western Blotting *(74)*

1. Assemble the tank blotting device as described by the supplier, ensuring that all the layers (Whatman paper, transfer membrane, and pads) are prewetted with the blotting buffer and that any air bubbles have been thoroughly removed. The membrane should be positioned closest to the anode. The connections should be checked for electrode orientation (*see* **Note 26**).
2. Run protein transfer for 1 h at 240 mA and 100 V.
3. Disassemble the blotting apparatus and check the transfer by staining the nitrocellulose membrane with the Ponceau solution. Apply a few mL of the Ponceau staining solution to the membrane (protein transfer side up), incubate for a few minutes by gently shaking, remove the staining solution, and wash the membrane with H_2O or PBS until protein bands are easily detectable. Mark the protein transfer side and migrating direction of the samples on the blotted membrane with a pencil. Excise the lane with the marker. Be careful, as the bands of the marker are not visible with Ponceau staining. Mark both membranes so that the marker lane can be repositioned during the ECL detection procedure (*see* **Note 27**).

4. Place the membranes in a petri dish or equivalent tray and incubate on a rocking shaker in a sufficient amount of blocking buffer (membrane should be well-covered and easily moving) for 1–2 h at room temperature or overnight at 4°C.
5. Proceed as outlined in the ECL brochure of the supplier. Use the antibodies as listed in the Materials section.

Bands corresponding to approx 30 kD molecular weight should be detectable in the induced samples as well as various steps of the purification procedure (*see* **Note 28**).

3.3.2. Enzyme-Linked Immunosorbent Assay (ELISA) *(75)*

1. Coat the wells of the microtiter plate with 0.5–1 µg gp96 in 100 µL dilution buffer and add 100 µL of dilution buffer alone in a corresponding well to each antigen-coated cavity. Incubate the plate overnight at 4°C or for 4 h at room temperature. Discard the coating solution and wash once with 200 µL PBS, pH 7.4.
2. Add 200 µL of blocking buffer (MPBS) to each well and incubate for 2–3 h at room temperature. Discard the blocking reagent and wash three times with PBS.
3. Add 100 µL of a dilution series of the expressed anti-gp96 scFv antibody samples and 100 µL of the rat-anti-Grp94 MAb to the antigen-coated and the corresponding uncoated wells. Incubate for 2 h at room temperature. Discard the antibody solutions and wash five times with 200 µL PBST.
4. To those wells incubated with scFv antibodies, add 100 µL of the secondary antibody mouse anti-human-c-myc MAb. Add 100 µL of MPBS to the remaining wells. Incubate at room temperature for 2 h. Discard the antibody solutions and wash five times with PBST.
5. Add 100 µL of the peroxidase-conjugated secondary antibodies to the appropriate wells. Incubate for 2 h at room temperature. Discard the solutions and wash five times with PBST.
6. Add 150 µL of the prepared TMB substrate solution (equal volumes of TMB peroxidase substrate and peroxidase solution B) and measure the kinetics of the absorbance at 595 nm in a microplate reader.

3.3.3. Dot-Blot Analysis *(76)*

1. Cut stripes of nitrocellulose membrane to fit 2 mL tubes and define three equal distinguishable sections on each with a pencil or scalpel. Mark the top for later interpretation of the results.
2. Dilute gp96 in the dilution buffers a, b, and c to a concentration of approx 250 ng/µL. Heat the sample in buffer c for 5 min at 95°C, cool shortly on ice, and spin quickly to recover all condensed liquid from the lid.
3. Place the prewetted (dilution buffer or PBS) membrane stripes on at least two layers of prewetted Whatman paper sheets. Apply 2 µL (=0.5 g) of the three different gp96 samples in the center of the appropriate premarked sections and let the sample buffers soak through the membrane (*see* **Note 27**).
4. Block the coated stripes with 1.5 mL MPBS in 2 mL tubes for at least 30 min at room temperature on a rotating device. Discard the blocking agent. Rinse once with approx 2 mL of TBS.
5. Add 500 µL of the anti-gp96 scFv samples (undiluted or diluted in MPBS, depending on the activity determined in the ELISA), the rat-anti-Grp94-antibody (positive control, 1:1000 or higher dilution in MPBS), and a scFv antibody nonreactive to gp96 to separate tubes. Incubate with gentle rotation at room temperature for 2 h.

6. Rinse once with 2 mL of TNT and then wash on a rotator three times for 15 min with 1.5 mL of TNT (only the scFv samples).

7. Add 1.5 mL of the mouse anti-human-c-myc antibody (1:5000 dilution in MPBS) and incubate for 1 h rotating at room temperature.

8. Repeat **step 6** for all membranes.

9. Incubate the membranes with 1.5 mL of the appropriate secondary peroxidase-conjugated antibodies (each diluted 1:5000 in MPBS) for 1 h at room temperature.

10. Rinse the tubes once with 1.5 mL of TNT, wash the membranes twice with 1.5 mL of TNT, and once with 1.5 mL of TBS (10 min each washing step).

11. Develop the membranes with 1.75 mL of horseradish peroxidase substrate solution in the tube or in small Petri dishes. Observe the developing signal and stop the reaction when the signals are significantly evident by rinsing shortly in H_2O or TBS. Dry on Whatman paper and store membranes in the dark (*see* **Note 29**).

3.3.4. Immunoprecipitation of Native gp96

The screening of the antibody library has been carried out with murine gp96. Therefore, one must check for the binding of the isolated scFv antibodies to the original antigen as well as to the human counterpart if vaccination protocols in man are considered. It is encouraged to use antigen of human origin for the antibody selection process where available.

3.3.4.1. PREPARATION OF CELL LYSATE

1. Wash 10^7 cells twice with PBS.

2. Add 35S-methionine (200 µCi) to 10 mL methionine-free RPMI 40 medium supplemented with 10% dialyzed FCS into a 250 mL tissue culture flask (*see* **Note 30**).

3. Incubate the cells at 37°C, and 5% CO_2 for 16 h.

4. Wash the cells twice with 20 mL ice-cold PBS in a 50 mL tube.

5. Transfer the cells into a 1.5 mL tube.

6. Wash the cells once with 1.5 mL of ice-cold PBS.

7. Add 500 µL of ice-cold lysis buffer (detergent or hypotonic) to the cell pellet.

8. Resuspend the pellet, vortex for 10 s, and incubate for 30 min on ice. If hypotonic lysis buffer is used, transfer the cell suspension after the incubation to the precooled douncer. The cells should then be dounced on ice with 15 strokes.

9. Spin the suspension for 30 s at 15,000g (13,000 rpm in Heraeus Biofuge fresco, Kendro) to remove cell debris.

10. Transfer the supernatant to a new precooled 1.5 mL tube and keep on ice.

3.3.4.2. PREPARATION OF BEADS

1. Pretreat the CNBr-activated sepharose beads for 15 min with 1 mM HCl at room temperature in a 50 mL tube. Use 20 mL of 1 mM HCl for 0.5 g of beads. The dry sepharose will swell immediately (0.5 g of dry beads correspond to 2 mL final volume of swollen beads). Spin down the beads at 700g (2000 rpm in Heraeus Megafuge) for 5 min and remove the supernatant. Wash beads again twice with 20–50 mL of 1 mM HCl. Alternatively, the 1 mM HCl wash solution can be applied in aliquots to the beads: add 3–4 times the bead volume of 1 mM HCl, mix gently by inverting the tube a few times, and then spin down the beads at 700g. Discard the supernatant and repeat wash procedure several times (*see also* instructions of supplier and **Note 31**).

2. Equilibrate the beads: add coupling buffer (20 mL for 0.5 g beads), mix gently, and spin for 5 min at 700*g*.
3. Change the buffer of the scFv antibody solution to coupling buffer by using a PD-10 desalting column. Dilute the antibody solution with coupling buffer to a concentration of about 0.5–1 mg/mL (*see* **Note 32**).
4. Add the antibody coupling solution to preswollen beads. The volume of the beads should represent approximately 20% of the coupling solution.
5. Gently rotate the suspension overnight at 4°C or for 1 h at room temperature (*see* **Note 33**).
6. Remove coupling solution. To determine the coupling efficiency measure the OD_{280} of the antibody coupling solution before the addition of the beads and at the end of the incubation. The coupling efficiency should be >50%.
7. Incubate the beads with 20 mL of the blocking buffer rotating for 1 h at room temperature.
8. Wash the beads as in **step 2** by alternating washing buffer, pH 4.0, with buffer, pH 8.0. Apply each buffer three times.
9. Wash the beads twice with PBS pH 7.4 as in **step 2**.
10. Add fresh PBS, pH 7.4, to obtain a 20% bead-suspension. Store the beads at 4°C. For long-term storage, add sodium azide to a final concentration of 0.02% (w/v) to prevent microbial growth (*see* **Note 3**).
11. Prepare control beads coupled with glycine as in **steps 1–10**. Use 0.2 *M* glycine, pH 8.0, instead of anti-gp96 scFv Abs.

3.3.4.3. IMMUNOPRECIPITATION

1. Preclear the lysate of proteins, which unspecifically bind to glycine beads, by adding 100 µL of the cold 20% glycine bead suspension to 500 µL of the lysate.
2. Vortex for 10 s and rotate overnight at 4°C.
3. Spin for 30 s at 15,000*g* (13,000 rpm in Heraeus Biofuge, Kendro) and transfer supernatant into a new precooled 1.5 mL tube.
4. Begin precipitation by adding 100 µL of the cold 20% anti-gp96 scFv Ab bead suspension to the precleared lysate.
5. Vortex and rotate for 2 h at 4°C.
6. Wash the beads five (!) times in PBS, pH 7.4, containing 0.5% NP-40 by adding the buffer, vortexing for 10 s, and spinning for 30 s at 15,000*g* (13,000 rpm in Heraeus Biofuge, Kendro).
7. After the addition of 2X SDS-PAGE loading buffer the beads can now be boiled for 5–10 min and the supernatant run on SDS-PAGE (as described in **Subheading 3.3.1**,) or frozen at –20°C.
8. Fix and dry the gel (as described in **ref. *66***).
9. For the detection of the radioactively marked proteins on the gel, follow the classical protocols using photographic films described in (*66*) or apply image plates to be read on a phosphoimager following the supplier's instructions (Fuji Photo Film).

3.4. Large Scale Expression and Purification of Soluble scFv Antibodies

3.4.1. Induction of Soluble scFv Fragments

The expression of soluble scFv fragments in a large scale shaking culture follows the same protocol as described for the small scale procedure because it represents an upscale of all steps. Ensure that larger flasks for the cultivation and centrifugation tubes are available. Be aware of the requirement for appropriate equipment such as centrifuges and shaking incubators as well as autoclaving capacities when producing proteins at a larger scale. The suggestion for expression of scFv in a total volume of 4–5 L bacterial culture is the result of the maximal scale volume that we are able to handle in our laboratory, by following the principles of each step, however, any scale can easily be performed according to the individual feasibility of the desired procedure.

3.4.2. Purification of the scFv Antibodies Using Immobilized Metal Ion Affinity Chromatography (IMAC)

The purification steps described in **Subheading 3.2.4.** also apply to the upscaled process, but ensure the chromatographic equipment such as pumping capacity, column size, and matrix volume are adjusted to the scale performed (*see also* instructions from the suppliers).

The main obstacle is the handling of large volumes of the bacterial culture and therefore the procedures of concentrating and dialysing the scFv containing culture supernatant. Be aware that all procedures should be performed at 4°C. A cold room or lab might be required!

Figure 1 shows a suggested scheme designed to handle larger volumes of supernatant (starting from 4–5 L) concerning the concentration and buffer exchange as a preparation for the chromatographic purification of the soluble scFv antibodies. Various filtration devices are available from several well-known suppliers. In each case the equipment can and should be optimally adjusted to the needs and scale of the laboratory.

Here, we briefly describe the procedure depicted in **Fig. 1**:

1. Follow the instructions provided by the manufacturer concerning the pretreatment, cleaning, and storage of the spiral membrane cartridge.
2. Prefilter the scFv containing solution consisting of the culture supernatant and the periplasmic preparation using a spiral-cap filter capsule.
3. Fill the round bottom flask (or similar three neck tank) with the filtered supernatant. The container with the remaining solution serves as the feed flask and the supernatant will be fed automatically to the main flask during the concentration process.
4. Assemble the system by connecting all in- and outlets with the appropriate tubing according to **Fig. 1**. Place the main process flask on top of a magnetic stirrer. Rotate the stir bar at a low to medium speed (*see* **Note 34**).
5. Start the pump and fill the cartridge slowly with the solution until a regular flow through the outlet tube back to the flask is observed.
6. Carefully close the outlet valve to create a slow permeate flow. Inlet pressure should be adjusted to approx 0.8–1.0 bar (12–15 psi). Make sure not to exceed a pressure drop of 0.7 bar (10 psi). Adjust the performance of the pump to keep a continuous recirculating flow through the cartridge back to the flask.
7. After the entire remaining supernatant has been fed to the process flask and has been concentrated to approx 2 L of the total volume, connect a flask containing dialysis buffer to the feeding line.
8. Allow diafiltration to proceed using dialysis buffer of at least 5 vol of initial concentrated supernatant at the start (*see* **Note 35**).

9. After complete diafiltration, proceed until the supernatant has been concentrated to about 1/5–1/10 of the original volume. Stop the pump slowly and disconnect the tubing.
10. Filter the concentrate in order to remove any aggregates before loading onto the chromatography column, and add protease inhibitors, e.g., Pefabloc (1:500).
11. Clean and store the cartridge as described by the manufacturer.

3.4.3. Determination of scFv Fragment Expression and Verification of the Binding Characteristics

Follow the steps in **Subheading 3.3.** described for the small scale expression procedure.

3.5. Purification of gp96 Using scFv Antibody Fragments Coupled to Sepharose Beads

3.5.1. Production of gp96-Specific Affinity Columns (77)

1. Follow the steps for the immobilization of the scFv antibodies to the CNBr-activated sepharose as described in **Subheading 3.3.4.1.** Use approx 5–10 mg scFv antibody to couple 0.5 g of beads. In addition, prepare control beads by coupling BSA or HSA (10–15 mg protein/0.5 g beads) to the matrix. The coupling can be carried out in the empty columns themselves (different sizes, MoBiTec). When using a batch procedure in separate 50 mL tubes, transfer the gel matrix to the appropriate empty column. Ensure that compression of the gel bed does not occur while adding the filter on top of the bed.
2. Equilibrate the gel matrix with 20% ethanol and store columns at 4°C until use.

3.5.2. One-Step Affinity Purification of gp96

1. Resuspend a 1 mL cell pellet, previously washed with cold PBS, in ice-cold hypotonic lysis buffer supplemented with protease inhibitors, using a total of 10 times the pellet volume.
2. Allow the cells to swell by incubating them with rotation for 1 h at 4°C.
3. Homogenize the cells by douncing on ice with approx 15 long and 10 short strokes.
4. Remove remaining cells and cell debris by spinning the cells at $2100g$ (3500 rpm in Heraeus Megafuge, Kendro) at 4°C for 20 min.
5. Transfer the supernatant to ultracentrifuge tubes and spin at $100,000g$ for 1 h.
6. During the ultracentrifugation step, equilibrate the scFv Sepharose column as well as the control BSA/HSA column with 5–10 column volumes of PBS, pH 7.4.
7. Apply the supernatant several times onto the columns by starting with the BSA column and allowing the supernatant to run directly onto the scFv column by gravity flow at 4°C. Repeat this at least 10 times (*see* **Note 36**).
8. Wash the columns separately with PBS, pH 7.4, followed by a wash with PBS, pH 7.4, containing 0.5 M NaCl and a final wash with PBS again. Use 5 bed volumes of washing buffer for each step. The washing procedure is carried out at room temperature. Collect the buffers in fractions in 1.5 or 2 mL tubes cooled on ice or in a cooling block (*see* **Note 37**).
9. Elute both columns at room temperature with 5 bed volumes PBS, pH 7.4, containing 1.3 M NaCl, collecting 1 mL aliquots into cooled tubes (*see* **Note 37**).
10. Prepare SDS-protein samples from the fractions and check for the presence of gp96 using SDS-PAGE and Western blot as described in **Subheading 3.3.1.**
11. Pool the fractions containing gp96 and determine the approximate protein concentration in a UV spectrophotometer by using the Warburg Christian formula (*56*). To get a quick

but rough estimation, the absorption of gp96 at 280 nm can be measured and the concentration calculated using an extinction coefficient ϵ_{280} of 1: protein concentration = A280 / ϵ_{280} × d (mg/mL) (*see* **Note 21**).

12. Concentrate the solution to approx 0.5–1 mg/mL in a concentrating device at 4°C (*see* **Note 38**). During this concentration step change the buffer by adding about five times the sample volume of 10 mM sodium phosphate, 0.38 M NaCl, pH 7.0, in small portions.
13. Quantify the protein by following **step 11** and/or by using a protein assay *(57,58)*.
14. Store the gp96 in aliquots at –80°C (*see* **Note 1**).
15. Regenerate the columns by applying about 5–10 bed volumes PBS, pH 7.4, containing 2 M NaCl.
16. Equilibrate the columns with 5 bed volumes 20% (v/v) ethanol in H$_2$O or PBS, pH 7.4 containing 0.02% (w/v) sodium azide. Store the columns at 4°C.

4. Notes

1. Thawed gp96 preparations are quite unstable and can be stored at 4°C for approx 1 wk. Therefore, prepare small aliquots that suit your experiments once the stock has been initially thawed and store them at –70°C. Avoid repeated freeze-thaw cycles.
2. Because EtBr is light-sensitive, store the stock solution in the dark. Caution: Wearing gloves while handling EtBr is imperative because of its mutagenic and toxic properties.
3. Be aware of the toxic properties of sodium azide. Wear gloves while handling it.
4. The solution is sensitive to light and should be stored tightly closed in the dark at 4°C.
5. Freshly prepare the substrate solution each time before use, and use the solution immediately!
6. Add a drop of mineral oil on top of the *Bst*NI reaction mixture in order to prevent evaporation during the incubation at 60°C.
7. Load an aliquot of the 100 bp ladder on both sides or within the gel for better interpretation of the pattern. Do not pour the agarose gels too thick, to ensure clear and sharp bands.
8. If possible, sequence more than two representatives of each group or even all single clones to catch each antibody sequence. Keep in mind that this might be very costly and time-consuming. If all clones are to be sequenced, you can skip the restriction digest procedure.
9. The following primers can be used for the sequencing in
   a. pHEN1 *(35)*:
      forward primer LMB3 (5'-CAGGAAACAGCTATGAC)
      reverse primer fd-SEQ1 (5'-GAATTTTCTGTATGAGG)
   b. pHOG21:
      forward primer DP-1 (5'-ATTAAAGAGGAGAAATTAACCA)
      reverse primer pSEXBn
      (5'-GGTCGACGTTAACCGACAAACAACAGATAAAACG)
10. Consider the following for the calculation of the DNA concentration:
    a. λ DNA = 48,502 bp
    b. For comparison with each insert and the pHOG21 sample, choose a band of the λ BstEII digestion marker that is most similar in size and intensity.
    c. Use the equation: Quantity of insert or vector DNA on gel = (base pairs of λ band to size-corresponding insert) × (the amount of λ DNA in chosen lane) / (48,502 bp).
    d. Calculate total amount and concentration of DNA in eluted samples.
11. The amount of 50 ng of DNA is needed for each *E. coli* transformation. Considering molecular weights of approx 0.750 kb for the scFv inserts and approx 2.85 kb for the

vector pHOG21 (ratio vector:insert = approx 1:4), as well as, the molar ratio of 1:2, the actual ratio of the amounts of vector to insert will be 1:8. This means that in this case 6.25 ng of vector and 43.75 ng of insert must be added to the ligation reaction mix.

12. Do not centrifuge at high speed, as a bacterial pellet that is not too dense will facilitate resuspension, and undamaged *E. coli* cells are necessary for the subsequent induction.

13. Ensure that no glucose had been added to the medium in order to guarantee induction via the *lac*-promoter.

14. Prior to use, add Pefabloc to a final concentration of 0.2 m*M* and dissolve a mini or regular protease inhibitor cocktail tablet in every 10 mL or 50 mL of shock solution, respectively.

15. Dialyzed samples can be loaded onto a metal chelate affinity chromatography column for purification. If the sample is to be purified by IMAC, imidazole can be added to the dialysis buffer up to a concentration of approx 10 m*M*. This may help to prevent the adsorption of *E. coli* proteins that would only weakly bind to the metal chelate complex and therefore block potential binding sites for the scFv fragments. The optimal concentration for the additional imidazole in the dialysis buffer must be determined for each his-tagged protein in order not to challenge the binding of the his-tagged protein to the matrix.

16. Do not use liquid nitrogen to freeze the samples as often recommended for intact immunoglobulin molecules. The shock-freezing procedure might lead to aggregation and inactivation of the scFv proteins after re-thawing (*see also* **Note 22**). Please take into account that in assays such as ELISA or dot blot the background might be higher with samples that have not been purified by IMAC due to unspecific binding of remaining *E. coli* proteins.

17. Use approx 5 mL of chelating resin for each liter of culture medium. Filter and degas all buffers before applying to the column. Simple filtration with vacuum driven filter units such as stericups (Millipore) is sufficient for this purpose. Do not use a vacuum-driven filter for the antibody solution because excessive foaming will occur, thereby destroying the properties of the protein to be purified.

18. Take samples of each flow-through, in order to determine the binding efficiency, so that a sufficient number of sample loadings to be repeated and the volume of the chelating resin can eventually be adapted.

19. If desired, collect the eluate in fractions in order to check for loss of scFv during the washing step.

20. Do not take fractions that are too large in order to avoid unnecessary dilution of the scFv antibody. To increase the concentration of the scFv antibody in the collected fractions, the elution flow can be paused, when approx one column void volume has been applied, and then be incubated for at least 30 min to loosen the binding of the scFv to the chelating complex. The eluted protein will be abundant in fewer fractions in a higher concentration. For the same reason, keep the flow rate relatively low at 1–2 mL/min during the elution step.

21. The Warburg Christian formula only provides an estimation of the protein concentration: $1,55 \times A_{280} - 0.757 \times A_{260} =$ protein concentration (mg/mL). If a more accurate determination is required, a protein assay such as the Bradford (Bio-Rad) assay may be performed using the IgG (for antibody samples) or the BSA standards provided to create the calibration curve (*71,72*).

22. For long-term storage, 10–50% (v/v) glycerol or BSA (final concentration of 10 mg/mL) may be added as protective agents. Remember that stabilizing proteins may interfere in

subsequent procedures, such as coupling to sepharose beads, and must be removed prior usage. As well, each scFv protein behaves differently in its environment, due to its amino acid sequence. Therefore, the optimal buffer composition for storage has to be determined empirically. Addition of imidazole at a concentration of approx 50 mM to the chosen basic buffer, such as PBS or Tris-HCl, seems to help stabilizing the scFv fragments.

23. Casting the polyacrylamide gels immediately before use results in better running conditions and clearer and sharper protein bands. For casting instructions refer to **ref. 66**.
24. Run two gels of the same sample composition in one chamber for detection via Coomassie staining and Western blotting in order to get the optimal results for further interpretation.
25. Though it may sound obvious, ensure correct connections of the anode and cathode.
26. For the transfer of the proteins from the gel to the carrier membrane both blotting techniques—wet in a liquid tank or semi-dry—can be performed.
27. Do not allow the membrane to dry at any step of the procedure.
28. After the incubation of the membrane with the ECL substrate, drain the substrate, and rinse quickly in H$_2$O, then drain the H$_2$O onto Whatman paper. This additional step will reduce potential background signals significantly.
29. The ECL chemiluminescent detection system, as described in **Subheading 3.3.1.**, can also be used with the dot blot procedure. The amounts of the antigen coated can be reduced and the antibodies may be applied in higher dilutions due to the increased sensitivity of this system. For sensitivity and documentation reasons, the ECL method may be the system of choice.
30. Precautions should be taken during storage, handling, and disposal of radioactive material according to appropriate national regulations.
31. Avoid applying high g forces to the beads in order to avoid breakage. When using larger volumes of resin, the beads can also be washed on a sintered glass filter (*see* supplier's protocol).
32. Remember that the original sample will be diluted 1.4 times. The coupling buffer should not contain any reactive amino groups itself that may interfere with the covalent linkage of the proteins to the resin. The abundant buffer substance Tris-HCl cannot be used in the coupling step.
33. Do not use a magnetic stirrer to avoid destruction of the Sepharose beads.
34. Tightly connect all parts in order to create a closed system, and ensure that the valves are open.
35. Ensure that the pressure does not become too high. Adjust the recirculating flow and inlet pressure, so that the dialysis buffer is continuously but slowly added to the supernatant. If the pressure is too high and too much buffer is added at once, precipitation may occur. Ensure that the stir bar thoroughly mixes the incoming dialysis buffer with the concentrated supernatant.
36. The solution may also be recycled over the columns overnight at 4°C using a peristaltic pump. Ensure that the flow rate is adjusted to prevent the columns from running dry.
37. The washing and elution buffers must be determined empirically for each scFv antibody. Choosing inappropriate conditions may result in impurity of the eluted fraction, lack of gp96 elution, or even loss of antigenic peptides from the heat shock protein-peptide complex. In consequence, the immunogenicity of the isolated gp96 may not be retained (*65*).
38. Pretreat the concentrator with 0.2 M glycine to block nonspecific adsorption of gp96 to the membrane.

Acknowledgments

We would like to thank Christoph Dufter for his efforts in helping with the creation of the figure and for his professional advice, Franziska Biellmann for preparing affinity columns and purifying gp96 from various cell lines, as well as Tania Simon for reading the manuscript and providing its linguistic refinement. Thanks to Ulrich Christ and Matthias Tremmel for the production of the sequencing primers (Department of Transplantation Immunology, Institute of Immunology, University of Heidelberg). Special acknowledgment also goes to Fiona Sait, Ahuva Nissim, and Greg Winter (Medical Research Council, Cambridge, UK) for kindly providing the synthetic scFv library (#1). We also thank Dr. Sergey Kipriyanov (Affimed Therapeutics AG, Ladenburg, Germany), Prof. Dr. Izumi Kumagai (Tohoku University, Sendai, Japan), and Dr. Olga Kupriyanova for helpful discussions about storing conditions for scFv proteins.

References

1. Udono, H. and Srivastava, P. K. (1993) Heat shock protein 70-associated peptides elicit specific cancer immunity. *J. Exp. Med.* **178,** 1391–1396.
2. Castelli, C., Ciupitu, A.-M. T., Rini, F., Rivoltini, L., Mazzocchi, A., Kiessling, R., and Parmiani, G. (2001) Human heat shock protein 70 peptide complexes specifically activate antimelanoma T cells. *Cancer Res.* **61,** 222–227.
3. Blachere, N. E., Udono, H., Janetzki, S., Li, Z., Heike, M., and Srivastava, P. K. (1993) Heat shock protein vaccines against cancer. *J. Immunother.* **14,** 352–356.
4. Wang, X.-Y., Kazim, L., Repasky, E. A., and Subjeck, J. R. (2001) Characterization of heat shock protein 110 and glucose-regulated protein 170 as cancer vaccines and the effect of fever-range hyperthermia on vaccine activity. *J. Immunol.* **165,** 490–497.
5. Udono, H., Levey, D. L., and Srivastava, P. K. (1994) Cellular requirements for tumor-specific immunity elicited by heat shock proteins: tumor rejection antigen gp96 primes CD8+ T cells *in vivo. Proc. Natl. Acad. Sci. USA* **91,** 3077–3081.
6. Basu, S. and Srivastava, P. K. (1999) Calreticulin, a peptide-binding chaperone of the endoplasmic reticulum, elicits tumor- and peptide-specific immunity. *J. Exp. Med.* **189,** 797–802.
7. Nair, S., Wearsch, P. A., Mitchell, D. A., Wassenberg, J. J., Gilboa, E., and Nicchitta, C. V. (1999) Calreticulin displays *in vivo* peptide-binding activity and can elicit CTL responses against bound peptides. *J. Immunol.* **162,** 6426–6432.
8. Tamura, Y., Peng, P., Liu, K., Daou, M., and Srivastava, P. K. (1997) Immunotherapy of tumors with autologous tumor-derived heat shock protein preparations. *Science* **278,** 117–120.
9. Navaratnam, M., Desphpande, M. S., Hariharan, M. J., Zatechka, D. S., and Srikumaran, S. (2001) Heat shock protein-peptide complexes elicit cytotoxic T-lymphocyte and antibody responses specific for bovine herpesvirus 1. *Vaccine* **19,** 1425–1434.
10. Zügel, U., Sponaas, A.-M., Neckermann, J., Schoel, B., and Kaufmann, S. H. E. (2001) gp96-peptide vaccination of mice against intracellular bacteria. *Infect. Immun.* **69,** 4164–4167.
11. Singh-Jasuja, H., Hilf, N., Arnold-Schild, D., and Schild, H. (2001) The role of heat shock proteins and their receptors in the acivation of the immune system. *Biol. Chem.* **382,** 629–636.
12. Anderson, K. M. and Srivastava, P. K. (2001) Heat, heat shock, heat shock proteins and death: a central link in innate and adaptive immune response. *Immunol. Lett.* **74,** 35–39.

13. Srivastava, P. K. (2000) Immunotherapy of human cancer: lessons from mice. *Nat. Immunol.* **1,** 363–366.
14. Srivastava, P. K., Ménoret, A., Basu, S., Binder, R. J., and McQuade, K. L. (1998) Heat shock proteins come of age: primitive functions acquire new roles in an adaptive world. *Immunity* **8,** 657–665.
15. Ménoret, A., and Chandawarkar, R. (1998) Heat-shock protein-based anticancer immuno-therapy: an idea whose time has come. *Semin. in Oncol.* **25,** 654–660.
16. Schild, H., Arnold-Schild, D., Lammert, E., and Rammensee, H. G. (1999) Stress pro-teins and immunity mediated by cytotoxic T lymphocytes. *Curr. Opin. Immunol.* **11,** 109–113.
17. Heike, M., Weinmann, A., Bethke, K., and Galle, P. R. (1999) Stress protein/peptide com-plexes derived from autologous tumor tissue as tumor vaccines. *Biochem. Pharmacol.* **58,** 1381–1387.
18. Suto, R. and Srivastava, P. K. (1995) A mechanism for the specific immunogenicity of heat shock protein-chaperoned peptides. *Science* **269,** 1585–1588.
19. Arnold, D., Faath, S., Rammensee, H.-G. R., and Schild, H. (1995) Cross-priming of minor histocompatibility antigen-specific cytotoxic T cells upon immunization with the heat shock protein gp96. *J. Exp. Med.* **182,** 885–889.
20. Nieland, T. J. F., Agnes, A., Tan, M. C., Monnee-Van Muijen, M., Koning, F., Kruisbeek, A. M., and Van Bleek, G. (1995) Isolation of an immunodominant viral peptide that is endogenously bound to the stress protein GP96/GRP94. *Proc. Natl. Acad. Sci. USA* **93,** 6135–6139.
21. Blachere, N. E., Li, Z., Chandawarkar, R. Y., Suto, R., Jaikaria, N. S., Basu, S., et al. (1997) Heat shock protein-peptide complexes, reconstituted in vitro, elicit peptide-specific cytotoxic T lymphocyte response and tumor immunity. *J. Exp. Med.* **186,** 1315–1322.
22. Lammert, E., Arnold, D., Nijenhuis, M., Momburg, F., Hämmerling, G., Brunner, J., et al. (1997) The endoplasmic reticulum-resident stress protein gp96 binds peptides translo-cated by TAP. *Eur. J. Immunol.* **27,** 923–927.
23. Ciupitu, A. M., Petersson, M., O'Donnell, C. L., Williams, K., Jindal, S., Kiessling, R., and Welsh, R. M. (1998) Immunization with a lymphocytic choriomeningitis virus pep-tide mixed with heat shock protein 70 results in protective antiviral immunity and specific cytotoxic T lymphocytes. *J. Exp. Med.* **187,** 685–691.
24. Ishii, T., Udono, H., Yamano, T., Ohta, H., Uenaka, A., Ono, T., et al. (1999) Isolation of MHC class I-restricted tumor antigen peptide and its precursors associated with the heat shock proteins hsp70, hsp90, and gp96. *J. Immunol.* **162,** 1303–1309.
25. Binder, R. J., Blachere, N. E., and Srivastava, P. K. (2001) Heat shock protein-chaperoned peptides but not free peptides introduced into the cytosol are presented efficiently by ma-jor histocompatibility complex I molecules. *J. Biol. Chem.* **276,** 17,163–17,171.
26. Meng, S. D., Gao, T., Gao, G. F., and Tien, P. (2001) HBV-specific peptide associated with heat-shock protein gp96. *Lancet* **357,** 528–529.
27. Arnold-Schild, D., Hanau, D., Spehner, D., Schmid, C., Rammensee, H.-G., de la Salle, H., and Schild, H. (1999) Cutting edge: receptor-mediated endocytosis of heat shock pro-teins by professional antigen-presenting cells. *J. Immunol.* **162,** 3757–3760.
28. Wassenberg, J. J., Dezfulian, C., and Nicchitta, C. V. (1999) Receptor mediated and fluid phase pathways for internalization of the ER Hsp90 chaperone GRP94 in murine mac-rophages. *J. Cell Sci.* **112,** 2167–2175.
29. Binder, R., Han, D. H., and Srivastava, P. K. (2000) CD91: a receptor for heat shock protein gp96. *Nature Immunol.* **1,** 151–155.

30. Singh-Jasuja, H., Toes, R. E., Spee, P., Munz, C., Hilf, N., Schoenberger, S. P., et al. (2000) Cross-presentation of glycoprotein 96-associated antigens on major histocompatibility complex class I molecules requires receptor-mediated endocytosis. *J. Exp. Med.* **191,** 1965–1974.
31. Singh-Jasuja, H., Hilf, N., Scherer, H. U., Arnold-Schild, D., Rammensee, H. G., Toes, R. E., and Schild H. (2000) The heat shock protein gp96: a receptor-targeted cross-priming carrier and acivator of dendritic cells. *Cell Stress Chap.* **5,** 462–470.
32. Basu, S., Binder, R. J., Ramalingam, T., and Srivastava, P. K. (2001) CD91 is a common receptor for heat shock proteins gp96, hsp90, hsp70, and calreticulin. *Immunity* **14,** 303–313.
33. Srivastava, P. K., Udono, H., Blachere, N. E., and Li, Z. (1994) Heat shock proteins transfer peptides during antigen processing and CTL priming. *Immunogenetics* **39,** 93–98.
34. Udono, H. and Srivastava, P. K. (1994) Comparison of tumor-specific immunogenicities of stress-induced proteins gp96, hsp90, and hsp70. *J. Immunol.* **152,** 5398–5403.
35. Nicchitta, C. V. (1998) Biochemical, cell biological and immunological issues surrounding the endoplasmic reticulum chaperone GRP94/gp96. *Curr. Opin. Immunol.* **10,** 103–109.
36. Linderoth, N. A., Popowicz, A., and Sastry, S. (2000) Identification of the peptide-binding site in the heat shock chaperone/tumor rejection gp96 (Grp94). *J. Biol. Chem.* **275,** 5472–5477.
37. Singh-Jasuja, H., Scherer, H. U., Hilf, N., Arnold-Schild, D., Rammensee, H. G., Toes, R. E., and Schild, H. (2000) The heat shock protein gp96 induces maturation of dendritic cells and down-regulation of its receptor. *Eur. J. Immunol.* **30,** 2211–2215.
38. Linderoth, N. A., Simon, M. N., Rodionova, N. A., Cadene, M., Laws, W. R., Chait, B. T., and Sastry, S. (2001) Biophysical analysis of the endoplasmic reticulum-resident chaperone/heat shock protein gp96/GRP94 and its complex with peptide antigen. *Biochemistry* **40,** 1483–1495.
39. Menoret, A., Niswonger, M. I., Altmeyer, S., and Srivastava, P. K. (2001) An ER protein implicated in chaperoning peptides to MHC class I is an aminopeptidase. *J. Biol. Chem.,* in press.
40. Janetzki, S., Palla, D., Rosenhauer, V., Lochs, H., Lewis, J. J., and Srivastava, P. K. (2000) Immunization of cancer patients with autologous cancer-derived heat shock protein gp96 preparations: a pilot study. *Int. J. Cancer* **88,** 232–238.
41. Winter, G. and Milstein, C. (1991) Man-made antibodies. *Nature* **349,** 293–299.
42. Lerner, R. A., Kang, A. S., Bain, J. D., Burton, D. R., and Barbas, C. F., III (1992) Antibodies without immunization. *Science* **258,** 1313–1314.
43. McCafferty, J., Griffiths, A. D., Winter, G., and Chiswell, D. J. (1990) Phage antibodies: filamentous phage displaying antibody variable domains. *Nature* **348,** 552–554.
44. Barbas, C. F., III, Kang, A. S., Lerner, R. A., and Benkovic, S. J. (1991) Assembly of combinatorial antibody libraries on phage surfaces: the gene III site. *Proc. Natl. Acad. Sci. USA* **88,** 7978–7982.
45. Breitling, F., Dübel, S., Seehaus, T., Klewinghaus, I., and Little, M. (1991) A surface expression vector for antibody screening. *Gene* **104,** 147–153.
46. Hoogenboom, H. R., Griffiths, A. D., Johnson, K. S., Chiswell, D. J., Hudson, P., and Winter, G. (1991) Multi-subunit proteins on the surface of filamentous phage: methodologies for displaying antibody (Fab) heavy and light chains. *Nucleic Acids Res.* **19,** 4133–4137.

47. Little, M., Breitling, F., Dübel, S., Fuchs, P., and Braunagel, M. (1995) Human antibody libraries in *Escherichia coli. J. Biotechnol.* **41,** 187–195.
48. Marks, J. D., Hoogenboom, H. R., Bonnert, T. P., McCafferty, J., Griffiths, A. D., and Winter, G. (1991) By-passing immunization: human antibodies from V-gene libraries displayed on phage. *J. Mol. Biol.* **222,** 581–597.
49. Rapoport, B., Portolano, S., and McLachlan, S. M. (1995) Combinatorial libraries: new insights into human organ-specific autoantibodies. *Immunol. Today* **16,** 43–49.
50. Griffiths, A. D., Malmquist, M., Marks, J. D., Bye, J. M., Embleton, M. J., McCafferty, J., et al. (1993) Human anti-self antibodies with high specificity from phage display libraries. *EMBO J.* **12,** 725–734.
51. Vaughan, T. J., Williams, A. J., Pritchard, K., Osbourn, J. K., Pope, A. R., Earnshaw, J. C., et al. (1996) Human antibodies with sub-nanomolar affinities isolated from a large non-immunized phage display library. *Nature Biotech.* **14,** 309–314.
52. Welschof, M., Terness, P., Kipriyanov, S. M., Stanescu, D., Breitling, F., Dörsam, H., et al. (1997) The antigen-binding domain of a human IgG-anti-F(ab')$_2$ autoantibody. *Proc. Natl. Acad. Sci. USA* **94,** 1902–1907.
53. Little, M., Welschof, M., Braunagel, M., Hermes, I., Christ, C., Keller, A., et al. (1999) Generation of a large complex antibody library from multiple donors. *J. Immunol. Methods* **231,** 3–9.
54. Waterhouse, P., Griffiths, A. D., Johnson, K. S., and Winter, G. (1993) Combinatorial infection and *in vivo* recombination: a strategy for making large phage antibody repertoires. *Nucleic Acids Res.* **21,** 2265–2266.
55. Hoogenboom, H. R. and Winter, G. (1992) By-passing immunization. Human antibodies from synthetic repertoires of germline VH gene segments rearranged *in vitro. J. Mol. Biol.* **227,** 381–388.
56. Barbas, C. F., Bain, J. D., Hoekstra, D. M., and Lerner, R. A. (1992) Semisynthetic combinatorial antibody libraries: a chemical solution to the diversity problem. *Proc. Natl. Acad. Sci. USA* **89,** 4457–4467.
57. Braunagel, M. and Little, M. (1997) Construction of a semisynthetic antibody library using trinucleotide oligos. *Nucleic Acids Res.* **25,** 4690–4691.
58. Nissim, A., Hoogenboom, H. R., Tomlinson, I. M., Flynn, G., Midgley, C., Lane, D., and Winter, G. (1994) Antibody fragments from a 'single pot' phage display library as immunochemical reagents. *EMBO J.* **13,** 692–698.
59. Bird, R. E., Hardman, K. D., Jacobson, J. W., Johnson, S., Kaufman, B. M., Lee, S.-M., et al. (1988) Single-chain antigen-binding proteins. *Science* **242,** 423–426.
60. Lindquist, S. (1988) The heat shock proteins. *Ann. Rev. Genet.* **22,** 631–677.
61. Robert, J., Ménoret, A., Basu, S., Cohen, N., and Srivastava, P. K. (2001) Phylogenetic conservation of the molecular and immunological properties of the chaperones gp96 and hsp70. *Eur. J. Immunol.* **31,** 186–195.
62. Skerra, A. and Plückthun, A. (1988) Assembly of a functional immunoglobulin Fv fragment in *Escherichia coli. Science* **240,** 1038–1041.
63. Kipriyanov, S. M., Moldenhauer, G., and Little, M. (1997) High level production of soluble single chain antibodies in small-scale *Escherichia coli* cultures. *J. Immunol. Methods* **200,** 69–77.
64. Kipriyanov, S. M. and Little, M. (1997) Affinity purification of tagged recombinant proteins using immobilized single chain Fv fragments. *Anal. Biochem.* **244,** 189–191.

65. Arnold-Schild, D., Kleist, C., Welschof, M., Opelz, G., Rammensee, H.-G., Schild, H., and Terness, P. (2000) One-step single-chain Fv recombinant antibody-based purification of gp96 for vaccine development. *Cancer Res.* **60,** 4175–4178.

66. Sambrook, J. and Russell, D. W. (2001) *Molecular Cloning: A Laboratory Manual,* 3rd ed., Cold Spring Harbor Laboratory Press, Cold Spring Harbor, NY.

67. Porath, J., Carlsson, J., Olsson, I., and Belfrage, G. (1975) Metal chelate affinity chromatography, a new approach to protein fractionation. *Nature* **258,** 598–599.

68. Lindner, P., Guth, B., Wülfing, C., Krebber, C., Steipe, B., Müller, F., and Plückthun, A. (1992) Purification of native proteins from the cytoplasm and periplasm of *Escherichia coli* using IMAC and histidine tails: a comparison of proteins and protocols. *Methods Compan. Methods Enzymol.* **4,** 41–55.

69. Sanger, F., Nicklen, S., and Coulson, A. R. (1977) DNA sequencing with chain-terminating inhibitors. *Proc. Natl. Acad. Sci. USA* **74,** 5463–5467.

70. Warburg, O. and Christian, W. (1941), Isolierung und Kristallisation des Gärungsferments Enolase. *Biochem. Z.* **310,** 384–421.

71. Stoschek, C. M. (1990) Quantitation of protein. *Methods Enzymol.* **182,** 50–68.

72. Bradford, M. M. (1976) A rapid and sensitive method for the quantitation of microgram quantities of protein utilizing the principle of protein-dye binding. *Anal. Biochem.* **72,** 248–254.

73. Laemmli, U. K. (1970) Cleavage of structural proteins during the assembly of the head of bacteriophage T4. *Nature* **227,** 680–685.

74. Towbin, H., Staehelin, T., and Gordon, J. (1979) Electrophoretic transfer of proteins from polyacrylamide gels to nitrocellulose sheets: procedure and some applications. *Proc. Natl. Acad. Sci. USA* **76,** 4350–4354.

75. Engvall, E. and Perlmann, P. (1971) Enzyme linked immunosorbent assay (ELISA): quantitative assay of immunoglobulin G. *Immunochem.* **8,** 871–874.

76. Beyer, C. F. (1984) A "dot-immunoblotting assay" on nitrocellulose membrane for the detection of the immunoglobulin class of mouse monoclonal antibodies. *J. Immunol. Methods* **67,** 79–86.

77. Berry, M. J. and Pierce, J. J. (1993) Stability of immunoadsorbents comprising antibody fragments. Comparison of Fv fragments and single-chain Fv fragments. *J. Chromatogr.* **629,** 161–168.

25

Recombinant Adenoviruses
for In Vivo Expression of Antibody Fragments

Roland E. Kontermann, Tina Korn, and Valérie Jérôme

1. Introduction

A growing number of recombinant antibodies is being developed for immuno-therapy of cancer *(1,2)* (*see* also Chapter 2). Although these recombinant antibodies can exhibit a potent anti-tumoral activity in vitro, efficacy in vivo is often limited by the short serum half-life of these molecules. Thus, repeated or continuous administrations are required to obtain a sufficiently high serum concentration. An alternative approach to the injection of the therapeutic molecules is the expression and secretion of these proteins in vivo, which leads to high levels of the molecules in the serum *(3–6)*. Furthermore, this approach obviates the need for the preparation of bulk amounts of pure protein. Recombinant adenoviruses are widely used vectors for the delivery of a transgene in gene therapy *(7)*. Recently, it was demonstrated that an anti-carcino-embryonic antigen (CEA) scFv-granulocyte/monocyte colony-stimulating factor (GM-CSF) fusion protein is expressed in vivo for a prolonged period of time after intravenous injection of recombinant adenoviruses *(8)*.

Here, we describe the generation of recombinant adenoviruses for the expression of recombinant antibodies, exemplified for bispecific single-chain diabodies (scDb). These scDbs have been successfully applied for the recruitment of effector molecules and the retargeting of effector cells and viral vectors *(9–12)*. Possible applications of in vivo expressed single-chain diabodies include the retargeting of cytotoxic T lymphocytes to tumor cells. Single-chain diabodies are generated by joining the four variable light and heavy chain domains of two antibodies either in the format V_HA-linkerA-V_LB-linkerM-V_HB-linkerB-V_LA (V_H-V_L orientation) or V_LA-linkerA-V_HB-linkerM-V_LB-linkerB-V_HA (V_L-V_H orientation) *(13)*. Linkers A and B are routinely chosen to be 5–6 residues and linker M 15–20 residues (*see* **Figs. 1** and **2**). In addition to the standard glycine/serine-rich linkers, we have isolated other nonrepetitive linkers from phage-displayed scDb libraries *(14)*. The following protocols describe the generation of a scDb in the V_H-V_L orientation (*see* **Fig. 2**). In the first step, the first antibody is

From: *Methods in Molecular Biology, vol. 207: Recombinant Antibodies for Cancer Therapy: Methods and Protocols*
Edited by: M. Welschof and J. Krauss © Humana Press Inc., Totowa, NJ

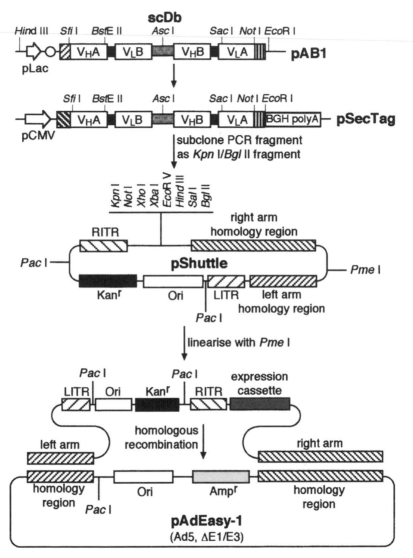

Fig. 1. Construction of a recombinant adenovirus for expression of a scDb. A bispecific single-chain diabody is assembled and cloned into a bacterial expression vector. After subcloning into a mammalian expression vector, the expression cassette is introduced into pShuttle. Co-transformation of the pShuttle plasmid DNA, which is linearized by *Pme*I digestion, and pAdEasy-1 DNA into BJ5183 leads to incorporation of the expression cassette into the adenoviral genome by homologous recombination. The pAdEasy-1 DNA is then linearized with *Pac*I to expose the inverted terminal repeat sequences and transfected into HEK293 producer cells. These cells contain the *E1* region missing in pAdEasy-1, which is essential for production of viral particles. Amp^r, ampicillin resistance; Kan^r, kanamycin resistance; LITR, left inverted terminal repeat; Ori, origin of replication; RITR, right inverted terminal repeat).

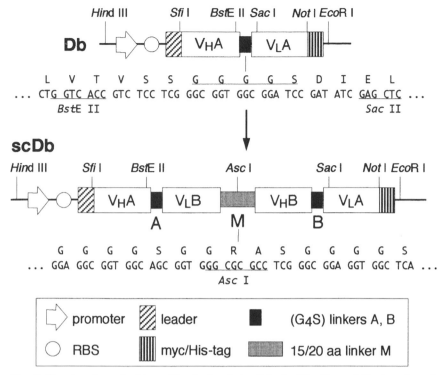

Fig. 2. Construction of a bispecific single-chain diabody. The V_H and V_L domains of antibody A are assembled after PCR amplification in form of a bivalent diabody, introducing *BstE*II and *Sac*I sites for subsequent cloning. The V_H and V_L domains of the second antibody are then cloned into this construct with the indicated linker sequences A, M, and B.

cloned as a bivalent diabody introducing a 5 residues linker as well as appropriate cloning sites at the C-terminal region of the V_H domain and the N-terminal region of the V_L domain. In the second step, the V_H and V_L domains of the second antibody are amplified separately introducing sequences encoding the middle linker M. The two fragments are then cloned into the diabody construct of step 1. The resulting scDb contained in a bacterial expression vector is then subcloned into a mammalian expression vector, such as pSecTag possessing the CMV promoter, an Igκ leader sequence and the bovine growth hormone (BGH) polyadenylation sequence (*see* **Fig. 1**). This expression cassette is subsequently cloned into the pShuttle vector and introduced by homologous recombination into pAdEasy-1. Recombinant adenoviruses are finally purified from the supernatant of transfected HEK293 producer cells (*see* **Fig. 1**).

2. Materials

2.1. Construction of a Single-Chain Diabody

1. Bacterial expression vector (e.g., pAB1 *[15]*).
2. Mammalian expression vector pSecTag (Invitrogen, Groningen, The Netherlands).

3. Thermocycler PTC 200 (MJ Research, Watertown, MA).
4. Thermostable DNA polymerases and reaction buffers: *Taq* polymerase (e.g., from Amersham-Pharmacia, Freiburg, Germany), *Pfu* polymerase, and herculase (Stratagene, Amsterdam, The Netherlands).
5. dNTPs (Amersham-Pharmacia).
6. Restriction enzymes *Asc*I, *Bst*EII, *Eco*RI, *Not*I, *Sac*I, *Sfi*I, and restriction enzyme buffers (New England Biolabs, Beverly, MA).
7. Luria-Bertani medium (LB): 5 g NaCl, 10 g bacto-tryptone, 5 g yeast extract per 1 L.
8. LB agar for plates: add 15 g agar/L LB.
9. LB/Ampicillin: LB agar/medium containing 100 µg/mL ampicillin.
10. TG1 (Stratagene).
11. Primers for amplification of individual V_H and V_L domains.

2.2. Generation of Recombinant Adenoviruses

1. Plasmids: pShuttle and pAdEasy-1 (Stratagene).
2. Bacterial strains: DH5α (Gibco-BRL, Karlsruhe, Germany) and BJ5183 (Stratagene).
3. Primers (restriction sites are underlined):
   CMV-BackKpn: 5'-GAC TCG GGT ACC CTG CTT CGC GAT GTA CGG GCC AGA TAT-3'
   scDb-ForHind (anneals at the DNA sequence encoding the C-terminal hexyhistidyl-tag):
   5'-T CAC AAG CTT TTA ATG GTG ATG ATG GTG ATG TGC CGC CCC-3'
   BGH-BackHind: 5'-CTG AGC AAG CTT TAA ACC CGC TGA TCA GCC TCG ACT GTG-3'
   BGH-ForBgl: 5'- G CAC AGA TCT ATC CCC AGC ATG CCT GCT ATT GTC TTC-3'
4. LB medium and plates (*see* **Subheading 2.1.**, **items 7** and **8**).
5. LB/Kanamycin: LB agar/medium containing 30 µg/mL kanamycin.
6. SOC medium (Gibco-BRL).
7. Restriction enzyme *Pme*I and buffer (New England Biolabs).
8. Gene Pulser electroporator (Bio-Rad).
9. Electroporation cuvets (2 mm width) (Bio-Rad).
10. 37°C incubator (Heraeus, Hanau, Germany) and shaker (INFORS AG, Botteningen, Germany).
11. DNA Maxi-prep kit and Midi-prep kit (Qiagen, Hilden, Germany).
12. Quickspin DNA purification kit (Qiagen).

2.3. Generation of Electrocompetent BJ5381

1. LB medium (*see* **Subheading 2.1.**, **item 7**).
2. Bacterial strain BJ5183 (Stratagene).
3. Wash-buffer: 10% ultra-pure glycerol, 90% bi-distilled H_2O, (v/v).
4. 50 mL Tubes (Falcon).
5. 37°C Shaker (INFORS AG).
6. 1-L Erlenmeyer flasks.
7. 250-mL Centrifuge tubes (Beckman, München, Germany).
8. Centrifuge and rotor (Beckman).

2.4. Preparation of Recombinant Adenoviruses

1. Restriction enzyme *Pac*I and buffer (New England Biolabs).
2. DNA Mini-prep kit and Maxi-prep kit (Qiagen).
3. Ethanol 100%.

4. 3 M Sodium acetate, pH 5.2.
5. HEK293 cells (Stratagene).
6. DMEM (Biowhitaker, Verviers, Belgium).
7. Fetal calf serum (FCS) (Biowhitaker).
8. OptiMEM™ (Gibco-BRL).
9. Lipofectamine™ (Gibco-BRL).
10. T-25 and T-175 cell culture flasks (Greiner, Frickenhausen, Germany).
11. Cell scraper (NUNC, Karlsruhe, Germany).
12. Pen/Strep stock solution: 10,000 U Penicillin/10 mg Streptomycin/mL (Biowhitaker).
13. Centrifuge CPKR (Beckman).
14. CO_2 incubator cytoperm (Heraeus).
15. Inverted microscope (Leitz, Heidelberg, Germany).
16. CsCl 1.4: 53 g + 87 mL of 10 mM Tris-HCl, pH 7.9.
17. CsCl 1.2: 26.8 g + 92 mL of 10 mM Tris-HCl, pH 7.9.
18. 1 M Tris-HCl, pH 7.9.
19. L8-60M ultracentrifuge (Beckman).
20. Swinging bucket rotor SW28 (Beckman).
21. Polyallomer centrifuge tubes 25 × 89 mM (Beckman).
22. 15 mL Falcon tubes (Becton-Dickinson, Le Pont De Claix, France).
23. PD-10 sephadex G25 columns (Amersham-Pharmacia).
24. PBS, pH 7.5: 137 mM NaCl, 3 mM KCl, 8 mM Na_2HPO_4, 1.5 mM KH_2PO_4.
25. 96-Well sterile cell culture plate (NUNC).
26. 5 mL and 1 mL Syringe (Braun, Melsungen, Germany).
27. 18G and 26 1/2G needle (Becton-Dickinson).

2.5. ELISA

1. 96-Well flat-bottom flexible Falcon microtiter plates (Becton-Dickinson).
2. PBS (*see* **Subheading 2.4.**, **item 24**).
3. 50 mM Carbonate buffer, pH 9.6.
4. Skimmed milk powder.
5. HRP-conjugated mouse anti-His-tag antibody (Santa Cruz Biotechnology, Santa Cruz, CA).
6. TMB substrate buffer: 100 mM sodium phosphate buffer, pH 6.0.
7. TMB substrate solution: add 100 µL of 10 mg 3,3'-5,5'-tetramethylbenzidine (TMB) in DMSO and 2 µL of 30% H_2O_2 per 10 mL of TMB substrate buffer.
8. Microtiter plate reader Spectromax 340 (MGW-Biotech, Ebersberg, Germany).

3. Methods

3.1. Generation of a Bispecific Single-Chain Diabody

1. PCR amplify DNA encoding the V_H domain of the first antibody (A) with primers introducing a *Sfi*I site at the N-terminus encoding region and a *BstE*II site at the C-terminus encoding region (if not already present) (*see* **Fig. 2** for details). Digest with *Sfi*I and *BstE*II. For polymerase chain reaction (PCR), we routinely use *Taq* polymerase as well as a proof-reading polymerase (*pfu*, herculase) and 25 cycles for amplification. The PCR reactions are performed in a total volume of 50 µL containing 250 µM dNTPs, 1.5 mM MgCl$_2$, 1 pmol of each primer, and 0.1 µg template DNA. Each cycle consists of 30 s, 94°C, 1 min, 50°C, 1 min, 72°C min.
2. PCR amplify DNA encoding the V_L domain of the first antibody (A) with a forward

primer introducing a *Not*I site at the C-terminus encoding and a backward primer encoding the C-terminus encoding region of the V_H domain (covering the *Bst*EII site), a five residue linker A, and introducing a *Sac*I site at the N-terminus encoding region of the V_L domain (*see* **Fig. 2** for details). Digest with *Bst*EII and *Not*I.

3. Clone into a bacterial expression vector (such as pAB1, *[15]*) digested with *Sfi*I and *Not*I and transform into TG1. The insert encodes a bivalent diabody Db-A. For further analysis the vector should also encode sequences for detection and purification, such as a C-terminal hexahistidyl-tag.

4. PCR amplify DNA encoding the V_H domain of the second antibody (B) with a backward primer encoding the C-terminal half of the linker *M* beginning with an *Asc*I site and a forward primer encoding a 5 residue linker B and a *Sac*I site. Digest fragment with *Asc*I and *Sac*I.

5. PCR amplify DNA encoding the V_L domain of the second antibody (B) with a forward primer encoding the N-terminal half of the linker M beginning with an *Asc*I site and a backward primer encoding a 5 residue linker A and a *Bst*EII site. Digest with *Bst*EII and *Asc*I.

6. Clone both fragments into Db-A digested with *Bst*EII and *Sac*I. Transform into TG1. The resulting sequence encodes a bispecific single-chain diabody (scDb). Check for correct expression of functional scDb *(2)*.

7. Subclone scDb-encoding DNA into a mammalian expression vector, such as pSecTag. This can be done in form of a *Sfi*I/*Eco*RI fragment. The vector contains the CMV promoter and substitutes the bacterial leader sequence by an Igk leader sequence. Furthermore, it contains a BGH (bovine growth hormone) polyadenylation sequence downstream of the coding sequence.

8. Confirm expression of the scDb by transient transfection of mammalian cells (e.g., HEK293, CHO, NIH3T3) and immunoblotting analysis or ELISA of cell culture supernatant *(2)*.

3.2. Generation of an Adenoviral Expression System

3.2.1. Cloning into pShuttle

The scDb expression cassette is cloned into pShuttle, which is then used to introduce the expression cassette into an adenoviral genome (pAdEasy-1) by homologous recombination. This step requires linearization of pShuttle with *Pme*I. Since the expression cassette contains an internal *Pme*I site in front of the BGH polyA sequence, cloning into pShuttle is performed by a two fragments ligation step.

1. Generate fragment 1, containing the promoter region and the scDb gene, by PCR amplification with primers CMV-BackKpn and scDb-ForHind. Digest with *Kpn*I and *Hin*dIII.

2. Generate fragment 2, containing the BGH polyA sequence, by PCR amplification with primers BGH-BackHind and BGH-ForBgl. This step also eliminates the internal *Pme*I site. Digest with *Hin*dIII and *Bgl*II.

3. Digest pShuttle with *Kpn*I and *Bgl*II and ligate with fragments 1 and 2. Transform DNA (pShuttle-scDb) into DH5α and prepare plasmid DNA by standard Maxi-preparation procedures.

3.2.2. Recombination into pAdEasy-1

pAdEasy-1 contains most of the adenovirus serotype 5 genome and is deleted for the *E1* and *E3* genes, which are dispensable. These genes are responsible for assembly of infectious virus particles (*E1*) and the evasion from the host immunity (*E3*). Recombination takes place at the right arm homology region and either the left arm homology region or the origin of replication.

1. Linearize 2 µg of pShuttle-scDb by digestion with 50 U *Pme*I overnight.
2. Separate digested DNA on a 0.5% agarose gel and isolate cut DNA by Quickspin purification. Elute with 50 µL H_2O.
3. Mix 1 µL of pAdEasy-1 (100 ng/µL) and 8 µL linearized pShuttle-scDb DNA with 55 µL of electrocompetent BJ5183 cells (*see* **Subheading 3.2.3.**) and incubate for 1 min on ice (*see* **Note 1**).
4. Transfer mixture into an electroporation cuvet (2 mm width) precooled on ice prior to use and perform the electroporation at 2500 V, 200 Ω, and 25 µFD in a Gene Pulser electroporator. Immediately transfer the transformed bacteria to a 50 mL Falcon tube containing 0.5 mL of SOC medium.
5. Incubate in a shaker at 37°C for 20 min. Then, plate 150 µL and 350 µL on LB/Kanamycin plates and grow at 37°C overnight.

3.2.3. Preparation of Electrocompetent Bacteria

Recombination between pShuttle and pAdEasy-1 takes place in the *E. coli* strain BJ5183, which has a high recombination capability and transformation efficiency.

1. Use a fresh colony of BJ5183 cells to inoculate 10 mL of LB medium in a 50 mL Falcon tube. Grow the cells in a shaker at 37°C overnight.
2. Dilute 0.5 mL of the cells into 500 mL of LB medium in four 1-L flasks (125 mL each). Grow for 4–5 h with vigorous shaking at 37°C until A_{550}~0.8.
3. Collect the cells in two centrifuge tubes (250 mL each) and incubate on ice 1 h.
4. Spin down the cells by centrifugation at 1200*g* at 4°C for 10 min.
5. Discard the supernatant, and wash the cells by resuspending in 500 mL of sterile, ice-cold wash-buffer (*see* **Note 2**).
6. Centrifuge the cell suspension at 1200*g* at 4°C for 30 min (pellet is unstable!).
7. Repeat **steps 5** and **6**.
8. Discard the supernatant, leaving about 20 ml, and transfer cell suspension into a prechilled 50 mL conical tube. Spin at 1200*g* at 4°C for 10 min, then pipet all but 2 mL of the supernatant out.
9. Resuspend the cells in the remaining wash-buffer. Aliquot 55 µL into prechilled tubes freeze immediately in liquid nitrogen. Store the aliquots at –80°C.

3.2.4. Screening of Positive Clones

Positive recombinants are identified by restriction digest of Mini-prep DNA of individual clones with *Pac*I. Positive clones produce a large fragment of approx 30 kb and, depending on whether recombination took place at the left arm homology region or at the origin of replication, a smaller fragment of either 4.5 or 3.0 kb.

1. Pick small clones and grow them overnight in 5 mL LB containing 30 µg/mL kanamycin (*see* **Note 3**).
2. Use 4 mL of the culture to perform the DNA Mini-preparation according to standard protocols (Alkaline lysis method).
3. Resuspend the pellet in 30 µL H_2O and analyze the DNA pattern by restriction digestion

with 2 U of *Pac*I. Positive clones (pAdscDb) yield a large fragment ~30 kb and a fragment of 3.0 kb or 4.5 kb.

4. Retransform 1 µL of the positive recombinant plasmid Mini-preparation DNA into DH5α and prepare plasmid DNA by standard Maxi-preparation procedures.

3.2.5. Transfection and Preparation of Virus Lysate

The pAdscDb DNA has to be linearized with *Pac*I in order to expose the two inverted terminal repeats (ITR). Virus particles are produced after transfection of the DNA into HEK293 cells, which complement the *E1* gene necessary for virus assembly. Recombinant viruses are then purified from the cell culture supernatant.

1. Digest 5 µg of pAdscDb with 8 U *Pac*I for 5 h at 37°C. Ethanol precipitate the plasmid DNA by adding 2.5 vol Ethanol and 1/10 vol 3 *M* sodium acetate, pH 5.2, and resuspend pellet in 20 µL sterile H_2O.
2. One day prior to transfection, plate HEK293 cells at a density 2×10^6 cells per T-25 flask. They should be 50–70% confluent at the time of the transfection.
3. Perform a Lipofectamine™ transfection: Mix the 20 µL of *Pac*I-digested pAdscDb with 230 µL OptiMEM™ and add 20 µL Lipofectamine™ in 230 µL OptiMEM™. Mix gently and incubate 15–30 min at room temperature. In between, wash cells once with OptiMEM™, add 2.5 mL OptiMEM™ per flask. Return to a 37°C CO_2 incubator for 15 min. Add the Lipofectamine™-DNA mix to the flask and incubate for 6 h in a 37°C CO_2 incubator before replacing the medium by 6 mL DMEM (10% FCS, 1% Pen/Strep). Incubate for 7–10 d. CPE or plaques are not observed after transfection.
4. Scrape the cells off the flask with a rubber policeman (**No trypsin!**), transfer to a 50 mL Falcon tube. Spin down the cells at 250*g* for 5 min at room temperature. Resuspend the pellet in 2 mL sterile PBS. Perform 4 cycles freeze/thaw/vortex. Spin the sample at 3500*g* at 4°C for 5 min and store the supernatant at –20°C.
5. Infect two 50–70% confluent T-25 flasks of HEK293 cells using half of the above viral supernatant per flask. CPE or cell lysis becomes evident at d 2–3 post-infection. Collect the viruses, as described above (**step 4**), when half of the cells are detached (3–5 d postinfection). At this stage you have ~10^7 particles/mL (*see* **Note 4**).

3.2.6. Large Scale Virus Production

A large scale production of high-titer recombinant viral particles involves a sequential increase in cell culture size and adenovirus infection cycles. Some viral particles will be left from each amplification step. These should be kept in case further steps fail. For further amplification, always start with the lowest passage of viral particles.

1. Plate HEK293 cells in three T-75 flasks (~5×10^6 cells/flask).
2. Take 0.5 mL of the viral stock from **step 5, Subheading 3.2.5.** and complete to 2 mL with DMEM-5% FCS (dilution ~5 MOI [multiplicity of infection]).
3. Remove the medium from the flasks and add carefully the 2 mL of diluted adenoviruses. Spread by rocking the flasks in cross shape. It is important not to disturb the cell monolayer. Incubate for 90 min at 37°C in a CO_2 incubator.
4. Add 9 mL of DMEM-5% FCS. When all the cells are rounded up and half are detached (3–4 d postinfection), harvest and combine the 3 flasks. Spin for 5 min at 250*g* at room temperature and remove the supernatant.
5. Resuspend the pellet in 3 mL sterile PBS and perform 4 cycles freeze/thaw/vortex. Spin the sample at 3500*g* at 4°C for 5 min and store the supernatant at –20°C (*see* **Note 5**).

6. Repeat **steps 1–5** using three T-175 flasks (~1 × 10^7 cells/flask). Complete 3 mL of the viral stock from **step 5** to 15 mL with DMEM-5% FCS (dilution ~25 MOI). Use 5 mL of this dilution for **step 3** and add 25 mL of DMEM-5% FCS in **step 4**. Use 5 mL sterile PBS to resuspend pellet in **step 5**.

7. Repeat **steps 1–5** using twenty T-175 flasks (~1 × 10^7 cells/flask). Take 0.25 mL of the viral stock from **step 6** and complete to 5 mL with DMEM-5% FCS (dilution ~50 MOI). Use 5 mL of this dilution for **step 3** and add 25 mL of DMEM-5% FCS in **step 4**. Use 8 mL sterile PBS to resuspend pellet in **step 5**.

3.2.7. Purification of Adenoviruses by Density Gradient Centrifugation

The viral particles are purified by cesium chloride (CsCl) discontinuous gradient centrifugation. A high concentration of CsCl can interfere with viral infection in cell or tissue. Therefore, the CsCl must be removed at the end of the run using a desalting column (PD-10 sephadex G25 column).

1. Precool an ultracentrifuge (Beckman; L8-60M) and a swinging bucket rotor (Beckman; SW 28) to 4°C.

2. Pour 8 mL of sterile CsCl 1.4 in the sterile centrifuge tubes. **Very gently** overlay with 6 mL of sterile CsCl 1.2.

3. Spin the sample from **Subheading 3.2.6.**, **step 7** at 3500g at 4°C for 5 min, collect the supernatant in a fresh 15 mL Falcon tube and complete to 14 mL with sterile PBS. Load very gently on the top of the discontinuous gradient. Gently overlay with 5 mL sterile mineral oil. Make sure that the tubes are balanced (*see* **Note 6**).

4. Centrifuge at 100,000g for 90 min at 4°C, deceleration rate = 0.

5. After the run, carefully remove the tubes from the rotor in a laminar flow hood and remove the mineral oil. Puncture the side of the tube, below the lowest bluish-white band containing the adenoviruses, using a 5 mL syringe with a 18G needle (*see* **Fig. 3**). Aspirate about 1 mL carefully to avoid collecting impurities. Aspirate sterile PBS in the syringe up to 2.5 mL total volume and store on ice.

6. Equilibrate the PD-10 column with 25 mL PBS.

7. Load the virions on the column. Elute with 3.5 mL PBS and collect 4 fractions in a 2 mL Eppendorf tube (F1: 0.5 mL; F2: 1 mL; F3: 1 mL; F4: 0.5 mL). Add 10% final concentration of sterile glycerol to each fraction. Mix gently. Before freezing the purified adenoviruses, take a 10 μL aliquot from each fraction, which will be used for the titration.

3.2.8. Determination of Virus Titer by TCID50 Assay

The Tissue Culture Infectious Dose$_{50}$ (TCID$_{50}$) method is a quick (10 d) technique to determine the virus titer (*16*). For accurate results, dilutions and titration should be performed in duplicate.

1. One day before infection, prepare 20 mL of HEK293 cell suspension at 10^5 cells/mL DMEM-2% FCS. Using a multi-channel pipet dispense 100 μL (10^4 cells) per well of 96-well flat-bottom plates.

2. Perform a predilution 1/10^4 of the virus stock you want to titrate. Then, prepare eight serial dilutions in 5 mL sterile polystyrol tubes. Dispense 1.8 mL of DMEM-2% FCS per tube. Add 0.2 mL of the viral stock (prediluted 1/10^4) into the first tube. Mix by pipeting up and down five times (dilution 10^{-1}). Change the tip after each dilution. Take 0.2 mL of 10^{-1} dilution and transfer to the second tube. Repeat dilutions up to 10^{-8} (*see* **Note 7**).

3. Discard the medium from the 96-well plates and dispense for each row 0.1 mL per well (wells #1 to #10) for each dilution mixture. Columns #11 and #12, which are used for the

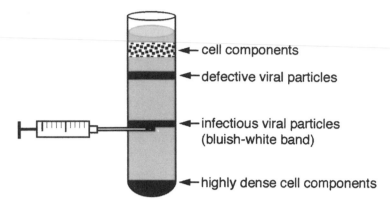

Fig. 3. Density gratient centrifugation of virus particles. After ultracentrifugation, the viral particles migrate as a bluish-white band below cell components and defective viral particles.

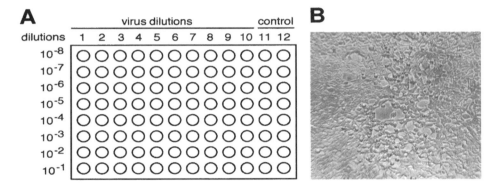

Fig. 4. Determination of virus titer. (**A**) Pipetting scheme for the determination of the virus titer. (**B**) cytopathic effects (CPE) after 7 d of incubation of HEK293 with adenoviruses.

negative control (to test the cells viability), contain 0.1 mL DMEM-2% FCS (*see* **Fig. 4A**). Leave the plates in the incubator for 10 d.

4. After 10 d read the plates under the microscope. Make sure first that the negative control (columns #10 and #11) do not show any cytopathic effects (CPE) or cell growth problem and second that the lowest dilution (10^{-1}) shows 100% infection and the highest dilution (10^{-8}) 0%. Determine the ratio of positive wells (presence of CPE; *see* **Fig. 4B**) per row (e.g., 5/10 = 5 wells displaying CPE in a row).

5. Calculation of the titer:
   For 100 µL of dilution, the titer is $T = 10^{1+d(S-0.5)}$ ($TCID_{50}$/mL)
   d = Log 10 of the dilution (corresponds to 1 for a 10-fold dilution between each row); S = the sum of the ratios of positive wells per row. The titer by $TCID_{50}$ (50% tissue culture infectious dose) method is 0.7 Log higher than the titer by standard plaque assay method.

Therefore, $T = 10^{(1+d\,(S-0.5))-0.7}$ PFU/mL. The calculated titer must be then multiplied by the predilution factor.

3.3. In Vivo Administration

Recombinant viral adenoviruses can, even in absence of the E1 function, express viral proteins leading to direct toxic effects to hepatocytes which can be detected in immune-deficient and immune-competent mice *(17,18)*. Therefore, it is important to keep the number of injected particles as low as possible. Liver toxicity in mice was observed after injection of 1.2×10^{10} viral particles *(18)*.

1. Prepare dilutions of 1×10^8 to 1×10^{10} adenovirus vectors in 200 µL PBS final volume and equilibrate 10 min at 37°C.
2. Use 26G 1/2 0.45 × 13 needles (Becton Dickinson) to inject **slowly** nude mice into the tail vein with the 200 µL dilution (*see* **Note 8**).
3. Take serum samples at appropriate time points.

3.4. Analysis of In Vivo Expression by ELISA

In vivo expression can be monitored by ELISA using the C-terminal tags for detection of antigen-bound antibody fragments. If no purified antigen is available other detection methods, such as FACS or immunoblotting, can be performed. We were able to detect down to 1–10 ng/mL antibody fragment in serum by a conventional ELISA.

1. Coat a microtiter plate with 100 µL/well antigen at a conc. of 1–10 µg/mL in PBS or 50 m*M* carbonate buffer, pH 9.6, overnight at 4°C.
2. The next day, wash plate once with PBS and block remaining binding sites with PBS, 2% skimmed milk powder (MPBS).
3. Dilute serum taken from the mice 1/2, 1/10, and 1/100 in MPBS.
4. Make also a serial dilution of purified antibody fragment (10 µg/mL to 1 ng/mL).
5. Add 100 µL of the diluted samples to the microtiter plate and incubate for 1 h at room temperature.
6. Wash plate six times with PBS
7. Add 100 µL/well HRP-conjugated anti-His-tag antibody diluted to 1 µg/mL in MPBS and incubate for 1 h at room temperature.
8. Wash plate six times with PBS
9. Develop ELISA by adding 100 µL of TMB substrate solution. Incubate until blue colour has developed (approx 5–30 min).
10. Stop reaction by adding 50 µL of 1 *M* H_2SO_4 and read plate at 450 nm.
11. Determine serum concentration using the values of the purified antibody fragments as a standard curve.

4. Notes

1. The pAdeasy-1 DNA must be >80% supercoiled to allow a good recombination in bacteria. The BJ5183 cells must be highly competent (>10^8 colonies/µg).
2. Use only ultra-pure glycerol (99.5% purity) to prepare the wash-buffer. Working in the cold room improves the quality of the electrocompetent bacteria. The BJ5183 bacteria must be kept concentrated (500 mL culture yields <1 mL competent bacteria). The bacteria lose their competence after 1 mo of storage at –80°C.
3. The presence of too many colonies (e.g., >100 clones per transformation) usually indi-

cates that too much pShuttle vector DNA was used for the co-transformation; it should be in the range from 100–500 ng.

4. The presence of recombinant adenoviruses can be controlled by PCR. Take 5 µL of virus supernatant, add 10 µL PCR-grade proteinase K, incubate at 56°C for 1 h, then boil samples for 5 min, spin for 5 min at 23,000g and use 5 µL for PCR.

5. To ensure a good amplification in the last round of infection, the HEK293 cells should not be infected at too low (e.g., no obvious cell lysis after 4–5 d) or too high titer (e.g., cells lysed less than 2 d postinfection).

6. To avoid overloading the gradient, the viral stock should result from less than 1×10^9 infected cells.

7. For the titration always start distributing the highest dilution in the top row. The pre-dilution of the purified viral stock can be in the range from $1/10^3$–$1/10^5$ depending on the titre. If CPE can be seen 2–3 d post-infection for the highest dilution (10^{-8}), perform a higher pre-dilution.

8. Mice can be injected into the tail vein with at most 200 µL of solution; when the adenoviruses display a high titer the injection volume can be decrease to 100 µL. Do not forget to take into consideration the dead volume of the syringe (~100 µL).

References

1. Kontermann, R. E. (2000) Recombinant antibodies for cancer therapy. *Mod. Asp. Immunobiol.* **1**, 88–91.
2. Kontermann, R. E. and Dübel, S. (eds.) (2001) *Antibody Engineering: a Lab Manual.* Springer, Heidelberg.
3. Chen, S.-Y., Yang, A.-G., Chen, J. D., Kute, T., King, R., Collier, J., et al. (1997) Potent antitumor activity of a new class of tumor-specific killer cells. *Nature* **385**, 78–80.
4. Oral, H. B., Larkin, D. F., Fehervari, Z., Byrnes, A. P., Rankin, A. M., Haskard, D. O., et al. (1997) Ex vivo adenovirus-mediated gene transfer and immunomodulatory protein production in human cornea. *Gene Ther.* **4**, 639–647.
5. Lee, C. T., Wu, S., Ciernik, I. F., Chen, H., Nadaf-Rahrov, S., Gabrilovich, D., and Carbone, D. P. (1997) Genetic immunotherapy of established tumors with adenovirus-murine granulocyte-macrophage colony-stimulating factor. *Human Gene Ther.* **8**, 187–193.
6. Kurata, H., Liu, C. B., Valkova, J., Koch, A. E., Yssel, H., Hirabayashi, Y., et al. (1999) Recombinant adenovirus vectors for cytokine gene therapy in mice. *J. Allergy Clin. Immunol.* **103**, S471–S484.
7. Zhang, W. W. (1999) Development and application of adenoviral vectors for gene therapy of cancer. *Cancer Gene Ther.* **6**, 113–138.
8. Whittington, H. A., Ashworth, L. J., and Hawkins, R. E. (1998) Recombinant adenoviral delivery for in vivo expression of scFv antibody fusion proteins. *Gene Ther.* **5**, 770–777.
9. Brüsselbach, S., Korn, T., Völkel, T., Müller, R., and Kontermann, R. E. (1999) Enzyme recruitment and tumor cell killing in vitro by a bispecific single-chain diabody. *Tumor Targeting* **4**, 115–123.
10. Kontermann, R.E . & Müller, R. (1999) Intracellular and cell surface displayed single-chain diabodies. *J. Immunol. Meth.* **226**, 179–188.
11. Alt, M., Müller, R., and Kontermann, R. E. (1999) Novel tetravalent and bispecific IgG-like antibody molecules combining single-chain diabodies with the immunoglobulin γ1 Fc or CH3 region. *FEBS Lett.* **454**, 90–94.
12. Nettelbeck, D. M., Miller, D. W., Jérôme, V., Zuzarte, M., Watkins, S. J., Hawkins, R. E.,

et al. (2001) Targeting of adenovirus to endothelial cells by a bispecific single-chain diabody directed against the adenovirus fiber knob domain and human endoglin (CD105). *Mol. Ther.* **3,** 882–891.

13. Korn, T., Völkel, T., and Kontermann, R. E. (2001) Bivalent and bispecific diabodies and single-chain diabodies, in *Antibody Engineering: a Lab Manual* (Kontermann, R. E. and Dübel, S., eds.), Springer, Heidelberg, pp. 619–636.

14. Völkel, T., Korn, T., Bach, M., Müller, R., and Kontermann, R. E. (2001) Optimised linker sequences for the expression of monomeric and dimeric single-chain diabodies. *Protein Eng.* **14,** 815–823.

15. Kontermann, R. E., Martineau, P., Cummings, C. E., Karpas, A., Allen, D., Derbyshire, E. & Winter, G. (1997) Enzyme immunoasssays using bispecific diabodies. *Immunotechnology* **3,** 137–144.

16. Precious, B. and Russell, W. W. (1985) Growth, purification and titration of adenoviruses, in *Virology: A Practical Approach* (Mahy, B. W. J., ed.), IRL, Oxford, UK.

17. Schiedner, G., Morral, N., Parks, R. J., Wu, Y., Koopmans, S. C., Langston, C., et al (1998) Genomic DNA transfer with high-capacity adenovirus vector results in improved in vivo gene expression and decreased toxicity. *Nature Genet.* **18,** 180–183.

18. Morral, N., Parks, R. J., Zhou, H., Langston, C., Schiedner, G., Quinones, J., et al. (1998) High doses of a helper-dependent adenoviral vector yield supraphysiological levels of α_1-antitrypsin with negligible toxicity. *Hum. Gene Ther.* **9,** 2709–2716.

V

Large Scale Production of Recombinant Antibodies for Clinical Application

26

Production of Antibody Fragments in a Bioreactor

Halldis Hellebust

1. Introduction

Clinical use of antibodies or antibody fragments is dependent on highly effective production systems. Antibody fragments like single-chain Fv or Fab have been successfully expressed in microorganisms for more than a decade, and the most commonly used host has been *Escherichia coli*. The ease of genetic manipulation in *E. coli* has made it the first choice for expression of antibody fragments, and by fusion of the protein to a signal sequence, antibody fragments are secreted to the periplasm of the bacteria, allowing correct folding and recovery of functionally active proteins. Finally, *E. coli* can be grown to high cell densities in an inexpensive medium allowing high volumetric yield of antibody fragments.

There are numerous examples of successful expression of functional antibody fragments in E. coli in shaker-flask cultures. However, it is a huge step from a shaker-flask culture to an industrial process for cost-effective production of large amounts of antibody fragments, and upon process development there are several points to consider. The first step would be to set up a cultivation technique that is possible to scale up, i.e., to grow the strain in a bioreactor (fermenter) under controlled conditions where it is possible to obtain high cell densities. Provided genetic stability of the host/vector system, it may be possible to obtain at least ten times higher volumetric yield in a bioreactor compared to a shaker flask. In the literature, there are a few examples of successful production of antibody fragments in bioreactors, and yields from hundred milligrams up to several grams per liter of culture have been reported *(1–7)*.

Some general strategies for obtaining high-level expression of recombinant proteins in E. coli have been described *(8,9)*, and these are also valid for antibody fragments. The host/vector used initially for cloning of a gene is not necessary useful for large-scale production of the protein. A vector that contains only the gene for ampicillin resistance (i.e., β-lactamase) as a selective marker is not suitable for scale up, because the β-lactamase leaks into the growth medium and degrades the ampicillin,

From: *Methods in Molecular Biology, vol. 207: Recombinant Antibodies for Cancer Therapy: Methods and Protocols*
Edited by: M. Welschof and J. Krauss © Humana Press Inc., Totowa, NJ

and thus plasmid-free cells will start to grow up. Vectors with kanamycin or tetracycline resistance are generally more stable than vectors with ampicillin resistance. Another approach to increase plasmid stability is to insert a suicide gene that cause cell death upon plasmid loss *(10–12)*.

A primary goal of moving from a shaker flask to a bioreactor is to increase the productivity, i.e., the amount of product formed per volume and time, and this is achieved both by increasing the culture volume and cell density. The main problems related to bacterial cultures are that the growth ceases because they run into substrate and oxygen limitation, and by-products like acetate accumulate. To overcome these problems, the cultivation is divided into two phases, a batch phase where the bacteria grow exponentially and utilize the nutrient present, and a feeding phase where various regimes of nutrient feed are imposed until the cultivation is complete *(13)*. The most commonly used cultivation technique for *E. coli* is glucose limiting fed-batch, and cell dry weights greater than 50 g per liter are routinely obtained. Nonlimiting fed-batch cultivations have also been described *(5)* where cell dry weights of more than 100 g per liter have been obtained. However, such cultivation technique requires special equipment.

In addition to the general considerations, there are some special features of antibody fragments that need to be taken into account. Antibody fragments are generally secreted to the periplasm of *E. coli* where they fold correctly and are soluble. However, many antibody fragments tends to form periplasmic inclusion bodies. This is dependent on the primary sequence of the antibody as well as growth and induction conditions, and it is a general rule to try to slow down the rate of synthesis. Lowering of the temperature in the induction phase to $25-30°C$ has been shown to increase the yield of soluble protein *(14,15)*.

Another point to consider is the promoter and the strength of induction. Many antibody fragments are harmful to *E. coli*, and it is therefore important to use a promoter with minimal leakiness during the growth phase. The most commonly used promoter for expression of antibody fragments have been the lac promoter, in addition the alkaline phosphatase *(1,4,6)* and the arabinose *(3)* promoters have also been used with success. To increase the fraction of correct folded and soluble protein, the promoter should not be fully induced, and the optimal induction strength needs to be determined for each individual antibody fragment.

Many antibody fragments influence the outer membrane of *E. coli* and leak into the medium. In some cases the antibody fragments also cause a certain degree of cell lysis. All this results in excess foaming in the induction phase.

A start-up protocol for a simple glucose-limiting fed-batch cultivation in a standard laboratory bioreactor (1–10 L) will be presented. The medium used in this protocol will give a cell dry weight of about 10 g/L (i.e., OD 30–40). It is important to get the cultivation to work with lower cell densities before moving into high cell density cultivations. The host/vector system is *E. coli* RV308 pHKK, which has been used with great success earlier *(5)*.

2. Materials

2.1. Preparation of Glycerol Stock and Inoculum Culture

1. *E. coli* RV308 (ATCC 31608) or similar strain that grow well on minimal medium.
2. pHKK vector (*see* **Note 1**).
3. LB (Luria Bertani) broth.
4. LB-A plates: LB agar plates containing 50 µg/mL ampicillin.
5. LB-GA: LB medium containing 2% glucose and 100 µg/mL ampicillin.
6. Glycerol (autoclave separately).

2.2. Cultivation in Bioreactor

1. Mineral medium: 1.8 g/L $(NH_4)_2$ SO_4, 1.6 g/L KH_2PO_4, 6.6 g/L $Na_2HPO_4 \times 2H_2O$, 0.5 g/L $(NH_4)_2$-H-citrate (autoclave in the bioreactor).
2. 20% glucose (autoclave separately) (*see* **Note 2**).
3. 1 M $MgSO_4$ (autoclave separately).
4. Trace element solution: 0.5 g/L $CaCl_2 \times 2H_2O$, 16.7 g/L $FeCl_3 \times 6 H_2O$, 0.18 g/L $ZnSO_4$ $\times 7 H_2O$, 0.16 g/L $CuSO_4 \times 5 H_2O$, 0.11 g/L $MnCl_2 \times 2H_2O$, 0.18 g/L $CoCl_2 \times 6 H_2O$, 50 mM Na-EDTA (sterile-filter and store at room temperature).
5. Ampicillin, 100 mg/mL (sterile-filter and store at –20°C).
6. Adecanol LG-109 (Asahi Denka Kogyo, Tokyo, Japan) or similar antifoam (autoclave separately) (*see* **Note 3**).
7. 12.5% NH_3 (*see* **Note 4**).
8. Glucose sticks (Diabur-Test 5000, Roche 647659).
9. IPTG, 100 mM (sterile filter and store at –20°C).

2.3. Periplasmic Extraction

1. 50 mM Tris-HCl, pH 8.0.
2. Sucrose solution: 40% sucrose, 2 mM EDTA, 50 mM Tris-HCl, pH 8.0.
3. Lysozym (Sigma L-6876), 100 mg/mL.
4. Ribonuclease A (Sigma R-5503), 10 mg/mL (*see* **Note 5**).

3. Methods

3.1. Preparation of Glycerol Stock and Inoculum Culture

1. Ligate your antibody fragment into the pHKK vector, transform *E. coli* RV308 cells and plate on LB-A plates. Incubate over night at 37°C.
2. Inoculate an individual colony into 10 mL LB-GA medium in a 50 mL tube. Let grow overnight in a rotary shaker at 37°C.
3. Add 4.5 mL of a solution of LB broth/glycerol (50/50) to the tube.
4. Aliquote into a number of tubes containing 0.1–1 mL suspension and store at –70°C.
5. Inoculum culture: Thaw one tube of the glycerol stock, and inoculate 100 µL into 100 mL LB-GA medium in a 500 mL Erlenmeyer flask equipped with a cotton plug. Discard the tube from the glycerol stock. Incubate the flasks in a rotary shaker at 30°C for about 7 h (until OD is about 0.4).
6. Centrifuge the culture at 3000*g* for 15 min and discard the supernatant.
7. Resuspend the cells in 10 mL mineral medium. This is enough inoculum culture for a 3-L bioreactor.

3.2. Preparation of Bioreactor and Cultivation

1. Prepare and sterilize the bioreactor containing the mineral medium according to the supplier recommendation.
2. Connect bottles with 20% glucose for feeding (*see* **Note 2**) and 12.5% NH₃ for maintenance of pH at 7.0 (*see* **Note 5**).
2. Add per liter of mineral medium: 100 mL of 20% glucose, 2 mL of trace element solution, 2 mL of 1 M MgSO₄, 1 mL of ampicillin (100 mg/mL) and 50 µL of Adecanol to the vessel.
3. Set temperature to 30°C.
4. Inoculate the fermenter to an OD of about 0.02–0.03 (*see* **Note 6**).
5. Maintain dissolved oxygen tension ≥20 % by adjusting airflow and stirrer speed.
6. Upon depletion of glucose, start feeding at a rate of about 25 mL/h of 20% glucose per liter of cultivation volume (*see* **Note 7**).
7. Induce the culture by addition of 1 mL IPTG per liter of cultivation volume about 2 h after the feeding of glucose has started and continue the cultivation for up to 10 h (*see* **Note 8**).
8. Add antifoam when necessary.

3.3. Sample Removal and Periplasmic Extraction

1. Remove a sample of about 10 mL from the bioreactor.
2. For measurement of OD, dilute the sample in 0.9% NaCl and read the absorbance at 600 nm. The reading should be between 0.1 and 0.4.
3. Centrifuge a sample of 1 mL at 20.000g for 5 min at 4°C. Remove the supernatant, i.e., medium and save for analysis.
4. Check that the glucose concentration in the medium with a glucose stick (*see* **Note 9**).
6. Resuspend the cell pellet in 0.5 mL 50 mM Tris-HCl, pH 8.0, and add 0.5 mL sucrose solution, 10 µL lysozyme and 10 µL RNase A, and incubate for 1 h with rotation.
7. Centrifuge a sample 20,000g for 5 min at 4°C. Remove the supernatant, i.e., periplasm, and save for analysis.

4. Notes

1. This vector has kindly been supplied by Dr. Uwe Horn, HKI, Jena, Germany *(5)*. The vector is covered by the Patent WO 97/21829. Important elements in this vector are ampicillin resistance, the hok/sok suicide gene, the lac repressor, the lac promoter, and the pelB leader sequence.
2. Concentration of glucose in the feeding solution will depend on the size of the reactor. Typically, a 20% glucose solution is appropriate for feeding for small reactors (1–2 L), while the concentration of glucose in the feeding solution may be increased up to 60% for culture volumes of 5–10 L and above. About 500 mL of 20% glucose will be needed per liter culture volume.
3. Different antifoams may interact in different ways with the subsequent purification process of the protein, and this needs to be checked for each individual process.
4. Prepare about 100 mL of per liter cultivation volume in a sterile bottle with sterile tubs for connection to the bioreactor. The solution itself needs not to be sterilized.
5. This RNase is contaminated with DNase and will serve as a general nuclease, and this is what we need in this step. If you use another RNase, it might be necessary to add DNase as well.
6. When the culture is inoculated at such low OD, it can be left to grow overnight and the feeding and induction phase will take place the next day. The generation time for *E. coli*

RV308 in this medium is about 1.5 h at 30°C, and the lag phase when moving from LB-GA medium to minimal medium is about 4–5 h.

7. The feeding rate during the induction phase might be a parameter of variation.

8. The concentration of IPTG needs to be optimised for each single antibody fragment, but 100 mM serves as a good start point.

9. The glucose concentration in the medium should remain zero throughout the cultivation.

References

1. Carter, P., Kelley, R. F., Rodrigues, M. L., Snedecor, B., Covarrubias, M., Velligan, M. D., et al. (1992) High level *Escherichia coli* expression and production of a bivalent humanized antibody fragment. *Bio/Technology* **10**, 163–167.

2. Pack, P., Kujau, M., Schroeckh, V., Knüpfer, U., Wendelroth, R., Riesenberg, D., and Plückthun, A. (1993) Improved bivalent miniantibodies, with identical avidity as whole antibodies, produced by high cell density fermentation of *Escherichia coli*. *Bio/Technology* **11**, 1271–1277.

3. Better, M., Bernhard, S. L., Lei, S. P., Fishwild, D. M., Lane, J. A., Carrol, S. F., and Horwitz, A. H. (1993) Potent anti-CD5 ricin A chain immunoconjugates from bacterially produced Fab' and F(ab')$_2$. *Proc. Natl. Acad. Sci. USA* **90**, 457–461.

4. Zapata, G., Ridgway, J. B. B., Mordenti, J., Osaka, G., Wong, W. L. T., Bennett, G. L., and Carter, P. (1995) Engineering linear F(ab')$_2$ fragments for efficient production in *Escherichia coli* and enhanced antiproliferate activity. *Protein Eng.* **8**, 1057–1062.

5. Horn, U., Strittmatter, W., Krebber, A., Knüpfer, U., Kujau, M., Wenderoth, R., et al. (1996) High volumetric yields of functional dimeric miniantibodies in *Escherichia coli*, using an optimized expression vector and high-cell-density fermentation under non-limited growth conditions. *Appl. Microbiol. Biotechnol.* **46**, 524–532.

6. Zhu, Z., Zapata, G., Shalaby, R., Snedecor, B., Chen, H., and Carter, P. (1996) High level secretion of humanized bispecific diabody from *Escherichia coli*. *Bio/Technology* **14**, 192–196.

7. Forsberg, G., Forsgren, M., Jaki, M., Norin, M., Sterky, C., Enhörning, Å., et al. (1997) Identification of framework residues in a secreted recombinant antibody fragment that control production level and localization in *Escherichia coli*. *J. Biol. Chem.* **272**, 12,430–12,436.

8. Markrides, S. C. (1996) Strategies for achieving high-level expression of genes in *Escherichia coli*. *Microbiol. Rev.* **60**, 512–538.

9. Hanning, G. and Makrides, S. C. (1998) Strategies for optimizing heterologous protein expression in *Escherichia coli*. *Trends in Biotechnol.* **16**, 54–60.

10. Summers, D. (1998) Timing, self-control and a sense of direction are the secrets of multicopy plasmid stability. *Mol. Microbiol.* **29**, 1137–1145.

11. Baneyx, F. (1999) Recombinant protein expression in *Escherichia coli*. *Curr. Opin. Biotechnol.* **10**, 411–421.

12. Gerdes, K. (1988) The parB (hok/sok) locus of plasmid R1: A general purpose plasmid stabilization system. *Bio/Technology* **6**, 1402–1405.

13. Lee, S. Y. (1996) High cell-density culture of Escherichia coli. *Trends in Biotechnol.* **14**, 98–105.

14. Plücktun, A. and Pack, P. (1997) New protein engineering approaches to multivalent antibody fragments. *Immunotechnology* **3**, 83–105.

15. Harrison, J. S. and Keshavarz-Moore, E. (1996) Production of antibody fragments in *Escherichia coli*. *Annu. NY Acad. Sci.* **782**, 143–158.

27

Large Scale Production of Recombinant Antibodies by Utilizing Cellulose-Binding Domains

Itai Benhar and Yevgeny Berdichevsky

1. Introduction

Many recombinant proteins, particularly proteins with diagnostic and therapeutic potential such as antibodies, lymphokines, receptors, enzymes, and enzyme-inhibitors, are being produced from transformed host cells containing recombinant DNA. The host cells are transformed with an expression vector containing genes encoding for the proteins of interest, and then are cultured under conditions that favor the production of the desired protein. When *Escherichia coli* is used for the expression of recombinant proteins, the heterologous protein produced often precipitates within the cell to form refractile (inclusion) bodies. For the isolation of the recombinant protein in the native (biologically active) state, it should be separated from cell debris, solubilized with a chaotropic agent such as high concentrations of urea or guanidinium hydrochloride, then refolded by gradual removal of the denaturant (reviewed in **ref. *1***). In cases where the native state of the protein is dependent on the formation of disulfide bonds, the protein is reduced while in the denatured state by addition of reducing agents. The formation of disulfide bonds of the protein during the refolding process is facilitated by redox-shuffling induced by the inclusion of reducing and oxidizing agents in the refolding buffer *(2)*.

The expression of antibody fragments in *E. coli* permits rapid access to engineered molecules with full antigen-binding properties. While the expression in a functional state by secretion to the periplasm is the standard method for the production of Fv and Fab fragments, single-chain Fv fragments and fusion proteins thereof are mainly produced by refolding from insoluble inclusion bodies *(3)*. Although all of these antibody fragments serve as valuable aids in the study of antigen binding, their different biochemical properties must be considered when using them as research tools or for medical applications. For such applications, scFvs are frequently fused to accessory proteins such as toxins *(4)*, cytotoxic drugs or radioactive isotopes *(5)*, or enzymes for prodrug

From: *Methods in Molecular Biology, vol. 207: Recombinant Antibodies for Cancer Therapy: Methods and Protocols*
Edited by: M. Welschof and J. Krauss © Humana Press Inc., Totowa, NJ

activation *(6)*. For such scFv-fusion proteins, denaturation followed by refolding from inclusion bodies is frequently the only means by which the protein may be recovered in an active form. However, refolding is an empirical process that has to be optimized for each particular protein of interest *(1)*. Under conventional folding conditions, the yield of renaturation is often exceedingly low owing to uncontrollable processes such as aggregation or formation of thermodynamically stable, but non-native folding intermediates. Furthermore, refolding should be performed at extremely low protein concentrations owing to the kinetic competition between correct folding and incorrect aggregation *(7)*. Aggregation during refolding may be reduced by the addition of co-solvents such as amino acids (arginine) or other salts, or by refolding in the presence of molecular chaperones *(8,9)*, but such remedies are inadequate, particularly for large industrial scale.

Aggregation during refolding may be prevented by immobilizing the denatured protein onto a solid support prior to initiation of refolding. Some proteins may be charged under refolding conditions, so that they may be immobilized onto ion-exchange matrices in a low-ionic strength denaturant. Refolding is then induced by gradual removal of denaturant, and release from the matrix by increasing the salt concentration *(10)*. This approach is not adequate for refolding proteins for which the net charge under pH conditions that are compatible with refolding is too low to allow efficient immobilization onto an ion-exchange matrix. This is the case with many single-chain antibodies and fusion proteins thereof (our unpublished observations). When immobilization of the denatured protein by itself is not an option, its possible to engineer an affinity tag linked to the N-terminus or to the C-terminus of the protein. Small affinity tags, such as a hexa-histidine tag or a hexa-arginine tag, were applied for such purposes. Histidine-tagged proteins may be immobilized and refolded on a metal-carrying support *(11)*, while arginine-tagged proteins may be immobilized and refolded on a support carrying polyanionic groups *(12)*. One must assume that the folding of the immobilized protein is not perturbed by its proximity to the matrix and that placing a short tagging peptide at its terminus does not divert it into a nonproductive folding pathway.

Refolding of an immobilized protein with fewer physical constraints may be achieved by its immobilization through a polypeptide fusion partner. In folding of fusion proteins, when the individual fusion partners are joined by a flexible peptide linker, the fusion partners fold independently of each other *(13)*. However, most known protein tags (such as glutathione-S-transferase, maltose-binding protein, staphylococcal protein A, and most bacterial and fungal cellulose and chitin-binding domains) will not be useful for the purpose of immobilization of a denatured fusion protein onto the appropriate affinity support. This is because the protein affinity tags themselves are denatured and not functional under such conditions. A possible solution is to use as an affinity tag a protein whose compact and stable structure prevents it from unfolding under the conditions where most other proteins are completely denatured. Such robust proteins are rare, but one example of such a protein is the cellulose-binding domain from *Clostridium thermocellum*.

Cellulose-binding domains (CBDs) are noncatalytic subunits of cellulose-degrading enzymes or enzyme-complexes proteins found in many cellulose metabolizing bacteria and fungi *(14)*. CBDs bind to and can be eluted from cellulose under mild conditions and specific reagents are not required. The CBDs retain their cellulose-binding properties when fused to heterologous proteins and as such are being applied as affinity tags for protein purification and for enzyme immobilization *(14–18)*. A unique property of the CBD from *Clostridium thermocellum* is that it maintains its specific cellulose binding properties under conditions where most proteins are denatured and nonfunctional. We found that this CBD, alone, or when fused to single-chain antibodies, will bind reversibly to cellulose in up to 6 *M* urea. This property makes *Clostridium thermocellum* CBD an ideal candidate for an affinity tag to be applied for matrix-assisted (in this case, cellulose-assisted) refolding of fusion proteins. When a protein-CBD fusion is denatured, allowed to bind cellulose, and then refolded, it is immobilized onto the cellulose matrix while the protein fused to CBD is still in the unfolded state. Gradual removal of the denaturant then facilitates the refolding of the protein into the native state. Finally, the refolded protein can be separated from the cellulose matrix by applying appropriate elution conditions. When necessary, the protein can be separated from CBD by proteolytic cleavage and chromatographic separation. In addition, after being refolded while bound to the cellulose matrix, the protein-CBD fusion may by recovered by digestion of the cellulose matrix by a cellulolytic enzyme *(19)*.

Recently we incorporated *Clostridium thermocellum* CBD into a phage-display system for efficient isolation of ligand-binding proteins, particularly single-chain antibodies, and for engineering the matrix-binding properties of CBD itself *(20)*. The modular design of our expression vectors makes it possible to proceed directly from isolation of the ligand-binding protein to its efficient production as described *(21)*. Our examples are of the production of single-chain antibodies (scFvs)-CBD fusion proteins, many of which are notoriously difficult to refold by standard refolding protocols *(22)*.

In this chapter we describe a method for the efficient large-scale isolation of recombinant single-chain antibodies in a biologically active form. The protocol is comprised of the following steps (*see* **Fig. 1**).

1. The DNA encoding for a scFv is fused to CBD coding DNA in one of a series of appropriate expression vectors.
2. Upon expression in *E. coli* the scFv-CBD fusion protein accumulates as insoluble inclusion bodies.
3. The inclusion bodies are recovered, then solubilized and denatured by an appropriate chaotropic solvent.
4. The solubilized inclusion bodies are reversibly immobilized onto a cellulose matrix via specific interaction of the matrix with the CBD moiety.
5. Refolding of the scFv-CBD fusion protein is induced by reducing with time the concentration of the denaturing solvent while in contact with the cellulose matrix.
6. The refolded scFv-CBD fusion protein is then recovered in its native state by releasing it from the cellulose matrix by applying a high pH buffer.
7. The scFv may be separated from the CBD by specific proteolytic cleavage.
8. Gel filtration is used as a final polishing step to recover the pure scFv.

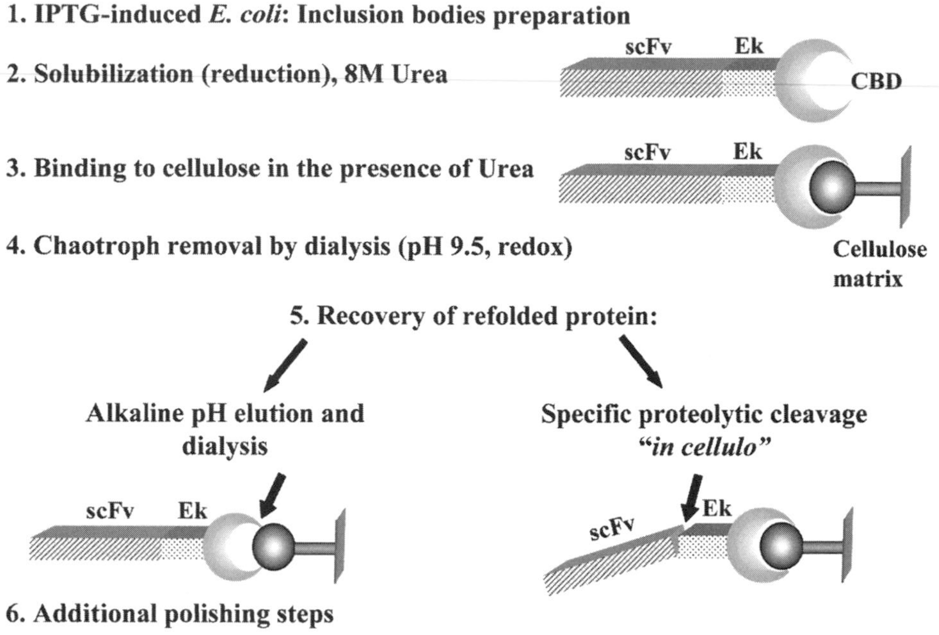

1. IPTG-induced *E. coli*: Inclusion bodies preparation

2. Solubilization (reduction), 8M Urea

scFv   Ek   CBD

3. Binding to cellulose in the presence of Urea

scFv   Ek

4. Chaotroph removal by dialysis (pH 9.5, redox)

Cellulose matrix

5. Recovery of refolded protein:

Alkaline pH elution and dialysis

scFv   Ek

Specific proteolytic cleavage *"in cellulo"*

scFv   Ek

6. Additional polishing steps

Fig.1. Overview of cellulose-assisted refolding protocol.

2. Materials and Equipment

2.1. Cloning Procedures

1. Vectors for subcloning of scFv DNA: pFEKCA3d-scFv and pH6T-FEKCA11c-scFv *(21)*, (*see* **Note 1**).
2. DNA modifying enzymes: *Nco*I, *Not*I, and T4 DNA Ligase (New England Biolabs, Beverly, MA).
3. TE buffer: 10 mM Tris-HCl, pH 8.0, 1 mM EDTA, pH 8.0 (*see* **Note 2**).
4. Bench-top centrifuge (Centrifuge 5417, Eppendorf, Hamburg, Germany).
5. Thermoblock (Thermolyne 17600 Dri-Bath, Duburue).
6. Minisart 0.22- and 0.45-µm filters (Sartorius AG, Germany).
7. Bovine albumin (BSA) (New England Biolabs).
8. Agarose (Sigma , Israel).
9. QIAquick™ Gel extraction kit (Qiagen, Valencia, CA).

2.2. Growing and Maintenance of Bacterial Strains

1. Incubator Shaker (New Brunswick Scientific Co., Inc., Edison, NJ).
2. Centrifuge (RC5, Sorvall, DuPont, Boston, MA).
3. Bench-top centrifuge (Centrifuge 5417, Eppendorf).
4. UV/visible spectrophotometer (Spectronic Genesys5, Milton Roy).
5. *E. coli* strain XL-1Blue (New England Biolabs).
6. *E. coli* strain BL21(DE-3) (Novagen, Madison, WI).
7. Sodium chloride (Merck, Darmstadt, Germany).

8. Tryptone (Difco, Becton Dickinson Microbiology Systems, MD).
9. Yeast extract (Difco, Becton Dickinson Microbiology Systems).
10. Bacto-agar (Difco, Becton Dickinson Microbiology Systems).
11. Antibiotics: 100 mg/mL ampicillin (Sigma).

2.3. Preparation of Inclusion Bodies

1. Mechanical homogenizer (Tissuemizer, Heidolph, Germany).
2. Lysozyme (Sigma).
3. 25% Solution of Triton X-100 (Sigma) (*see* **Note 3**).
4. Urea (Merck).
5. Trizma base (Sigma).
6. 2,3,-Dihydroxybutane-1,4-dithiol (DTE) (Sigma).
7. Buffers: (*see* **Note 2**).
   a. Buffer A: 50 mM Tris-HCl, pH 8.0, 20 mM EDTA.
   b. Buffer B: 50 mM Tris-HCl, pH 8.0, 20 mM EDTA, 1% Triton X-100.
   c. Buffer C: 8 M urea, 50 mM Tris-HCl, pH 8.0, 20 mM EDTA.
   d. Buffer D: 8 M urea, 50 mM Tris-HCl, pH 8.0, 20 mM imidazole.
   e. Buffer E: 8 M urea, 50 mM Tris-HCl, pH 8.0, 250 mM Imidazole.

2.4. Cellulose-Assisted Refolding, Sodium Dodecyl Sulfate Polyacrylamide Gel Electrophorese (SDS-PAGE), and Chromatography Matrices

1. Mixer (Rotomix RM-1, ELMI, Riga, Latvija).
2. Cellulose (20- and 50-μm particles) (Sigma).
3. FPLC system equipped with absorbance detector (Pharmacia, Sweden).
4. Centricon-30 (Amicon, Beverly, MA).
5. Dialysis tubing (30 kDa cutoff, GibcoBRL Life Technologies, MD).
6. Coomassie Plus Protein Assay Reagent (Pierce, Rockford, IL).
7. 2-Mercaptoethanol (2-ME) (Sigma) (*see* **Note 4**).
8. Sodium dodecyl sulfate (SDS) (BDH Laboratory Supplies, UK) (*see* **Note 5**).
9. EC 120 Mini Vertical Gel system, E-C Apparatus Corporation.
10. Tris-buffered saline (TBS) 20 mM Tris-HCl, pH 7.5, 1 mM EDTA, 250 mM NaCl.
11. Enterokinase light chain (New England Biolabs)
12. Enterokinase buffer: 20 mM Tris-HCl, pH7.4, 50 mM NaCl, 2 mM CaCl$_2$.
13. Ni-NTA agarose and Ni-NTA superflow (Qiagen).
14. Superose 12 HR (Pharmacia).

3. Methods

3.1. Construction of scFv-CBD Bacterial-Expression Vectors

3.1.1. Background

For construction of scFv-CBD bacterial expression vectors, we introduced by polymerase chain reaction (PCR) the sequence encoding for Asp-Tyr-Lys-Asp-Asp-Asp-Asp-Lys-Leu between the C-terminus of the scFv to the N-terminus of the *Clostridium thermocellum* CBD (GenBank Accession number X68233) *(21)* (*see* **Note 6**). This sequence comprises a FLAG epitope *(23)*, followed by an Enterokinase cleavage site. A complete expression cassette was then assembled by PCR and cloned into pET3d

(Novagen, Madison WI) for intracellular expression. A scheme of the constructed expression vector pFEKCA3d-scFv is shown in **Fig. 2A**. A second expression vector, pH6T-FEKCA11c-scFv (*see* **Fig. 2B**) was constructed by linking the sequence encoding for Met-(His)$_6$-Leu-Val-Pro-Arg-Gly-Ser to the 5' end of the scFv-CBD cassette and subsequent subcloning into pET11c (Novagen). When expressed from the latter plasmid, the scFv-CBD fusion protein is preceded by a metal-binding His-tag followed by the thrombin cleavage site (*see* **Fig. 2**). For bacterial expression, the plasmids are introduced into *E. coli* strain BL21(DE3) (Novagen), carrying the T7 RNA polymerase gene on its chromosome under the control of an IPTG-inducible *lac*UV5 promoter.

3.1.2. Cloning of scFv's Genes into Expression Vectors

1. To replace the resident scFv, digest 10 µg of the scFv-CBD cassette-containing vectors DNA with 10 units each of *Nco*I and *Not*I restriction enzymes. Incubate 2 h at 37°C (*see* **Notes 1**, **7**, and **8**).
2. Digest the gene coding for your scFv of interest with the same restriction enzymes. Incubate 2 h at 37°C (*see* **Note 9**).
3. Separate the restriction fragments on 1% agarose gel by standard agarose gel electrophoresis.
4. Cut out and purify the restriction fragments from the agarose gel applying QIAquick™ Gel Extraction Kit, or a gel extraction kit of your choice.
5. Ligate the digested DNA fragments (200 ng each) with 400 U of T4 DNA Ligase in an appropriate buffer for 12 h at 16°C.
6. Transform *E. coli* XL-1Blue cells (*see* **Note 7**). Spread the *E. coli* cells on LB plates supplemented with 100 µg/mL Ampicillin.
7. Pick well-isolated single colonies and grow 5-mL cultures for 16 h in LB supplemented with 100 µg/mL Ampicillin. Purify the plasmid DNA utilizing QIAprep® Spin Miniprep kit, or a plasmid isolation kit of your choice.
8. Confirm the scFv gene insertion by digestion with *Nco*I and *Not*I restriction enzymes for 2 h at 37°C followed by separation on 1% agarose gel.
9. Transform *E. coli* BL21(DE-3) cells. Grow the *E. coli* cells on LB plates supplemented with 100 µg/mL Ampicillin.

3.2. Growing of Bacterial Strains

1. Grow the pFEKCA3d-scFv or pH6T-FEKCA11c-scFv containing *E. coli* BL21(DE-3) cells in Superbroth medium (35 g/L Tryptone, 20 g/L yeast extract, 5 g/L NaCl, supplemented with 1% glucose and 100 µg/mL ampicillin) at 37°C to an OD$_{600}$ of 2–3.
2. Induce the protein expression by addition of IPTG to 1 mM final concentration for 3 h.
3. Harvest cells by centrifugation 6000 rpm (5000g) at 4°C for 15 min at Sorvall Centrifuge (GSA rotor) or its equivalent. Decant the supernatant.
4. Weight the cell pellet and store at –20°C.

Induction of pFEKCA3d-scFv or pH6T-FEKCA11c-scFv carrying cells will result in the accumulation of the recombinant proteins as insoluble inclusion bodies.

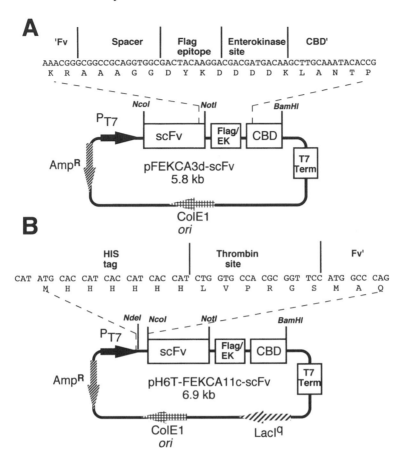

Fig. 2. Expression vectors pFEKCA3d-scFv (**A**) and pH6T-FEKCA3d-scFv (**B**) used for expression of scFv-CBD fusion proteins. The nucleotide and amino acid sequence of the scFv-Flag-Enterokinase-CBD region in A and of the His tag-thrombin site-scFv in B are shown at the top.

3.3. Recovery of Inclusion Bodies

3.3.1. Preparation of Inclusion Bodies

1. Suspend the bacterial paste (typically, 5 g from 500 mL of induced culture) in 70 mL of buffer A.
2. Lyse the bacterial cells by addition of 20 mg lysozyme for 1 h at room temperature (*see* **Note 10**).
3. Add 5 mL of 5 *M* NaCl and 5 mL of 25% Triton X100 (*see* **Note 3**).
4. Incubate 30 min at room temperature, shaking often and well.

5. Disrupt the cells with a mechanical homogenizer.
6. Collect the insoluble fraction of the disrupted cells by centrifugation at 20,000g for 40 min at 4°C (Sorvall, GSA rotor).
7. Resuspend the pellet in buffer B.
8. Collect the insoluble fraction by centrifugation at 20,000g for 30 min at 4°C.
9. Resuspend the inclusion bodies in 40 mL of buffer A.
10. Collect the insoluble fraction by centrifugation as in **step 6** above.

3.3.2. Solubilization of Insoluble scFv-CBD Fusion Protein

The collected insoluble material in **Subheading 3.3.1.** should be enriched in its scFv-CBD fraction, which accounts for 60–80% of the inclusion bodies protein as can be judged by SDS-PAGE (*see* **Fig. 3**, lane 3).

1. Solubilize the inclusion bodies in buffer C for 1 h at room temperature (*see* **Note 11**).
2. Reduce the insoluble protein by addition of 50 mM 2,3,-dihydroxybutane-1,4-dithiol (DTE) for 1 h at room temperature (*see* **Note 12**).
3. Remove the urea-insoluble material by centrifugation at 22,000g at 4°C for 10 min (SS-34 rotor).

3.3.3. Purification of scFv-CBD Fusion Protein
Under Denaturing Conditions

When the scFv-CBD fusion protein is made from pH6T-FEKCA11c-scFv (*see* **Fig. 2**), the urea-solubilized inclusion bodies can be purified under denaturing conditions by metal-chelate affinity chromatography on a Ni-NTA resin (Qiagen) (*see* **Fig. 3**):

1. Load the urea-solubilized inclusion bodies onto a Ni-NTA column (*see* **Note 13**).
2. Wash the column with 10 column volumes of buffer D.
3. Elute the scFv-CBD fusion protein with 2 column volumes of buffer E.
4. Reduce the eluted protein by addition of 50 mM DTE for 1 h at room temperature prior to refolding.

3.4. Cellulose-Assisted Refolding and Purification
of scFv-CBD Fusion Proteins

3.4.1. Cellulose-Assisted Refolding

Cellulose-assisted refolding is carried out as follows:

1. Mix the solubilized reduced inclusion bodies with an equal volume of 20% suspension (w/v) of crystalline cellulose in TBS.
2. Stir the suspension 1 h at room temperature to allow for binding to cellulose.
3. Transfer the suspension into dialysis tubes of a 30,000-kDa cutoff.
4. Refold the scFv-CBD fusion protein by dialysis for 24 h at 4°C against 100 vol of TBS adjusted to pH 9.5 with NaOH.

3.4.2. Purification of Cellulose-Bound scFv-CBD Protein

1. Recover the cellulose composite into a 50-mL centrifuge tube and collect the cellulose by low-speed centrifugation (1000g at 4°C for 10 min).
2. Wash twice by adding 40 mL of TBS adjusted to 1 M NaCl, vortex mixing and cellulose recovery by low-speed centrifugation.

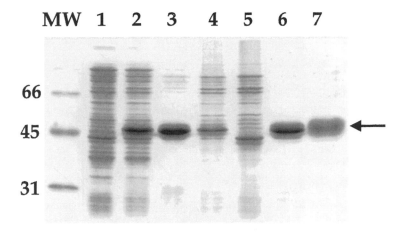

Fig. 3. Purification of Gal6(Fv)-CBD. Gal6(Fv) is a single-chain antibody derived against *E. coli* β-galactosidase. Lane 1, total cell extract from uninduced BL21(DE3) cells carrying plasmid pH6T-FEKCA3d-Gal6(Fv). Lane 2, total cell extract from BL21(DE3) cells carrying plasmid pH6T-FEKCA3d-Gal6(Fv) induced for 3 h with 1 m*M* IPTG. Lane 3, Washed, solubilized, and reduced inclusion bodies that were used in Ni-NTA purification. Lane 4, Inclusion bodies protein that did not bind to the Ni-NTA resin. Lane 5, Proteins released from the Ni-NTA column by 8 *M* urea/50 m*M* Tris-HCl, pH 8.0, 20 m*M* imidazole. Lane 6, Purified inclusion bodies recovered from the column by EDTA. Lane 7, Purified and neutralized crystalline cellulose-assisted refolded Gal6(Fv)-CBD. 5–10 μg protein were loaded in each lane of a 14% SDS polyacrylamide gel. Proteins were visualized by staining with Coomassie brilliant blue. The arrow marks the position of the scFv-CBD fusion protein.

3. Wash once with 40 mL of distilled water.
4. Elute the cellulose-bound scFv-CBD twice with 10 mL of 100 m*M* NaOH/100 m*M* NaCl (*see* **Note 14**).
5. Combine the eluates and neutralize them by dialysis against 100 vol of TBS at 4°C for 16 h.
6. Concentrate the purified protein using a Centricon microconcentrator with a 30,000-kDa cutoff (this step is optional).
7. As a polishing step, apply gel-filtration chromatography on a Superose 12 HR column to finally purify the scFv-CBD fusion protein. (This step is optional.)
8. Store the purified protein at –20°C.

3.4.3. Recovery of Purified scFv by Proteolytic Digestion While Immobilized

As an alternative to basic pH elution of scFv-CBD fusion proteins from cellulose, the scFv can be liberated from the fusion protein by utilizing the enterokinase site we engineered at the 3' end of the scFvs in the pFEKCA expression system (**Figs. 2** and **4**). Here, the protein is subjected to proteolytic cleavage while immobilized onto the cellulose matrix. The protease will have to be removed after digestion is completed.

1. Immobilize and refold 20 mg of scFv-CBD fusion protein onto 2 g of crystalline cellulose.
2. Wash and equilibrate the cellulose bound protein in enterokinase buffer.
3. Add 200 U of enterokinase light chain.

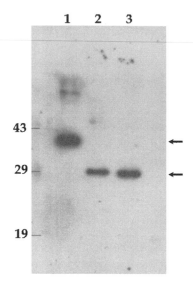

Fig. 4. Immunoblot analysis of Gal6(Fv) liberated by digestion of cellulose-immobilized Gal6(Fv)-CBD. Lane 1, Undigested protein immobilized on cellulose, boiled in Laemmli sample buffer before loading the SDS polyacrylamide gel. Lane 2, supernatant of Gal6(Fv)-CBD that had been digested while immobilized. Lane 3, Gal6(Fv)-CBD digested in solution. The scFv-CBD and free scFv were detected with an anti FLAG monoclonal antibody followed with HRP-conjugated rabbit-anti-mouse antibodies and an ECL HRP substrate. The upper arrow indicates the undigested scFv-CBD. The lower arrow indicates the free Gal6(Fv). The numbers on the left indicate the size of molecular-weight markers in kDa.

4. Incubate for 8 h at 23°C.
5. Centrifuge the cellulose matrix 5000*g* at 4°C for 5 min.
6. Recover the liberated scFv in the supernatant.
7. Remove the protease applying conventional gel-filtration chromatography procedures.

4. Notes

1. The expression vectors pFEKCA3d-scFv and pH6T-FEKCA11c-scFv are available upon request.
2. Buffers are made in distilled, deionized water (Milli-Q biocel, Millipore).
3. 25% Solution of Triton X-100 in deionized water should be prepared in advance.
4. 2-Mercaptoethanol is a highly toxic chemical. Wear suitable protective clothing, gloves, and eye/face protection.
5. SDS is harmful if swallowed. Causes irritation to eyes and skin.
6. Details regarding PCR primer sequences and PCR conditions are available upon request.
7. For detailed protocols for DNA fragments digestion and separation, as well as for plasmid DNA purification and transformation, *see* Sambrook et al. *(24)*.
8. Supercoiled plasmids require up to fivefold more *Not*I for complete digestion than linear DNAs. Therefore the simultaneous digestion with *Nco*I and *Not*I ensures the complete digestion by *Not*I.

9. The scFv-CBD bacterial expression vectors are designed for direct subcloning of the antibody genes from phage-display vectors such as pCANTAB-5E (Pharmacia Biotech [Uppsala, Sweden] Recombinant Phage Antibody System) and pHEN *(25)*. Alternatively, use PCR with *Nco*I and *Not*I restriction-site tagging primers to subclone an antibody gene.

10. Prepare 4 mL of 5 mg/mL lysozyme in deionized water.

11. Due to the dissociation of urea, the pH of this buffer should be adjusted immediately prior to use. Do not autoclave.

12. If metal-chelate affinity chromatography on a Ni-NTA resin is chosen as a purification step before cellulose-assisted refolding, reduce the scFv-CBD fusion protein after the purification, because DTE will reduce nickel ions.

13. Omit EDTA from the wash buffers because EDTA will strip nickel ions from the resin.

14. Elution conditions may vary for different fusion partners and different cellulose batches. The NaOH concentration may be between 10 and 100 mM. The elution conditions we apply to recover the refolded proteins from the cellulose matrix are rather harsh (100 mM NaOH, pH 13.0). Although the scFvs we have produced by this method tolerated the elution conditions, other fusion partners may be less tolerant to such conditions. We overcame this difficulty by re-engineering the elution properties of CBD so that it may be recovered under milder conditions *(21,26)*. One CBD mutant, having Asp56 and Trp118 both mutated to alanine, binds to cellulose with the same high capacity. However, its dissociation constant is increased about 20-fold. We incorporated this mutant CBD into our expression vectors described herein, and found that the scFv-CBD fusion protein can be eluted by 0.01 M NaOH or 3% triethylamine. Such conditions are milder and acceptable for numerous protocols for the elution of proteins from affinity columns.

References

1. Lilie, H., Schwarz, E., and Rudolph, R. (1998) Advances in refolding of proteins produced in *E. coli. Curr. Opin. Biotechnol.* **9**, 497–501.

2. Buchner, J., Pastan, I., and Brinkmann, U. (1992) A method for increasing the yield of properly folded recombinant fusion proteins: single-chain immunotoxins from renaturation of bacterial inclusion bodies. *Anal. Biochem.* **205**, 263–270.

3. Skerra, A. (1993) Bacterial expression of immunoglobulin fragments. *Curr. Opin. Immunol.* **5**, 256–262.

4. Kreitman, R. J. and Pastan, I. (1997) Immunotoxins for targeting cancer and autoimmune disease, in *Antibody Therapeutics* (Harris, W. J. and Adair, J. R., eds.) CRC Press, Boca Raton, FL, pp. 33–52.

5. Yarranton, G. (1997) Antibodies as carriers for drugs and radioisotopes, in *Antibody Therapeutics* (Harris, W. J. and Adair, J. R., eds.) CRC Press, Boca Raton, FL, pp. 53–72.

6. Benhar, I. and Pastan, I. (1997) Tumor targeting by antibody-drug conjugates, in *Antibody Therapeutics* (Harris, W. J. and Adair, J. R., eds) CRC Press, Boca Raton, FL, pp. 73–85.

7. Kiefhaber, T., Rudolph, R., Kohler, H. H., and Buchner, J. (1991) Protein aggregation *in vitro* and *in vivo*: a quantitative model of the kinetic competition between folding and aggregation. *Biotechnology* (NY) **9**, 825–829.

8. Guise, A. D., West, S. M., and Chaudhuri, J. B. (1996) Protein folding *in vivo* and renaturation of recombinant proteins from inclusion bodies. *Mol. Biotechnol.* **6**, 53–64.

9. Fenton, W. A., and Horwich, A. L. (1997) GroEL-mediated protein folding. *Protein Sci.* **6**, 743–760.

10. Creighton, T. E. (1985) Folding of proteins adsorbed reversibly to ion-exchange resins, in *UCLA Symposia on Molecular and Cellular Biology New Series*, vol. 39 (Oxender D. L., ed.), Liss, Inc., New York, pp. 249–258.

11. Glansbeek H. L., van Beuningen, H. M., Vitters, E. L., van der Kraan, P. M., and van den Berg, W. B. (1998) Expression of recombinant human soluble type II transforming growth factor-beta receptor in *Pichia pastoris* and *Escherichia coli*: two powerful systems to express a potent inhibitor of transforming growth factor-beta. *Protein Exp. Purif.* **12**, 201–207.

12. Stempfer, G., Holl-Neugebauer, B., and Rudolph, R. (1996) Improved refolding of an immobilized fusion protein. *Nat. Biotechnol.* **14**, 329–34.

13. Garel, J-R. (1992) Large multidomain and multisubunit proteins, in *Protein Folding* (Creighton, T. E., ed.), W. H. Freeman and Company, NY, pp. 405–454.

14. Bayer, E. A., Morag E., and Lamed, R. (1994) The cellulosome: a treasure-trove for biotechnology. *Trends Biotechnol.* **12**, 379–386.

15. Ong, E., Greenwood, J. M., Gilkes, N. R., Kilburn, D. G., Miller , R. C. J., and Warren, R. A. J. (1989) The cellulose-binding domains of cellulases: tools for biotechnology. *Trends Biotechnol.* **7**, 239–243.

16. Assouline, Z., Shen, H., Kilburn, D. G., and Warren, R. A. J. (1993) Production and properties of a Factor-X-cellulose binding domain fusion protein. *Protein Eng.* **6**, 787–792.

17. Ramirez, C., Fung, J., Miller, R. C. J., Warren, R. A. J., and Kilburn, D. G. (1993) A bifunctional affinity linker to couple antibodies to cellulose. *Bio/Technology* **11**, 1570–1573.

18. Shoseyov, O. and Karmely, Y. (1995) Kits and methods of detection using cellulose binding domain fusion proteins. US Patent Application No. 460,458.

19. Morag, E., Bayer, E. A., and Lamed, R. (1992) Affinity digestion for the near-total recovery of purified cellulosome from *Clostridium thermocellum. Enzyme Microb. Technol.* **14**, 289–292.

20. Berdichevsky, Y., Ben-Zeev, E., Lamed, R., and Benhar, I. (1999) Phage display of a cellulose binding domain from *Clostridium thermocellum* and its application as a tool for antibody engineering. *J. Immunol. Methods* **228**, 151–162.

21. Berdichevsky, Y., Lamed, R., Frenkel, D., Gophna, U., Bayer, E. A., Yaron, S., et al. (1999). Matrix-assisted refolding of single-chain Fv-cellulose binding domain fusion proteins. *Protein Expr. Purif.* **17**, 249–259.

22. Tsumoto, K., Shinoki, K., Kondo, H., Uchikawa, M., Juji, T., and Kumagai, I. (1998) Highly efficient recovery of functional single-chain Fv fragments from inclusion bodies overexpressed in *Escherichia coli* by controlled introduction of oxidizing reagent-application to a human single-chain Fv fragment. *J. Immunol. Methods* **219**, 119–129.

23. Brizzard, B. L., Chubet, R. G., and Vizard, D. L. (1994) Immunoaffinity purification of FLAG epitope-tagged bacterial alkaline phosphatase using a novel monoclonal antibody and peptide elution. *Biotechniques* **16**, 730–735.

24. Sambrook, J. L., Fritsch, E. F., and Maniatis, T. (1989) *Molecular Cloning: A Laboratory Manual*, 2nd ed. 1989. Cold Spring Harbor Laboratory Press, Cold Spring Harbor, NY.

25. Hoogenboom, H. R. and Winter, G (1992) By-passing immunisation. Human antibodies from synthetic repertoires of germline VH gene segments rearranged *in vitro. J. Mol. Biol.* **227**, 381–388

26. Benhar, I., Tamarkin, A., Marash, L., Berdichevsky, Y., Yaron, S., Shoham, Y., et al. (2001). Phage display of cellulose binding domains for biotechnological application, in *Glycosyl Hydrolases for Biomass Conversion. ACS Symposium Series 769* (Himmel, M.E., Baker, J. O., and Saddler, J. N., eds.), American Chemical Society, Washington, DC, pp. 168–189.

28

Production of Tumor-Specific Antibodies in Tobacco

Carmen Vaquero-Martin and Rainer Fischer

1. Introduction

1.1. Plants as a Recombinant Antibody Expression and Production System

Fundamental changes in plant molecular biology have taken place during the past decade. Together with the enormous advances made in recombinant DNA technology, protein engineering, plant transformation and tissue culture, plant molecular biology is giving rise to an agricultural revolution. Biotechnology is adding unique uses to the traditional uses of plants, such as phytoremediation—the use of plants to remove pollutants from the environment *(1)*—and molecular farming—the use of plants as bioreactors for the production of medically valuable organic compounds and recombinant proteins and antibodies *(2–5)*.

Plants represent an inexpensive, safe and efficient alternative to most conventional systems for the production of recombinant proteins and antibodies, such as microbial or mammalian expression systems *(6,7)* and are becoming more important for the pharmaceutical industry. This interest is based on the advantages of molecular farming for the production of therapeutic and diagnostic recombinant antibodies. Molecular farming brings together the advantages of the cost-effectiveness and low-technology requirements of the microbial systems with the cell biology of a eukaryotic expression system that allows the processing of most complex proteins into their native structure *(2–5)*.

Since Hiatt reported the first expression of a recombinant antibody in tobacco *(8)*, a large number of reports have demonstrated the suitability of several plant species (both monocots and dicots) for the functional expression of recombinant antibodies and antibody fragments (i.e., **refs. *9–11***). Further progress has made possible to produce chimeric mouse-human therapeutic antibodies in plants in sufficient quantities for preclinical trials *(12,13)*. This has implications for molecular medicine because it permits the production of large amounts of proteins for disease therapy and diagnosis.

From: *Methods in Molecular Biology, vol. 207: Recombinant Antibodies for Cancer Therapy: Methods and Protocols*
Edited by: M. Welschof and J. Krauss © Humana Press Inc., Totowa, NJ

Bacterial, yeast, insect and mammalian expression systems have been employed for the expression of recombinant antibodies and antibody fragments. Each of the systems has its own advantages and disadvantages (reviewed in **ref.** *14*). Plants have emerged as an attractive alternative expression system for the production of recombinant antibodies because, first, they have a eukaryotic protein synthesis pathway, very similar to animal cells with only minor differences in protein glycosylation *(15)*. This allows the expression of correctly folded IgG and secretory IgA antibodies (i.e., **refs.** *10,13*). Second, antibodies produced in plants accumulate to high levels and plant material can be stored over long periods of time without loss of antibody activity *(16)*. Third, contamination of expressed proteins with human or animal pathogens (HIV, hepatitis) or the co-purification of blood-borne pathogens (prion diseases) and oncogenic sequences are avoided.

Classical methods of protein expression often require a significant investment in recombinant protein purification (bacteria) or require expensive growth media (animal cells). Bacteria produce contaminating endotoxins that are difficult to remove and bacterially expressed recombinant proteins often form inclusion bodies, making labor- and cost-intensive in vitro refolding necessary. Mammalian cell cultivation requires sophisticated equipment and expensive media supplements, such as fetal calf serum (FCS). In addition, the use of transgenic animals *(18)* as a source of recombinant antibodies is becoming limited by legal and ethical constraints.

In contrast, molecular farming only requires transgenic plants, water, mineral salts, and sunlight *(2–5)*. Current applications of the plant-based expression systems in biotechnology include the production of recombinant antibodies (rAbs) *(12,18)*, enzymes *(19,20)*, hormones, interleukins *(21)*, plasma proteins *(22)* and vaccines *(23,24)*. Chimeric plant viruses, produced in plants, can also be used for the presentation of vaccines on the viral surface *(25)*. The ease with which plants can be genetically manipulated, and grown in single-cell suspension culture or scaled up for field-scale production is a great advantage over the more commonly used microbial methods, mammalian-cell culture, and transgenic animal technology.

1.2. Plant Expression Strategies

Transient expression systems are very useful to obtain an early indication about the expression properties of a genetically engineered construct in plants. This is particularly important for engineered antibodies where loss or reduction of affinity can occur and should be detected and corrected at an early stage.

There are three major transient expression systems used to deliver a gene into plant cells: delivery of projectiles coated with "naked DNA" by particle bombardment, infiltration of intact tissue with recombinant *Agrobacteria* (agroinfiltration), or infection with modified viral vectors. The overall level of transformation varies between these three systems. Particle bombardment usually reaches only a few cells and for transcription the DNA has to reach the cell nucleus *(26)*. Agroinfiltration targets many more cells than particle bombardment and the T-DNA harboring the gene of interest is actively transferred into the nucleus with the aid of bacterial proteins *(27)*. A viral vector can systemically infect most cells in a plant and transcription of the introduced gene in RNA viruses is achieved by viral replication in the cytoplasm, which transiently generates many transcripts of the gene of interest.

Although particle bombardment can be used to test recombinant protein stability, it is unsuitable for the production of larger amounts of foreign proteins. In contrast the other two systems, agroinfiltration and recombinant virus infection, produce antibodies in amounts that allow purification and rapid characterization of the plant-expressed protein *(13,28,29)*. This is an important issue because it permits the rapid analyses of a large number of antibody constructs prior to generation of transgenic plants. A major advantage of agroinfiltration is that multiple genes present in different populations of *Agrobacteria* can be simultaneously expressed. Thus, the assembly of complex multimeric proteins such as IgG or IgA can be tested in *planta (13)*.

Generation of a stably transformed plant involves the chromosomal integration of a heterologous gene followed by the regeneration of fully developed plant from the transformed plant cells or cell material. Transformation can be achieved by in vitro methods such as micro-injection, direct DNA uptake into protoplasts and particle bombardment, or by methods based on *Agrobacterium* T-DNA mediated transformation. Despite the first successful transformation of a plant cell in vitro was reported only 17 yr ago *(30)*, transformation of many plant species is now possible. However, there are still technical and logistical hurdles to be overcome, such as developing efficient transformation techniques for all major crop species. Novel transformation technologies are being developed to combine the benefits of *Agrobacterium*-mediated transformation and particle bombardment *(31)*. Developing plant lines expressing recombinant proteins is time-intensive, and in the best case 8–12 wk are needed for transgenic plants to be available, but this depends on the plant species.

Protein expression studies in transgenic plants have demonstrated that recombinant antibodies and antibody fragments can be functionally expressed in plants. These studies have covered many plant species including tobacco, pea, wheat, rice, petunia, soybean, and potato *(8–12,32–34)*. For the successful production of an antibody, a high level of expression should be achieved in the transgenic plant cell. For that several factors have to be considered, i.e. the efficiency of transcriptional control elements as promoters and enhancers, the subcellular targeting of the protein, or the tissue-specific expression of the protein *(35)*. Although in general recombinant antibody expression in plants is very efficient, each antibody has unique expression characteristics and yields are difficult to predict.

1.3. Production of Therapeutic and Diagnostic Antibodies in Plants: Development and Examples in the Market

The first clinical trial of plant-based immunotherapy was reported by Planet Biotechnology, Inc. (Mountain View, CA). The novel drug CaroRx™ is based on sIgA antibodies produced in transgenic tobacco plants and is designed to prevent the oral bacterial infection that contributes to dental caries *(36)*. Planet Biotechnology has demonstrated that CaroRx™ can effectively eliminate *Streptococcus mutans*, the bacteria that causes tooth decay in humans *(37)*. Planet Biotechnology is also engaged in the design and development of novel sIgA-based therapeutics to treat infectious diseases and toxic conditions affecting oral, respiratory, gastrointestinal, genital, and urinary mucosal surfaces and skin.

Monsanto (formerly Agracetus, Middleton, WI) created a corn line producing human antibodies at yields of 1.5 kg of pharmaceutical-quality protein per acre of corn. Given that the yield per acre of corn is on the range of 4–8 tons, there is considerable room for improvement in yields. A pharmaceutical partner plans to begin injecting cancer patients with doses of up to 250 mg of the antibody-based cancer drug purified from corn seeds. The company is also cultivating transgenic soybeans that produce humanized antibodies against herpes simplex virus 2 (HSV-2). These antibodies were shown to be efficient in preventing of vaginal HSV-2 transmission in mice. The ex vivo stability and in vivo efficacy of the plant and mammalian cell-culture produced antibodies were similar *(12)*. Plant-produced antibodies are likely to allow development of an inexpensive method for mucosal immuno-protection against sexually transmitted diseases.

ProdiGene (College Station, TX) and EPIcyte Pharmaceuticals (San Diego, CA) have entered into a strategic partnership to produce antibodies in corn (www.prodigene.com/news.html). Their interest is the production of human mucosal antibodies for passive immunization by exploiting ProdiGene's expertise in protein expression *(36–41)* together with EPIcyte's academic and patent position.

1.4. Production of Tumor-Specific Antibodies and Antibody Fragments in Plants: scFv, Diabody, Fusion Proteins, and Mouse-Human Chimeric Antibodies Derived from a CEA-Specific Murine Monoclonal Antibody

Antibodies specific for the carcino-embryonic antigen (CEA) antibodies are commercialized as a diagnostic tool for colon cancer. Chemical and molecular engineered CEA-specific antibodies are being evaluated for their use in diagnosis and clinical treatments of colorectal cancer *(41,42)*. Bispecific diabodies coupling CEA-specificity with a second specificity, such as CD3 are being developed to improve the clinical performance of these scFvs *(43)*.

In our group, we have evaluated the feasibility of producing CEA-specific recombinant antibodies in plants (*see* **Figs. 1** and **2**). Using the genes encoding the heavy and light chains of a murine monoclonal antibody (MAb) (mT84.66), several recombinant antibody constructs were engineered for their expression in plants. Those include a single chain Fv (scFvT84.66) (*see* **Fig. 1**), a diabody (diaT84.66) (*see* **Fig. 2**), a mouse-human chimeric antibody (cT84.66), and scFv and diabody fused to interleukin-2 (IL-2). The constructs were initially tested and characterized using an *Agrobacterium*-mediated transient expression assay in tobacco *(13)*. The protocol of this assay has been described in detail *(13,28)*. The recombinant tumor-specific antibodies expressed transiently in tobacco leaves were shown to be functional, therefore we proceeded to develop stable transgenic plants expressing the MAbs. Although the transient system allows for upscaling and purification, large-scale production of Ab can be achieved only through use of transgenic plants.

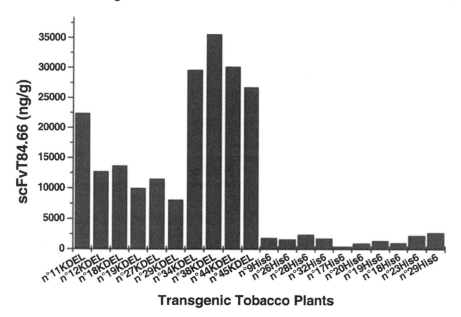

Fig. 1. Levels of functional scFvT84.66 in transgenic T_0 tobacco plants. Expression of recombinant protein in regenerated plants was analyzed by competition ELISA. Presented are the levels for the highest expressing regenerated plants for the constructs scFvT84.66-KDEL and scFvT84.66-H_6.

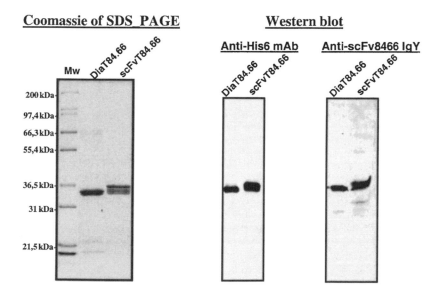

Fig. 2. Protein purification of scFvT84.66his6-KDEL and diabodyT84.66-His6 from transgenic plants. Recombinant antibodies were purified from transgenic leaf material as described above and analyzed by Coomassie staining of SDS-PAGE gels and immunoblotting.

ScFvT84.66 was shown to be functionally expressed in all monocots and dicots tested including: tobacco *(13)* *(see also* **Figs.** **1** and **2**), pea *(33)*, rice *(34)*, wheat *(11)*, and tomato. The addition of the ER retrieval signal KDEL at the C-terminus of the protein increased the level of functional protein in all plant species and tissues (seeds, leaves, and fruits) analyzed.

His6-tagged scFvT84.66 or diaT84.66 were readily purified by immobilized metal affinity chromatography (IMAC) from tobacco leaves. The full-size cT84.66 antibody was purified from plant material by protein A chromatography. Protein purification protocols from plant material are described in **Subheading 3.5.** CEA-specific antibodies produced in plants were fully active after purification as demonstrated by the capacity of binding to the A3 domain of CEA in ELISA and to immuno-label CEA-expressing cells (LS174T). We conclude that plants represent an excellent production system for recombinant antibodies derived from mT84.66, a valuable molecule for clinical imaging of CEA-positive tumors.

Protocols will be described in Materials and Methods for the following assays:

1. Transformation and regeneration of transgenic tobacco.
2. Analysis of antibody expression in transgenic plants.
3. Protein purification for the characterization of recombinant protein(s) (IMAC, protein A).

2. Materials

2.1. Generation of Explants
of Nicotiana tabacum Cultivar Petit Havana SR1

1. Autoclave and bake Weck glasses (preserving jars).
2. Vitamin solution: 4 µg/L glycine, 1 µg/L nicotinic acid, 1 µg/L pyridoxine. Filter-sterilize and store at 4°C.
3. MS agar, pH 5.8: 4.43 g/L Murashige and Skoog basal salt with minimal organics (MSMO+), 20 g/L sucrose, 0.4 mg/L thiamine-HCl. Adjust pH to 5.8, add 8 g/L agar, and autoclave. Add 0.5 mL/L of vitamin solution.
4. MS II agar: MS agar supplemented with 1 mg/L 6-Benzylaminopurine, 0.1 mg/L 1-naphthalene acetic acid (NAA) and 100 mg/L kanamycin, 200 mg/L claforan, 200 mg/L betabactyl.
5. MS III agar: MS medium supplemented with 100 mg/L kanamycin, 200 mg/L claforan, 200 mg/l betabactyl.

2.2. Growth and Induction of Agrobacterium tumefaciens

1. Autoclave Erlenmeyer conical bottles and centrifuge tubes.
2. YEB medium: pH 7.4: 5 g/L beef extract, 1 g/L tryptone, 1 g/L yeast extract, 5 g/L sucrose. Adjust pH and autoclave. Add sterile $MgSO_4$ to a final concentration of 2 mM.
3. Induction medium: YEB medium, 10 mM 2-(*N*-morpholino) ethanesulfonic acid (MES). Adjust pH to 5.6 and autoclave. Add Acetosyringone (3',5'-dimethoxy-4-hydroxyacetophenone) to a final concentration of 20 µM and sterile $MgSO_4$ to a final concentration of 2 mM.
4. MMA medium: 4.43 g/L MS salts, 10 mM MES, 20 g/L sucrose. Adjust the pH to 5.6 and autoclave. Add Acetosyringone to a final concentration of 200 µM.

2.3. Analysis of Antibody Expression in Transgenic Tobacco Plants

1. Autoclave mortars, pestles, and centrifuge tubes.
2. Liquid nitrogen.
3. Extraction buffer (EB): PBS, pH 6.0, 5 mM β-Mercaptoethanol, 5 mM EDTA.
4. Electrophoresis extraction buffer (ESB): 75 mM Tris-HCl, pH 6.8, 9 M Urea, 4.5% (w/v) SDS, 7.5% (v/v) β-Mercaptoethanol.

2.4. Purification of Recombinant Antibody from Transgenic Tobacco Plants

1. Disposable columns (BIORAD), adapters, and tubes.
2. Extraction buffer for protein A purification: PBS, 5 mM β-Mercaptoethanol, 10 mM ascorbic acid (vitamin C), 5 mM EDTA, pH 6.0 (*see* **Note 1a**).
3. Extraction buffer for IMAC purification: PBS, 5 mM β-Mercaptoethanol, 10 mM ascorbic acid, pH 6.0 (*see* **Note 1a**).

3. Methods

3.1. Preparation of Agrobacteria for Tobacco Transformation

1. Grow the recombinant *Agrobacteria* strain transformed with the appropriate plant expression vector, in 50 mL of YEB medium containing the appropriate antibiotics. These are depending on the bacterial strain and recombinant plasmid used (e.g., for strain GV3101: 100 µg/mL Rifampicin, 25 µg/mL Kanamycin, and 100 µg/mL Carbenicillin). Incubate at 28°C with shaking until OD$_{600}$ reaches ~1.0 (*see* **Notes 2** and **3**).
2. Transfer the culture to Falcon tubes or sterile centrifuge tubes. Pellet *Agrobacteria* cells by centrifugation at 5000g for 20 min at 15°C.
3. Resuspend the cells in 2–5 mL of induction media using a sterile pipet and transfer to a new Erlenmeyer flask containing 200 mL of induction media. Grow the culture at 28°C with shaking overnight to OD$_{600}$ ~0.8.
4. Transfer the culture to a GS3 tube and pellet the cells by centrifugation at 5000g for 10 min at 15°C.
5. Resuspend the cells in 2–5 mL of MMA media and increase the volume with MMA medium until the OD$_{600}$ reaches ~1.0.
6. Keep the *Agrobacterium* suspension at 22°C room temperature (RT) for 2 h.

3.2. Transformation and Regeneration of Tobacco Plants (see also Note 4)

1. Work all the time under sterile conditions on a continuous-flow chamber. Regularly sterilize the dissecting instruments by dipping in alcohol and flaming.
2. Incubate seeds of *Nicotiana tabacum* (cultivar Petit Havana SR1) in 70% ethanol for 2 min, then wash with sterile water.
3. Transfer surface sterilized seeds to Weck glasses (preserving jars) containing ~100 mL of MS medium. Close the glasses tightly with parafilm and incubate in a phytochamber at 22°C and 16 h photoperiod during germination of seeds and growth of plantlets.
4. Cut young ~5 cm long leaves in small pieces (0.5 cm^2) and transfer to Weck glasses containing ~100 mL of *Agrobacterium* suspension culture. Incubate at RT for 30 min.
5. Transfer the leaf pieces onto sterile water-wetted Whatman paper in Petri plates. Seal them with Saran wrap and incubate at 22°C in the dark for 2 d.

6. Wash leaf pieces with sterile distilled water containing 100 mg/L kanamycine, 200 mg/L claforan, 200 mg/L Betabactyl (Ticarcillin:Clavulanic acid = 25:1).
7. Transfer leaf pieces onto MS II plates and incubate them at 25° C under 16 h photoperiod for 3–4 wk until of shoots develop.
8. Cut the shoots and transfer them to MS III-plates. Incubate plates at 25°C and 16 h photoperiod for ~2 wk until roots develop.
9. Transfer the small plants to Weck glasses containing MS III media and follow the incubation until plants are strong enough to be planted into soil.
10. Transfer plants to soil and cultivate them in a greenhouse or phytochamber. For analysis of antibody expression young developing leaves should be used.

3.3. Extraction of Total Soluble Protein from Tobacco Leaves for Analysis of Transgene Expression by ELISA

1. Remove midrib from the leaf and weigh the material.
2. Grind the leaf material in liquid nitrogen to a fine powder with a mortar and pestle.
3. Add 2 mL of extraction buffer per gram of fresh leaf material and grind until a green homogenate is obtained.
4. Transfer extracts to Eppendorf tubes and centrifuge 20 min at 13,000 rpm at 4°C.
5. Transfer supernatants to new tubes and centrifuge as in **step 4** above.
6. Transfer supernatants to new tubes and keep samples at 4°C for short-term storage (~24 h) or at –20°C supplemented with 10% glycerol for longer storage.

3.4. Extraction of Total Protein from Tobacco Leaves for Analyses of Transgene Expression by Immunoblotting

1. Remove midrib from leaf and weigh the material.
2. Grind the leaf material in liquid nitrogen to a fine powder with a mortar and pestle.
3. Add 1 mL of ESB per gram fresh leaf material and grind until a homogenate is obtained.
4. Transfer sample to an Eppendorf tube and boil for 10 min in a water bath.
5. Centrifuge samples at 13,000 rpm at room temperature and transfer supernatant to new tubes. Use immediately for immunoblot analyses or store samples at –20°C.

3.5. Purification of Recombinant Antibodies from Transgenic Tobacco (see Notes 4 and 5)

3.5.1. Protein A Purification

1. Grind leaves at 4°C using a blender and two volumes of ice-cold extraction buffer (*see* **Notes 1a** and **1b**).
2. Filter the extract through Miracloth and centrifuged at 20.000*g* for 30 min at 4°C.
3. Add NaCl to the supernatant to a final concentration of 500 m*M*, adjust the pH to 8.0 and incubate the solution for 30 min at 4°C with stirring. Check the pH again and readjust if necessary.
4. Centrifuge at 20.000*g* for 30 min at 4°C.
5. Filter supernatant through Miracloth and Whatman paper.
6. Pack a column with protein A (Pharmacia) and equilibrate the matrix by washing with three volumes of PBS, pH 8.0.
7. Apply filtered plant extract to the column at a flowrate of ~5 mL/min.
8. Wash extensively with PBS, pH 8.0, 100 m*M* NaCl. All green pigments should be washed away.
9. Elute bound protein with 100 m*M* glycine, pH 2.0.

10. Adjust the pH of elution fractions to pH 7.5–8.0 by addition of 1:5 of the volume of 1 *M* Tris-HCl. Check pH with pH paper sticks.
11. Immediately dialyze against PBS, pH 7.4, and store at 4°C (*see* **Note 1c**).
12. Regenerate and store the matrix as recommended by the manufacturer.
13. Analyze the samples by standard procedures, i.e., ELISA and immunoblotting.

3.5.2. IMAC Purification Procedure

1. Work at 4°C throughout the whole procedure (*see* **Note 1b**).
2. Grind leaves using a blender and two volumes of ice-cold extraction buffer (*see* **Note 1a**).
3. Filter the extract through Miracloth and centrifuge at 20.000*g* for 30 min at 4°C.
4. Collect the supernatant and add to final concentrations 0.05% Tween20, 500 m*M* NaCl and 10 m*M* imidazole. Adjust the pH to 8.0 and incubate 30 min at 4°C with stirring. Check the pH and readjust if necessary.
5. Centrifuge at 20.000*g* for 30 min at 4°C.
6. Filter the supernatant through Miracloth and Whatman paper.
7. Pack a column with Ni^{2+}-NTA resin (Qiagen) and equilibrate the matrix by washing with 3 vol of PBS, pH 8.0.
8. Apply plant filtrate to the column at a flowrate of ~1–2 mL/min.
9. Wash matrix with PBS, pH 8.0, 500 m*M* NaCl, 0.05% Tween-20, 10 m*M* imidazole.
10. Elute bound protein with PBS, 250 m*M* imidazole, pH 4.5.
11. Immediately dialyze against PBS, pH 7.4, and store at 4 °C (*see* **Note 1c**).
12. Regenerate and store the matrix as recommended by the manufacturer.
13. Analyze the samples by standard procedures, i.e., ELISA and immunoblotting (*see* **Fig. 2**).

4. Notes

1. Yields of purified protein are dependent on the expressed protein. Different proteins might require adjustment of extraction and purification protocols. Things to consider for optimizing the protein purification are:
   a. Extraction buffer. Choose a buffer where a maximum amount of active recombinant protein and a minimum amount of contaminants are extracted. Although the aforementioned buffer is suitable for extracting active antibodies from tobacco leaves, other buffers may yield better results for different proteins, plant species, or plant tissues.
   b. Time employed and working temperature. We observed higher degradation problems when protein extracts were kept at 4°C overnight. It is very important to proceed with the purification immediately after tissue disruption in order to obtain a good-quality preparation. Also the whole procedure should be carried out at low temperatures (cold room).
   c. Storage of proteins. Purified protein fractions should be dialyzed directly after elution against a stabilizing storage buffer, i.e., PBS, pH 7.4, 5 m*M* EDTA, and stored at 4°C, or at –20°C containing 10% glycerol.
2. Depending on the plant species, different *Agrobacteria* strains are suitable for their use in transformation. For tobacco transformation we have used *A. tumefaciens* strain GV3101 (pMP90RK, Gm^R Km^R Rif^R) (*13*).
3. For inoculation of YEB media with *Agrobacteria* glycerol stocks should be used for faster growth. When cultures are initiated from a single colony, sterile plastic tips have to be used for inoculation of 5–10 mL YEB media, but not toothpicks, which can inhibit *Agrobacteria* growth. Cultures have to be incubated longer, typically for 2–3 d.

4. Antibody expression in stable transgenic plants has been achieved not only in different Nicotiana species (*N. tabacum* cultivar Petit Havana SR1, *N. tabacum* Xanthi NC, *N. tabacum* cultivar Samsun, *N. Benthamiana*), but also in several other crops, for example in rice, wheat, pea, soybean and petunia. Transformation protocols for each different plant specie can be found elsewhere *(11,12,32–34)*.

5. Protein purification can be carried out once enough plant material is available. For storage of leaves from transgenic plants, the material is weighted and frozen at –80°C. We have observed no significant loss of activity or storage-related degradation of antibodies over a period of a few months.

References

1. Gleba, D., Borisjuk, N. V., Borisjuk, L. G., Kneer, R., Poulev, A., Skarzhindskaya, M., et al. (1999) Use of plant roots for phytoremediation and molecular pharming. *Proc. Natl. Acad. Sci. USA* **96**, 5973–5977.

2. Franken, E., Teuschel, U., and Hain, R. (1997) Recombinant proteins from transgenic plants. *Curr. Opin. Biotechnol.* **8**, 411–416.

3. Hood, E. E. and Jilka, J. M. (1999) Plant–based production of xenogenic proteins. *Curr. Opin. Biotechnol.* **10**, 382–386.

4. Fischer, R., Liao, Y.-C., Hoffmann, K., Schillberg, S., and Emans, N. (1999) Molecular farming of recombinant antibodies in plants. *Biol. Chem.* **380**, 825–839.

5. Whitelam, G. C. and Cockburn, W. (1996) Antibody expression in transgenic plants. *Trends Plant Sci.* **1**, 268–271.

6. Taticek, R. A., Lee, C. W. T., and Shukler, M. L. (1994) Large scale insect and plant cell culture. *Curr. Opin. Biotechnol.* **5**, 165–174.

7. Skerra, A. (1993) Bacterial expression of immunoglobulin fragments. *Curr. Opin. Biotechnol.* **5**, 256–262.

8. Hiatt, A., Cafferkey, R., and Bowdish, K. (1989) Production of antibodies in transgenic plants. *Nature* **342**, 76–78.

9. Voss, A., Niersbach, M., Hain, R., Hirsch, H., Liao, Y., Kreuzaler, F., and Fischer, R. (1995) Reduced virus infectivity in *N. tabacum* secreting a TMV–specific full size antibody. *Mol. Breeding* **1**, 39–50.

10. Ma, J. K., Hiatt, A., Hein, M., Vine, N. D., Wang, F., Stabila, P., van Dolleweerd, C., Mostov, K., and Lehner, T. (1995) Generation and assembly of secretory antibodies in plants. *Science* **268**, 716–719.

11. Stöger, E., Vaquero, C., Torres, E., Sack, M., Nicholson, L., Drossard, J., et al. (2000) Cereal crops as viable production and storage system for pharmaceutical scFv antibodies. *Plant Mol. Biol.* **42**, 583–590.

12. Zeitlin, L., Olmsted, S. S., Moench, T. R., Co, M. S., Martinell, B. J., Paradkar, V. M., et al. (1998) A humanized monoclonal antibody produced in transgenic plants for immunopro-tection of the vagina against genital herpes. *Nat. Biotechnol.* **16**, 1361–1364.

13. Vaquero, C., Sack, M., Chandler, J., Drossard, J., Schuster, F., Schillberg, S., and Fischer, R. (1999) Transient expression of a tumor–specific single chain fragment and a chimeric antibody in tobacco leaves. *Proc. Natl. Acad. Sci. USA* **96**, 11,128–11,133.

14. Verma, R., Boleti, E., and George, A. J. T. (1998) Antibody engineering: comparison of bacterial, yeast, insect and mammalian expression systems. *J. Immun. Methods* **216**, 165–181.

15. Cabanes-Macheteau, M., Fitchette-Laine, A. C., Loutelier-Bourhis, C., Lange, C., Vine, N., Ma, J., et al. (1999) N–Glycosylation of a mouse IgG expressed in transgenic tobacco plants. *Glycobiology* **9,** 365–372.
16. Fiedler, U. and Conrad, U. (1995). High–level production and long–term storage of engineered antibodies in transgenic tobacco seeds. *Biotechnology* (NY) **13,** 1090–1093.
17. Echelard, Y. (1996) Recombinant protein production in transgenic animals. *Curr. Opin. Biotechnol.* **7,** 536–540.
18. Ma, J. and Hein, M. (1995) Immunotherpeuic potential of antibodies produced in plants. *Trends Biotechnol.* **13,** 522–527.
19. Hogue, R. S., Lee, J. M., and An, G. (1990) Production of a foreign protein product with genetically modified plant cells. *Enzyme Microb. Technol.* **12,** 533–538.
20. Witcher, D., Hood, E., Peterson, D., Bailey, M., Bond, D., Kusnadi, A., et al. (1998) Commercial production of β–glucoronidase (GUS): a model system for the production of proteins in plants. *Mol. Breed.* **4,** 301–312.
21. Magnuson, N. S., Linzmaier, P. M., Reeves, R., An, G., HayGlass, K., and Lee, J. M. (1998) Secretion of biologically active human interleukin–2 and interleukin–4 from genetically modified tobacco cells in suspension culture. *Protein Exp. Purif.* **13,** 45–52.
22. Sijmons, P. C., Dekker, B. M. M., Schrammeijer, B., Verwoerd, T. C., van den Elzen, P. J. M., and Hoekema, A. (1990) Production of correctly processed human serum albumin in transgenic plants. *Bio/Technology* **8,** 217–221.
23. Mason, H. S. and Arntzen, C. J. (1995) Transgenic plants as vaccine production systems, *Trends Biotechnol.* **13,** 388–392.
24. Walmsley, A. and Arntzen, C. (2000) Plants for delivery of edible vaccines. *Curr. Opin. Biotech.* **11,** 126–129.
25. Johnson, J., Lin, T., and Lomonossoff, G. (1997) Presentation of heterologous peptides on plant viruses: genetics, structure and function. *Ann. Rev. Phytopathol.* **35,** 67–86.
26. Christou, P. (1996) Transformation technology. *Trends Plant Sci.* **1,** 423–431.
27. Kapila, J., De Rycke, R., van Montagu, M., and Angenon, G. (1996) An Agrobacterium mediated transient gene expression system for intact leaves. *Plant Sci.* **122,** 101–108.
28. Fischer, R., Vaquero–Martin, C., Sack, M., Drossard, J., Emans, N., and Commandeur, U. (1999) Toward Molecular Farming in the future: Transient protein expression in plants. *Biotechnol. Appl. Biochem.* **30,** 117–120.
29. McCormick, A. A., Kumagai, M. H., Hanley, k., Turpen, T. H., Hakim, I., Grill, L. K., et al. (1999). Rapid production of specific vaccines for lymphoma by expression of the tumor–derived single–chain Fv epitopes in tobacco plants. *Proc. Natl. Acad. Sci. USA* **96,** 703–708.
30. Herrera-Estralla. L., De Block, M., Messens, E., Hernalsteens, J. P., Van Montagu, M., and Schell. J. (1983). Chimeric genes as dominant selectable markers in plant cell. *EMBO J.* **2,** 987–995.
31. Gelvin, S. B. (1998) The introduction and expression of transgenes in plants. *Curr. Opin. Biotechnol.* **9,** 227–232.
32. De Jaeger, G., Buys, E., Eeckhout, D., De Wilde, C., Jacobs, A., Kapila, J., et al. (1999). High level accumulation of single–chain variable fragments in the cytosol of transgenic Petunia hybrida. *Eur. J. Biochem.* **259,** 426–434.
33. Perrin, Y., Vaquero C., Gerrard I., Sack M., Drossard J., Stöger E., e tal. (2000) Transgenic pea seeds as bioreactors for the production of a single–chain Fv fragment (scFv) antibody used in cancer diagnosis and therapy. *Molecular Breeding* **6,** 345–352.

34. Torres, E., Vaquero, C., Nicholson, L., Sack, M., Stoger, E., Drossard, J., et al. (1999) Rice cell culture as an alternative production system for functional diagnostic and therapeutic antibodies. *Transgenic Res.* **8,** 441–449.
35. Gallie, D. (1998) Controlling gene expression in transgenics. *Curr. Opin. Plant Biol.* **1,** 166–172.
36. Ma, J. K., Hikmat, B. Y., Wycoff, K., Vine, N. D., Chargelegue, D., Yu, L., et al. (1998) Characterization of a recombinant plant monoclonal secretory antibody and preventive immunotherapy in humans. *Nat Med.* **4,** 601–606.
37. Larrick, J. W., Yu, L., Chen, J., Jaiswal, S., and Wycoff, K. (1998) Production of antibodies in transgenic plants. *Res. Immunol.* **149,** 603–608.
38. Witcher, D., Hood, E., Peterson, D., Bailey, M., Marchall, L., Bond, D., et al. (1998) Commercial production of β–glucuronidase (GUS): a model system for the production of proteins in plants. *Mol. Breeding* **4,** 301–312.
39. Hood, E. E., Kusnadi, A., Nikolov, Z., and Howard, J. A. (1999) Molecular farming of industrial proteins from transgenic maize. *Adv. Exp. Med. Biol.* **464,** 127–147.
40. Hood, E., Witcher, D., Maddock, S., Meyer, T., Baszczynski, C., Bailey, M., Fet al. (1997) Commercial production of Avidin from transgenic maize: characterization of transformation, production, processing, extraction and purification. *Mol. Breeding* **3,** 291–306.
41. Kusnadi, A. R., Hood, E. E., Witcher, D. R., Howard, J. A., and Nikolov, Z. L. (1998) Production and purification of two recombinant proteins from transgenic corn. *Biotechnol. Prog.* **14,** 149–155.
42. Zhong, G.-Y., Peterson, D., Delaney, D., Bailey, M., Witcher, D., Register, J., et al. (1999) Commercial production of Aprotinin in transgenic maize seeds. *Mol. Breeding* **5,** 345–356.
43. Wu, A. M., Chen, W., Raubitschek, A., Williams, L. E., Neumaier, M., Fischer, R., et al. (1996). Tumor localization of anti–CEA single–chain Fvs: improved targeting by non–covalent dimers. *Immunotechnology* **2,** 21–36.
44. Mayer, A., Chester, K. A., Flynn, A. A., and Begent, R. H. J. (1999) Taking engineered anti–CEA antibodies to the clinic. *J. Immmunol. Methods* **231,** 261–273.
45. Holliger, P., Manzke, O., Span, M., Hawkins, R., Fleischmann, B., Qinghua, L., et al. (1999) Carcinoembryonic antigen (CEA)–specific T–cell activation in colon carcinoma induced by anti–CD3 × anti–CEA bispecific diabodies and B7 × anti–CEA bispecific fusion proteins. *Cancer Res.* **59,** 2909–2916.

Index